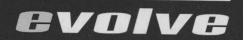

W9-CLV-752

The Latest *Evolution* in Learning.

Evolve provides online access to free learning resources and activities designed specifically for the textbook you are using in your class. The resources will provide you with information that enhances the material covered in the book and much more.

Visit the Web address listed below to start your learning evolution today!

▶▶ **LOGIN:** *http://evolve.elsevier.com/Chitty/professional/*

Evolve Online Courseware for Chitty: *Professional Nursing: Concepts & Challenges, fourth edition* offers the following features:

- ## WebLinks

  An exciting resource that lets you link to hundreds of websites carefully chosen to supplement the content of the textbook. The WebLinks are regularly updated with new ones added as they develop.

- ## Sample Critical Path for Congestive Heart Failure

  A multidisciplinary care plan designed to guide the care of patients with congestive heart failure.

- ## State Boards of Nursing

  Contains addresses, phone and fax numbers, and websites of the state boards of nursing for all 50 states.

- ## NANDA-Approved Nursing Diagnoses 2003-2004

  A comprehensive listing of 167 NANDA, International nursing diagnoses.

Think outside the book...*evolve.*

Professional Nursing

Concepts & Challenges

fourth edition

KAY KITTRELL CHITTY
RN, EdD
Adjunct Faculty
College of Nursing
Medical University of South Carolina

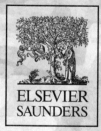

ELSEVIER
SAUNDERS

11830 Westline Industrial Drive
St. Louis, Missouri 63146

PROFESSIONAL NURSING: Concepts and Challenges   ISBN 0-7216-0695-4
Copyright © 2005, 2001, 1997, 1993 by Elsevier Inc.

NOTICE

Nursing is an ever-changing field. Standard safety precautions must be followed, but as new research and
clinical experience broaden our knowledge, changes in treatment and drug therapy may become necessary
or appropriate. Readers are advised to check the most current product information provided by the
manufacturer of each drug to be administered to verify the recommended dose, the method and duration
of administration, and contraindications. It is the responsibility of the licensed prescriber, relying on
experience and knowledge of the patient, to determine dosages and the best treatment for each
individual patient. Neither the publisher nor the author assumes any liability for any injury and/or damage
to persons or property arising from this publication.

Previous editions copyrighted 2001, 1997, 1993.

International Standard Book Number 0-7216-0695-4

Senior Acquisitions Editor: Tom Wilhelm
Managing Editor: Jeff Downing
Production Services Manager: John Rogers
Senior Project Manager: Cheryl A. Abbott
Designer: Julia Dummitt

Printed in the United States of America

Last digit is the print number: 9 8 7 6 5 4 3 2

The fourth edition of this book is dedicated
to the nursing students who use it.
Welcome to a proud and honorable profession.

Martha Raile Alligood, RN, PhD
Dean and Professor
School of Nursing
Palm Beach Atlantic University
West Palm Beach, Florida

Virginia Trotter Betts, RN, MSN, JD, FAAN
Commissioner of Mental Health
  and Developmental Disabilities
State of Tennessee
Nashville, Tennessee

Carol T. Bush, RN, PhD
Manager, Mental Health Utilization
  Review
Georgia Regional Hospital at Atlanta
Atlanta, Georgia

Pamela S. Chally, RN, PhD
Dean and Professor
School of Nursing
College of Health
University of North Florida
Jacksonville, Florida

M. Catherine Hough, RN, PhD
Assistant Professor
School of Nursing
College of Health
University of North Florida
Jacksonville, Florida

Jennifer E. Jenkins, RN, MBA
National Client Relations Manager
LifeMasters Supported Healthcare
Golden, Colorado

Arlene W. Keeling, RN, PhD
Professor and Director ANCP Program
Director, Center for Nursing Historical
  Inquiry
School of Nursing
University of Virginia
Charlottesville, Virginia

Judith K. Leavitt, RN, MEd, FAAN
Associate Professor
School of Nursing
University of Mississippi Medical
  Center
Jackson, Mississippi

Diane J. Mancino, RN, EdD, CAE
Executive Director
National Student Nurses' Association,
  Inc. and
Foundation of the National Student
  Nurses' Association, Inc.
Brooklyn, New York

Frances A. Maurer, RN, MS
Community Health Educator
  and Consultant
Baltimore, Maryland

Elaine F. Nichols, RN, EdD
Nursing Education Consultant
Medina, Ohio

PREFACE

Professions exist to serve society. When society changes, as ours has done in so many ways since September 11, 2001, professions must also change. So it is with nursing. To maintain our relevance and dynamism today, nurses must possess a skill set far more complex than ever before in the history of the profession.

To be effective, nurses must master more information than ever before available about human health and disease; they must be good leaders and good team members; they must think critically and creatively; they must communicate and collaborate with a diverse array of patients, families, and health care colleagues; they must be caring and businesslike; they must grapple with practical, ethical, and legal dilemmas not dreamed of even a decade ago; and they must practice their profession in both traditional settings and in nontraditional community settings. Needless to say, to be an effective nurse today is a daunting undertaking.

The fourth edition of this text is designed to assist students to understand what it means to be a professional; to appreciate the history of nursing; to understand and prize nursing's values, standards, and ethics; to recognize and deal effectively with the social and economic factors that influence how the profession is practiced; and to appreciate the need to be lifelong learners. It addresses concepts underlying the elements of the American Association of Colleges of Nursing's 1998 document, The Essentials of Baccalaureate Education for Professional Nursing Practice.

Feedback from users of earlier editions reveals that this text is used in RN to BSN "bridge" courses, in early courses in generic baccalaureate curricula, and as a resource for practicing nurses and graduate students. Students in nursing programs are increasingly second-degree students, midcareer adults, and others who bring considerable life experience to the learning situation. Accordingly, every effort has been made to present material that is comprehensive enough to challenge users at all levels without overwhelming the novice. The text has been designed to be "student friendly," and care has been taken to keep jargon to a minimum yet to provide a comprehensive glossary to assist in developing and refining a professional vocabulary. The visual features of the book have been carefully improved with today's visual learner in mind.

To faculty who have used the book before, this edition should feel and look familiar, with many of the successful features maintained and updated. For example, assisting users of all levels to greater self-awareness has been a goal of all four editions of this text. Therefore self-assessment exercises were retained and expanded in this revision. Upon close examination, however, differences from the previous edition will emerge. In some instances chapter headings have been modified to reflect current emphases. In addition to updating, new content has been added to every chapter. New content includes the following:

- The emphasis on critical and creative thinking and clinical decision making has been enhanced.

- The focus on men in nursing has been expanded.
- Cultural competence has been emphasized.
- Managed care content has been expanded.
- The impact of violence in society and the workplace has been enhanced.
- Content on classification systems (NANDA, NIC, and NOC) has been expanded, and a discussion of unified nursing language systems has been added.
- Distance learning and its impact on professionalism have been added.
- The spiritual aspects of patient care have been increased.
- Evidence-based practice content has been enhanced.
- The importance of caring for self, including a discussion of the Magnet Recognition Program, has been added.
- An introduction to reconceptualizing the nurse-patient relationship to conform to today's short-term nurse-patient interactions has been added.
- Content on communication and collaboration has been improved and expanded.
- New roles in the community, such as palliative care nursing and telehealth nursing, have been added.
- Where appropriate, clinical examples and vignettes have been expanded.
- Information about HIPAA and the Nurse Licensure Compact has been introduced.
- Interviews with association presidents, practicing nurses, and other experts have been increased.
- The challenge of creating and maintaining a healthy work environment has been emphasized.
- WebLinks for each chapter have been added to the Evolve website (**www. evolve.elsevier.com/Chitty/professional/**) to assist students to do independent research using reliable, pertinent sites online.
- The Evolve website also features:
  A sample critical path for congestive heart failure
  Contact information for all state boards of nursing
  A comprehensive listing of NANDA-approved Nursing Diagnoses for 2003-2004

The Instructor's Electronic Resource, which will be available online through the Evolve website, has been revised based on user feedback to contain activities for both small and large groups. It contains in-class and out-of-class activities designed to enhance students' learning and to enrich classroom experiences. The Instructor's Electronic Resource also includes chapter outlines, chapter objectives, and suggested readings. Contact your Elsevier Sales Representative or call our Sales Support Team at 1-800-222-9570 to obtain access to Evolve.

As with earlier editions, it continues to be my heartfelt hope that the students and faculty who use this new edition will find it even more stimulating, enjoyable, and enlightening than the first three editions and that it will continue to contribute to the positive development of our profession.

Kay Kittrell Chitty

A C K N O W L E D G M E N T S

The successful completion of any major project brings both a sense of accomplishment and of relief. The completion of the fourth edition of *Professional Nursing: Concepts & Challenges* also brings overwhelming gratitude to the many individuals who participated in what has truly been a great team effort:

- To the faculty and students who used earlier editions and provided me with their suggestions for revisions
- To the reference librarians at the Charleston County Library and the Medical University of South Carolina for their unselfish donation of time, talents, and energy
- To nursing colleagues who freely shared their profound expertise and contacts
- To the nurses and other experts who shared their experiences and perceptions in interviews
- To all who assisted in gathering photographs—especially Arlene Keeling and the Center for Nursing Historical Inquiry at the University of Virginia, The American Nurses Association, the Tennessee Nurses Association, Diane Mancino and the National Student Nurses Association, Judy Leavitt, Jeff Downing, and Sarah Winfrey
- To all who contributed definitions and philosophies of nursing from their schools and hospitals—the University of North Florida School of Nursing in Jacksonville, Florida; Hamilton Medical Center Department of Nursing in Dalton, Georgia; St. Vincent's Medical Center Department of Nursing in Jacksonville, Florida; The University of Akron College of Nursing in Akron, Ohio; the University of Rochester School of Nursing in Rochester, New York; Beth Israel-Deaconess Medical Center Department of Nursing in Boston, Massachusetts; Central Missouri State University Department of Nursing in Warrensburg, Missouri; Memorial Health Care System Department of Nursing in Chattanooga, Tennessee; and Palm Beach Atlantic University School of Nursing in West Palm Beach, Florida
- To Jeff Downing, Managing Editor, and Cheryl Abbott, Senior Project Manager, at Elsevier for their patience, attention to detail, and support

Special thanks are due the contributors to this edition, who took on this extra responsibility in spite of already over-full personal and professional lives. Their recompense will not be tangible, for academia is sadly lacking in rewards for textbook writing. In spite of this obstacle, these contributors rose to the occasion. Their love of the nursing profession and commitment to its hopeful future will serve as their remuneration. I am deeply indebted to them, one and all.

Finally, I wish to express my appreciation to Tom Wilhelm, my optimistic and encouraging Acquisitions Editor, who provided the support and resources for the efficient and (relatively) painless completion of this revision.

CONTENTS

CHAPTER 1

Professional Nursing Comes of Age: 1859-2004,   1

Arlene W. Keeling

Nursing in Early Nineteenth-Century America,   2

Mid–Nineteenth-Century Nursing in England: The Influence of Florence
Nightingale,   2

1861-1873: The American Civil War—An Impetus for "Trained Nursing,"   4

1874-1900: The Roots Take Hold,   8

1900-1917: A Young Profession Faces New Challenges,   13

1917: The Flu Epidemic and World War I Bring New Challenges to a Young
Profession,   15

1920-1930: The Roaring Twenties,   17

1931-1945: The Profession Responds to the Great Depression and
World War II,   18

1945-1960: The Rise of Hospitals—Bureaucracy, Science, and Shortages,   21

1961-1985: New Roles for Nurses,   23

1986-2004: Managed Care and Its Challenges for Nursing,   26

Lessons of History,   27

References,   28

CHAPTER 2

Educational Patterns in Nursing,   31

Elaine F. Nichols and Kay Kittrell Chitty

Development of Nursing Education in the United States,   33

Educational Pathways to Becoming a Registered Nurse,   35

Influences on the Growth of Baccalaureate Education,   37

Baccalaureate Programs Today,   38

Alternative Educational Programs in Nursing,   42

Practical Nursing Programs (LPN or LVN),   43

Accreditation of Educational Programs,   44

Graduate Education in Nursing,   45

History of Doctoral Education in Nursing,   48

Current Status of Doctoral Education in Nursing,   49

Certification Programs,   49

Continuing Education,   52

Future Directions for Nursing Education,   53

Challenges in Nursing Education,   55

References,   60

CHAPTER 3

The Social Context for Nursing,   63
Kay Kittrell Chitty

Traditional Socialization of Women,   64
Nursing, Feminism, and Women's Movements,   67
Men in Nursing,   70
Image of Nursing,   76
Social Phenomena Affecting Nursing,   85
Imbalance in Supply and Demand for Nurses,   96
References,   101

CHAPTER 4

Professional Associations,   105
Diane J. Mancino

Work of Nursing Associations,   106
Types of Associations,   113
Benefits of Belonging to Professional Associations,   117
Deciding Which Associations to Join,   120
Becoming an Involved Association Member,   120
Perspectives of Nursing Leaders About Professional
    Associations,   120
Analysis of Selected Issues Addressed by Nursing
    Associations,   127
References,   133

CHAPTER 5

Nursing Today,   135
Kay Kittrell Chitty

Current Status of Nursing in the United States,   136
Nursing Opportunities Requiring Higher Degrees,   154
Employment Outlook in Nursing,   159
References,   162

CHAPTER 6

The Professionalization of Nursing,   163
Kay Kittrell Chitty

Historical Review: Characteristics of a Profession,   164
The Evolution From Occupation to Profession,   166
Barriers to Professionalism in Nursing,   168
Nursing's Pathway to Professionalism,   170
Collegiality as an Attribute of the Professional Nurse,   177
Need for a New Paradigm,   178
References,   181

CHAPTER 7

Defining Nursing and Nursing's Scope of Practice,　183
Kay Kittrell Chitty
Defining Nursing: Harder Than It Seems,　184
Defining Nursing's Scope of Practice,　194
Four Documents You Should Possess,　195
References,　196

CHAPTER 8

Professional Socialization,　197
Kay Kittrell Chitty
Education and Professional Socialization,　198
Models of Professional Socialization,　200
Postgraduate Resocialization to the Work Setting,　209
References,　220

CHAPTER 9

Philosophies of Nursing,　222
Kay Kittrell Chitty
Beliefs,　223
Values,　225
Philosophies,　229
Developing a Personal Philosophy of Nursing,　237
References,　239

CHAPTER 10

Major Concepts in Nursing,　241
Kay Kittrell Chitty
Systems,　242
Person,　244
Environment/Suprasystem,　248
Health,　254
Putting It All Together: Nursing,　266
References,　269

CHAPTER 11

Nursing Theory: The Basis for Professional Nursing,　271
Martha Raile Alligood
What is Theory?,　271
Nursing Conceptual Models,　279
Theories of Nursing,　286

Theoretical Challenges for Nursing Education, Practice,
   and Research,   289
References,   295

CHAPTER 12

The Scientific Method, Nursing Research, and Evidence-Based Practice,   299

Carol T. Bush

Science and the Scientific Method,   300
Nursing Research Based on the Scientific Method,   303
What is Nursing Research?,   306
Interviews With Nurse Researchers,   315
Relationship of Nursing Research to Nursing Theory and Practice,   315
Collaboration in Nursing Research,   319
Support for Nursing Research,   321
Roles of Nurses in Research,   322
Evidence-Based Practice: Bridging the Gap Between Research
   and Practice,   323
References,   327

CHAPTER 13

The Health Care Delivery System,   329

Jennifer E. Jenkins

Major Categories in Health Care Services,   331
Classifications of Health Care Agencies,   333
Traditional Internal Structures of Health Care Agencies,   338
The Health Care Team,   341
Forces Changing the Health Care Delivery System,   346
Health Care's Response to Managed Care and Consumer Expectations,   350
Maintaining Quality in Health Care Agencies,   354
References,   359

CHAPTER 14

Nursing Roles in the Health Care Delivery System,   360

Jennifer E. Jenkins

Types of Nursing Care Delivery Systems Historically Used in
   Acute Care Settings,   361
How Patients Define Excellent Nursing Care,   371
Differentiating Levels of Practice: An Ongoing Debate,   371
The Nurse's Role on the Health Care Team,   373
Nursing Organization Governance,   378
Nurses and Interdisciplinary Teams,   381
References,   384

CHAPTER 15

Critical Thinking, the Nursing Process, and Clinical Judgment,   386

Kay Kittrell Chitty

Critical Thinking in Nursing,   387
The Nursing Process in Historical Perspective,   390
Phases of the Nursing Process,   393
Dynamic Nature of the Nursing Process,   404
Unified Nursing Language Systems,   404
Developing Clinical Judgment in Nursing,   406
References,   412

CHAPTER 16

Financing Health Care,   413

Frances A. Maurer

Basic Economic Theory,   415
Is Basic Economic Theory Applicable to Health Care?,   416
Current Methods of Payment for Health Care,   418
History of Health Care Finance,   420
Continued Escalation of Health Care Costs,   423
Cost-Containment Measures Revisited,   424
Recent Legislative Efforts in Health Care Reform,   427
Current Issues of Concern,   430
Impact of Managed Care on Health Services,   435
Economics of Nursing Care,   439
Cost Containment and Quality Management,   443
Health Care Reform and National Health Insurance,   443
References,   451

CHAPTER 17

Illness and Culture: Impact on Patients, Families, and Nurses,   455

Kay Kittrell Chitty

Illness,   456
Stages of Illness,   458
Impact of Illness on Patients and Families,   470
Impact of Caregiving on Nurses,   484
References,   489

CHAPTER 18

Communication and Collaboration in Nursing,   491

Kay Kittrell Chitty

Therapeutic Use of Self,   492
Communication Theory,   499

How Communication Develops,   502
Criteria for Successful Communication,   502
Becoming a Better Communicator,   504
Communication With Professional Colleagues,   512
Collaboration Skills,   513
References,   519

CHAPTER 19

Nursing Ethics,   521

Pamela S. Chally and M. Catherine Hough

Nursing Codes of Ethics,   523
Ethical Theories,   526
Ethical Principles,   528
Theories of Moral Development,   532
Understanding Ethical Dilemmas in Nursing,   534
Patient Self-Determination Act,   538
Ethical Decision Making,   543
References,   549

CHAPTER 20

Legal Aspects of Nursing,   551

Virginia Trotter Betts

American Legal System,   552
Nursing as a Practice Discipline,   553
Special Concerns in Professional Nursing Practice,   558
Evolving Legal Issues and the Nurse,   566
Preventing Legal Problems in Nursing Practice,   572
References,   577

CHAPTER 21

Nurses and Political Action,   579

Judith Kline Leavitt and Virginia Trotter Betts

Policy and Politics: What They Are and What
   They Are Not,   580
Politics and Power,   583
A Lesson in Civics Comes Alive,   586
Health Care Legislation and Regulation,   590
Getting Involved,   594
We Were All Once Novices,   597
A Nurse Who Knew How to Use Political Power,   598
Nursing Awaits Your Contribution,   598
References,   600

CHAPTER 22
Nursing's Future Challenges,   601
Kay Kittrell Chitty

Societal Challenges,   602
Challenges in Nursing Practice,   614
Challenges in Nursing Education,   619
A Challenge to the Entire Nursing Profession: Focus, Unite, Act!,   623
References,   625

Epilogue,   627

Glossary,   628

Professional Nursing

Concepts & Challenges

Professional Nursing Comes of Age: 1859-2004

Arlene W. Keeling

Key Terms

Clara Barton
Mary Ann ("Mother")
  Bickerdyke
Mary Breckinridge
Cadet Nurse Corps
Mary E. Davis
Dorothea L. Dix

Lavinia Lloyd Dock
Lorretta Ford
Florence Nightingale
Mary Adelaide Nutting
Sophia Palmer
Phoebe Pember
Isabel Hampton Robb

Margiaret Sanger
Jessie Sleet Scales
Sojourner Truth
Harriet Tubman
Lillian Wald

Learning Outcomes

After studying this chapter, students will be able to:

- Identify the social, political, and economic factors that influenced the rise of professional nursing in the United States.
- Describe the influence of Florence Nightingale on the development of the nursing profession in the United States.
- Discuss major medical events that affected the nursing profession.
- Identify early nursing leaders.
- Explain the effect that wars have had on the nursing profession.
- Describe the struggles and contributions of African-American and male nurses in the development of the nursing profession.
- Trace the rise of advanced practice nursing in the United States.

To understand the challenges facing professional nursing today, readers must know something of the history of the nursing profession. The rise of nursing as a profession in the United States is a complex story of opportunities, challenges, struggles, and the search for identity within the context of larger social forces. From the work of Florence Nightingale in the Crimea (1854) to the present, the profession has been influenced by the social, political, and economic climate of the times and by technological advances and theoretical shifts in medicine and science. Early in its development, nursing was influenced by the ideology of the Victorian Era and the Progressive Era. By the mid-twentieth century, its evolution was imbedded in an emerging context of change—in attitudes toward minorities, the women's movement, advances in technology and science, and the rise of medical specialization. Since the 1980s, health care reform, politics, the Internet, emerging infectious diseases, and an emphasis on global awareness have all played a part in shaping nursing's development. More recently, an aging population, threats of bioterrorism, and nursing shortages are affecting the profession's future. This chapter presents a brief overview of some of the highlights of nursing's history and several of its leaders. The history of nursing education, discussed in Chapter 2, is introduced in this section. Since an in-depth analysis of nursing's history is beyond the scope of this textbook, the reader is encouraged to use the references at the end of the chapter for further reading.

NURSING IN EARLY NINETEENTH-CENTURY AMERICA

Before 1873, when the first "training schools" for nursing opened in the United States, nursing care was provided in the home by mothers, wives, daughters, and sisters of the sick. From the earliest years of settlement in the colonies and during the growth and development of the United States as it expanded westward, the care of the sick was directed by physicians and managed by family members outside of hospitals. Only those who were destitute, orphaned, or chronically incapacitated were admitted to hospitals, which were essentially almshouses. Care in these places was of poor quality and provided by other inmates, who were equally destitute and untrained.

MID–NINETEENTH-CENTURY NURSING IN ENGLAND: THE INFLUENCE OF FLORENCE NIGHTINGALE

In 1820 Florence Nightingale, extolled as the most influential nurse in the history of modern nursing, was born into the aristocratic social sphere of Victorian England, a heritage that would become critical to her success. At an early age, Nightingale received a classic education directed by her father. This education, combined with her personal characteristics of sensitivity, compassion, and restlessness, along with the perspective she gained through extensive travel on the European continent, provided her with the foundation for the role she would play in the future.

As a young woman, Nightingale (Figure 1-1) often felt stifled by her privileged and protected social position in upper-class Victorian England. In addition, because she had often accompanied her mother on visits to the poor, Nightingale became aware of the disease and disability caused by poverty, as well as the horrible conditions in public hospitals. As a result, she took it upon herself to visit the sick in her community.

By 1850, rebelling against her strict Victorian culture and convinced that she wanted to be a nurse, Nightingale entered the nurses' training program in Kaisersworth, Germany, where she spent 3 years learning the basics of nursing under the guidance of the Protestant deaconesses. After completion of her training,

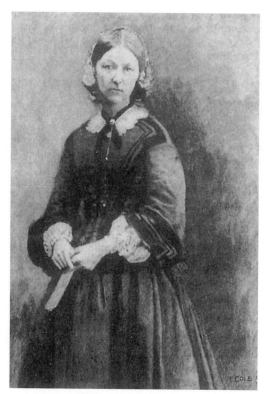

Figure 1-1
Florence Nightingale, (1820-1910).

Florence Nightingale studied under the Sisters of Charity in Paris. Only a year later, she would have the opportunity to use her newly acquired skills when Britain went to war in the Crimea.

Nightingale in the Crimea, 1854-1856

On hearing of the horrible conditions suffered by the sick and wounded British soldiers in Turkey during the Crimean War, Nightingale took a small band of untrained women to the British hospital in Scutari. There she found a hospital "totally lacking in equipment. … There were no medical supplies. There were not even the basic necessities of life …" (Woodham-Smith, 1949, p. 162). With great compassion and despite the opposition of military officers, Nightingale set about the task of organizing and cleaning the hospital and providing care to the wounded soldiers. She boldly made use of her personal power and political and social connections, writing to influential government officials, including her close friend Sir Sidney Herbert, the British Secretary of War. Armed with excellent training in statistics, Nightingale gathered data on morbidity and mortality of the soldiers in Scutari. Using this supportive evidence, she effectively argued the case for reform of the entire British Army medical system.

The Nightingale School

Following the Crimean War, Nightingale founded the first training school for nurses at St. Thomas's Hospital in London (1860), which would become the model for nursing education in the United States. Through the publication of numerous articles and papers, Nightingale promulgated her ideas about nursing and nursing education. In her most famous publication, the 1859 *Notes on Nursing: What It Is and What It Is Not,* Nightingale stated clearly for the first time that learning a unique body of knowledge was required of those wishing to practice professional nursing.

Nightingale held the firm belief that good nursing care was essential to the healing process and that the art of nursing included attention to the symptoms of the disease and factors in the environment. According to Nightingale, "[Nursing] has been limited to signify little more than the administration of medicines and the application of poultices. It ought to signify the proper use of fresh air, light, warmth, cleanliness, quiet and the proper choosing and giving of diet—all at the least expense of vital power to the patient" (Nightingale, 1946, p. 6). Moreover, Nightingale specifically rejected the theory that microorganisms, rather than filth and dampness, caused disease (Nightingale, 1946, p. 7) and held fast to this notion despite evidence to the contrary being provided by such notable scientists as Joseph Lister and Louis Pasteur in the latter part of the century.

Historical NOTE 1

Lister's original work on antisepsis was published in the 1860s. It would take another 10 years for the ideas of antiseptic surgery and the germ theory to be accepted by medicine.

These widely published beliefs, along with Nightingale's dedication to hospital reform, to upgrading conditions for the sick and wounded in the military, and to establishing training schools for nurses, greatly affected the development of nursing in the United States.

1861-1873: THE AMERICAN CIVIL WAR—AN IMPETUS FOR "TRAINED NURSING"

There were no professional nurses in America in 1861, when the first shots were fired on Fort Sumter, South Carolina, initiating the War Between the States. Furthermore, there was no organized system of medical or nursing care in either the Union or the Confederacy and no plan to cope with the deluge of wounded men who poured into Washington and Richmond following the Battle of Bull Run in northern Virginia on July 21, 1861. No provision had been made for field hospitals, and hospital tents were located at the rear of the fighting, too far from the front. As a result, conditions on the battlefield were horrible: everywhere wounded and dying men lay in agony while the stench of chloroform and blood-soaked blankets filled the air (Young, 1959, p. 134).

Mary Livermore, writing about conditions at the front after the Battle of Bull Run, related:

> Mrs. Hoge and myself were sent to the hospitals and to medical headquarters at the front, with instructions to obtain any possible information that would lead to better preparations for the wounded of another great battle (Livermore, 1867, p. 187).

Immediately the appeal for nurses was made, and women on both sides responded. Most significant perhaps was the response by the Catholic orders, particularly the Sisters of Charity, the Sisters of Mercy, and the Sisters of the Holy Cross, who had a long history of providing care for the sick (Wall, 1995). Doubtless the most skillful and devoted of the women who nursed in the Civil War, these religious sisters were highly disciplined, organized, and efficient.

Union Nursing: 1861-1865

As word of the shocking conditions spread, northern women responded immediately. The Women's Central Relief Committee, formed in New York City early in the Civil War, sent a committee to Washington, D.C., to mobilize volunteer support and to pressure the government to provide care for the soldiers. An entire medical system was needed. President Lincoln heeded their recommendations and created the United States Sanitary Commission (Figure 1-2), immediately appointing **Dorothea L. Dix,** an avid reformer of care for the mentally ill, as superintendent of Women Nurses of the Army. Unfortunately, Dix had no official corps of trained nurses to lead. She was faced with the task of supplying nurses when there were none, because in 1861 there were no training schools for nurses in the United States. As a substitute for professional training, Dix focused on the criteria of good health, high moral character, and a matronly, "plain" appearance as qualifications for service. She soon enlisted 100 women to train for a month under physicians at Bellevue Hospital and New York Hospital to prepare them to supervise the care of the sick and wounded throughout the Union.

As the year progressed, thousands of women volunteered to help, challenging social mores and the Victorian ideology that a woman's place was in the home. Black and white, rich and poor, married and single women left their homes to care for soldiers in hospital tents and in hastily converted schools, churches, and warehouses. Among the African-American women who served were **Sojourner Truth,** a famous abolitionist, and **Harriet Tubman,** a former field slave who had escaped to the North in 1849. Defying the boundaries of time, place, gender, and race, both of these women not only cared for the soldiers but also smuggled slaves to freedom using the complex Underground Railroad system.

Meanwhile, Soldier's Aid Societies sprang into existence as women used their social organizations to serve the war effort. Employing their domestic skills, the women stitched garments, rolled bandages, made blankets, knitted socks, and prepared boxes of food and supplies to be sent to the front.

The Western Front

In the early months of the war, the deplorable conditions in the Washington, D.C., camps were repeated everywhere troops were stationed, and accounts of outbreaks

SANITARY COMMISSION.

No. 39.

THIRD REPORT

CONCERNING THE

Aid and Comfort given by the Sanitary Commission

TO

SICK SOLDIERS PASSING THROUGH WASHINGTON.

BY FREDERICK N. KNAPP, Special Relief Agent.

WASHINGTON, *March* 21, 1862.

To FRED. LAW OLMSTED,
    Secretary Sanitary Commission:

SIR:—My last report bore date of October 21. Since that time to the present, the work upon our hands has steadily increased. More room, more money, more time, more medical attendance, have all been demanded. Fewer new regiments have arrived of late, but the regiments already in the field having become more generally acquainted with our plans for rendering help, are now in the habit of sending directly to our care sick and discharged men, who come to the city from the various regimental hospitals to obtain their pay and to start for home.

During the last two months quite a number of men have been sent to us thus, even from the more distant regiments at Poolsville and at Budd's Ferry, with letters from their surgeons, or other officers, requesting us to receive them and render them such assistance as they might demand. These men frequently reach here just at night, and are much exhausted, and need, peculiarly, the shelter and the helping hand which we give to them.

A large number of men have also come to us from the hospitals at Philadelphia, Baltimore, and Annapolis. These hospitals receive by hundreds the convalescents from the general hospitals in and around Washington. When these convalescents are well enough to join their regiments, or else, while partially recovered, they are so far diseased as to call for their discharge from the service, they return to Washington, all needing more or less care; some of them almost entirely helpless.

Figure 1-2
Sanitary Commission—Third Report. (Reproduced with permission of the Keeling Collection, the Center for Nursing Historical Inquiry, University of Virginia, School of Nursing.)

of pneumonia and typhoid fever, poor food, and numerous deaths from injuries, amputations, and gangrene soon reached families back home. In response to one letter reporting such chaos to a church in Illinois, the congregation sent **Mary Ann ("Mother") Bickerdyke,** an uneducated, widowed housekeeper known locally for her nursing ability, to the Western Front to investigate the situation. Bickerdyke found appalling conditions. Cairo, Illinois, was filled with thousands of previously robust soldiers, now suffering from fevers, dying of measles and dysentery, and living in filth. Undaunted by her lack of authority and despite the strong objections of the surgeons in the camp, "Mother Bickerdyke" rallied the men, ordering them to chop kindling, build fires, and heat large kettles of water. In a whirlwind of activity, Bickerdyke arranged for many tasks to be done: the clothes washed, the soldiers bathed, the bedding fumigated, and the garbage removed. In fact, she made such an impact in so short a time that one surgeon complained that "a cyclone in calico" had struck the camp (Young, 1959, p. 92).

Other nurses who served on the Western Front included Mary Safford, a rich, frail, educated woman, and Emily Haines Harrison, a young widow who served as a nurse in Ohio from 1861 to 1865 (Ganger, 1988). Like Bickerdyke, these young women worked tirelessly to attend to the needs of the sick and injured, ignoring the opposition of the surgeons (Livermore, 1867).

Clara Barton

Soon after the Civil War broke out in 1861, **Clara Barton,** a Massachusetts woman who was working as a copyist in the U.S. Patent Office, began an independent campaign to provide relief for the soldiers. Appealing to the nation for supplies of woolen shirts, blankets, towels, lanterns, camp kettles, and other necessities (Barton, 1862), she established her own system of distribution, refusing to enlist in the military nurse corps headed by Dorothea Dix (Oates, 1994). Working outside of the government's official organization, Barton did not receive her first army pass authorizing her to take supplies to the battlegrounds of Virginia until August 12, 1862. Then, having taken a leave of absence from her patent job, she made her way to Culpeper, Virginia. At the scene of the battle, she set up a makeshift field hospital and cared for the wounded and dying. During this battle, Barton gained her famous title, "Angel of the Battlefield." Her efforts did not end with the war. Barton went on to found an organization whose name is synonymous with compassionate service: the American Red Cross.

Nursing in the Confederacy

Like their sisters in the North, the women of the South responded to the news of war with an outpouring of support for the soldiers. Among those who served were Kate Cumming, Phoebe Pember, and Sally Thompkins. However, unlike the women in the North, southern women worked without the benefit of an official government organization. In contrast to Lincoln's rapid response to organize the provision of medical care, the Confederate government did not assume control and partial support of all southern military hospitals until the last months of 1861 and early 1862. Until this time, many hospitals were staffed only with female volunteers or wounded soldiers. With the advent of government control, some aspects of hospital organization changed dramatically, and several women were appointed as superintendents of hospitals. Superintendent Sallie Thompkins, who had earlier established a private hospital in Richmond, Virginia, was commissioned a "captain of Cavalry, unassigned" by President Davis, and was the only woman in the Confederacy to hold military rank.

While thousands of women supported the war effort, only a few were appointed as matrons of hospitals. One of the earliest to be placed in charge was **Phoebe Pember.**

When she was assigned to Chimborazo Hospital, a sprawling government-run institution on the western boundary of Richmond, Virginia, in September 1862, Pember noted that the care was provided by "sick or wounded men, convalescing and placed in that position, however ignorant they might be—until strong enough for field duty" (Pember, 1959, p. 18). Not only was there inadequate help, but there were also shortages in supplies throughout the South as a result of blockaded seaports. In Chimborazo, fuel was inadequate, food was skimpy, soap was unavailable, and bandages were reused without being cleansed (Pember, 1959). Pember remedied this situation as best she could, imposing order, discipline, and cleanliness on hospital operations.

Change in the American Military Medical System

By the end of the Civil War both the physical and administrative structure of the military hospitals had been transformed. In the North and South, women volunteers, religious orders, and newly appointed matrons and superintendents had made a significant impact. The hospitals were orderly, clean, and well ventilated, and the death rate was surprisingly low. Moreover, it had become clear that women as nurses and organizers had played a major role in these reforms. The Civil War, for all of its horror, had helped to advance the cause of professional nursing. The success in the reform of military hospitals would open the doors for reform of civilian hospital facilities throughout the country (Rosenberg, 1987).

1874-1900: THE ROOTS TAKE HOLD

During the years following the Civil War, a number of events exerted a positive influence on the founding of training schools for nurses. In 1869, Dr. Samuel Gross, a progressive physician, recommended to the American Medical Association that large hospitals begin the process of developing training schools for nurses. He proposed that the students in these schools be taught by medical staff and resident physicians. Simultaneously, members of the United States Sanitary Commission, who had served during the war and learned its lessons, began to lobby for the creation of nursing schools. Support for their efforts gained momentum as advocates of social reform reported the shockingly inadequate conditions that existed in many hospitals. Another voice for nursing's cause belonged to Sarah J. Hale, editor of the popular and widely read *Godey's Lady's Book and Magazine*. Hale advocated formal training for nurses in an editorial entitled "Lady Nurses" in February 1871:

> Much has been lately said of the benefits that would follow if the calling of the sick nurse were elevated to a profession which an educated lady might adopt without a sense of degradation, either of her own part or in the estimation of others. . . . There can be no doubt that the duties of the sick nurse, to be properly performed, require an education and training little, if at all, inferior to those possessed by members of the medical profession. To leave these duties to untaught and ill-trained persons is as great a mistake as it was to allow the office of surgeon to be held by one whose proper calling was that of a mechanic of the humblest class. The manner in which a reform may be effected is easily pointed out. Every medical college should have a course of study and training especially adapted for ladies who desire to qualify themselves for the profession of nurse; and those who had gone through the course,

and passed the requisite examination, should receive a degree and a diploma, which would at once establish their position in society. The "graduate nurse" would in general estimation be as much above the ordinary nurse of the present day as the professional surgeon of our times is above the barber-surgeon of the last century (Donahue, 1996).

Together, these influential men and women paved the way for the formal establishment of nurse training schools.

𝓗𝑖𝑠𝑡𝑜𝑟𝑖𝑐𝑎𝑙 NOTE 2

In 1882 to 1883, Koch discovered tuberculosis and cholera organisms. Laboratory findings were gaining credibility. From this point on, medicine would be increasingly based on scientific evidence rather than on tradition or hypothesis.

The First Training Schools for Nurses and the Feminization of Nursing

The first three training schools for nurses, modeled after Nightingale's famous school at St. Thomas's Hospital in London, were Bellevue Training School for Nurses in New York City, Connecticut Training School for Nurses in New Haven, Connecticut, and the Boston Training School for Nurses at Massachusetts General Hospital in Boston (Dock, 1907). The widely held Victorian belief in women's innate sensitivity and high morals led to the early requirement that applicants to these programs be female, for it was thought that only these feminine qualities could improve the quality of nursing care. Thus sensitivity, breeding, intelligence, and "ladylike" behavior, including submission to authority, were highly desired personal characteristics for applicants. The feminization of the profession took root. The number of training schools increased steadily during the last decades of the nineteenth century, and by 1900 they played a critical role in providing hospitals with a stable, subservient, female workforce, as hospitals came to be staffed primarily by students (Figure 1-3). According to historian Rosenberg, "no single change transformed the hospital's day to day workings more than the acceptance of trained nurses and nurse training schools, which brought a disciplined corps of would-be professionals in the wards" (Rosenberg, 1987, p. 344). See Chapter 2 for a thorough description of the history of nursing education.

The 1893 Chicago World's Fair Promotes Professionalization

The 1893 Chicago World's Fair, a shining monument to the ideals of the Progressive Movement, was the setting for dramatic steps in the professionalization of nursing. There, some of the most influential nursing leaders of the century, including Isabel Hampton (later Isabel Hampton Robb), Lavinia Lloyd Dock, and Bedford Fenwick of Great Britain, gathered to share ideas and discuss issues pertaining to nursing education. In this setting, **Isabel Hampton Robb,** organizer of the Johns Hopkins School of Nursing and one of the greatest early leaders of nursing, presented a paper

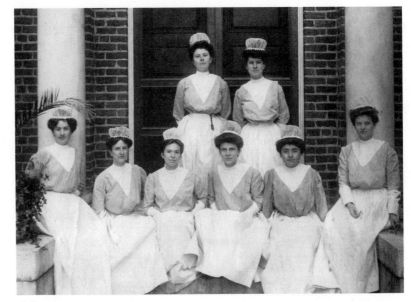

Figure 1-3
University of Virginia student nurses, circa 1910. (Reproduced with permission of the School of Nursing Collection, the Center for Nursing Historical Inquiry, University of Virginia, School of Nursing.)

"protesting the lack of uniformity in nursing school curricula and the inadequacy of nursing education." A paper by Florence Nightingale addressing the need for scientific training of nurses was also read. The very next day, these visionary women began to transform ideas into action, establishing the American Society of Superintendents of Training Schools for Nurses to begin to address issues in nursing education. The society changed its name in 1912 to the National League of Nursing Education (NLNE); in 1952 it was again reorganized and given its current name, the National League for Nursing (NLN) (Christy, 1984).

Isabel Hampton Robb, a visionary and influential leader, recognized the need "to unite practitioners of nursing" as well as nursing educators. In 1896 she founded the Nurses' Associated Alumnae of the United States and Canada, which in 1911 became officially known as the American Nurses Association (ANA) (Christy, 1969, p. 38).

At the close of the decade, in 1899, this small group of American nursing leaders, along with nursing leaders from abroad, collaborated again with Bedford Fenwick of Britain to found the International Council of Nurses (ICN). The ICN was dedicated to uniting nursing organizations of all nations, and, fittingly, the first meeting was held at the World Exposition in Buffalo, New York, in 1901. At that meeting, a major topic of discussion was the need for state registration of nurses.

Visiting Nursing: The Henry Street Settlement

It was also during this final decade of the century that urbanization, immigration, and industrialization had begun to create huge social problems. Chief among these were the overcrowding and filth of cities, the emergence of sweat shops and child labor, and the spread of infectious diseases. Typically, immigrant families lived in crowded, suffocating, rat-infested tenements, with the central air chutes filled with garbage. Responding to the needs of the immigrant communities, **Lillian Wald** and her colleague Mary Brewster moved into a tenement on New York's Lower East Side and, with the help of private philanthropists, established the Henry Street Settlement. This highly organized agency provided both visiting nursing care and civic and social services, including playgrounds and country camps, to inner city residents. Lillian Wald, writing in July 25, 1893, noted some aspects of the care and services she provided:

> My first call was on the Goldberg baby whose pulse and improved condition had been maintained after our last night's care. After taking the temperature, washing and dressing the child, I called on the doctor who had been summoned before, told him of the family's tribulations and he offered not to charge them for the visit. Then I took Hattie Issacs, the consumptive, a big bunch of flowers and while she slept I cleaned out the window of medicine bottles. Then I bathed her … made the bed, cooked a light breakfast of eggs and milk which I had brought with me, fed her and assisted the mother to straighten up and then left … After luncheon, I saw the O'Brien's and took the little one, with whooping cough, to play in the back of our yard. On the next floor, the Costra baby had a sore mouth for which I gave the mother borax and honey and little cloths to keep it clean … (Wald, 1893).

Lavinia Lloyd Dock

Lavinia Lloyd Dock, a fiery political and social activist who became a central figure in American and international nursing history during the Progressive Era (Estabrooks, 1995), soon joined the Henry Street Settlement to work with her colleagues.

🏛 *Historical* NOTE 3

In describing Lavinia Dock, Isabel M. Stewart, a colleague, said "… this suffrage thing—it was the whole thing for her; she wanted not only to work for it, but really to suffer for it … [S]he was a member of the advanced wing of the Suffrage Party, and they were having a meeting in Washington at the time that Wilson was beginning to think of the possibility of war … and Lavinia got up and seized the flag and on she marched, out of the door, and they followed her … and they picketed the White House …! Anyway, they all went into the cooler [jail] for the night. I think it just pleased her to no end" (Stewart, 1961).

Dock (Figure 1-4) was not only a nurse but also a militant suffragist, who linked the future of nursing to the greater women's movement. In one early article she wrote:

> As the modern nursing movement is emphatically an outcome of the original and general woman's movement … it would be a great pity for them [nurses] to allow one of the most remarkable movements of the day to go on under their eyes without comprehending it … Unless we possess the ballot we shall not know when we may get up in the morning to find all that we had gained has been taken from us (Dock, 1907, p. 897).

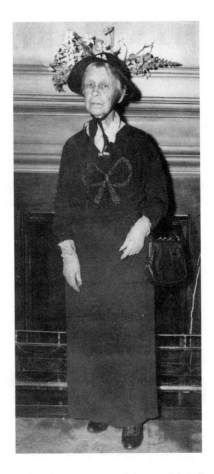

Figure **1-4**
Lavinia L. Dock. (Reproduced with permission of the Special Collections, Milbank Memorial Library, Teachers College, Columbia University.)

War Crystallizes the Need for Nurses: Spanish American War—1898

In 1898 the United States Congress declared war on Spain, and once again, as in the Civil War, nursing would have a major role to play. Immediately, Cuban camps were devastated by typhoid fever and other infectious diseases, and a call for nurses was sent out. In response, Isabel Hampton Robb, president of the Nurses' Associated Alumnae of the United States and Canada, offered the services of trained nurses (Wall, 1995). Instead of accepting this offer, the surgeon general appointed an ad hoc Hospital Corps, formed by the Daughters of the American Revolution (DAR) to recruit nurses. Anita N. McGee, a physician and DAR member, was granted the authority to head this group. McGee required that only graduates of nurse training schools be recruited as contract nurses for the army. However, when typhoid fever became epidemic and there were thousands of soldiers who needed care, others, including the Sisters of the Holy Cross and untrained African-American nurses who had had typhoid fever in the past, were accepted for service (Wall, 1995). Significant for the first use of trained nurses in war, the Spanish-American War would set the stage for the development of a permanent Army Nurse Corps (1901) and Navy Nurse Corps (1908) in the future.

1900-1917: A YOUNG PROFESSION FACES NEW CHALLENGES

In October 1900, after years of dedicated work by Isabel Hampton Robb, Mary Adelaide Nutting, Lavinia L. Dock, **Sophia Palmer,** and **Mary E. Davis,** the first issue of the *American Journal of Nursing* was published (Christy, 1984). Sophia Palmer, the director of nursing at Rochester City Hospital, New York, was appointed as the first editor. Nurses now had both a professional organization and an official journal through which they could communicate with one another. According to the editorial in the first issue:

> It will be the aim of the editors to present month by month the most useful facts, the most progressive thought and the latest news that the profession has to offer in the most attractive form that can be secured ... (Palmer, 1900, p. 64).

State Licensure: A Milestone for the Profession

In 1903, state legislatures in North Carolina, New Jersey, New York, and Virginia passed licensure laws for nursing, all within a span of 2 months. Lavinia Dock noted the significance of these laws:

> We all understand that these little bills are only an opening wedge. We all know that the idea for which we are working is a state examination, to be passed, fixed upon a stated basis of work. I think our ideal bill would demand a specified time for graduates, I mean a certain amount of work to be done before they enter upon the study of nursing; then a specified time for practice in the work constituting the nurses' work ... and make a compulsory examination before practice ... (New York State Nurses Association, 1903).

Within the next decade, many other states followed with a plan for licensure of professional nurses. The roots of professional nursing had taken hold.

⬚ *Historical* NOTE 4

The state of the art of medicine grew dramatically after the turn of the century. Science was well respected, and data were being collected on patients' conditions. Temperature graphs were routinely kept, the microscopic examination of urine and blood was an established procedure, and the x-ray was now widely available in hospitals (Howell, 1996).

"A Successful Experiment": African-American Clinic Nursing in New York City

At the same time that nursing was addressing these professional issues, tuberculosis was a major health problem in the teeming slums of the newly developing cities.

Dr. Edward T. Devine, president of the Charity Organization Society, noted the high incidence of tuberculosis among New York City's African-American population. Aware of racial barriers and cultural resistance to seeking medical care, Dr. Devine determined that a "Negro" district nurse should be hired to work in the African-American community to persuade people to accept treatment. **Jessie Sleet Scales,** an African-American nurse who had been trained at Providence Hospital in Chicago, a hospital exclusively for "colored people," was chosen to work on a trial basis. Her report to the Charity Organization Society was published in the *American Journal of Nursing* in 1901, entitled "A Successful Experiment":

> I beg to render to you a report of the work done by me as a district nurse among the colored people of New York City during the months of October and November ... I have visited forty-one families and made 156 calls in connection with these families, caring for nine cases of consumption, four cases of peritonitis, two cases of chickenpox, two cases of cancer, one case of diphtheria, two cases of heart disease, two cases of tumor, one case of gastric catarrh, two cases of pneumonia, four cases of rheumatism, and two cases of scalp wound. I have given baths, applied poultices, dressed wounds, washed and dressed newborn babies, cared for mothers ... (Sleet, 1901, p. 729).

Jessie Sleet Scales (Figure 1-5) was in fact so successful in community health work that she became legendary (Mosley, 1996). Scales later recommended to Lillian Wald that Elizabeth Tyler, a graduate of Freedmen's Hospital Training School for Nurses, work with African-American patients at the Henry Street Settlement. Working within the confines of a racist society, she and Tyler established the Stillman House, a branch of the Henry Street Settlement serving "colored people" in a small store on West 61st Street.

For community health nursing, the addition of these pioneer African-American nurses to the ranks of the Henry Street Settlement signified activism, expansion, and growth. Despite the ever-present racial barriers and deplorable living and health conditions, these courageous young women succeeded in providing excellent nursing care to underserved families with spiraling health care needs.

In 1912, the ideas associated with the Henry Street Settlement won widespread acceptance. District and visiting nursing services proliferated, and national standards were needed. As a result, the National Organization of Public Health Nursing (NOPHN) was established with Lillian Wald as its first president.

Historical NOTE 5

Margaret Sanger and the Birth Control Movement: **Margaret Sanger,** a nurse who worked on the Lower East Side of New York City in 1912, was struck by the ignorance of immigrant women about pregnancy and contraception. After witnessing the death of Sadie Sachs from a self-attempted abortion, Sanger was inspired to action by the tragedy and became determined to teach women about birth control. A radical activist in her early years, Sanger devoted her life to the birth control movement (Kennedy, 1970).

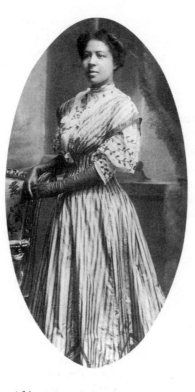

Figure 1-5
Jessie Sleet Scales, a visionary African-American nurse who was among the first to bring community health nursing principles to the slums of New York City around 1900. (Reproduced with permission of the E. M. Carnegie Collection, Archives of Hampton University.)

1917: THE FLU EPIDEMIC AND WORLD WAR I BRING NEW CHALLENGES TO A YOUNG PROFESSION

Two significant events coincided in 1917 to provide nursing with new challenges. The United States entered World War I, and an influenza epidemic swept across the country. The concept of using trained female nurses to care for soldiers had been proved on the field of battle and accepted (Figure 1-6). Therefore, when the United States entered the war in Europe, a Committee on Nursing was formed under the Council of National Defense (Dock and Stewart, 1920). This committee was chaired by **Mary Adelaide Nutting,** Professor of Nursing and Health at Columbia University (see Chapter 2 for further discussion of Nutting, a leader in nursing education), and included Jane A. Delano, Director of Nursing in the American Red Cross (Figure 1-7), among others. Charged with supplying an adequate number of trained nurses to U.S. Army hospitals abroad, the committee initiated a national publicity campaign to recruit young women to enter nurses training, established the Army School of Nursing with Annie Goodrich as dean, introduced college women to nursing in the Vassar Training Camp for Nurses, and began widespread public education in home nursing and hygiene through Red Cross nursing.

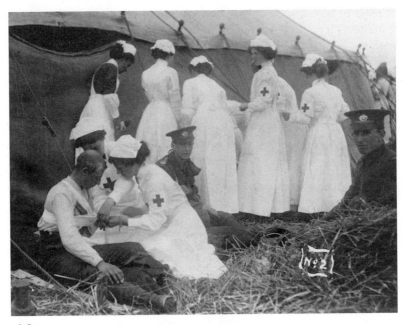

Figure **1-6**
World War I Red Cross Nursing. (Reproduced with permission of the Keeling Collection, the Center for Nursing Historical Inquiry, University of Virginia, School of Nursing.)

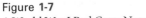

Figure **1-7**
A World War I Red Cross Nursing certificate, signed by Jane A. Delano, an early director of the American Red Cross.

On the home front, the flu epidemic of 1917 to 1919 increased the public's awareness of the necessity of public health nursing. Across the nation, the public health service, American Red Cross, and Visiting Nursing Associations mobilized to provide care for the thousands of citizens struck with influenza. In Richmond, Virginia, in 1918, the burden of home visits fell to the Instructive Visiting Nurse Association (IVNA). According to the director, Nannie Minor, RN:

> For many days our office was a nightmare ... from early morning until late at night we sat at the telephone with the receiver rarely out of our hands, listening to heartrending stories and appeals for aid to which we could so inadequately respond. For about two weeks we were receiving about 180-250 calls a day and the nurses were manning between 450-500 visits (Minor, 1918).

In spring 1919, the second wave of the flu epidemic struck the East Coast and swept across the country. Although not as lethal as the first, widespread illness among Americans closed businesses, schools, and churches and increased demands for nursing services.

1920-1930: THE ROARING TWENTIES

By the time World War I ended, nursing again had demonstrated the effectiveness of using young, trained, professional nurses to care for soldiers during war. Moreover, the profession had also made clear the need for nurses to have both the responsibility for and the authority to manage the care of their patients. As a result, in 1920 Congress passed a bill that provided nurses with military rank (Dock and Stewart, 1920). This bill followed the passage of the Nineteenth Amendment to the U.S. Constitution, a bill that granted women the right to vote. Both acts of Congress opened the decade of the "Roaring Twenties" and the beginning of unheard freedom for American women. Shortened hairstyles, rising hemlines, and the use of cosmetics, all part of the "flapper" era, reflected these new-found freedoms.

The twenties also saw increased use of hospitals and an acceptance of the scientific basis of medicine. Most major surgical procedures were now being done in hospitals, and penicillin was discovered in 1928. This drug profoundly affected the treatment of infection, and antibiotic use for the prevention of postoperative infections became routine.

In the early part of the decade, Congress passed the Shephard-Towner Act to provide services for mothers and children in cities and counties throughout the nation. Amidst all of these changes, nursing was progressing in two divergent areas. The Goldmark Report, a study of nursing education, advocated the establishment of collegiate schools of nursing rather than hospital-based diploma programs (see Chapter 2), and programs in rural midwifery were being organized.

1925: The Frontier Nursing Service

In 1925, **Mary Breckinridge,** a nurse and certified midwife who had family social-connections with Kentucky's health commissioner, established the Kentucky Committee for Mothers and Babies, later to be known as the Frontier Nursing

Service (FNS). This service provided the first organized midwifery program in the United States. Nurses of the FNS worked in Leslie County, Kentucky, an isolated rural area in the Appalachian Mountains. There they traveled by horseback to reach the families of each district. In 1930 alone, the FNS reported 22,347 visits to 8,563 families and 10,459 visits to their nursing centers (Pletsh, 1981). Serving the health needs of the poverty-stricken mountain community, the FNS nurses delivered babies and provided pre- and postnatal care, educated mothers and their families about nutrition and hygiene, and cared for the sick. Through this rural midwifery service, Breckenridge demonstrated that nurses could play a significant role in providing primary rural health care.

Historical NOTE 6

The concept of the postoperative recovery room staffed by graduate nurses, introduced in the late 1930s, would set the precedent for the development of intensive care units in the future (Lynaugh and Fairman, 1992).

1931-1945: THE PROFESSION RESPONDS TO THE GREAT DEPRESSION AND WORLD WAR II

The crash of the stock market in 1929, along with the resulting economic depression and unemployment, was to have a profound impact on the nursing profession. Until this time, most nurses worked as private duty nurses in patient's homes, for hospitals were largely staffed by nursing students. As businesses failed and unemployment spread, families without incomes could no longer afford private duty nurses when they needed them, and many nurses joined the growing ranks of the unemployed. The creation of the Civil Works Administration (CWA) in 1933 by President Roosevelt was particularly important for unemployed nurses, especially for public health nurses. Under the CWA, nurses participated in providing rural and school health services and took part in specific projects conducting surveys to determine service needs related to communicable disease and nutrition of children (Fitzpatrick, 1975).

During these economically shattered times, many hospitals were forced to close their schools of nursing. As a result, they no longer had a reliable, cheap student workforce and faced a shortage of staff to care for patients. At the same time there was a dramatic increase in the number of patients who needed charity care. The solution soon became apparent: the unemployed graduate nurses, willing to work for minimum pay, could be recruited to work in the hospitals rather than in private duty. This change in staffing hospitals with graduate nurses rather than students would have lasting implications for the profession.

World War II: New Opportunities for Nursing

By 1938 German and Italian expansionism in Europe threatened to involve the United States in war. Organized nursing began to prepare to meet the need for nurses should that occur. The Army Nurse Corps increased its numbers, and in 1940 Julia C. Stenson, the ANA president, convened a meeting of representatives of the major nursing organizations to coordinate the efforts of the profession to prepare for war (Bullough, 1976). By 1941, when the Japanese bombing of Pearl Harbor drew the United States into war, nurses were vigorously recruited to serve at the battlefront.

Historical NOTE 7

From Tressa Cates's diary, Sternberg General Army Hospital in Manila, in the days immediately following the attack on Pearl Harbor: "Today was a ghastly dream. Beds that were empty yesterday were now occupied by mangled and horribly burned patients. In a few hours, the simple routine of our lives was completely changed. We worked twelve to fourteen hours at a time and felt no exhaustion—only numbness. We couldn't quite believe what happened … our wounded and dying continued to fill the beds" (Cates, 1957, pp. 18-19).

Nurses who a few months earlier had not even thought of wartime nursing found themselves accompanying troops to Europe, landing in Normandy a few days after the invasion. Dressed in army fatigues, they cared for troops in field and evacuation hospitals in North Africa, Italy, France, and the Philippines, while Navy nurses gave care aboard hospital ships.

While soldiers were receiving care on the front, there were severe shortages of nurses at home. One of the most significant programs initiated as a result of the shortage of nurses for the war effort was the **Cadet Nurse Corps,** founded by Frances Payne Bolton, the congresswoman from Ohio. The Bolton Act became law on June 15, 1943. Headed by Lucile Petry Leone, the Cadet Corps sought to recruit 65,000 new students in 1944 and another 60,000 in 1945, about twice the number entering schools in peacetime (Petry, 1945). Admission to the Cadet Corps could not be refused on the basis of race or marital status. Of further note, the Corps had minimum educational standards. These policies, combined with federal assistance to nursing schools and the requirement that schools have budgets that were separate from the hospitals, had a significant impact on the profession's growth and development as it sought to integrate African-American students and to break from the hospital-affiliated apprenticeship model of nursing education. By the end of the war, the Cadet program had subsidized the education of about 179,000 nursing students (Figure 1-8). The Bolton Act also provided funds to graduate nurses for advanced study in order to increase the number of nursing instructors and prepare nurses to practice in psychiatry and in public health nursing.

Over 100,000 nurses volunteered and were certified for military services in the Army and Navy Nurse Corps (Nurses' Contribution, 1945, p. 683). Nursing made great strides in its professional development during the war and immediately afterward. In the field hospitals at the front, nursing and medical boundaries blurred as members of both professions worked together to save as many of the wounded as

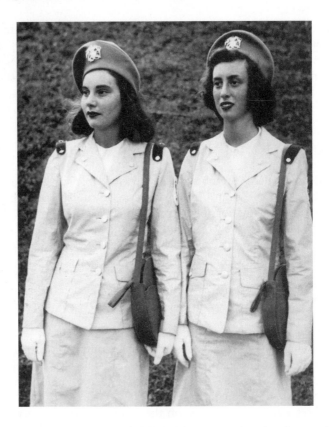

Figure **1-8**
Cadet nurses Peggy and Barbara Bishop, 1944. (Reproduced with permission of the School of Nursing Collection, the Center for Nursing Historical Inquiry, University of Virginia, School of Nursing.)

they could. As a result, nurses took on new responsibilities and learned new skills. As Virginia G. Shannon of the U.S. Army recalled:

> In October 1944 we were ready for the invasion of Southern France … We expected to be based at Lyon but just kept going until we were only 10 miles behind the lines. Again, we were in a hospital that had not been finished but had a big red cross on it … There were so many casualties from the battles. Wounded and injured were brought in from the Rhine, and as fast as we could evacuate them, more were brought in. We had to learn a lot of things right on the spot. When there wasn't a doctor to do it, the nurses did it. I did blood transfusions, intravenous medications and even sewed up secondary closure wounds (Fessler, 1996, p. 185).

After the war, further progress toward professionalization was made. In 1947, military nurses were awarded full commissioned officer status, and segregation of African-American nurses was ended. In 1948, The Brown Report recommended establishing schools of nursing in universities and colleges, enhancing the educational standards for professional nurses (Figure 1-9; see Chapter 2). By 1954 discrimination against

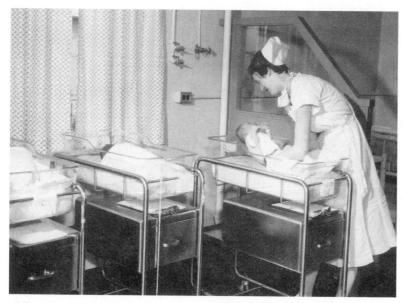

Figure **1-9**
Pediatric nursing student, 1959. (Reproduced with permission of the School of Nursing Alumni Association Collection, the Center for Nursing Historical Inquiry, University of Virginia, School of Nursing.)

male nurses was also reduced when men were finally admitted into military nursing (Bullough, 1976).

1945-1960: THE RISE OF HOSPITALS—BUREAUCRACY, SCIENCE, AND SHORTAGES

Numerous technological and scientific advances were made in medicine in the period from 1945 to 1960. Following World War II, federal budget appropriations for medical research increased enormously, resulting in a surge of research in many of the specialized areas. Dramatic innovations in medical care followed. Sulfa drugs transformed the care of infectious diseases. New cardiac drugs were developed. Cardiac surgeries were performed, and in 1941 Dr. Claude S. Beck, a surgeon at Western Reserve School of Medicine in Cleveland, Ohio, reported the first two attempts of defibrillation for ventricular fibrillation during surgery.

At the same time, postwar economic resurgence, an expansion in private health care insurance, and the "baby boom" all had an impact on the medical system (Figure 1-10). In 1946, the Hill Burton Act, providing funds to construct hospitals, led to a surge in the growth of new facilities. This rapid expansion in the number of hospital beds resulted in an acute shortage of nurses and increasingly difficult working conditions for those who were employed. Long hours, inadequate salaries, and increasing patient loads made many nurses unhappy with their jobs, and threats of strikes and collective bargaining ensued. For years, heated

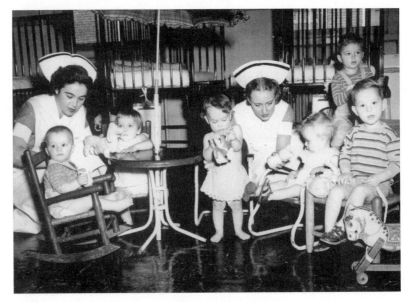

Figure 1-10
Student nurses in pediatrics, circa 1945. (Reproduced with permission of the School of Nursing Collection, the Center for Nursing Historical Inquiry, University of Virginia, School of Nursing.)

debates would continue about whether or not professional nurses should go on strike.

In response to the shortages, "team nursing" was introduced. This method of care delivery utilized licensed practical nurses (LPNs), nursing assistants, and nurses aides under the supervision of a registered nurse. Although efficient, the method fragmented patient care and removed the registered nurse from the bedside. Another response to the shortage was the institution of the associate degree program, an abbreviated 2-year program designed by Mildred Montag (discussed in more detail in Chapter 2).

The 1950s saw additional changes in health care. During this decade the profession advocated clinical nursing research, and the *Journal of Nursing Research* was first published. Military corpsmen entered nursing programs, the number of male nurses increased, and more nurses sought advanced degrees. State units of the American Nurses Association accepted African-American nurses for membership, as did the national organization, thereby ending racial discrimination in nursing organizations. As a result the National Association of Colored Graduate Nurses was dissolved in 1951 (to be replaced in 1972 by the formation of the National Black Nurses Association). In 1957, challenged by the launch of Sputnik to keep pace with the Russians in science and technology, America moved swiftly toward the development of space-age technology. The accompanying scientific advances in medical and nursing research would continue to revolutionize nursing and medical care for the remainder of the twentieth century.

Historical NOTE 8

MASH units in Korea: In 1950, when the Korean War broke out, nurses were once again required for combat. This time, Army nurses were stationed as close to the front as possible in Mobile Army Surgical Hospital (MASH) units that could be set up quickly to provide emergency trauma care. Once again, nurses at the front faced new challenges as the injured were flown in by helicopter only minutes after being wounded in combat.

1961-1985: NEW ROLES FOR NURSES

Although the first nursing specialists—nurse anesthetists at the Mayo Clinic and public health nurses in New York City—date back to the late 19th century, the 1960s is more often noted as the era of the rise in specialty care and clinical specialization for nurses. The impressive development of the clinical specialist role in psychiatric nursing in the early sixties, combined with the rise of intensive care units and technological advances of the period, fostered the growth of clinical specialization in other areas of nursing, including cardiac-thoracic surgery and coronary care.

Coronary Care Nursing

One of the most significant events of the 1960s was the establishment of the coronary care unit (CCU), a subspecialty unit, created by Dr. Hughes Day in Kansas City and Dr. Lawrence Meltzer in Philadelphia, working independently between 1962 and 1963. Several factors culminated in the development of this subspecialty care. Electrocardiograms were available, the defibrillator had recently been shown effective in saving lives, the concept of intensive care had been established and was already in place in many hospitals, and physicians were interested in subspecialty care. Furthermore, during the recent wars, nurses had accepted new responsibilities and roles as the need arose.

In the coronary care units (Figure 1-11), nurses began to share with physicians the emerging medical knowledge about the diagnosis and treatment of cardiac arrhythmias. Soon they began to be recognized for their expertise in the care

Historical NOTE 9

In 1965, Medicare and Medicaid became law under Title XVIII of the Social Security Act, ensuring access to health care for elderly, poor, and disabled Americans. That same year, the American Nurses Association approved its first position paper on nursing education, which called for all nursing education for professional practice to take place in colleges and universities (ANA, 1965). Had that position been acted upon, it would have been critical in uniting the profession on the issue of preparation for entry into practice.

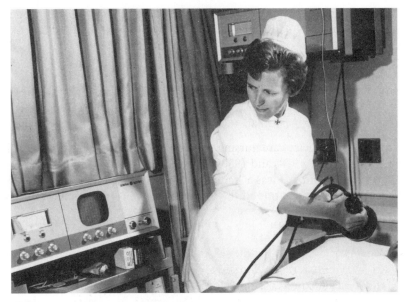

Figure **1-11**
Rose Pinneo, RN, Director of the Coronary Care Unit at Presbyterian Hospital in Philadelphia, demonstrating the use of an early cardiac defibrillator, circa 1965. (Reproduced with permission of the Pinneo Collection, Center for Nursing Historical Inquiry, University of Virginia, School of Nursing.)

of critically ill cardiac patients and were permitted to administer intravenous drugs and defibrillate patients according to written protocols. Gaining acceptance as colleagues, the CCU nurses set the stage for more autonomous practice in a variety of specialty areas, including burn, dialysis, and oncology units, as well as in medical and surgical ICUs.

Nurse Practitioners

The rise in medical specialization in the sixties, along with the concurrent shortage of primary care physicians and the public demand for improved access to health care that grew out of Lyndon Johnson's "Great Society" reforms, fostered the emergence of the nurse practitioner (NP) in primary care. In 1965, **Lorretta Ford,** RN, and Henry Silver, MD, opened the first pediatric nurse practitioner program at the University of Colorado. This collaborative project, designed to prepare professional nurses to manage common childhood illnesses and provide well-child care, demonstrated that nurse practitioners were competent in managing 75 percent of pediatric patients in community clinics (Ford and Silver, 1967). Their research subsequently attracted considerable attention across the United States and led to federal and state support for the nurse practitioner role. In 1971, Idaho became the first state to recognize diagnosis and treatment as part of the legal scope of practice for NPs. Other states, including Alaska and North Carolina, authorized NPs to write prescriptions in 1975 (Safriet, 1992). By the mid-1980s, nurse practitioner programs had been developed in schools of nursing throughout the country, and nurse practitioners were employed in a wide variety of outpatient settings. By the mid-1990s, programs for acute care nurse practitioners were developed, and jobs became available in tertiary care settings (Figure 1-12).

Historical NOTE 10

The concept of primary care nursing, introduced by Manthey in 1968, was implemented in many hospitals during the 1970s and 1980s. This method of care delivery advocated "total patient care" done by the registered nurse. It was a "return to the bedside" for experienced nurses and an attempt to combat the depersonalization of the bureaucratic delivery system of care (Lynaugh and Brush, 1996).

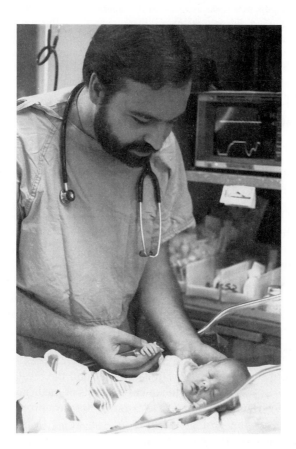

Figure **1-12**
Tom Buckley, RN, BSN, Clinician V, circa 1990. (Reproduced with permission of the School of Nursing Collection, the Center for Nursing Historical Inquiry, University of Virginia, School of Nursing.)

Nursing in Vietnam

The war in Vietnam, one of America's longest and most controversial wars, provided nurses once again with opportunities to stretch the boundaries of the discipline as they did whatever needed to be done to provide immediate care to the massive numbers of casualties coming into the field hospitals. Working in inflatable medical units in the jungles of Vietnam, these nurses fought to save lives. They performed emergency tracheotomies, inserted chest tubes, administered blood, and gave morphine without orders when there were not enough physicians to meet the demands. One nurse wrote of how terrified and helpless she felt while transporting the critically ill:

> Whenever we had someone who had a bad head injury, we'd have to send them to one of the hospitals on the coast, like the 85th Evac. Most of the time, the Air Force would do our evaking [sic] for us, but if it was just one person going down, then a lot of times the dust-off choppers would take him and they'd have one of us nurses ride along to take care of him. I went very often, because I was assigned to the emergency room. I remember just how desperate I used to feel during these nights; there was really nothing in the helicopter to take care of them with in case anything should happen. We did have a suction apparatus we could work with our foot, but that was about the only thing that we could really use. I remember praying all the way down that they wouldn't die before they got there and feeling so afraid that something was going to happen. There was so little I could do (Walker, 1985, pp. 60-61).

Another nurse described the stress of the war:

> I still remember my baptism into the realities of war: the nausea and revulsion that spilled all over me; my shaking hands as I examined the wounded, took vital signs, and fought to get control of my brain. I still see the face of the first soldier I reached: brown eyes staring wide in death, the back of his head and neck blown away (Boulay, 1989, p. 272).

As the nurses faced these external challenges, they also fought the emotional battles that rose within themselves as they struggled to comprehend the lack of support for their work from large segments of the American public. By 1967, after a massive military build-up by President Johnson, demonstrations against the war were a common occurrence throughout the United States. Later, after the nurses returned home, the trauma of the battlefield would be intensified by this lack of support, and many nurses suffered posttraumatic stress disorder (PSTD).

1986-2004: MANAGED CARE AND ITS CHALLENGES FOR NURSING

With the advent of managed care in the late 1980s and the resulting emphasis on health care reform as a way to continue to cut the costs of medical care, nursing was caught up in the whirlwind of change. Determined to take a proactive stance in the reform effort, the nursing profession wrote its *Agenda for Health Care Reform* in 1992. The plan for reform was comprehensive and focused on restructuring the health care system in the United States to reduce costs and improve access to care. Challenges for nursing in the managed care era included (1) providing quality, cost-effective care; (2) continuing to care, in a culture that did not value caring

(Reverby, 1987); and (3) obtaining third-party reimbursement for nurses in advanced practice roles in both primary and acute care.

LESSONS OF HISTORY

The nursing profession cannot meet the challenges of the twenty-first century without an accurate understanding of its past. The classic reason for studying history is to avoid repeating its mistakes. However, some issues and problems facing the profession could be addressed using "recycled" solutions. For example, today there are challenges in providing care to inner-city communities. Earlier, in the twentieth century, this challenge was met quite aptly by Lillian Wald in the creation of the Henry Street Settlement, in which she addressed not only the physical but also the psychological needs of children and their families (Buhler-Wilkerson, 1993). Today, the nursing profession often struggles to explain how nurse practitioners differ from physician's assistants. Yesterday's answer, by Lavinia Dock and Maitland Stewart, might be considered:

> The nurse often acts as the physician's assistant, but she has many duties apart from this function, the most important being her own distinct art of nursing. In this field it is she, and not the physician, who is expert (Dock and Stewart, 1920, p. 340).

Since September 11, 2001, we are all too aware of the challenges of relating to a global community in which the threats of war, bioterrorism, and emerging epidemics such as severe acute respiratory syndrome (SARS) are a reality. Dock's emphasis on maintaining a world perspective and addressing nursing issues within the context of global women's issues may be instructive. Moreover, we recognize the need for culturally sensitive care. In the past, African-American nurses met the needs of their patients by being sensitive to cultural differences while challenging racial barriers.

The nursing profession must adjust to the continually changing roles for nurses and expectations of what duties nurses can assume. In the past, especially during war, nurses have demonstrated flexibility and competence in the face of change. Cognizant of our heritage, we look to meet the challenges of the present and plan for the future.

Summary of Key Points

- In 1860 Florence Nightingale founded a school for nurses at St. Thomas's Hospital, London, that would become the model for nursing education in the United States.
- Volunteer Civil War nurses played a major role in reform of military hospitals, thereby opening the door for reform of civilian hospitals nationwide and advancing the cause of professional nursing.
- Formal educational programs for U.S. nurses were established in 1873 in hospitals in New York City, New Haven, and Boston.
- American nursing's first professional organization, the American Society of Superintendents of Training Schools for Nurses, was founded during the 1893 Chicago World's Fair. This organization became the National League for

Nursing Education (NLNE) in 1912 and the National League for Nursing (NLN) in 1952.
- The forerunner of the American Nurses Association (ANA) was founded in 1896 by Isabel Hampton Robb.
- In 1899 the International Council of Nurses (ICN) was formed to unite nursing organizations of all nations.
- The development of nursing and the general women's movement, including the right to vote, paralleled each other.
- The initiation of state licensure in 1903 heralded standardization of nursing education programs that, until this time, had varied widely.
- The establishment of the Henry Street Settlement and the rise of community health nursing played a major role in the widespread public acceptance of nurses, particularly African-American nurses.
- World War I and the influenza epidemic of 1917-1919 created a strong demand for nursing services. Many nursing schools were opened in response, mostly in hospitals.
- The Great Depression and World War II created new opportunities for nurses, including the Cadet Nurse Corps, which added 179,000 new registered nurses to the profession by the end of the war.
- Since World War II, hospital expansion, technological advances, and social changes have created new and progressively autonomous roles for nurses, especially advanced practice nurses.
- Nursing history can inform the present.

CRITICAL THINKING QUESTIONS
1. Florence Nightingale is often credited with being the first nurse researcher. Why do you think this is so?
2. Discuss the significance of the events that occurred during the Chicago World's Fair, 1893, to the advancement of the nursing profession.
3. Do you agree with L. L. Dock's view that nursing is inevitably tied to the greater issues of the women's movement throughout the world? Why or why not? How has this attitude affected the entry of men into nursing?
4. Wars have often been the driving force in creating social change. How did wars influence the profession of nursing?
5. Identify some emerging trends in health care and explain how they will affect the practice of professional nursing.

REFERENCES

Army nurses in ETO, *Am J Nurs* 45(9):386-387, 1945a.

The nurses' contribution to American victory: facts and figures from Pearl Harbor to VJ Day, *Am J Nurs* 45(9):683-686, 1945b.

American Nurses Association: ANA's first position on education for nursing, *Am J Nurs* 65:106-111, 1965.

Barton C: Diary: the papers of Clara Barton (1812-1912), Washington, DC, 1862, Library of Congress, Manuscript Division.

Boulay DM: A Vietnam tour of duty, *Nurs Outlook* 37(6):271-273, 1989.

Buhler-Wilkerson K: Guarded by standards and directed by strangers, *Nurs Hist Rev* 1:139-154, 1993a.

Buhler-Wilkerson K: Bringing the care to the people: Lillian Wald's legacy to public health nursing, *Am J Pub Health* 83(12):1778-1786, 1993b.

Bullough B: The lasting impact of WW II in nursing, *Am J Nurs* 76(1):118-120, 1976.

Carnegie ME: *The path we tread: blacks in nursing, 1854-1984,* Philadelphia, 1986, JB Lippincott.

Cates TR: *The drainpipe diary,* New York, 1957, Vantage Press.

Christman L: The influence of specialization on the nursing profession, *Nurs Science* 3(6):446-453, 1965.

Christman L: The nurse specialist as a professional activist, *Nurs Clin N Am* 6(2):231-235, 1971.

Christy TE: Portrait of a leader: Lavinia Lloyd Dock, *Nurs Outlook* 17(6):72-75, 1969.

Christy TE: The fateful decade: 1890-1900, *Am J Nurs* 75(7):1163-1165, 1975.

Dock LL: What we may expect from the law, *Am J Nurs* I: 8-12, 1900.

Dock LL: Some urgent social claims, *Am J Nurs* 7:895-901, 1907.

Dock LL: Mountain medicine, *Am J Nurs* 9:181-183, 1908.

Dock LL, Stewart IM: *A short history of nursing,* New York, 1920, Putnam.

Donahue MP: *Nursing: the finest art,* ed 2, Philadelphia, 1996, Mosby.

Eastabrooks CA: Lavinia Lloyd Dock: the Henry Street years, *Nurs Hist Rev* 3:143-172, 1995.

Fessler DB: *No time for fear: voices of American military nurses in World War II,* East Lansing, MI, 1996, Michigan State University Press.

Fitzpatrick ML: Nursing and the Great Depression, *Am J Nurs* 75(12):2188-2190, 1975.

Ford LC: A nurse for all settings: the nurse practitioner, *Nurs Outlook* 27(8):516-521, 1979.

Ford LC, Silver HK: The expanded role of the nurse in childcare, *Nurs Outlook* 15(8):43-45, 1967.

Ganger CW: A sketch of Emily Haines Harrison: Civil War nurse, spy and nurse on the Kansas prairie, *J Nurs Hist* 3(2):22-35, 1988.

Griffon DP: Crowning the edifice: Ethel Fenwick and state registration, *Nurs Hist Rev* 3:201-212, 1995.

Howell J: *Technology in the hospital,* Baltimore, 1996, The Johns Hopkins University Press.

Kennedy D: Birth control in America: the career of Margaret Sanger, New Haven, 1970, Yale University Press.

Livermore M: *My story of the war,* Hartford, CT, 1867, SS Scranton.

Lynaugh J, Fairman J: New nurses, new spaces: a preview of the AACN history study, *Am J Crit Care* 1(1):19-24, 1992.

Lynaugh J, Brush B: *American nursing: from hospitals to health systems,* Cambridge, MA, 1996, Blackwell Publishers.

Mayo A: Advanced courses in clinical nursing, *Am J Nurs* 44:580, 1944.

Minor N: Instructive Visiting Nurses Association papers. In Chauf K: *Richmond, Virginia, nursing and the influenza epidemic of 1918,* Charlottesville, VA, 1918, University of Virginia, Center for Nursing Historical Inquiry manuscript collection.

Mosley M: Satisfied to carry the bag, *Nurs Hist Rev* 4:65-82, 1996.

New York State Nurses Association: Remarks made by Lavinia Dock [Jan 20], New York, 1903, New York State Nurses Association.

Nightingale F: *Notes on nursing: what it is and what it is not,* Reprint, Philadelphia, 1946, JB Lippincott (originally published in 1859).

Norman EM: A study of female military nurses in Vietnam during the years 1965-1973, *J Nurs Hist* 2(1):43-60, 1986.

Oates SB: *A woman of valor,* New York, 1994, The Free Press.

Palmer S: The editor, *Am J Nurs* 1(1):64, 1900.

Pember PY: *A Southern woman's story,* Atlanta, 1959, Bill Wiley.

Petry L: The U.S. Cadet Nurse Corps: a summing up, *Am J Nurs* 45(12):1027-1028, 1945.

Pletsch PK: Mary Breckinridge: a pioneer who made her mark, *Am J Nurs* 81(12):2188-2190, 1981.

Reverby SM: *Ordered to care: the dilemma of American nursing,* 1850-1945, Cambridge, 1987, Cambridge University Press.

Reiter F: The nurse clinician, *Am J Nurs* 66(2):274-280, 1966.

Rosenberg CE: *The care of strangers,* New York, 1987, Basic Books.

Safriet BJ: Health dollars and regulatory sense: the role of advanced practice nursing, *Yale J Reg* 9:149-220, 1992.

Sandelowski M: Making the best of things: technology in American nursing, 1870-1940, *Nurs Hist Rev* 5:3-22, 1997.

Sarnecky MT: Nursing in the American Army from the Revolution to the Spanish-American War, *Nurs Hist Rev* 5:49-69, 1997.

Simpkins F, Patton J: *The women of the Confederacy,* Richmond, VA, 1936, Garrett & Massis.

Sleet J: A successful experiment, *Am J Nurs* 2:729, 1901.

Smoyak SA: Specialization in nursing: from then to now, *Nurs Outlook* 24(11):676-681, 1976.

Starr P: *The social transformation of American medicine,* New York, 1982, Basic Books.

Smith FT: Florence Nightingale: early feminist, *Am J Nurs* 81(5):1021-1024, 1981.

Stevens R: *In sickness and in wealth: American hospitals in the twentieth century,* New York, 1989, Basic Books.

Stewart IM: *Reminiscences of Isabel M. Stewart,* New York, 1961, New York Oral History Research Office, Columbia University.

Wald LD: Letter to Jacob Schiff, July 25, New York, 1893, LD Wald Collection, Manuscript Division, New York Public Library.

Walker K: *A piece of my heart: the story of twenty-six American women who served in Vietnam,* New York, 1985, Ballantine.

Wall BM: Courage to care: the Sisters of the Holy Cross in the Spanish-American War, *Nurs Hist Rev* 3:55-77, 1995.

Woodham-Smith C: *Florence Nightingale,* London, 1949, Constable & Company LTD.

Woodham-Smith C: *Florence Nightingale,* New York, 1951, McGraw-Hill.

Young A: *The women and the crisis: women of the north in the Civil War,* New York, 1959, McDowell, Obolensky.

Educational Patterns in Nursing

Elaine F. Nichols and Kay Kittrell Chitty

Key Terms*

Accreditation
Advanced Degrees
Advanced Practice Nurses (APNs)
Alternative Educational Programs
American Association of Colleges of Nursing (AACN)
American Nurses Credentialing Center (ANCC)
Articulation
Associate Degree in Nursing (ADN)
Baccalaureate Degree in Nursing (BSN)
Basic Programs

Brown Report
Certification
Commission on Collegiate Nursing Education (CCNE)
Contact Hour
Continuing Education (CE)
Diploma Program
Distance Learning (DL)
External Degree Programs
Generic Master's Degree
Generic Nursing Doctorate (ND)
Goldmark Report
Licensure
Lysaught Report
Mandatory Continuing Education

Mildred Montag
National Council Licensing Examination for Practical Nursing (NCLEX-PN)
National Council Licensing Examination for Registered Nurses (NCLEX-RN)
National League for Nursing (NLN)
National League for Nursing Accreditation Commission (NLNAC)
Position Paper (American Nurses Association)
Practical Nurses (LPNs/LVNs)
RN-to-Baccalaureate in Nursing

Learning Outcomes

After studying this chapter, students will be able to:

- Trace the development of basic and graduate education in nursing.
- Discuss the influence of early nursing studies on today's nursing education.
- Discuss traditional and alternative ways of becoming a registered nurse.
- Discuss program options for registered nurses and students with nonnursing baccalaureate degrees.
- Differentiate between licensed practical/vocational nurses and registered nurses.
- Explain the difference between licensure and certification.

---

*Educational terms and definitions used in this chapter are congruent with those used by the American Association of Colleges of Nursing, as defined in *Enrollment and Graduations in Baccalaureate and Graduate Programs in Nursing, 2002-2003* (Berlin, Stennett, and Bednash, 2003).

- Define accreditation and its influence on the quality and effectiveness of nursing education programs.
- Discuss the significance of the 1965 American Nurses Association position paper to today's types of nursing programs.
- Discuss similarities and differences among three reports projecting nursing education for the twenty-first century.
- Identify current and future challenges in nursing education.

Diversity is the major characteristic of nursing education today. Influenced by a variety of factors—societal changes, efforts to achieve full professional status, women's issues, historical factors, public expectations, professional standards, legislation, national studies, and constant changes in the health care system—many different types of nursing education programs currently exist.

In 2004, there were 1,634 programs preparing registered nurses (RNs) in the United States (Figure 2-1). Of these, 54.1 percent were associate degree programs, 40.5 percent were baccalaureate programs, and 5.4 percent were diploma programs (National League for Nursing Accrediting Commission, 2004). In addition to the basic registered nurse programs, there were also 398 master's programs and 83 doctoral programs. Also included in the educational system of nursing are a large number of practical nursing programs (LPN/LVN programs), continuing education programs, and advanced practice certification programs.

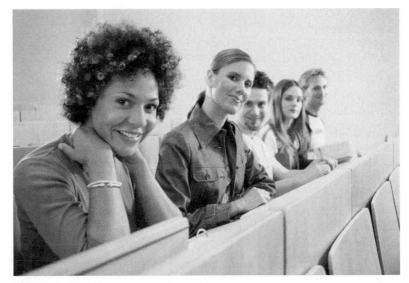

Figure 2-1
In 2004, there were 1,634 programs preparing registered nurses in the United States and its territories. Students entering nursing today are diverse in terms of age, sociocultural background, and gender.

This chapter provides an orientation to the multiple and sometimes confusing nursing educational pathways in existence today. This coverage includes the history behind educational programs, descriptions of the various programs, and trends and future issues.

DEVELOPMENT OF NURSING EDUCATION IN THE UNITED STATES

As mentioned in Chapter 1, Florence Nightingale is credited with founding modern nursing and creating the first educational system for nurses. After hospitals came into existence in western Europe, and before the influence of Florence Nightingale, nurses had no formal preparation in giving care, because there were no organized programs to educate nurses until the late 1800s. Until this time, nursing care was administered by relatives or self-trained persons who were often held in low regard by society.

Nightingale revolutionized and professionalized nursing by stressing that nursing was not a domestic, charitable service but a respected occupation requiring advanced education. In 1860 she opened a school of nursing at St. Thomas's Hospital in London and established the following highly innovative principles:

1. The nurse should be trained in an educational institution supported by public funds and associated with a medical school.
2. The nursing school should be affiliated with a teaching hospital but also independent of it.
3. The curriculum should include both theory and practical experience.
4. Professional nurses should be in charge of administration and instruction and should be paid for their instruction.
5. Students should be carefully selected and should reside in "nurses' houses" that form discipline and character.
6. Students should be required to attend lectures, take quizzes, write papers, and keep diaries. Student records should be maintained (Notter and Spalding, 1976).

Nightingale also believed that nursing schools should be financially and administratively separate from the hospitals in which the students trained. This was not the case, however, when nursing schools were first established in the United States.

The first training schools for nurses in the United States were established in 1872. Located at Bellevue Hospital in New York, the New England Hospital for Women and Children in New Haven, Connecticut, and Massachusetts General Hospital in Boston, the course of study was one year in length. These schools became known as the "famous trio" of nursing schools. In October 1873, Melinda Anne (Linda) Richards became the first "trained nurse" educated in the United States. By 1879 there were 11 U.S. nursing training schools. Other schools rapidly developed, and by 1900, there were 432 hospital-owned and hospital-operated programs in the United States (Donahue, 1985). These early training programs differed in length from 6 months to 2 years, and each school set its own standards and requirements. Upon graduation from these programs, students were given a diploma. The term **diploma program** was, and still is, used to identify these hospital-based nursing eucation programs. The primary reason for the schools' existence was to staff the hospitals that operated them. The education of student nurses was not always a primary concern.

Early Studies of the Quality of Nursing Education

Nursing leaders of the early 1900s were concerned about the poor quality of many of the recently-formed nurse training programs. They initiated studies about nursing and nursing education to prompt changes. October 1899 marked the culmination of some 4 years of work by the American Society of Superintendents of Training Schools for Nurses. Isabel Hampton Robb chaired a Society-selected committee to investigate a means to prepare nurses better for leadership in schools of nursing. Teachers College, which had opened in New York 10 years earlier for the training of teachers, seemed the logical location for the leadership training of nurses. The program was originally designed to prepare administrators of nursing service and nursing education and began as an 8-month course in hospital economics (Donahue, 1985).

Mary Adelaide Nutting came to Teachers College in 1907 as the first nursing professor in the world. Under her direction, the department progressed and became a pioneer in nursing education. The school became known as the "Mother House" of collegiate education because it fostered the initial movements toward undergraduate and graduate degrees for nurses (Donahue, 1985). In 1912, Nutting conducted a nationwide investigation of nursing education, "The Educational Status of Nursing," which focused on the living conditions of students, the material being taught, and the teaching methods being used (Christy, 1969).

One of the first major studies on the status of nursing education was published in 1923. Titled "The Study of Nursing and Nursing Education in the United States" and referred to as the **Goldmark Report,** the study focused on the clinical learning experiences of students, hospital control of the schools, the desirability of establishing university schools of nursing, the lack of funds specifically for nursing education, and the lack of prepared teachers (Kalisch and Kalisch, 1995).

The year 1924 marked another first in nursing education, when the Yale School of Nursing was opened as the first nursing school to be established as a separate university department with an independent budget and its own dean, Annie W. Goodrich. The school demonstrated its effectiveness so markedly that in 1929 the Rockefeller Foundation ensured the permanency of the school by awarding it an endowment of $1 million (Kalisch and Kalisch, 1995).

In 1934, a study entitled "Nursing Schools Today and Tomorrow" reported the number of schools in existence, gave detailed descriptions of the schools, described their curricula, and made recommendations for professional collegiate education (National League of Nursing Education, 1934). In 1937, *A Curriculum Guide for Schools of Nursing* was published, outlining a 3-year curriculum and influencing the structure of diploma schools for decades after its publication (National League of Nursing Education, 1937).

Although published over a 30-year period and undertaken by different groups, these early studies consistently made five similar recommendations:

1. Nursing education programs should be established within the system of higher education.
2. Nurses should be highly educated.
3. Students should not be used to staff hospitals.
4. Standards should be established for nursing practice.

5. All students should meet certain minimum qualifications upon graduation.

These studies set the stage for the development of the educational programs that exist today.

EDUCATIONAL PATHWAYS TO BECOMING A REGISTERED NURSE

Today, preparation for a career as a registered nurse usually begins in one of three ways: in an associate degree program, a baccalaureate degree program, or a hospital-based diploma program. These **basic programs** vary in the courses offered, length of study, and cost. Following the completion of a basic program for registered nurses, graduates are eligible to take the **National Council Licensing Examination for Registered Nurses (NCLEX-RN).** Upon successful completion of the licensing examination, graduates may legally practice as registered nurses and use the initials RN after their names. Employment and career advancement vary depending on the basic program attended (Figure 2-2).

Having three different educational routes to achieve RN licensure is confusing to the public—and even to many nurses themselves. In the following sections, each type of basic program is described, along with its history, unique characteristics, and special issues. These basic programs are discussed in the chronological order in which they appeared in nursing education history.

Diploma Program

The hospital-based diploma program was the earliest form of nursing education in the United States. At the peak of diploma education in the 1920s and 1930s, approximately 2,000 programs existed, with numerous programs in almost every state.

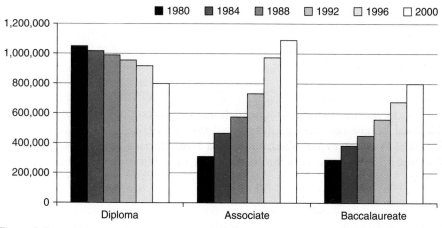

Figure 2-2

Distribution of the RN population according to basic nursing education, 1980-2000. (From U.S. Department of Health and Human Services: *The registered nurse population, March 2000: findings from the national sample survey of registered nurses,* Washington, DC, 2001, Government Printing Office, p 6.)

Since their numbers peaked in the first third of that century, the number of diploma programs has decreased, with a dramatic decline since the mid-1960s as nursing education moved rapidly into collegiate settings. In 1960, there were approximately 800 diploma programs in the United States. By 1980, that number had decreased to approximately 300. By 1997, only 100 diploma programs remained in 20 states (National League for Nursing, 1999c). Today there are only[67] (National League for Nursing Accrediting Commission, 2004). This decline in the number of diploma programs is due to several factors: the growth of associate degree and baccalaureate degree programs in nursing, the inability of hospitals to continue to finance nursing education, accreditation standards that have made it difficult for diploma programs to attract qualified faculty, and the increasing complexity of health care, which has required nurses to have greater academic preparation.

Despite the significant decrease in the number of diploma programs, many outstanding nurses practicing today received their basic nursing education in these programs. In the early days of formal nurses "training" in this country—that is, during the late 1800s and early 1900s—diploma programs provided one of the few avenues for women to obtain formal education and jobs. Most of the early programs followed a modified apprenticeship model. Lectures were given by physicians, and clinical training was supervised by head nurses and nursing directors. Nursing courses paralleled medical areas and included surgery, obstetrics, pediatrics, and operating room experience. Students were sometimes sent to affiliated institutions where they could obtain experiences that were not available at the home hospital.

The schedule was demanding, with classes being held after patient care assignments were completed. Critics charged that students were used as inexpensive labor to staff the hospitals and that education was given a lower priority. The truth of those charges varied, depending on which hospital was scrutinized, but there is no question that early nursing students virtually ran the hospitals. Programs lasted 3 years, and at graduation, students were awarded diplomas in nursing. Today, most diploma programs are about 24 months in duration.

A problem that many diploma program graduates faced was that hospitals were not part of the higher education system in the United States. Therefore most colleges and universities did not recognize the nursing diploma as an academic credential and often refused to give college credit for courses taken in diploma programs, regardless of the quality of the courses, students, and faculty. Most diploma programs today have established agreements with colleges and universities that allow students to earn college credit in courses such as English, psychology, and the sciences, thereby enabling them to attain advanced standing in a baccalaureate program upon completion of the diploma program.

During nursing shortages, diploma programs generally have experienced increased enrollments. When the nursing profession has faced periods of job shortages, however, diploma graduates have found it necessary to return to school for further education to advance within today's complex health care system.

Baccalaureate Programs

Armed with the early studies of nursing education, nursing leaders continued to push for nursing education to move into the mainstream of higher education, that is, into colleges and universities where other professionals were educated. Their belief was that nurses needed the **baccalaureate degree in nursing (BSN)** to qualify nursing as a recognized profession and to provide leadership in administration, teaching, and public health.

By the time the first baccalaureate nursing program was established in 1909 at the University of Minnesota, diploma programs were numerous and firmly entrenched as the system for educating nurses. This first baccalaureate program was part of the University's School of Medicine and followed the 3-year diploma program structure. Despite its many limitations, it was the start of the movement to bring nursing education into the recognized system of higher education.

Seven other baccalaureate programs in nursing were established by 1919 (Conley, 1973). Most of the early baccalaureate programs were 5 years in duration. This structure provided for 3 years of nursing education and 2 years of liberal arts. The growth in the numbers of these programs was slow both because of the reluctance of universities to accept nursing as an academic discipline and because of the power of the hospital-based diploma programs. The theoretical, scientific orientation of the baccalaureate program was in marked contrast to the "hands on" skill and service orientation that was the hallmark of hospital-based diploma education.

INFLUENCES ON THE GROWTH OF BACCALAUREATE EDUCATION

National studies of nursing and nursing education stated and restated the need for nursing education and practice to be based on knowledge from the sciences and humanities. Chief among these studies was Esther Lucille Brown's report *Nursing for the Future*, more commonly known as the **Brown Report.** Published in 1948, the Brown Report recommended that basic schools of nursing be placed in universities and colleges and that efforts be made to recruit men and minorities into nursing education programs. This report, sponsored by the Carnegie Foundation, was widely reviewed, discussed, and debated.

In 1965 the **American Nurses Association (ANA)** published a **position paper** entitled "Educational Preparation for Nurse Practitioners and Assistants to Nurses." Although not all nursing historians agree, this paper, which subsequently created conflict and division within nursing, had a significant influence on the growth of baccalaureate education in nursing. In preparing the position paper, the ANA studied nursing education, nursing practice, and trends in health care. It concluded that baccalaureate education should become the basic foundation for professional practice. The ANA position paper made four major recommendations:

1. Education for all those who are licensed to practice nursing should take place in institutions of higher learning.
2. Minimum preparation for beginning professional nursing practice should be the baccalaureate degree in nursing.
3. Minimum preparation for beginning technical nursing practice should be the associate degree in nursing.
4. Education for assistants in the health service occupations should consist of short, intensive preservice programs in vocational education institutions rather than on-the-job training programs (American Nurses Association, 1965).

Despite tremendous opposition from proponents of diploma and associate degree programs, in 1979 the ANA further strengthened its resolve by proposing three additional positions:

1. By 1985, the minimum preparation for entry into professional nursing practice should be the baccalaureate degree in nursing.
2. Two levels of nursing practice should be identified (professional and technical) and a mechanism to devise competencies for the two categories established by 1980.
3. There should be increased accessibility to high-quality career mobility programs that use flexible approaches for individuals seeking academic degrees in nursing (American Nurses Association, 1979).

The controversy created by the initial ANA position paper and the additional 1979 resolutions continued for many years. Practicing nurses across the United States, who were mainly diploma program graduates, as well as hospitals that supported diploma programs, vehemently protested the recommendations.

In 1970, the National Commission for the Study of Nursing and Nursing Education published a report entitled "An Abstract for Action" (Lysaught, 1970). Also known as the **Lysaught Report,** it made recommendations concerning the supply and demand for nurses, nursing roles and functions, and nursing education. Among the priorities identified by this study were (1) the need for increased research into both the practice and education of nurses and (2) enhanced educational systems and curricula (Lysaught, 1970).

In the early 1980s, the National Commission on Nursing published two reports suggesting that the major block to the advancement of nursing was the ongoing conflict within the profession about educational preparation for nurses. These studies recommended establishing a clear system of nursing education, including pathways for educational mobility and development of additional graduate education programs.

Another major national nursing group supporting the baccalaureate as the entry credential was the **National League for Nursing (NLN).** The organization's membership is made up of nurses, faculty members, health care agencies, all types of nursing programs, and nonnursing citizens who are supportive of nursing. In 1982, after much debate, the NLN board of directors approved the "Position Statement on Nursing Roles: Scope and Preparation," which affirmed the nursing baccalaureate degree as the minimum educational level for professional nursing practice and the associate degree or diploma as the preparation for technical nursing practice (National League for Nursing, 1982).

In 1996, the **American Association of Colleges of Nursing (AACN)** board approved a position statement, "The Baccalaureate Degree in Nursing as Minimal Preparation for Professional Practice." This document supports, among other things, articulated programs, which enable associate degree nurses to attain the baccalaureate degree. This document was updated in 2000.

BACCALAUREATE PROGRAMS TODAY

Today, baccalaureate programs provide education for both basic students who are preparing for licensure and registered nurses returning to school to obtain a baccalaureate degree in nursing. This section focuses on the program characteristics of prelicensure baccalaureate education, sometimes called basic programs. Baccalaureate programs for registered nurses are discussed later in this chapter.

Basic baccalaureate programs combine nursing courses with general education courses in a 4- or 5-year curriculum in a senior college or university. Students may be admitted to the nursing program as entering freshmen or after completing certain liberal arts courses. Students meet the same admission requirements to the university as other students and often must meet additional requirements to be admitted to the nursing major.

Courses in the nursing major focus on nursing science, communication, decision making, leadership, and care to persons of all ages in a wide variety of settings. Because this education takes place in senior universities, nursing students interact with the larger student population, which promotes diverse thinking, cultural awareness, and broad socialization.

Faculty qualifications in baccalaureate programs are usually higher than in other basic nursing programs. A minimum of a master's degree (or, increasingly, a doctorate in nursing or a related field) is required. The requirement of a doctorate ensures that nursing faculty members are able to meet the teaching, research, and service requirements expected of faculty in universities.

Baccalaureate graduates are prepared to take the National Council Licensing Examination for Registered Nurses and, after licensure, assume beginning practice and ultimately leadership positions in any health care setting, including hospitals, community agencies, schools, clinics, and homes (National League for Nursing, 1997b). Graduates with baccalaureate degrees are also prepared to move into graduate programs in nursing and advanced practice certification programs. Programs granting a baccalaureate are the most costly of the basic programs in terms of time and money, but such an investment results in long-term professional advancement. Today, there is great demand for baccalaureate graduates, and they enjoy the greatest career mobility of all basic program graduates in nursing.

An early criticism of baccalaureate preparation involved the perception that new baccalaureate graduates had fewer clinical skills than their diploma-educated counterparts. Contemporary baccalaureate programs have responded to this concern by increasing students' time in clinical practice (Figure 2-3). Additional time spent in clinical settings and preceptorships, in which students are paired with practicing registered nurses and work intensively in clinical settings, has been successful in enhancing the clinical skills of baccalaureate students.

Associate Degree Programs (ADN)

Associate degree in nursing (ADN) education represents the most recent form of basic preparation for registered nurse practice. Begun in 1952 as a result of research conducted by Dr. **Mildred Montag,** and fueled by the community college movement of the 1950s, associate degree programs are now the most common type of basic nursing education program in the United States and graduate the most registered nurses of all the basic programs.

The popularity of ADN programs is due to several features: accessibility of community colleges, low tuition costs, part-time and evening study opportunities, shorter

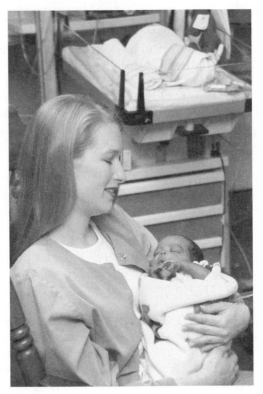

Figure **2-3**
Clinical experience is a vitally important aspect of every basic nursing program.

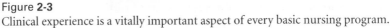

duration of programs, and graduates' eligibility to take the licensure examination for registered nurses.

When first designed by Dr. Montag, associate degree programs were to prepare nurse technicians who functioned under the supervision of professional nurses. Associate degree nurses were to work at the bedside, performing routine nursing skills for patients in acute and long-term care settings. The original associate degree program, as outlined by Montag (1951), offered general education courses in the first year and nursing courses in the second year. Montag originally viewed the associate degree as a final, end-point degree, not a stepping stone to the baccalaureate degree in nursing.

In practice, Montag's original conceptions of associate degree programs have been greatly modified. Associate degree curricula now offer more nursing credits than she suggested. They also include content on leadership and clinical decision making, abilities that Montag did not foresee in technical nurses. Owing to additions to the curriculum, few students can complete an associate degree in only 2 years. Associate degree graduates are employed in a wide variety of settings and usually function autonomously alongside baccalaureate and diploma graduates.

In the educational system of nursing today, the associate degree can be a step in the progression to the baccalaureate degree or master's degree.

In 1990, the NLN Council of Associate Degree Programs prepared a document entitled "Educational Outcomes of Associate Degree Nursing Programs: Roles and Competencies." This document was written in response to a national effort to differentiate the competencies of the associate degree nurse from those of the baccalaureate nurse. The document identified associate degree competencies in three roles: provider of care, manager of care, and member within the discipline of nursing. The further development of these competencies has had a direct effect on the associate degree programs that exist today.

External Degree Programs

External degree programs in nursing are different from traditional basic nursing education in that students attend no classes and follow no prescribed methods of learning. Learning is independent and is assessed through highly standardized and validated examinations. Students are responsible for arranging their own clinical experiences in accordance with established standards.

Excelsior College, formerly known as the New York Regents External Degree Nursing Program, is the most well-recognized external degree model. Beginning in 1972 with an associate degree program, Excelsior College now offers associate degree, baccalaureate, and master's degrees in nursing. All the nursing programs are accredited by the National League for Nursing Accreditation Commission (NLNAC).

Since 1981 the California State University Consortium has offered a statewide external degree baccalaureate program in nursing. The California program is for registered nurses already holding current licenses to practice in the state.

There are numerous external degree programs in existence today, many of which are marketed online and by direct mail. Prospective students must exercise caution to choose only bona fide accredited programs that are affiliated with recognized colleges and universities.

Articulated Programs

In response to the demand for educational mobility, **articulation** (movement) between programs has become much more common in today's nursing education system. The purpose of articulation is to facilitate opportunities for nurses to move up the educational ladder. An example of a fully articulated system is the licensed practical nurse/associate degree in nursing/bachelor of science in nursing/master of science in nursing (LPN/ADN/BSN/MSN) program in which students spend the first year preparing to be an LPN and the second year completing the associate degree. If desired or necessary, students can "stop out" of the program at the end of the first year, take the licensure examination for practical nursing, and return to the associate degree program at a later time. On the other hand, they may continue study in the program after the initial 2 years to earn a baccalaureate degree and even continue for a master's or doctoral degree.

Multiple-entry, multiple-exit programs are difficult to develop. A tremendous amount of joint institutional planning is needed to work out equivalent courses and to keep the programs congruent with one another. A change in one curriculum dictates changes in all the others. These challenges explain why fully articulated programs have been slow to develop. In increasing numbers, however, articulation agreements between baccalaureate and ADN programs and between ADN and LPN programs are being established that facilitate student movement between programs and accept transfer credit between institutions. These requirements often result in acceleration or advanced placement within the higher-degree school.

ALTERNATIVE EDUCATIONAL PROGRAMS IN NURSING

In addition to the basic programs leading to entry-level nursing practice, several **alternative educational programs** exist.

Baccalaureate Programs for Registered Nurses

After nursing organizations of the 1960s and 1970s publicly advocated for the baccalaureate degree to be the minimum education level for professional practice, the demand for the nursing bachelor's degree increased. Employers of nurses recognized that broadly educated nurses matched well with the complexities of health care. As a result, many supported the baccalaureate as a requirement for career mobility. Diploma and associate degree graduates returned to school in increasing numbers. Today, many associate degree nurses enter ADN programs with plans to earn a baccalaureate degree ultimately. Baccalaureate programs for RNs allow them, as well as diploma nurses, to accomplish this goal.

Registered nurses with diplomas and associate degrees were not always welcomed into baccalaureate programs. In the early years of baccalaureate education for RNs, many schools required these students to take courses in areas the students believed they had already mastered. For a number of years, there were barriers for these nurses in completing their baccalaureate degrees. In the past two decades, however, the majority of baccalaureate programs have recognized the legitimacy and importance of **RN-to-baccalaureate in nursing** education and have developed alternative tracks to accommodate the unique learning needs of the registered nurse student.

Baccalaureate programs for registered nurses are most often offered by universities that also offer a basic baccalaureate program for nonnurses. The registered nurse students may be integrated with the basic students, or they may be enrolled in a separate or partially separate sequence. Some baccalaureate programs for registered nurses are found in colleges that do not have a basic baccalaureate nursing program.

Most 4-year colleges and universities allow the transfer of general education credits from associate degree nursing programs. With increasing frequency, transfer credit is given for nursing courses as well, or there is the option of receiving credit for previous nursing courses through a variety of advanced placement methods such as examinations, demonstrations, and portfolios.

For diploma graduates, transfer credit is usually given for previous college courses, such as English, if they were included as part of the diploma program and taught by college faculty. Options for advanced placement of diploma graduates into baccalaureate programs are extremely variable, and prospective registered nurse students should seek information from several baccalaureate programs to select a program that fits individual needs and goals.

It is clear that the demand for the baccalaureate degree by large numbers of associate degree and diploma graduates continues to be strong. More nurses are returning to school to prepare for the wider opportunities offered by the baccalaureate degree. With broad preparation in clinical, scientific, community health, and patient education skills, the baccalaureate nurse is well positioned to move across community-based settings such as home health care, outpatient centers, and neighborhood clinics, where opportunities are fast expanding.

Programs for Nonnursing Postbaccalaureate Students

A more recent trend is a significant increase in the number of students with baccalaureate degrees in other fields making a career change to nursing. The educational system in nursing has responded to this group of students by offering options to the traditional basic baccalaureate education. Some baccalaureate programs offer these students an accelerated sequence, which results in a second baccalaureate degree. Many individuals with one baccalaureate degree, however, prefer to pursue a graduate degree.

This desire for graduate degrees has led to the development of an accelerated master's degree in nursing for individuals with nonnursing bachelor's degrees. These programs, known as **generic master's degree** programs, usually require about 3 years to complete. Graduates take the registered nurse licensure examination after completing the generic master's program.

Another educational track for students with baccalaureate degrees in other fields is the **generic nursing doctorate (ND).** This degree is discussed later in this chapter (see "Current Status of Doctoral Education in Nursing").

PRACTICAL NURSING PROGRAMS (LPN OR LVN)

Nursing education includes a large number of programs preparing practical nurses. **Practical nurses (LPNs/LVNs)** are differentiated from registered nurses by education and licensure and have a limited scope of practice. Licensed practical nurses (LPNs) or licensed vocational nurses (LVNs) are considered technical workers in nursing.

Practical nursing programs became a significant component of the nursing field during World War II. These programs were created to satisfy the demand for nurses and programs that could produce nurses quickly. The first planned curriculum for practical nursing was developed in 1942. Although national accreditation is available for practical nursing programs, the majority of LPN/LVN programs have state approval rather than national accreditation.

Practical nursing education typically lasts 12 months and takes place in a variety of settings: vocational/technical schools, community colleges, and high schools. Many LPN/LVN programs now offer credit for prior learning to health care workers such as hospital aides, orderlies, paramedics, emergency medical technicians, and military corps personnel. These individuals often enter nursing through practical nursing programs.

Graduates of practical nursing programs must pass the **National Council Licensing Examination for Practical Nursing (NCLEX-PN)** to become licensed.

The scope of their practice focuses on meeting basic patient needs in hospitals, long-term care facilities, and homes. They must practice under the supervision of a physician or registered nurse.

Many newly licensed practical nurses plan to become registered nurses, with the majority of these individuals either taking courses or planning to begin registered nurse courses in 1 to 2 years. National statistics show that 9.5 percent of all licensed RNs have practiced previously as LPNs or LVNs, indicating that many are achieving their goal of becoming registered nurses (U.S. Department of Health and Human Services, 2001).

When the demand for nurses and nursing education is greater than basic registered nurse programs can meet, practical nurse programs flourish. Currently, significant employment opportunities exist for licensed practical nurses because their lower salaries fit well with the cost-containment requirements of today's health care system. Practical nurses are not, however, a substitute for registered nurses.

ACCREDITATION OF EDUCATIONAL PROGRAMS

The concept of **accreditation** of educational programs in nursing is important. Although all nursing programs must be approved by their respective state boards of nursing for graduates to take the licensure examination, nursing programs may also seek accreditation, which goes beyond minimum state approval. Accreditation refers to a voluntary review process of educational programs by a professional organization. The organization, called an accrediting agency, compares the educational quality of the program with established standards and criteria. Accrediting agencies derive their authority from the U.S. Department of Education.

Prospective nursing students should inquire about the accreditation status of any nursing program they are considering. Qualifying for certain scholarships, loans, and military service usually depends on being enrolled in an accredited program. Acceptance into graduate programs in nursing may also depend on graduation from an accredited baccalaureate program. Employers of nurses are usually interested in hiring nurses who are graduates of accredited programs.

From 1952 through 1996, the National League for Nursing was the official professional accrediting organization for master's, baccalaureate, associate degree, diploma, and practical nursing programs in the United States. In 1997, as a result of a mandate from the U.S. Department of Education, a separate division of the NLN was created. The new division, the **National League for Nursing Accreditation Commission (NLNAC),** assumed responsibility for all national program accreditation activity. Accreditation is conducted through four NLNAC councils: the Council of Associate Degree Programs, the Council of Diploma Programs, the Council of Baccalaureate and Higher Degree Programs, and the Council of Practical Nursing Programs. Each council develops its own accreditation program and criteria and revises them periodically.

Accreditation of nursing schools grew out of concerns repeatedly expressed by members of the profession about the quality of and standards for nursing education. An accredited program voluntarily adheres to standards that protect the quality of education, public safety, and the profession itself. Accreditation provides both a mechanism and a stimulus for programs to initiate periodic self-examination and self-improvement. It assures students that their educational program is accountable for offering quality education.

Accrediting bodies establish standards by which they measure each program's effectiveness. Programs under review prepare reports, known as self-studies, that show how the school meets each standard. The self-study is reviewed by a volunteer team composed of nursing educators from the type of program being reviewed, and an on-site program review is conducted by the same team. Following the site visit, the visitors' report and the program's self-study are reviewed by the appropriate NLNAC council, and a decision is made about the accreditation status of each nursing program.

Once accredited and in good standing, continuing accreditation reviews take place every 8 to 10 years. Programs that do not meet standards may be placed on warning and given a specific time period to correct deficiencies. Accreditation can be withdrawn if deficiencies are not corrected within the specified time.

In 1996, the American Association of Colleges of Nursing (AACN) organized the **Commission on Collegiate Nursing Education (CCNE)** and began the process of acquiring recognition from the U.S. Department of Education as the national accrediting body for baccalaureate and higher degree nursing programs. Officially, CCNE began operation in 1998 and has subsequently established an organizational structure, policies and procedures, and accreditation standards and criteria. In December 1999, CCNE received a recommendation from the National Advisory Committee on Institutional Quality and Integrity, a panel of the U.S. Department of Education, that the Secretary of Education grant initial recognition of CCNE as a national agency for the accreditation of baccalaureate and graduate nursing education programs. This status was renewed in 2002. The establishment of a second national accrediting body for nursing education represents a significant development in the evolution of the nursing profession.

GRADUATE EDUCATION IN NURSING

A variety of economic, educational, and professional trends are fueling the demand for registered nurses with **advanced degrees.** The rapidly changing health care system requires nurses to possess increasing knowledge, clinical competency, greater independence, and autonomy in clinical judgments. Trends in community-based nursing centers, case management, complexity of home care, sophisticated technologies, and society's orientation to health and self-care are rapidly causing the educational needs of nurses to grow.

According to projections made by the federal government, 200,000 additional master's and doctorally prepared registered nurses will be needed by the year 2005 (U.S. Department of Health and Human Services, 1990). Nurses who have advanced education can become researchers, nurse practitioners, clinical specialists, educators, and administrators. Many open their own clinics, where they provide direct care and serve as consultants to businesses and health care agencies. Chapter 5 describes some of the opportunities open to nurses with advanced degrees. Certainly, having highly educated nurses will further strengthen the profession.

Master's Education

The purpose of master's education is to prepare persons with advanced nursing knowledge and clinical practice skills in a specialized area of practice. Teachers College, Columbia University, is credited with initiating graduate education in nursing. Beginning in 1899, the college offered a postgraduate course in hospital economics, which prepared nurses for positions in teaching and hospital administration. From this limited beginning, there has been consistent growth in the number of master's nursing programs in the United States.

Over the last 30 years, the growth in numbers of master's programs in nursing has been dramatic. In 1970, there were 70 programs; in 1980, 142 programs; in 1990, 212 programs; and in 2002, 398 programs prepared nurses at the master's level. Enrollment in master's nursing degree programs grew from 19,958 in 1986 to 34,181 in 2002. A majority of these students (63 percent) were attending school part-time (Berlin, Stennett, and Bednash, 2003).

Most individuals in the 1950s and 1960s viewed the master's degree in nursing as a terminal (final) degree. The master's degree was considered the highest degree nurses would ever need. Early master's programs were longer and more demanding than master's programs in other disciplines. Master's programs in the 1950s and 1960s prepared students for careers in nursing administration and nursing education.

With the rapid development of doctoral programs for nurses during the 1970s, however, the master's degree could no longer be considered a terminal degree. Programs were shortened from as long as 2 years to the approximate 1-year length of master's study in most other disciplines. Advanced practice through clinical specialization became the emphasis. Master's programs in nursing are most often found in senior colleges and universities that have basic baccalaureate programs in nursing. These programs may also seek voluntary accreditation from the NLNAC Council of Baccalaureate and Higher Degree Programs or from the CCNE.

Entrance requirements to master's programs in nursing usually include the following: a baccalaureate degree from an NLN-accredited program in nursing, licensure as a registered nurse, completion of the Graduate Record Examination (GRE) or other standard aptitude test, a minimum undergraduate grade point average (GPA) of 3.0, often recent work experience as a registered nurse in an area related to the desired area of specialization, and specific goals for graduate study.

The average program length is 18 to 24 months of full-time study. The curriculum includes theory, research, clinical practice, and courses in other disciplines. Master's students generally select both an area of clinical specialization, such as adult health or gerontology, and an area of role preparation, such as informatics, administration, or teaching. Students are often required to write a comprehensive examination or to complete a thesis or research project (or both).

Major areas of role preparation offered in 2002 included administration, case management, informatics, health policy/health care systems, teacher education, clinical nurse specialist, nurse practitioner, nurse-midwifery, nurse anesthesia, and other clinical and nonclinical areas of study. The majority of master's enrollees (53 percent) were preparing for advanced clinical practice as nurse practitioners (NPs) or combined NP/CNS (clinical nurse specialist) roles.

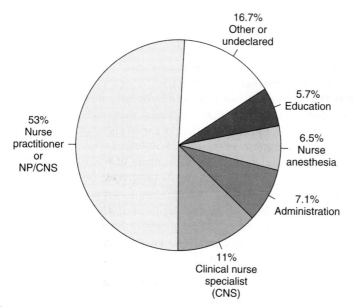

Figure 2-4

By a large margin, the majority of master's students in 2002 selected role preparation as nurse practitioners. The small number of students choosing teacher education is cause for concern about the future supply of nursing faculty. (Data from Berlin LE, Stennett J, Bednash GD: *Enrollment and graduations in baccalaureate and graduate programs in nursing*, Washington, DC, 2003, American Association of Colleges of Nursing.)

As illustrated in Figure 2-4, all other role preparation fields trailed nurse practitioner preparation in popularity, with 11 percent preparing for clinical specialist roles, 7.1 percent for administration/management, 6.5 percent for nurse anesthesia, and 5.7 percent for teaching. The balance of master's students were specializing in various other majors or undeclared (Berlin, Stennett, and Bednash, 2003). Clinical specialization choices for NP graduates included (in descending order of popularity) family NP, adult NP, pediatric NP, gerontological NP, women's health NP, neonatal NP, adult acute care NP, adult psychiatric/mental health NP, family psychiatric/mental health NP, and dual or combined tracks (Berlin, Stennett, and Bednash, 2003).

With the increasing demand for nurse practitioners, master's programs have expanded their practitioner tracks. Master's programs offering nurse practitioner options rose from 108 in 1992 to 355 in 2002 (Berlin, Stennett, and Bednash, 2003).

The master of science (MS) and the master of science in nursing (MSN) are the two most common degrees offered. A recent option in master's education is the RN/MSN track, which allows registered nurses who are prepared at the associate degree or diploma level and who meet graduate admission requirements to enter a program leading to a master's degree rather than a baccalaureate degree. Other recent graduate program options are combined degrees such as the master of science in nursing/master of business administration (MSN/MBA) for nurse administrators or the master of science in nursing/doctor of law (MSN/JD) for nurse attorneys. Clearly, diversity in nursing education extends to the graduate as well as the basic level.

Doctoral Education

Doctoral programs in nursing prepare nurses to become faculty members in universities, administrators in schools of nursing or large medical centers, researchers, theorists, and advanced practitioners. Doctoral programs in nursing offer several degree titles; the most common are the doctor of nursing science (DNS) and the doctor of philosophy (PhD).

HISTORY OF DOCTORAL EDUCATION IN NURSING

Formal doctoral education for nurses began at Columbia University's Teachers College in 1910 with the creation of the Department of Nursing and Health. The first student completed her work for the doctor of education (EdD) with a major in nursing education and was awarded her doctorate in 1932. Seventy years later in 2002, Teachers College was still granting an EdD in nursing education.

In 1934, New York University initiated the first PhD program for nurses. The programs at Teachers College and New York University provided many of the profession's early leaders, who worked over the years for improvement in nursing education (Parietti, 1990).

From 1934 through 1953, no new nursing doctoral programs were opened. In 1954, the University of Pittsburgh opened the first PhD program in clinical nursing and clinical research in the United States. As the 1950s drew to a close, a total of only 36 doctoral degrees had been awarded in nursing (Parietti, 1990).

Owing to the limited number of nursing doctoral programs, most nurses in the 1950s and 1960s earned doctorates in nonnursing fields, such as education, sociology, and physiology. Doctoral education for nurses moved into a new phase when the federal government initiated nurse scientist programs in 1962. These programs were created to increase the research skills of nurses and provide faculty for the development of doctoral programs in nursing. The nurse scientist programs were discontinued in 1975 after more universities began offering doctoral programs in nursing.

A program offering the nursing doctorate (ND) to students as their first nursing degree was begun at Case Western Reserve University in 1979. As mentioned earlier, the ND program is designed for students with baccalaureate degrees in fields other than nursing. The program was based on that school's philosophy that professional nursing education should begin at the postbaccalaureate level. Following completion of 900 clinical hours, ND graduates are eligible to take the registered nurse licensure examination before continuing to the postlicensure portion of the program. Graduates are prepared for leadership positions in practice, business, management, research, and education.

The 1970s saw a major increase in the number of doctoral programs in nursing. In that decade alone, 15 new doctoral programs were established. Between 1970 and 1980, the number of programs increased to 22, and between 1980 and 1990, the number more than doubled, from 22 to 48 (Parietti, 1990). In 1996, the number of doctoral programs stood at 66 (National League for Nursing, 1997a). By 2002, that number had risen to 83 (Berlin, Stennett, and Bednash, 2003).

CURRENT STATUS OF DOCTORAL EDUCATION IN NURSING

Doctoral degrees for students with prior degrees in nursing include the Doctor of Nursing Science (DNS) and the Doctor of Philosophy (PhD). Both of these degrees build on master's preparation in nursing. The DNS is viewed as a professional practice degree. Conceived as an advanced practice degree with an emphasis on clinical research, the DNS is intended to bridge the gap between practice and research (Allen, 1990). In contrast, the PhD is considered an academic degree and prepares scholars for research and the development of theory.

A continuing issue is the relative merit of these two degrees. As currently structured in most universities, the two programs are more similar than different. In the major job market for nurses with doctorates (that is, colleges and universities), the PhD is more widely understood and accepted by the academic community and therefore is favored by many doctorate-seeking nurses. The percentage of PhDs awarded in nursing remained stable between 1996 and 2002 at about 85 percent (National League for Nursing, 1997a; Berlin, Stennett, and Bednash, 2003).

Enrollment trends indicate that there is continued support for doctoral education in nursing. During the 1990s, the number of programs, as well as the number of requests for admission to these programs, greatly increased. This trend has partially stemmed from the requirement of a doctorate for academic advancement and tenure for university nursing faculty. Nurses also desire the doctorate to become competent researchers and to advance the profession as a whole. Doctoral programs that prepare nurses predominantly for research and teaching reported 3,098 students enrolled in 2002. Far fewer students complete their doctoral programs, however, with many students enrolled only part-time. For example, in 2002, only 457 actually completed research-focused doctorates in 81 of the 83 existing doctoral programs (Berlin, Stennett, and Bednash, 2003). It is projected that large numbers of nurses with doctoral degrees will be needed in the future as positions requiring this degree expand in universities and throughout the health care system.

CERTIFICATION PROGRAMS

Certification and licensure are both forms of regulation of a profession. **Licensure** refers to state regulation of the practice of nursing at the entry point to practice. **Certification** is a regulatory mechanism for advanced practice and is voluntarily pursued by individual nurses.

Certification is a credential that has professional but not legal status. Specialized programs developed to recognize nurses for advanced practice often lead to certification. Some certification programs are part of degree-granting programs such as a master's program; others are considered part of continuing education.

Certification means that a certificate is awarded by a professional group as validation of specific qualifications demonstrated by a registered nurse in a defined area of practice. Certification programs that exist today include nurse practitioner preparation in programs such as pediatrics, gerontology, family health, women's health care, nurse midwifery, and nurse anesthesia. These programs provide concentrated study in specific areas and last from several months to several years. A comprehensive examination is required to become certified, as well as documentation of experience, letters of reference, and other documents. Currently, more than 40 organizations offer advanced practice certification (Wise, 2003). Box 2-1 lists some of the professional associations that currently grant certification.

Certified nurses may have greater earning potential, wider employment opportunities, status, and prestige than noncertified nurses, and in some states, they are eligible for insurance reimbursement, along with physicians. Requirements for admission to certification programs vary, with some requiring only registered nurse licensure and others requiring either a baccalaureate or a master's degree.

The **American Nurses Credentialing Center (ANCC),** a subunit of the ANA, provides a number of certification programs for registered nurses. **Advanced practice nurses (APNs)** certified by the ANCC must have master's degrees and demonstrate successful completion of a certification examination based on nationally recognized standards of nursing practice and designed to test their special knowledge and skills. For certain specialties, APNs also must show evidence of specified clinical practice experience. Once granted, certification is effective for 3 to 5 years, whereupon the individual must apply for recertification based on either a retest or demonstration of continuing education credits and evidence of ongoing clinical practice.

In response to the need for a more formally organized national peer review program for advanced practice nursing certification bodies, the ANCC and more than a dozen other certification boards formed the American Board of Nursing

---

Box 2-1 A Sample of Certifying Organizations in Nursing*

- American Association of Critical Care Nursing
- American Association of Diabetes Educators
- American Association of Nurse Anesthetists
- American Association of Spinal Cord Injury Nurses
- American Board for Occupational Health Nurses, Inc.
- American Psychiatric Nurses' Association
- American College of Nurse Midwives
- American Nurses Credentialing Center (multiple specialties)
- American Organization of Nurse Executives
- National Association of Neonatal Nurses
- National Association of Nurse Practitioners
- Board of Certification for Emergency Nursing
- National Certification Board of Pediatric Nurse Practitioners
- National Certification Corporation for Obstetric, Gynecologic, and Neonatal Specialties
- National Board for Certification of School Nurses
- Rehabilitation Nursing Certification Board

*A complete list of certifying boards can be obtained by writing to the *Journal of Continuing Education in Nursing*, Slack, Inc., 6900 Grove Drive, Thorofare, NJ 08086. Ask for the Annual Continuing Education Survey. Also available online (*www.slackinc.com/allied/jcen/jcenhome.htm#survey*).

Specialties (ABNS). This umbrella board, established in 1991, approves membership of those APN-certifying bodies that have met the standards and principles of ABNS.

Nurses holding ANCC certification at the associate degree/diploma level can be identified by the initials RN, C (Registered Nurse, Certified) after their names. Certified baccalaureate nurses are entitled to use RN, BC (Registered Nurse, Board Certified). Those certified as clinical specialists use APRN, BC (Advanced Practice Registered Nurse, Board Certified). Box 2-2 lists the areas in which the ANCC offers certification.

Although certification is a desirable concept, several challenges must be overcome in regard to the current methods of certification. For example, the lack of uniformity

---

Box 2-2 **Areas of Certification Offered by the American Nurses Credentialing Center (ANCC) in 2003 and Their Corresponding Credentials**

Advanced Practice Exams—APRN, BC (Advanced Practice Registered Nurse, Board Certified)

- Acute Care Nurse Practitioner
- Adult Nurse Practitioner
- Family Nurse Practitioner
- Gerontological Nurse Practitioner
- Pediatric Nurse Practitioner
- Adult Psychiatric and Mental Health Nurse Practitioner*
- Family Psychiatric and Mental Health Nurse Practitioner*
- Clinical Nurse Specialist in Gerontological Nursing
- Clinical Nurse Specialist in Medical-Surgical Nursing
- Clinical Nurse Specialist in Pediatric Nursing*
- Clinical Nurse Specialist in Adult Psychiatric and Mental Health Nursing
- Clinical Nurse Specialist in Child and Adolescent Psychiatric and Mental Health Nursing
- Clinical Nurse Specialist in Community Health Nursing
- Clinical Nurse Specialist in Home Health Nursing
- Advanced Diabetes Management—Clinical Specialist
- Advanced Diabetes Management—Nurse Practitioner
- Advanced Diabetes Management—Registered Dietitian
- Advanced Diabetes Management—Registered Pharmacist
- Advanced Practice Palliative Nurse

Baccalaureate-Level Exams—RN, BC (Registered Nurse, Board Certified)

- Cardiac/Vascular Nurse
- College Health Nurse
- Community Health Nurse
- General Nursing Practice
- Gerontological Nurse
- Home Health Nurse
- Informatics Nurse: Baccalaureate degree in nursing
- Informatics Nurse: Baccalaureate degree in other relevant field of study

Continued

> **Box 2-2** **Areas of Certification Offered by the American Nurses Credentialing Center (ANCC) in 2003 and Their Corresponding Credentials—cont'd**
>
> - Medical-Surgical Nurse
> - Nursing Professional Development
> - Pediatric Nurse
> - Perinatal Nurse
> - Psychiatric and Mental Health Nurse
> - Nursing Administration (RN, CNA, BC)
> - Nursing Administration, Advanced (RN, CNAA, BC)
>
> **Associate Degree/Diploma-Level Exams—RN, C**
>
> - Cardiac/Vascular Nurse Registered Nurse, Certified
> - Gerontological Nurse
> - Medical-Surgical Nurse
> - Pediatric Nurse
> - Perinatal Nurse
> - Psychiatric and Mental Health Nurse

*These exams have not yet gone through ABNS and NCCA accreditation.
From American Nurses Credentialing Center: Online, 2003, Accessed August 29, 2003
(www.nursingworld.org/ancc/certification/certs.html).

of programs, testing, and practice requirements must be examined. How the profession can ensure certification standards and who should be responsible for certification of nurses are major issues in the nursing education system today.

To address these issues, the American Association of Colleges of Nursing issued position statements in 1994 and 1998 on the certification and regulation of advanced practice nurses. These position statements emphasized that the nursing profession must develop a standardized national advanced practice nursing certification process by the year 2000. The statements recommended that all advanced practice nurses hold a graduate degree in nursing and be certified in a manner standardized by *one* nationally recognized certifying board. This stipulation of a single certifying board is particularly important because professional certification validates and standardizes the qualifications and practice competencies of advanced practice nurses, thereby ensuring the public's health and safety (American Association of Colleges of Nursing, 1998). Judging from the proliferation of certifying bodies listed in Box 2-1, this is a goal the profession has yet to attain.

CONTINUING EDUCATION

Continuing education (CE) is a term used to describe informal ways in which nurses maintain expertise during their professional careers. Continuing education for nurses takes place in a variety of settings: colleges, universities, hospitals, community agencies, professional organizations, and professional meetings. Continuing education is available in many formats, such as workshops, institutes, conferences, short courses, evening courses, telecourses, and instructional modules offered through professional journals and online.

The ANA Council on Continuing Education was established in 1973. This council is responsible for standards of continuing education, accreditation of programs offering continuing education, transferability of CE credit from state to state, and development of guidelines for recognition systems within states.

In the 1970s, the continuing education unit (CEU) was created as a method of recognizing participation in nonacademic credit offerings. One CEU was given for every 10 hours of participation in an organized, approved, continuing education offering. Today the **contact hour** has replaced the CEU, and nurses receive one contact hour of credit for each 50 or 60 minutes they spend in a continuing education course.

A major nationwide trend is **mandatory continuing education.** Before renewing their licenses in states with mandatory continuing education, nurses must provide evidence that they have met that state's contact hour requirements. This requirement is the government's way of ensuring that nurses remain up to date in their profession. In 2002, mandatory continuing education credit as a prerequisite for license renewal was required in 25 states and U.S. territories (Wise, 2003). Box 2-3 lists those states and territories.

FUTURE DIRECTIONS FOR NURSING EDUCATION

In 1993, three major organizations issued statements and reports about nursing education for the twenty-first century. Their reports addressed the new direction nursing education needed to take in the future. The reports included the NLN's "Vision for Nursing Education" (1993, see also National League for Nursing, 1995), the AACN's "Nursing Education's Agenda for the 21st Century" (1999), and the Pew Health Professions Commission's "Health Professions Education for the Future: Schools in Service to the Nation" (O'Neil, 1993). Although the three organizations advocated somewhat different approaches and strategies, several common themes emerged in their reports. Common emphases included the following eight points:

1. Schools should recruit diverse students and faculties that reflect the multicultural nature of society.
2. Curricula and learning activities should develop student's critical thinking skills.
3. Curricula should emphasize students' abilities to communicate, form interpersonal relationships, and make decisions collaboratively with patients, their families, and interdisciplinary colleagues.
4. The number of advanced practice nurses should be increased, and curricula should emphasize health promotion and health maintenance skills for all nurses.
5. Emphasis should be placed on community-based care, increased accountability, state-of-the-art clinical skills, and increased information management skills (Figure 2-5).
6. Cost-effectiveness of care should be a focus in nursing curricula.
7. Faculty should develop programs that facilitate program articulation and career mobility.
8. Continuing faculty development activities should support excellence in practice, teaching, and research.

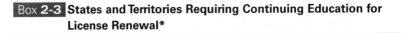

Box **2-3** States and Territories Requiring Continuing Education for License Renewal*

- Alabama
- Alaska
- Arkansas
- California
- Delaware
- Florida
- Iowa
- Kansas
- Kentucky
- Louisiana
- Massachusetts
- Michigan
- Minnesota
- Nebraska
- Nevada
- New Hampshire
- New Mexico
- North Mariana Islands
- Ohio
- Puerto Rico
- Texas
- U.S. Virgin Islands
- Utah
- West Virginia
- Wyoming

*A current list of states and territories requiring continuing education for license renewal can be obtained by writing to the *Journal of Continuing Education in Nursing,* Slack, Inc., 6900 Grove Drive, Thorofare, NJ 08086. Ask for a reprint of their Annual Continuing Education Survey. Also available online (*www.slackinc.com/allied/jcen/jcenhome.htm#survey*).

These eight areas of emphasis remain as important today as they were when first identified in 1993.

The Rise in Distance Learning (DL)

Now that the technology is available to create virtual universities, nursing education has recognized the value of distance learning. **Distance learning (DL)** is an umbrella term used to describe courses offered by electronic means, such as on television or online. DL offers several major positive features:

- It increases access to nursing education for adults in midcareer, who represent a growing proportion of the undergraduate nursing population.
- It increases access to nursing education in rural areas underserved by higher education.

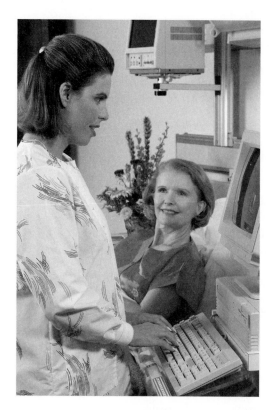

Figure 2-5
Information management is more important than ever in nursing. This nursing student is developing information technology skills in order to manage multiple sources of patient information successfully.

- It increases the efficiency of the shrinking number of nursing faculty members by allowing them to reach larger audiences than in traditional nursing classes on campuses.

As more colleges of nursing offer coursework through distance learning, the issue of adequate and properly supervised clinical experience arises. Technology may again provide at least a partial answer to this dilemma through the use of virtual reality. Virtual reality "employs computers and other multimedia peripherals to produce a simulated (i.e., virtual) environment that users perceive as comparable to real-world objects and events" (Simpson, 2003). Until the time that colleges can afford to implement virtual reality technology, DL students validate their clinical competence in a number of traditional ways, including preceptorships, clinical examinations, demonstrations, and clinical portfolios.

CHALLENGES IN NURSING EDUCATION

A number of challenges face nursing education. Three major challenges discussed in this section are declining numbers of nursing graduates, the faculty shortage, and the need to transform nursing education to meet the health care needs of the nation in the future.

Declining Numbers of Nursing Graduates

One way to measure growth in the number of new RN graduates is by the number of candidates taking the NCLEX-RN. After growing steadily during the first half of the 1990s, the number of new RN exam candidates fell annually in the last half of the decade. This resulted in 26 percent fewer RNs graduating in 2000 than in 1995 (U.S. Department of Health and Human Services, 2001). Declines were seen in all programs—diploma, associate degree, and baccalaureate—as illustrated in Figure 2-6. Although diploma graduates have gradually declined over several decades, as hospital-based diploma programs have closed, the declines in associate degree and baccalaureate graduates represent a recent and disturbing trend. Complicating the picture is the fact that declining enrollments foreshadow continued declines in graduations as students make their way through the educational pipeline.

On a positive note, the AACN (Berlin, Stennett, and Bednash, 2003) reported a 8.1 percent increase in generic (entry-level) baccalaureate enrollment between 2000 and 2001; however, lengthier baccalaureate programs increase the time before these students will emerge as licensed RNs. Associate degree graduations are declining somewhat faster than baccalaureate graduates, meaning that baccalaureate graduates have begun to comprise a greater share of total graduates. This one fact alone constrains the growth in supply of nurses, because baccalaureate-prepared RNs take twice as long to complete their schooling and enter the workforce. Although increasing the number of baccalaureate-prepared nurses is expected to strengthen the profession, it also has the effect of creating further delay in the growth in RN supply, even as enrollments increase. Figure 2-7 depicts the distribution of RN graduates by type of educational preparation.

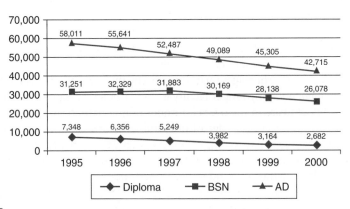

Figure 2-6

Total number of RN graduates by educational preparation, 1995-2000. (From U.S. Department of Health and Human Services: *Projected supply, demand, and shortages of registered nurses: 2000-2020*, Washington, DC, 2002, Government Printing Office.)

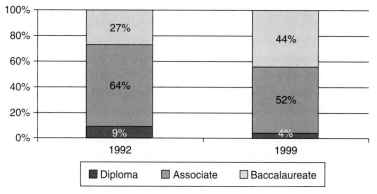

Figure 2-7

Distribution of RN graduates by educational preparation: 1992 and 1999. (From U.S. Department of Health and Human Services: *Projected supply, demand, and shortages of registered nurses: 2000-2020,* Washington, DC, 2002, Government Printing Office.)

Faculty Shortage

As the nursing profession ages, so does the nurse faculty population. Nationally, the mean age for faculty members was 49.7 years in 1993. By 2002, this average had risen to 51.1 years. This trend will result in increasing numbers of faculty retirements in the next decade. The faculty shortage, already affecting some areas of the country, is predicted to become severe in the majority of the nation's schools of nursing by the year 2010 (AACN, 2003).

Recognizing that the shortage of faculty was reaching critical proportions, the AACN in April 2003 issued an official report, known as a white paper, outlining the problem (AACN, 2003). Among their findings were the following:

- A 2000 national sample of schools reported 7.4 percent faculty vacancies, with only 20 of 220 schools reporting no vacancies. Although this may not seem like a large vacancy rate, it has a considerable impact because of teacher:student ratios mandated by nursing accreditation bodies.
- More than 5,000 qualified applicants to nursing programs at baccalaureate, master's, and doctoral levels were refused admission because of faculty shortages in 41.7 percent of schools in 2002.
- Reasons for faculty shortages include the following: age and retirement timelines; an inadequate pool of younger faculty for replacement; resignations for nonacademic jobs; decrease in the overall number of graduates from both master's and doctoral programs; average age of doctoral graduates (46.2 years) as compared with graduates of all professions (33.7 years), meaning that the number of productive work years for these older faculty members are curtailed; plans of new doctoral graduates to work outside education; average academic salaries lower than those in clinical areas and continuing budgetary constraints within most higher education systems, making salary increases unlikely; and expanding expectations of the faculty role. Furthermore, faculty members are challenged more and more by nontraditional students who demand more individual attention—at the same time as they are increasingly required to do research, service, and publishing.

The AACN (2003) white paper suggested numerous additional strategies for dealing with the faculty shortage, but these go beyond the scope of this chapter. Suffice it to say that the problem is real and severe and it will ultimately affect the nation's supply of registered nurses if solutions are not found (see the entire 2003 report at *www.aacn.nche.edu/publications/whitepapers/facultyshortages.htm*).

Need to Transform Nursing Education

Major nursing professional organizations recognize the need to reshape nursing education to meet the challenges of future patient care through improved nursing practice. In 1999, the National League for Nursing launched a 5-year project, "Transforming the Landscape for Nursing Education." The purpose of this project was to begin a national dialogue on skills and competencies, types of programs and curricula, academic and community partnerships, standards for future program types, and research initiatives for nursing education. Plans for this transformation include discovering the core knowledge needed to bridge education and practice; differentiating between knowledge and outcome competencies for a continuum of practice; identifying research on curricula, methods, and instructional strategies for core curricula common to basic preparation for health professions; developing seamless program articulation along the continuum of nursing education; and creating infrastructures that provide for ongoing communication among leaders in education and practice (National League for Nursing, 1999).

In April 2002, the ANA issued another visionary document entitled "Nursing's Agenda for the Future: The Future Vision for Nursing." The vision for nursing education articulated in this paper included the valuing of nursing education by the public; education programs that are accessible, affordable, and flexible; adequate faculty with high qualifications who engage in innovative teaching, clinical practice, and research; learning environments conducive to the creativity of faculty and students; evidence-based education; safe, quality care; and partnerships to enhance clinical experiences, meet the needs of special populations, and promote professional involvement. The following five strategies were outlined for achieving the vision: (1) establish congruence between the educational enterprise and societal needs; (2) enrich the high caliber of nursing faculty; (3) attain clarity in education about nursing roles and scopes of practice; (4) work for universal excellence in nursing education; and (5) promote the value of nursing education to the profession and the public (see the entire ANA 2002 report at *www.nursingworld.org/naf/*).

There is no question that the transformation of nursing education over the next two decades will be significant. The thoughts of a seasoned nursing education leader, Vernice Ferguson, about the factors that create this need for a transformation of nursing education are provided in Box 2-4.

Other Challenges

In addition to the three major challenges discussed above, nursing education must address a variety of other issues, including job market fluctuations; diminishing clinical sites with increasing competition for clinical learning sites by all health profession schools; diminishing resources in institutions of higher education and the perception of the high cost of operating nursing education

Box **2-4** Education of Nurses Must Change

As we shift from the centrality of the hospital which remains notable for illness care, we soon recognize that the education of nurses must change to accommodate the increased expectations of nurses as practitioners, educators, researchers, managers and administrators as well as policy shapers. No longer must the professional nurse feel frustrated as the profession's independent function is compromised. The opportunity is now afforded to enhance collaborative and satisfying relationships between and among other health care providers and to form partnerships with those being served assuring their maximum independence and empowerment. As new partnerships are forged with the recipients of nursing services, the helping model so well known to nurses who practice in rehabilitation, mental health and substance abuse programs is replacing the medical model as more appropriate.

A variety of practice settings await tomorrow's nurse including the rapidly growing home care arena, nurse managed centers and integrated managed care systems. Programmatic emphasis on subacute and chronic care, primary prevention, family centered care, sophisticated information and communications technology, coupled with a culturally responsive care provider, offer unparalleled opportunities for nursing. With the diversity in nursing roles, we are challenged to think creatively as we make unprecedented contributions to improving the public's health at a time of great chaos and opportunity. Linking educational efforts and research priorities to reform goals can position nursing as an essential player in the change process.

—Vernice L. Ferguson

Ferguson VL: *Educating the 21st century nurse: challenges and opportunities,* Introduction, Sudbury, MA, 1997, NLN Press and Jones and Bartlett.

programs; and the inability of some nursing programs to meet new accreditation standards.

Summary of Key Points

- The development of nursing education has been influenced by a number of factors leading to a diverse array of program offerings.
- First provided in hospitals, basic entry-level nursing education has evolved into three major types of programs: diploma, baccalaureate, and associate degree, each of which has a range of features.
- Alternatives such as baccalaureate degree programs for registered nurses, external degree programs, and accelerated options for postbaccalaureate students contribute to a complex educational picture for registered nurses.
- Masters and doctoral degrees are needed to meet the health care needs of society.
- Voluntary accreditation is designed to ensure the quality of nursing education programs.
- Schools have found it necessary to restrict enrollments because of faculty shortages, lack of clinical sites, and budget constraints.
- Life-long learning through continuing education is considered essential for all professionals, particularly in practice-based disciplines such as nursing. Continuing education is now mandated as a prerequisite for relicensure in 25 states and U.S. territories, and this number is expected to increase.
- The problem of reduced resources in nursing education may soon reach crisis proportions, and weaker schools may close. This is a result of underfunding of higher

education in general and, in particular, diminishing sources of federal funding for schools of nursing.

- Graduate programs in nursing are not preparing adequate numbers of nursing educators to meet current and future needs. Faculty shortages are already developing, and a severe faculty shortage is expected nationwide by 2010.
- In response to changes in higher education and the health care system, national organizations have suggested initiatives to revise educational requirements and program emphases for the twenty-first century that will enable future registered nurses at all levels to meet the changing health care needs of society.

CRITICAL THINKING QUESTIONS

1. What factors did you use to determine the type of basic nursing program you entered? Knowing what you know now, what changes, if any, would you make in your choice?
2. How would you advise a high school student interested in nursing to select a program?
3. Should the nursing profession have only one basic program that leads to a career in nursing? Discuss the pros and cons of a single program. Where should this basic program be located? What academic credential should be awarded at the completion of the program?
4. What content areas and skills should be included in basic nursing programs to prepare graduates for contemporary nursing practice? What should be eliminated to make room for this content?
5. Offering complete articulation of all types of nursing education from practical nursing through doctoral study seems like a logical course of action. Should states mandate program articulation? Why or why not?
6. Discuss the merits and drawbacks of mandatory continuing education from the viewpoints of nurses and consumers of nursing care.
7. What unique contributions to nursing are possible by nurses with master's-level education? With doctoral-level degrees?
8. Find out which of the national accrediting bodies, NLNAC or CCNE, accredits your school or college. Research their standards online (visit Evolve for WebLinks related to the content of this chapter: **http://evolve.elsevier.com/Chitty/ professional/**) and prepare a brief analysis of how your school meets those standards.

REFERENCES

Allen J, editor: *Consumer's guide to doctoral degree programs in nursing,* New York, 1990, National League for Nursing.

American Association of Colleges of Nursing: *The baccalaureate degree in nursing as minimal preparation for professional practice,* Position statement, Washington, DC, 1996, American Association of Colleges of Nursing.

American Association of Colleges of Nursing: *Nursing education's agenda for the 21st century,* Position statement, Washington, DC, 1993, revised 1999, American Association of Colleges of Nursing.

American Association of Colleges of Nursing: *Certification and regulation of advanced practice nurses,* Position statement, Washington, DC, 1994, revised 1998, American Association of Colleges of Nursing.

American Association of Colleges of Nursing: *Faculty shortages in baccalaureate and graduate nursing programs: scope of the problem and strategies for expanding the supply,* Washington, DC, 2003, American Association of Colleges of Nursing.

American Nurses Association: *Educational preparation for nurse practitioners and assistants to nurses,* Position paper, Kansas City, MO, 1965, American Nurses Association.

American Nurses Association: *A case for baccalaureate preparation in nursing,* Kansas City, MO, 1979, American Nurses Association.

American Nurses Association: *Nursing's agenda for the future: the future vision for nursing,* Washington, DC, 2002, American Nurses Association.

American Nurses Credentialing Center: Online, 2003, Accessed August 29, 2003 *(www. nursingworld.org/ancc/certification/certs.html).*

Berlin LE, Stennett J, Bednash GD: *Enrollment and graduations in baccalaureate and graduate programs in nursing,* Washington, DC, 2003, American Association of Colleges of Nursing.

Brown EL: *Nursing for the future,* New York, 1948, Russell Sage Foundation.

Christy T: Portrait of a leader: M. Adelaide Nutting, *Nurs Outlook* 17(1):20-24, 1969.

Conley V: *Curriculum and instruction in nursing,* Boston, 1973, Little, Brown.

Donahue MP: *Nursing: the finest art: an illustrated history,* St. Louis, 1985, Mosby.

Ferguson VL: *Educating the 21st century nurse: challenges and opportunities,* Sudbury, MA, 1997, NLN Press and Jones and Bartlett.

Kalisch P, Kalisch B: *The advance of American nursing,* ed 3, Boston, 1995, Little, Brown.

Lysaught J: *An abstract for action,* New York, 1970, McGraw-Hill.

Montag M: *The education of nursing technicians,* New York, 1951, Putnam.

National League for Nursing: *Scope and preparation,* Position statement on nursing roles, New York, 1982, National League for Nursing.

National League for Nursing, Council of Associate Degree Programs: *Educational outcomes of associate degree nursing programs: roles and competencies,* New York, 1990, National League for Nursing.

National League for Nursing: *A vision for nursing education,* New York, 1993, National League for Nursing.

National League for Nursing: *Emerging environment for nursing education and practice examined during two-year vision campaign: news from the National League for Nursing,* New York, 1995, National League for Nursing.

National League for Nursing, Center for Research in Nursing Education and Community Health: *Annual guide to graduate nursing education, 1997,* Sudbury, MA, 1997a, NLN Press and Jones and Bartlett.

National League for Nursing, Center for Research in Nursing Education and Community Health: *NLN guide to undergraduate RN education,* ed 5, Sudbury, MA, 1997b, NLN Press and Jones and Bartlett.

National League for Nursing: *Transforming the landscape: executive summary,* Biennial Convention, June 5, 1999, Miami Beach, Florida.

National League for Nursing: *RN state-approved schools of nursing,* 1998, ed 56, Sudbury, MA, 1999, NLN Press and Jones and Bartlett.

National League for Nursing Accrediting Commission Personal communication, 2004.

National League of Nursing Education: *Nursing schools today and tomorrow,* New York, 1934, National League of Nursing Education.

National League of Nursing Education: *A curriculum guide for schools of nursing,* New York, 1937, National League of Nursing Education.

Notter L, Spalding E: *Professional nursing, foundations, perspectives and relationships,* ed 9, Philadelphia, 1976, JB Lippincott.

O'Neil EH: *Health professions education for the future: schools in service to the nation,* San Francisco, 1993, Pew Health Professions Commission.

Parietti E: The development of doctoral education in nursing: a historical overview. In Allen J, editor: *Consumer's guide to doctoral degree programs in nursing,* New York, 1990, National League for Nursing, p 1532.

Simpson R: Welcome to the virtual classroom, *Nurs Admin Quart* 27(1):83-86, 2003.

U.S. Department of Health and Human Services: *Seventh report to the President and Congress on the status of health personnel in the United States,* Washington, DC, 1990, Government Printing Office.

U.S. Department of Health and Human Services: *The registered nurse population, March 2000: findings from the national sample survey of registered nurses,* Washington, DC, 2001, Government Printing Office.

U.S. Department of Health and Human Services: *Projected supply, demand, and shortages of registered nurses: 2000-2020,* Washington, DC, 2002, Government Printing Office.

Wise P: Annual CE survey: State and association/certifying boards CE requirements, *J Cont Ed Nurs* 34(1):5-13, 2003.

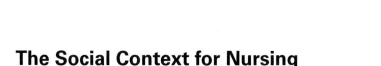

C H A P T E R

3

The Social Context for Nursing

Kay Kittrell Chitty

Key Terms

American Assembly for Men in
  Nursing (AAMN)
Androcentric
Biomedical Technology
Caring Technology
Consumerism
Cultural Competence
Demographics
Dominant Culture
Emotional Intelligence

Feminism
Gender Role Stereotypes
Information Technology (IT)
Knowledge Technology
Medical Paternalism
Nursing Information System
Patient Acuity
Point of Care Technology
Posttraumatic Stress Disorder
  (PTSD)

Role Strain
Sexual Assault Nurse Examiner
  (SANE)
Socialization
Stereotypes
Transcultural Nursing
Woodhull Study on Nursing
  and the Media

Learning Outcomes

After studying this chapter, students will be able to:

- Describe how individuals are socialized.
- Identify patterns of socialization and their effect on personal development.
- Analyze the traditional roles of women and how these have affected the development of the nursing profession.
- Discuss social trends affecting the development of nursing as a profession.
- Explain the impact of the media on the image of nursing.
- Evaluate the continuing development of technology and the implications for nursing.
- Describe the impact of societal violence on nursing.
- Describe the causes and effects of imbalances in supply of and demand for nurses in the United States.

Every profession is profoundly affected by the society it serves, and nursing is no exception. The social context has shaped nurses' attitudes, nursing practice, and the attitudes of the public toward nursing over the years. The social context also influences who chooses nursing as a career.

As you read this chapter, think about what drew you into the profession of nursing. What is the story of your individual journey into nursing? One nurse's story is found in the Critical Thinking Exercise below. This woman entered nursing nearly 30 years ago, perhaps before you were born. Can you identify some of the social forces that influenced her career choice? Are any of these forces still operating today? What are some of the social forces you are responding to as you enter or advance in nursing? How are they similar or different from this nurse's concerns? Take a few minutes now to reflect on your own individual journey toward nursing.

CRITICAL THINKING *Exercise*

One Nurse's Journey Into Nursing

Instructions: Analyze the story below and determine the social forces behind this nurse's decision to enter the profession. What assumptions did she make about the profession before entering it? Were her assumptions accurate or inaccurate? How would her assumptions hold up today?

"I was always interested in the sciences and did quite well in those subjects during my early years of school. In junior high I had an excellent biology teacher and thought I would like to be a biology teacher someday. In about the ninth grade, however, I questioned how I could combine my love of sciences and teaching with another goal—having a husband and children. The answer for me was to become a nurse. I believed that I could have the 'best of both worlds.' I wanted a career, but I also definitely wanted to get married and have children.

"Another motivation was my realization that my mother had wanted to become a nurse and never did. I know I entered nursing because of an intense interest in sciences, teaching, and doing something that would help my future family. But I believe my mother's unfulfilled wish to become a nurse also entered into my career choice."

Nurses need to understand how nursing is related to society as a whole. What impact does society have on the practice of nursing? Does the fact that nursing is a female-dominated profession have a bearing on the way the profession is developing? How have the women's movement and feminism influenced the practice of nursing? Since greater numbers of men are entering nursing, what issues face them, and how has society reacted to their increasing presence in a traditionally female profession? How do **demographics** (population trends) affect nursing? How does the public view nurses? Should this public image be changed? If so, how? What causes periodic imbalances in supply of and demand for nurses? These questions are explored in this chapter.

TRADITIONAL SOCIALIZATION OF WOMEN

Socialization is the process whereby values and expectations are transmitted from generation to generation. Lessons about appropriate gender roles are taught intentionally and unintentionally by parents, older siblings, and other adults, such as grandparents and teachers. From birth, males and females are treated differently. Today, many parents know the gender of their child even *before* birth and make purchasing and decorating decisions based on what they consider masculine or feminine.

Learning the Female Role

Historically in Western culture, girls learn to be "feminine," which has traditionally meant passive, dependent, affectionate, emotional, and expressive. They learn that beauty and charm make one desirable to men—and that catching a man is a major life goal. Caring for him and his children is life's work. This is considered an **androcentric,** or male-centered, cultural bias. Children learn, too, that the female role is less active, often less enjoyable, and certainly less valued than is the male role. Women have generally been socialized to avoid risk-taking and conflict and to acquiesce to authority. Traditionally, feminine attributes included an orientation toward security, peacekeeping, and submissiveness. Although there have been major changes in the female role since the mid-twentieth century, these feminine "traits" have been remarkably persistent.

Women have also been socialized to be self-sacrificing to parents, husbands, and children. When women subordinate their own needs for the sake of others, they can avoid unpleasantness and conflict. They also avoid the appearance of aggressiveness, for which assertive behavior has often been mistaken in the past.

An outcome of traditional female socialization was to prepare women for primary allegiance to families, not to succeed in careers. The socialized female traits of dependency, passivity, and need for approval unconsciously restrict women's choices in life to traditional family roles and certain "female" professions. Often, young girls have been encouraged to enter nursing because nursing was considered to be especially good training for marriage and motherhood. This attitude was reflected by the nurse whose story appears in the Critical Thinking Exercise.

Gender Role Stereotyping

Stereotypes are biased attitudes developed through interactions with family, friends, and others in an individual's social and cultural system. **Gender role stereotypes** deal with prejudiced ideas of how men and women should behave in a cultural group. Some common gender role stereotypes of women identified by Cummings (1995) are found in Box 3-1.

Gender role stereotyping can be subtle. It begins early in life and can easily be overlooked unless one is attuned to the forms in which it can occur. The Research Note on p. 67 describes a study by two researchers of popular children's television programs that analyzed gender messages aimed at 1- through 5-year-old children.

Female Stereotyping in Nursing

In the early days of modern nursing, the roles assigned to women were those of healer, caretaker, and nurturer, none of which was highly valued by society. The first formal schools of nursing in the United States were developed to attract "respectable women" into nursing, which may have helped to increase the value society put on

Box **3-1** Common Gender Role Stereotypes of Women

Mother

- Subrogates own needs
- Freely gives advice
- Becomes the peacemaker
- Fosters dependence
- Is passive, wants recognition

Iron Maiden

- Is competitive versus collaborative
- Possesses the ability to "be in charge"
- Gives critical feedback
- Sets rigid interpersonal boundaries
- Can be unapproachable

Superwoman

- Demands perfection
- Will not delegate
- Overcommits her time
- Assumes multiple roles
- Feels isolated, not supported

Based on Cummings SH: Attila the Hun versus Attila the hen: gender socialization of the American nurse, *Nurs Admin Quart* 19(2):25, 1995.

nursing. By replacing untrained hospital "nurses" with students who worked in the hospital in return for room, board, and training, however, one powerless labor pool was simply exchanged for another. Hospitals have been described as patriarchal "families," with nurses behaving as obedient "daughters" to administrator "daddies" or acting as helpful "wives" to physician "husbands" and loving "mothers" to patient "children" (Muff, 1988a).

For decades, middle-class American women were raised with expectations of being supported financially by their husbands. This expectation freed them from the need to choose a profession that offered long-term financial security. Instead, they could make a career choice with a focus on their present needs while realizing that, with any luck at all, they would not always need to support themselves. They entered nursing with a "now-but-not-necessarily-forever" attitude. This affected both salary expectations and commitment to nursing as a career (Cummings, 1995).

Approximately 94.6 percent of nurses in the United States in 2000 were women (HRSA, 2000). Like other traditionally female occupations, such as teaching and social work, nursing has been historically plagued with low status, low pay, and general subordination to higher-status men such as male physicians and hospital and clinic administrators. Nurses face a double challenge of being predominately female and operating within the stereotypic boundaries of a traditionally "female" profession (Moss, 1995).

RESEARCH note

Kimberly Powell and Lori Abels are researchers who examined children's television programs to assess the manner in which gender roles were presented. They defined sex-role as "a set of activities deemed appropriate for one sex but not the other" and sex-role stereotypes as existing when "actions are thought of as simply masculine or feminine and tend to be resistant to change" (p. 14). Powell and Abels decided to focus on two popular television programs aimed at preschool (ages 2 to 5) children—*Barney & Friends* and *Teletubbies*—for gendered themes, characteristics, and messages within the programs. For a theme to be identified, both researchers must have spotted it and it had to appear in at least half the episodes, which they viewed separately to avoid influencing each other.

After studying 10 episodes of each program, these researchers found that gendered messages and behaviors were presented in a number of ways. For example, female characters were usually followers; they looked feminine, that is, small or petite; they were underrepresented in the occupations portrayed; they played feminine roles such as caretaker or peacemaker; and they were shown in activities such as braiding hair, cooking, and washing dishes. Male characters were usually leaders; appeared in a variety of masculine occupations and roles, such as playing basketball, driving a bulldozer, or building a wall; were larger physically; and were stereotypically male in appearance. Socially, males were active and females passive.

The researchers concluded that both programs did well at opening up acceptable behavior choices for boys, such as being cooperative and social, yet they maintained sex-role stereotypes such as caretaker and follower for girls. They made three suggestions for improving gender representation in preschool television programs:

1. Depict women as construction workers or men as child care providers to present children with more options in learning what men and women can do.
2. Alternate males and females as leaders.
3. Design some programs that show females in action with males observing, or better yet, all working together and equally active.

Powell KA, Abels L: Sex-role stereotypes in TV programs aimed at the preschool audience: an analysis of Teletubbies and Barney & Friends, *Women & Language* 25(2):14-22, 2002.

NURSING, FEMINISM, AND WOMEN'S MOVEMENTS

Nursing, feminism, and women's movements have an uneasy relationship. Contemporary feminists have criticized nursing for failing to change the culture of nursing to a feminist one. For example, the relatively young American Nurses Association (ANA) refused to endorse women's suffrage until 1915, although the fight for women's right to vote had been going on for the previous 40 years. Decades later, the more mature ANA chose not to endorse the passage of the Equal Rights

Amendment (ERA) until the late 1970s, citing the ANA leadership's belief that biological differences between men and women demanded special legislative attention that the more generic ERA did not address.

Given this and other examples, it is not surprising that nursing has been viewed by some feminists as a traditional and even oppressive female occupation. There is some validity to this criticism, because nurses have tended to build their own power bases on connections with governmental agencies and strong, male-dominated professions such as medicine rather than on identification with other nurses and other women's groups (Bunting and Campbell, 1990). Many nurses have inadvertently contributed to this stereotype by passively looking to others outside nursing to improve conditions in nursing rather than working with other nurses to strengthen the profession from within.

What Is Feminism?

What exactly is **feminism**? Gray's (1994) explanation is brief, simple, and still relevant today: "The primary focus of feminism is an examination of gender privilege, that is, privilege that accrues or is denied because of one's biologically determined sexual characteristics" (p. 506). Gray further explained that feminism values women, their experiences, knowledge, and ways of knowing in a **dominant culture** in which everyone lives, grows, and participates.

The feminist perspective is not the exclusive property of women. Feminism is concerned with the advancement of all people by eliminating the dominance-submission model of relating; placing value on the worth and dignity of all people; eliminating hierarchies based on one group's domination of others; eliminating health disparities based on gender, age, ethnicity, or social status; and creating a healthier and safer society (Gary, Sigsby, and Campbell, 1998). These are goals that can be embraced by every thoughtful person.

Nursing and the Women's Movement

The women's movement that began in the 1960s has had a profound effect on society and has both hurt and helped the nursing profession. As women of the 1960s and 1970s sought career opportunities beyond the traditional female ones of teaching and nursing, bright and able women who formerly might have become nurses pursued careers in accounting, architecture, engineering, computer science, and a variety of other fields. This meant that nursing faced more competition for students than it once did.

There is no question that the almost endless array of career options now open to women accounts in part for declining interest in nursing by traditional, that is, 18-year-old, students. When women can freely choose any professional field of study, they often seek opportunities elsewhere. An interesting recent phenomenon has occurred, however. Deans and directors of schools of nursing in the United States report that applications are increasing from women and men who were originally educated to be attorneys, computer programmers, accountants, and other occupations more recently open to them. It seems that in spite of a vast number of career choices now available to men and women, nursing's appeal is strong to people of both genders who want to make a difference in the lives of others.

The women's movement helped nursing by bringing economic issues such as low salaries and poor working conditions into the open. The movement provoked a conscious awareness that equality and autonomy for women were inherent rights, not privileges, and stimulated the passage of legislation to ensure those rights.

Nursing also benefited from the women's movement in more subtle ways. As nursing students were increasingly educated in colleges and universities, they were exposed to campus activism, protest, and organizations that were trying to change the status of women. Learning informal lessons about power and how to bring about change had a positive effect on students, who later used this knowledge to improve the status of nursing.

Despite these positive directions, the nursing profession has been slow to internalize the women's movement message of self-determination and commitment. As mentioned earlier, many nurses have looked on nursing as a useful way to occupy themselves until marriage. To others, nursing has served simply as a "job" used to supplement the major breadwinner's income or to pay for a family vacation, new car, or camp for the kids. Sometimes nurses worked only to tide the family over temporarily rough economic waters, returning to home and family when the family's financial situation improved. This "stepping in" and "stepping out" of the profession has meant that these nurses' energies and loyalties were divided. The result is that nursing has not prospered as it might have if all of its members were committed to long-term careers and worked together to improve conditions in the profession.

It is unfortunate that there are registered nurses (RNs) who have not fully accepted the necessity for long-term professional commitment, which not only enhances personal growth but also strengthens the profession from within. Feminism and women's movements have helped nurses learn that women can be autonomous and assertive. With the firm commitment of all its members, male and female, to lifelong full participation, nursing can grow to its maximum potential, expand opportunities for its members, give voice to all its members, male and female, and ultimately contribute to the advancement of society at large. Shea (1994) encouraged nurses to contribute to contemporary feminism in the following four areas (pp. 577-578):

1. By endorsing feminism in their practice and sharing their passionate conviction about feminism and nursing with family members, friends, co-workers, and community members, so that the message reaches decision makers and desired changes take place.

2. By expressing themselves in public through letters to the editors of professional journals and daily newspapers; by telling nursing's stories, which the public wants and needs to hear.

3. By creating good public role models in the main vehicle for change in American society and on television. Nursing needs a television series that is "updated and reflective of what nurses really do, and how they think and feel. ... In order for these things to happen, some nurses will have to devote their full attention to 'nonnursing things' such as writing scripts, performing on the stage, taking photographs, developing artwork, and making feature-length films and documentaries featuring nurses" (p. 578).

4. By caring for nursing's young, both female and male. Socialization into nursing has to change toward becoming a more empathic, nonhierarchical, mutually beneficial process. There must be tolerance of different learning styles and cultural values, reflecting the diversity of the nursing population.

Even individuals who do not consider themselves feminists can agree that these are important goals for nursing.

MEN IN NURSING

In 1992, 4.3 percent (79,557) of practicing registered nurses in the United States were men. By 1996 that figure had risen to 5.4 percent (113,683) (U.S. Department of Health and Human Services, 1996). This represents an increase of nearly 70 percent in only 4 years. This trend did not continue, however, because the March 2000 survey by the Division of Nursing of the U.S. Department of Health and Human Services revealed that approximately 146,902 of the 2,694,540 RNs in this country were men. Although the number of men in nursing was considerably higher in 2000, growth in the profession in general meant that men represented exactly the same percentage, 5.4 percent, as in 1996.

The number of men in nursing is expected to rise as currently enrolled students graduate. The American Association of Colleges of Nursing (AACN) reported that in 2002, 9.6 percent of students in baccalaureate nursing programs, 9.6 percent in master's programs, and 10.3 percent in nursing doctoral programs were men (AACN, 2002). The male nurse, when compared with his female counterpart, is likely to be younger, to be employed full-time in nursing, to have more nonnursing education, and to have chosen nursing as a second career. Their motivations for entering nursing, however, are similar to those of their female counterparts. Most men enter nursing to help people (Boughn, 2001; Figure 3-1).

The American Assembly for Men in Nursing (AAMN)

The **American Assembly for Men in Nursing (AAMN)** was founded in 1974 with the stated purpose of providing "a framework for nurses, as a group, to meet, to discuss and influence factors which affect men as nurses" (AAMN, 2003). The organization's objectives are as follows (AAMN, 2003):

- Encourage men of all ages to become nurses and join together with all nurses in strengthening and humanizing health care.
- Support men who are nurses to grow professionally and demonstrate to one another and to society the increasing contributions being made by men within the nursing profession.
- Advocate for continued research, education, and dissemination of information about men's health issues, men in nursing, and nursing knowledge at the local and national levels.
- Support members' full participation in the nursing profession and its organizations and use this assembly for the limited objectives stated above.

The fact that the members of this group thought a separate organization was necessary to achieve their objectives raises the question, "Have men in nursing

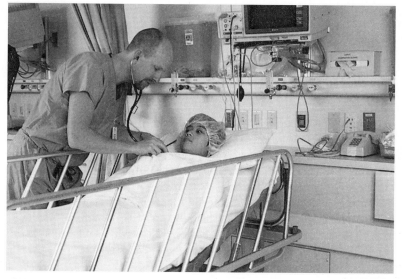

Figure **3-1**
Male registered nurses are becoming more visible as their numbers increase.

suffered discrimination because of their gender?" Let us now examine how men have fared in a profession traditionally dominated by women.

A Brief History of Men in Nursing

Men are not new to the profession of nursing. They supplied much of the nursing care during the eleventh, twelfth, and thirteenth centuries. It was not until late in the nineteenth century that nursing became a predominately female profession.

Despite all the positive things she did, Florence Nightingale played a major role in excluding men from the profession by asserting that nursing was a female discipline. She worked hard to establish nursing as a worthy career for "respectable women" and largely ignored the historical contributions of men. She saw the male role as confined to supplying physical strength, such as lifting or moving patients, when needed.

The Industrial Revolution also influenced the exit of men from nursing. During this time, the accepted professional areas for men were science, technology, and business. Men chose medicine, and women chose nursing (Black and Germaine-Warner, 1995).

The first two schools of nursing for men were established in the late 1800s. They were the Mills School of Nursing for Men at New York's Bellevue Hospital and McLean Asylum Training School in Massachusetts. The purpose of these training programs was to prepare men for psychiatric nursing, a field that in those days often required physical stamina and strength and was therefore considered appropriate for men.

In 1901, the U.S. Congress created the Army Nurse Corps for female nurses only. The Navy Nurse Corps followed 7 years later and was also restricted to women (Black and Germaine-Warner, 1995). Because of the lack of training programs and the gender restrictions placed on military nurses, it was difficult for men to enter nursing before World War II. Cummings (1995) reported that in 1941 only 68 of the 1,303 schools of nursing accepted men.

After World War II, the GI Bill helped to increase the number of male nursing students by providing funding for education. Military corpsmen entered nursing schools in large numbers, as they have following every major military conflict since. Nevertheless, as late as 1990, 8.3 percent of American baccalaureate nursing programs still had no male students (Villeneuve, 1994).

Why Men Enter Nursing

As mentioned earlier, most men enter nursing for the same reasons women do: they are motivated by their desire to care for others (Boughn, 2001). Men also have a variety of practical reasons: job security, career opportunity, stable income, and job flexibility. Traditionally, men tend to choose challenging and active areas of nursing, such as intensive care units, cardiac care units, emergency departments, trauma units, flight nursing, or anesthesiology, among others. Men are frequently drawn to the technological aspects of acute care specialties and are stimulated by the challenge created by the machines used in those units.

There has been concern that some men may look at nursing as a springboard to other professions and that they might not stay in nursing long because of the low status and low pay (Williams, 1989). This concern was borne out by a 2002 study by a University of Pennsylvania researcher, J. Solchalski, who found that 7.5 percent of new male nurses left the profession within 4 years of graduating from nursing school (Solchalski, 2002). This is compared with 4.1 percent of new female nurses.

Several issues face the large number of men who do choose to stay in nursing. These men often feel **role strain,** an emotional reaction that may be felt by a person in a profession that has a social structure dominated by members of the opposite sex. For men raised in the androcentric American culture, unused to anti-male gender discrimination, this can create anxiety and discontent. Increasingly, however, leadership roles in nursing organizations are filled by men.

Attitudes Toward Men in Nursing

As mentioned earlier, in American society men interested in health care historically became physicians, whereas women became nurses. Men entering the profession of nursing have crossed over traditional gender lines, and their masculinity may be questioned as a result. One negative assumption men in nursing encounter is that male nurses have problems with gender role identity (Kelly, Shoemaker, and Steele, 1996). Although the pervasive homophobia in our society and the belief that nursing is strictly a feminine profession may be changing, these attitudes are still pervasive enough to affect the decisions of teenage boys making career choices (Villeneuve, 1994).

Another issue men deal with is lack of public awareness that men can be as well suited for nursing as women. People commonly assume that a man delivering health care is either a physician or a medical student. One male pediatric nurse commented:

It's very funny, working in pediatrics even today. I have 3-year-old patients and I always introduce myself as, "I'm Bill, and I'm going to be your nurse." And they say, "You can't be a nurse." And I say, "Well, why?" [And they say,] "Well, because you're a guy" (Williams, 1995, p. 68).

Male nursing students may face discrimination from practicing nurses, physicians, and the public. Female nurses often ask male counterparts for assistance in lifting and turning patients, emphasizing physical strength rather than professional expertise. It is all too common for male students to find themselves unwelcome in prenatal clinics, delivery rooms, and other settings in which male physicians have free access.

One male obstetrician in a midsize southeastern community refused to allow a male nursing student in the delivery suite, explaining, "My patients are uncomfortable with a man in the room." The irony of one male health professional restricting the access of another male health professional student based on the student's gender did not escape the notice of the student. Unfortunately, the nurse in charge of the unit chose not to advocate for the student, and the student's clinical instructor was unsuccessful in doing so. He had to transfer to a different clinical group in another hospital to complete his clinical objectives.

This type of incident is not uncommon, as evidenced by News Note 1. Legal cases are being tried in the courts challenging these practices. Ketter (1994) interviewed a man involved in a recent court case who made the observation, "It makes no sense. Men doctors have been treating women for years. What's the difference if

news
note 1

The Following Letter Appeared in Hundreds of U.S. Newspapers in February, 1999.

Dear Ann Landers: I read your column about the woman who needed a breast exam and was offended that the technician was male. The ignorance of the American public about male nurses is shameful.

I am a male nurse who chose this field because I want to make a difference in people's lives. I want to ease their suffering and do what I can for the sick and dying. Male nurses take the same classes as our female counterparts. We have the same training and lose the same amount of sleep, which is considerable. We work right alongside our female colleagues and are licensed by the same state board. When I am assigned to a female patient, it would never occur to me to make a pass or derive any sexual pleasure from that individual. Believe me, a hospital is not the romantic setting that the TV shows project. Please let all the female patients who read your column know that we are there only to make their hospital stay, medical tests and surgery as easy and comfortable as possible. —Everywhere, USA

DEAR EVERYWHERE: Thank you for speaking so eloquently about a subject that needs airing. TV has indeed portrayed hospitals as places where romances flourish and love affairs abound. The shows may romanticize the hospital setting, but the people who work there know it is serious business.

Reprinted with permission of Ann Landers.

it's a doctor or a nurse?" Sometimes it is patients themselves who refuse to be cared for by male nurses even though they have male physicians. Rejection, whether by a patient or a fellow health care professional, is a painful experience for any nurse (Hood, 2002).

Being a male in the nursing profession may have a positive side, however. Williams (1995) discussed some of what she termed "hidden advantages" for men in nursing. She asserted that men are preferred in hiring because of their strength and a perceived potential for better leadership. According to Williams, because of their "renegade status" in a female-dominated profession, men are given more respect and encouraged to increase their education and enter the most prestigious specializations. Many male physicians tend to treat male nurses as equals, as do men in management positions. This may serve as a hidden advantage to men in nursing (Evans, 1997).

Williams also reported that men tend to earn more money than their female counterparts in nursing and that married male nurses are viewed as the traditional breadwinners of their families and are considered more permanent, reliable employees. A study in 2002 revealed that male nurses *do* earn about 12 percent more than female nurses but identifying the reasons for this disparity from among the countless possible variables has proven difficult (Sex Discrimination, 2002).

How can the presence of men in nursing strengthen the profession? Some believe men might help female nurses become more assertive. A male nurse commented on what he believes will have to happen for nursing to gain more respect:

> Women will have to fight and stick up for who they are and what they do, and women do not do that. So many times women in nursing do not support each other, for one thing; more likely they tear each other apart. … I don't think women are strong enough, they're not vocal enough, they're not demanding enough. I'm sure that men are more demanding and will be over the years (Williams, 1989, p. 126).

Another male nurse commented on the lack of career commitment of female nurses:

> The reason I feel career conditions in nursing are so poor is because from the hospital's standpoint, nurses are short-term employees. They come and go. They have babies. They change careers. For whatever individual reason, they're not there long enough to treat them as permanent employees. … Until women as a group treat it [nursing] as a career and insist upon equal benefits as they have in other careers, it's going to stay as it is (Williams, 1989, p. 127).

These attitudes were validated in a study of men in nursing by Cyr (1992). Most female respondents thought of nursing as a "job," whereas male respondents tended to view nursing as a "professional career."

Encouraging Men to Enter Nursing

What can be done to attract more men to nursing? Boughn (1994, p. 31) recommends the following strategies:

1. Correct public misconceptions about males' capacity for doing "caring work" such as nursing.
2. Reeducate high school guidance counselors to target appropriate populations for the rigors of nursing education and nursing practice not previously considered, such as academically capable male students.

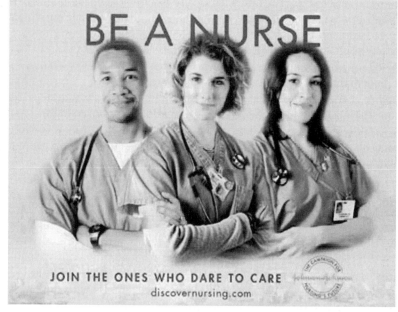

Figure 3-2
An example of an advertisement that depicts men in nursing in a favorable way. (Reprinted with permission from Johnson & Johnson, The Campaign for Nursing's Future.)

3. Involve male nursing students in recruitment efforts and make them visible in recruitment materials. Figure 3-2 is an example of a recruitment ad favorable to gender diversity in nursing.
4. Encourage national occupation publications to present nonsexist information regarding career options for males.
5. Encourage editors of professional journals and other literature to portray male nurses in advertisements depicting nurses.

In support of these ideas, a male nursing professor pointed out that the absence of male role models for students in colleges and universities is a discouragement to potential students. He reported on an initiative to provide mentoring for male nursing students to prepare them for full participation in a profession overwhelmingly dominated by women (Sowell, 1999).

Suggestions from other male nurses for attracting men into nursing include (Hilton, 2002):

1. Create a new title and image, recognizing that the name "nurse" carries a strictly female connotation.
2. Advertise nursing to men in the places they frequent, such as during ballgames and other nationally televised sporting events.
3. Be aware at all times that you are marketing to men, as well as women. For example, at career fairs and recruitment events, avoid giving away pink stethoscope covers or similar feminine favors.

4. Set goals for the percentage of men there will be in the profession in 5 years, 10 years, and so on. Challenge each school to set goals for male enrollment that can lead to the desired percentage being attained nationally.
5. Market the challenges and remunerative aspects of nursing.
6. Provide role models and mentors for male students and new graduates.
7. Promote higher job satisfaction throughout nursing.

Whether men in nursing experience disadvantages or advantages or some of both, one thing is certain: The increasing number of men in nursing will make the profession different. This should be seen as a positive trend, for both feminine and masculine qualities and abilities are needed to strengthen the profession and to treat whole human beings (Figure 3-3).

IMAGE OF NURSING

When you think of a nurse, what image comes to mind? Is it Florence Nightingale floating through the ward carrying her lamp to attend the wounded soldiers? Perhaps you remember a humorous "get well" card depicting a burly, unattractive woman carrying a bedpan under one arm and a huge hypodermic needle in the other hand? Or do you remember seeing soap opera nurses with big hair, lots of makeup, and tight white dresses flirting with the doctors? Nursing has been, and continues to be, colorfully presented and distorted in all forms of expression in society.

Why is image so important? First impressions say a lot about a particular group of people. These perceptions affect attitudes toward the profession of nursing.

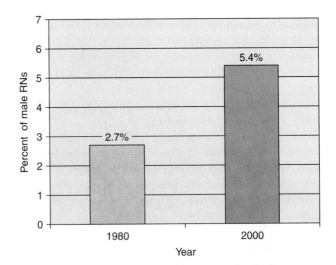

Figure 3-3
Although men still comprise a small percentage of the total RN population, the rate increased 226 percent in the two decades between 1980 and 2000. (Data from U.S. Department of Health and Human Services, Division of Nursing: *The registered nurse population, March 2000: findings from the national sample survey of registered nurses*, Washington, DC, 2001, Government Printing Office, p 8.)

According to studies of public opinion, the public views nurses as highly nurturing and concerned for others but only moderately well educated. In the public's view, physicians cure diseases, whereas nurses are nice and caring (Campbell-Heider, Hart, and Bergren, 1994).

Nursing is difficult for the public to define. As part of a class project in 1998, prenursing students at Auburn University in Alabama surveyed over 800 nonnursing individuals on campus to evaluate their perceptions of nursing. The overwhelming majority of participants responded that nursing is a "caring, helping profession" performed by persons mainly in hospitals or doctors' offices. These global descriptors demonstrate that respondents' understanding of the exact nature of nursing and the qualities required to be a nurse is limited (Huffstutler, Stevenson, Mullins, et al., 1998).

Where Did All the Uniforms Go?

Since most people come into contact with nurses from time to time, why does the public not better understand nursing? An image problem that the nursing profession has had a role in creating is the difficulty in knowing who exactly *are* the registered nurses. Gone are the traditional white caps and uniforms of yesteryear that made registered nurses instantly identifiable. In their place are the ubiquitous scrubs, in which everybody looks alike. While a stethoscope worn around the neck or tucked into a pocket serves to some degree to identify those in direct patient care, even name badges today may not include full names and rarely give titles.

Some hospitals and other health care organizations have contributed to the difficulty in identifying registered nurses by requiring all nursing staff to wear name badges with ambiguous titles such as "Patient Caregiver." This trend coincided with cost cutting by reducing the number of registered nurses employed in direct patient care. This practice is seen by many thoughtful nurses as an attempt to mask the relatively low number of registered nurses remaining in some settings by making everyone look the same.

Perhaps many nurses were glad to see the demise of the traditional caps and white uniforms. It is possible that uniforms projected a stereotypic image rather than a realistic perception of nurses as autonomous providers with a high level of education and scientific expertise (Campbell-Heider, Hart, and Bergren, 1994). Uniforms, however, did help identify registered nurses and differentiate them from the ever-increasing numbers of nonnursing assistive personnel. And it certainly made it easier for patients to identify various personnel. News Note 2 describes one hospital's attempts to redesign nursing attire with the assistance of a fashionable sportswear designer.

Formal or Informal Styles of Address?

Another area of concern for the image of nursing is the use of language and how health professionals address one another. Campbell-Heider and colleagues (1994) speak to this issue by noting that nurses often use their first names when introducing themselves to patients, whereas physicians use their professional titles. These authors believe that this practice reinforces gender role stereotypes and promotes social distance and hierarchical relations between the two disciplines. If formal titles are used for physicians,

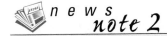

news note 2

After investing large sums of money in redecorating the hospital, administrators at Valley Hospital in Ridgewood, New Jersey, engaged New York clothing designer Yeohlee Teng to create attractive clothing for the more than one thousand Valley Hospital nurses. One goal was to make it possible for patients to distinguish nurses from the other hospital employees. Following 8 months of meetings, design reviews, fabric selections, and workroom fittings, Yeohlee, as she is known professionally, presented muslin prototypes of the new designs to a group of hospital managers and nurses. As nurses modeled one new uniform after another to the assembled group, each was critiqued for function, fit, comfort, and general appeal. In the end, the nurses remained convinced that scrubs were still the most practical, comfortable, and popular choice for nurses at Valley Hospital, disappointing both administrators and the designer.

Seabrook J: The white dress: What should nurses wear? *The New Yorker* 78(4):122-128, 2002.

they should be used for nurses. By using parallel styles of addressing one another, interdependence and mutual respect would be fostered. Campbell-Heider and colleagues (1994) conclude by stating, "Attention to personal symbols of language and dress advance the actuality and image of the professional nurse. Those who respect themselves will convey this attitude to their colleagues and patients" (p. 228).

Nurses cannot and should not attribute their image problems to any other group, including physicians. The nursing profession has major responsibility for improving its own image. Black and Germaine-Warner (1995) suggested a variety of things nurses can do, including the following:

- Recognizing that every nurse can and should work to improve nursing's image
- Participating in professional organizations
- Becoming politically active
- Writing for local media
- Offering technical assistance to the media
- Taking advantage of public speaking opportunities
- Sharing positive aspects of nursing with others

The Public's Perception of Nurses

In spite of internal and external challenges facing the nursing profession, "nurses are generally well thought of by the public and their image is very positive" (Ulmer, 2000). Results of a Harris poll in July 2000, which surveyed more than 1,000 people about their attitudes toward nursing, showed the following results: 92 percent trusted information given by nurses and 85 percent would be "pleased" if their child became a nurse. The accuracy of this high public regard was reinforced by annual Gallup polls from 1999 to 2003. Nurses came out on top of these polls on honesty and ethics in the professions: "Eighty-three percent of the people polled [in 2003] rated the honesty and ethics of nurses as high or very high. In four of the last five years since the nursing profession was added to the poll, nursing has rated No. 1. The only exception was in 2001, when nursing ranked second to firefighters in the wake of the September 11 attacks" (Ulrich, 2003).

Influence of the Media on Nursing's Image

The influence of the media's portrayals of nurses is extremely powerful, and this causes great concern for nursing because the image portrayed has often been negative and demeaning.

Seven major nursing stereotypes commonly portrayed by the media are as follows:
- Angel of mercy
- Handmaiden to the physician
- Woman in white
- Sex symbol
- Unintelligent
- Battle-axe
- Torturer

Muff (1988b) pointed out that almost all forms of media choose to depict nurses as females. They are generally portrayed as unintelligent women in traditional, even obsolete, roles. One probable result of this misrepresentation of nurses in the media is a negative impact on the recruitment of future nurses (Muff, 1988b), especially when this image is contrasted with the generally respectful treatment of physicians in the media.

Aber and Hawkins (1992) studied the portrayal of nurses in advertisements in medical and nursing journals. They found that in both professions' journals, nurses were presented in ways that were stereotypical and demeaning, often wearing long-outdated attire or being portrayed as sex objects and handmaidens to physicians. Aber and Hawkins concluded their report with the following thoughts:

> If we continue to accept an image of nurses as portrayed in our print media as dependent, passive and minor figures in the health care system, then that is what we will continue to be. If we demand that the image be changed to that of active participants in the delivery of care, as independent and interdependent professionals and as major figures in the health care drama, then that is what we will become (p. 293).

Initiatives to Improve Nursing's Image in the Media

A number of initiatives have been undertaken by foundations, corporations, and private individuals and groups to analyze and/or improve nursing's image in the media. Several of the major initiatives in the past 20 years are discussed here.

Nurses of America

From 1988 to 1991, a grant from the Pew Charitable Trusts provided support for an organization known as Nurses of America (NOA). NOA was sponsored by the four Quad-Council Organizations: the American Association of Colleges of Nursing (AACN), the American Nurses Association (ANA), the American Organization of Nurse Executives (AONE), and the National League for Nursing (NLN). Nurses of America initiated a multimedia project designed to inform the public, legislators, and business community about the contributions of contemporary nursing and nursing practice in the delivery of high-quality, cost-effective health care. A result of this project was publication of three Media Watch newsletters to more than 200,000 readers.

Nurses of America also sponsored a 1991 study entitled "Who Counts and Who Doesn't in News Coverage of Health Care." The study found that nurses were "virtually silent" as sources of health care news. Even though nurses represented the largest profession in the health care system, persons in every other "occupational" category (out of 12 categories) were quoted more frequently than nurses about health care issues. Following physicians, the most frequently quoted persons were government officials, business people, patients, family members, other white-collar health professionals, and nonprofessional hospital workers.

According to the NOA report, this study has several implications for the nursing profession:

> In terms of nursing, it is difficult for a group to have influence in the development of public policy and the allocation of resources unless it can be seen and heard as part of the public discussion. The role of nursing as a contributor to the health care system is limited if the press, for whatever reason, does not consider nursing a legitimate or credible source or subject (Nurses of America, 1991, p. 17).

Kalisch and Kalisch

Another study of interest was a comparative analysis of nurse and physician characters in the entertainment media, made by Kalisch and Kalisch (1986). This study revealed that while the role of physicians was presented in an exaggerated, idealistic, and heroic light, "media nurses" were shown in substantially less desired roles:

> Even basic intelligence, rationality, problem-solving abilities and clinical skills are absent in most nurse portrayals. Nurse characters are presented as generally unimportant in health care, largely occupying the background rather than playing an instrumental role in health care. Media nurses are viewed less positively than physicians by other characters, and show little commitment to their careers. The central and diverse role the nurse actually plays in the delivery of health care to the American public is virtually absent in the entertainment media (p. 185).

The Kalisches asserted that these images of nurses not only affect consumers' opinions of nurses but also affect the images nurses hold of themselves. They called for an improvement in the manner in which nurses are portrayed in the media "even if this does require a diminishment of the intensity of the halo that the media physician has worn in recent decades" (p. 193).

Mikulencak; Buresh and Gordon

Mikulencak gave mixed reviews to popular television shows in 1995, pointing out that nurses either loved or hated television medical dramas such as *ER* and *Chicago Hope*. These shows had large audiences. A Neilsen survey published in the *Wall Street Journal* on January 5, 1996, reported that *ER* ranked first in the top 10 prime-time programs with a 30 percent share of the viewing audience. This meant that

30 percent of all switched-on sets during that Neilsen Media Research survey period were tuned to *ER*.

According to Buresh and Gordon (1995), *ER* received high positive reviews from nurses themselves. This was probably due to the fact that a past president of the Emergency Nurses Association, consisting of 24,000 members, was, for a time, an advisor for the producers of *ER*. She conveyed feedback from nurses, suggested story ideas, and helped construct realistic scenarios.

This type of cooperation between nurses and the producers of *ER* was a new phenomenon. In the past, organized nursing struggled with television producers over the image being portrayed. Interestingly, in 2003 the Center for Nursing Advocacy, discussed below, anounced a campaign to convince the producers of ER to portray the nursing profession accurately.

It was the unified power of nurses that launched a successful campaign to eliminate the television program *The Nightingales* in the late 1980s. This program outraged nurses by its depiction of nursing students as sex objects in demeaning situations. Pressure, in the form of a letter-writing campaign by nurses, was coordinated by NOA. This led the producers of this series to cancel the short-lived program.

Another 1980s television series, *China Beach,* depicted nurses as intelligent, autonomous health professionals. This series, which received critical acclaim, was an award-winning drama about nurses in Vietnam. The program was widely praised by nursing groups, and its star became a media spokesperson and advocate for nursing. Unfortunately, the series was canceled, and a letter-writing campaign by nurses calling for the renewal of the series was unsuccessful.

The Woodhull Study on Nursing and the Media

A more recent comprehensive study of nursing in the print media was conducted in September 1997 by 17 students and 3 faculty coordinators from the University of Rochester (New York) School of Nursing (URSN). In this study, sponsored by Sigma Theta Tau International (STTI) and URSN, students examined approximately 20,000 articles from 16 newspapers, magazines, and trade publications. The **Woodhull Study on Nursing and the Media,** as it was called, was named in honor of the late Nancy Woodhull, a founding editor of *USA Today.* Woodhull became an advocate of nursing following her diagnosis of lung cancer when she was impressed with the comprehensive nursing care she received. She suggested the study and assisted in the design of the survey after she became concerned about the absence of media attention to nurses and nursing.

In December 1997, the students presented their findings and recommendations to a mixed audience of nurses and national media representatives at the STTI Biennial Convention. The key finding was "Nurses and the nursing profession are essentially invisible to the media and, consequently, to the American public" (Sigma Theta Tau, 1998, p. 8). The purpose of the Woodhull Study, its major findings, and strategies to guide the nursing profession's collective response are found in Box 3-2.

The Center for Nursing Advocacy

In 2001 a group of graduate students at Johns Hopkins University School of Nursing formed The Center for Nursing Advocacy. Among other concerns, they

Box 3-2 **The Woodhull Study at a Glance: Purpose, Findings, and Recommendations**

Purpose of the Study

The Woodhull Study was designed to survey and analyze the portrayal of health care and nursing in U.S. newspapers, news magazines, and health care industry trade publications.

Key study findings

Nurses and the nursing profession are essentially invisible in media coverage of health care and, consequently, to the American public.

1. Nurses were cited only 4 percent of the time in the over 2,000 health-related articles culled from 16 major news publications.
2. The few references to nurses or nursing that did occur were simply mentioned in passing.
3. In many of the stories, nurses and nursing would have been more germane sources to the story subject matter than the references selected.
4. Health care industry publications were no more likely to take advantage of nursing expertise, focusing more attention on bottom-line issues such as business or policy.

Key study recommendations

1. Both media and nursing should take more proactive roles in establishing an ongoing dialogue.
2. The often-repeated advice in media articles and advertisements to "consult your doctor" ignores the role of nurses in health care and needs to be changed to "consult your primary health care provider."
3. Journalists should distinguish researchers with doctoral degrees from medical doctors to add clarity to health care coverage.
4. To provide comprehensive coverage of health care, the media should include information by and about nurses.
5. It is essential to distinguish health care (the umbrella) from medicine as subject matter in the media.

Adapted from Sigma Theta Tau International: *The Woodhull Study on nursing and the media: health care's invisible partner,* Indianapolis, IN, 1998, Sigma Theta Tau International's Center Nursing Press.

believed that the inadequate and inaccurate portrayal of nurses in the media contributed to public misconceptions about the profession and thereby to the nursing shortage. Since forming, they have engaged in a number of campaigns to improve nursing's image, including commissioning a script for a pilot of a nurse-centered hospital-based television show. You can learn more about this organization and read the pilot script on their website *(http://www.nursing-advocacy.org)*.

What *you* can do to improve nursing's image in the media

Nursing organizations and associations are well equipped to implement the recommended response strategies found in the Woodhull Report and others. But what about individuals? What can individual nurses do to improve the image of nursing portrayed in the media? Box 3-3 presents a checklist for monitoring media images of nurses and nursing. Use this checklist as you view television, watch movies, read

Box 3-3 Checklist for Monitoring Media Images of Nurses and Nursing

Prominence in the Plot

1. Are nurse characters seen in leading or supportive roles?
2. Are nurse characters shown taking an active part in the proceedings, or are they shown primarily in the background (handing instruments, carrying trays, pushing wheelchairs)?
3. To what extent are nurse characters shown in professional roles, engaged in nursing practice?
4. Do nurse characters or other characters provide the actual nursing care?
5. In scenes with nonnursing professionals (physicians, hospital administrators), who does most of the talking?

Demographics

6. Does the portrayal show that men, as well as women, may aspire to a career in nursing?
7. Are nurse characters shown to be of varying ages?
8. Are some nurse characters single and others married?

Personality Traits

9. Are nurse characters portrayed as:

a. Intelligent	e. Sophisticated	i. Nurturant
b. Rational	f. Problem solvers	j. Empathic
c. Confident	g. Assertive	k. Sincere
d. Ambitious	h. Powerful	l. Kind

10. If other health care providers are included in the program, what differences are seen in their personality traits as compared with nurse characters?
11. When nurse characters exhibit personality traits 9a through 9h listed above, do such portrayals show them to be abnormal in some way?

Primary Values

12. Do nurse characters exhibit values for:

    a. Service to others, humanism   b. Scholarship, achievement

13. If other health care providers are included in the program, what differences are seen in their primary values as compared with nurse characters?
14. When nurse characters exhibit the primary values of scholarship and achievement, do such portrayals show them to be abnormal in some way?

Sex Objects

15. Are nurse characters portrayed as sex objects?
16. Are nurse characters referred to in sexually demeaning terms?
17. Are nurse characters presented as appealing because of their physical attractiveness or "cuteness" as opposed to their intellectual capacity, professional commitment, or skill?

Role of the Nurse

18. Is the profession of nursing shown to be an attractive and fulfilling long-term career?
19. Is the work of the nurse characters shown to be creative and exciting?

Continued

Box 3-3 Checklist for Monitoring Media Images of Nurses and Nursing—cont'd

Career Orientation

20. How important is the career of nursing to the nurse character portrayed?
21. How does this compare with other professionals depicted in the program?

Professional Competence

22. Are nurse characters praised for their professional capabilities by other characters?
23. Do nurse characters praise other professionals?
24. Do nurse characters exhibit autonomous judgment in professional matters?
25. Is there a gratuitous message that a nurse's role in health care is a supportive rather than central one?
26. Do nurse characters positively influence patient/family welfare?
27. Are nurse characters shown harming or acting to the detriment of patients?
28. How does the professional competence of nurse characters compare with the professional competence of other health care providers?
29. When nurse characters exhibit professional competence, are they shown to be abnormal in some way?

Education

30. Who actually teaches the nursing students?
31. Who appears to be in charge of nursing education?
32. Is there evidence that the practice of nursing requires special knowledge and skills?
33. What is actually taught to nursing students?

Administration

34. Are any roles filled by nurse administrators or managers, or are all nurse characters shown as staff nurses or students?
35. Is there evidence of an administrative hierarchy in nursing, or are nurses shown answering to physicians or hospital administrators?
36. Are nurse characters shown turning to other nurses for assistance, or are they depicted as relying on a physician or other character (generally male) for guidance, strength, or rescuing?

Overall Assessment and Comments

37. Overall, is this a positive or negative portrayal of nursing? Why or why not?

From *The Changing Image of the Nurse* by Kalisch and Kalisch, ©1987. Adapted by permission of Prentice-Hall, Inc., Upper Saddle River, NJ.

books and newspapers, and look at advertisements. Then take action:

- Write letters to those responsible for negative nursing images on television and in films.
- Write to the companies that sponsor television programs with negative images of nurses.
- Write letters to the editors of publications that present nursing in a less than favorable light.
- Boycott programs, films, and products that promote negative images of nurses and nursing.

In the final analysis, it is the professional responsibility of each and every nurse to reinforce positive images of nursing and, as important, to speak out against negative ones.

SOCIAL PHENOMENA AFFECTING NURSING

Because nursing is an integral part of the social context in which it functions, it is affected by and responds to changes in that larger social environment. Over the course of American nursing history, nurses have responded as individuals to wars and other social phenomena. Contemporary nursing, however, seeks to respond as a profession to social changes that shape our nation.

Although not an exhaustive list, five major social phenomena have been identified for discussion: the aging population, the rise of consumerism, increasing cultural diversity, technological advances, and violence. Each of these issues profoundly affects nursing practice.

Graying of America

Growth in the number of elderly Americans is proceeding at a dramatic rate. In 1990, there were approximately 13 million people 75 years of age or older in the United States. By 1995, that number had risen to nearly 15 million, and in 2000 reached 16.5 million. Demographic projections of the U.S. Bureau of the Census (2002) anticipate the proportion of elderly will grow rapidly in the next few decades. The number of people 75 years of age or older in 2005 is expected to be 17.7 million, and by 2020—well within the working lives of most of today's nursing students—the number is expected to reach 21.8 million. The very old, those 85 and over, represent the fastest growing segment of the total population (Figure 3-4), and they are major users of health services provided by nurses. In contrast, the number of 35- to 44-year-old Americans is expected to decline from 44.7 million in 2000 to 39.6 million by 2020. This phenomenon is often referred to as "the graying of America."

People over age 75 are more likely than younger people to be poor, widowed, female, living alone, and suffering from chronic conditions such as arthritis (50 percent), hypertension (36 percent), and heart disease (32 percent). As a consequence of these and other factors, this age-group uses a disproportionately higher share of health services than other age-groups, with people over 65 having twice as many contacts with the health care system than those under 65 (U.S. Department of Health and Human Services, 2002).

The oldest "baby boomers," those Americans born between 1946 and 1964, will create a bulge in the aging population between the years 2010 and 2030. As these postwar babies age, their large numbers are expected to create an additional strain on the health care system. Up until this point in the history of the United States, the elderly population has always been vastly outnumbered by younger people. The disproportion between healthy, young adults and more fragile elderly adults expected in the next 20 years will create stress on the economic and social systems of our nation. The graying of America will have a profound impact on the health care system and the nursing profession, which will stretch our already-challenged capacity to provide adequate medical and nursing care.

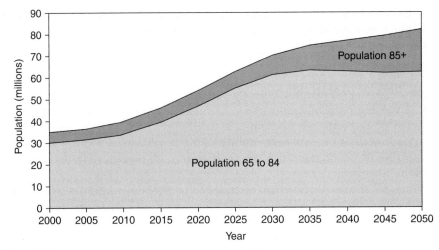

Figure 3-4
Population projections, ages 65 to 84 and ages 85 and over: 2000-2050. (From U. S. Department of Health and Human Services, Health Resources and Services Administration: *Projected supply, demand, and shortages of registered nurses: 2000-2020*, Washington, DC, 2002, Government Printing Office.)

The nursing profession has responded to the aging population by increasing the number of courses offered in gerontological nursing to prepare nurses to care for elders more effectively. Gerontological nursing is now a full-fledged speciality, as evidenced by certification at the generalist, specialist, and nurse practitioner levels offered by the American Nurses Credentialing Center. Colleges of nursing now offer master's-level preparation for gerontological clinical specialists and nurse practitioners. In spite of these responses, much remains to be done to prepare nurses for the dramatic increase in the number of aging patients they will encounter in the next few decades.

Consumer Movement

Since the 1960s, there has been a movement by consumers to make all businesses, including the health care system, more accountable for their actions. The American public, fueled by the principles of **consumerism,** criticized the dehumanization of health care. This led to the development in 1972 of the American Hospital Association's (AHA) document "A Patient's Bill of Rights," which guaranteed certain rights and privileges to every hospitalized patient. "A Patient's Bill of Rights" was revised in 1992, and in 2003 the AHA replaced it with a five-page brochure entitled "The Patient Care Partnership: Understanding Expectations, Rights, and Responsibilities." These brochures are meant to simplify and make more accessible the essentials of the former Patient's Bill of Rights and are available in several languages free of charge through the AHA *(http://www.hospitalconnect.com:80/aha/ptcommunication/partnership/partnership/index.html)*.

Many people believe the 1972 AHA document was the first formal declaration of patients' rights. A little-known fact is that in 1959, 14 years before the AHA action, the NLN issued a statement about patients' rights. Until the AHA's "A Patient's Bill of Rights" was published, however, the prevailing attitude in health care was that providers knew best, and good patients simply followed directions without asking questions. This is known as **medical paternalism.**

The rise of consumerism in health care led to the involvement of consumers in pressing Congress for legislation protecting the public from inadequate care, experimental drugs, poor nutrition, and many other health-related issues. Consumer groups have demanded controls on spiraling health care costs and gained participation on boards of health planning agencies, accrediting bodies, and professional licensing boards. Most state boards of nursing have at least one consumer member.

The emphasis on consumerism is enhanced by the development of community partnerships designed to address health-related issues of concern to citizens. Farley (1994) stated that community partnerships are an outgrowth of an attempt to shift power from health professionals to citizens. The goal of community partnerships is not to eliminate all problems; the goal is to focus the community's energies toward those health-related problems that they are willing to work together to solve. Citizens in every community must be involved in their own health care decisions.

Nurses can play an instrumental role in taking the decision making closer to the consumer. The traditional physician-patient relationship has been a dominant-subordinate one, and the role of consumers in the health care system has been subordinate and passive. To change this traditional relationship, consumers must actively participate in the health care system, be responsible for their own health maintenance, and demand high quality and cost-effectiveness. In 1994 Fagin and Binder pointed out that this is the nursing model of care. They stated that for change to occur, a shift in the locus of control in health matters away from the physician and to the consumer must occur. They recommended that consumers develop personal accountability for their health and medical choices. They further asserted that:

> The time is ripe for transformation in the health care system that will bring consumers into the fold as equals in the delivery of health care and leaders in the promotion of their own care. It will be up to nurses and others to couple health promotion efforts and traditional public health messages with a campaign to empower consumers within the delivery system and expose the mythology of enforced passivity that many Americans believe is endemic to receiving health services. So far only nurses have stepped forward to promote such changes in the delivery of health care (Fagin and Binder, p. 458).

By 1999, these changes were seemingly under way. The 106th United States Congress, responding to the reaction of health care consumers to limited choices and restrictions brought about by managed care, debated a Federal Patient's Bill of Rights. This document, the result of lobbying efforts of nursing organizations, consumers, organized medicine, the American Association of Retired People (AARP), and many others, was designed to ensure that every American had a basic level of care. A version of this legislation was expected to receive Congressional approval shortly after the turn of the century.

As expected, the 107th Congress revisited patient protections. After many months, much debate, and innumerable modifications, the McCain/Edwards/Kennedy Bipartisan Patient Protection Act (S. 1052) was passed by the United States Senate on June 29, 2001. A similar bill, also with numerous modifications, the Ganske/Dingle/Norwood Bipartisan Patient Protection Act (H.R. 2563), passed the House of Representatives on August 2, 2001. As of the press date of this book in 2004, federal patient protection provisions had not yet been passed by the United States Congress.

Cultural Diversity

Since its founding, the United States has been a melting pot of people from many cultures. At one time, most newly immigrated residents were anxious to become assimilated and assumed American names, dress, manners, language, and ways as soon as possible. This is no longer the case. A more accurate description of the United States today would be a "tossed salad." Instead of blending, as in a melting pot, individuals from other countries are increasingly appreciated for the uniqueness and flavor they bring to life in the United States, and many prefer to preserve their own cultural heritage rather than becoming "Americanized."

Diversity in the nation

Measuring the population with accuracy is a challenge the U.S. Census Bureau has faced for its entire history. As the racial diversity of the nation has grown, however, it has become even more difficult. In considering census data, it is important to recognize that the concept of race used by the Census Bureau depends on "self-identification by respondents; that is, the individual's perception of his/her racial identity" (U.S. Bureau of the Census, 2002, p. 5).

The population of most minority racial/ethnic groups in the United States is growing. In 2002 the total population was 284,797,000. Of this number, non-Hispanic whites were the largest group with 196,219,000, or 68.9 percent of the total. The second largest and fastest growing minority group was persons of Hispanic origin, with 36,972,000, or 13 percent. Next in size was the African-American population, numbering 36,247,000 (12.7 percent). Asians numbered 10,983,000 (3.9 percent) followed by Native Americans at 2,726,000 (less than 1 percent). The group identified as "other," which includes anyone who does not mark one of the five major categories on the Census form, was reported at 4,552,000, or 1.6 percent of the total population (U.S. Bureau of the Census, 2002).

Although the size of minority populations varies from state to state, it is expected that within the lifetimes of most students reading this book, the historically dominant Anglo-American (white) culture will become a minority group. This represents a radical change in the demographics and attitudes of the nation. Nursing must also change.

Diversity in the profession

How well are racial/ethnic minorities represented in the nursing profession? The answer is a cause of concern for nursing and governmental leaders nationwide. The fact is that although the number of minority nurses is growing, in 2000 they represented only 12 percent of all registered nurses, up from 10 percent in 1996 and 8 percent in 1980 but still far less than the overall population minority percentage, which stood at 30 percent in 2000 (U.S. Department of Health and Human Services, 2001). Although the number of minority RNs increased 35 percent from 1996 to 2000, whereas nonminority RNs increased only 2 percent, to address the needs of a more culturally diverse society, nursing must increase its recruitment and retention of minority students. Barriers perceived by potential nursing students from minority groups must be eliminated so that the nursing profession can reflect the rich cultural diversity of the population. Nursing leaders recognize that it is necessary to increase the number of people in the profession who have differing worldviews (Buerhaus and Auerbach, 1999; Figure 3-5).

Initiatives to support diversity in nursing

What is nursing doing to respond to the increasing cultural diversity? The response actually began in 1955, when Dr. Madeleine Leininger, a visionary nurse and cultural anthropologist, founded the field of **transcultural nursing.** She defined transcultural nursing as a

> [H]umanistic and scientific area of formal study and practice in nursing which is focused upon differences and similarities among cultures with respect to human care, health (or well-being), and illness based upon the people's cultural values, beliefs, and practices ... [Nurses] use this knowledge to provide culturally specific or culturally congruent nursing care to people (Leininger, 1991, p. 60).

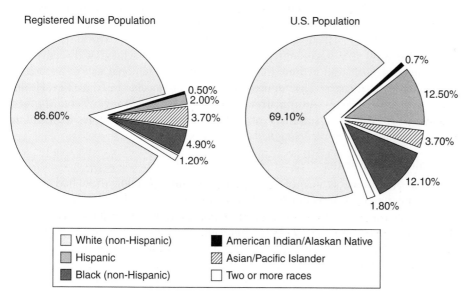

Figure 3-5

Distribution of registered nurses by racial/ethnic background, March 2000. (From U.S. Department of Health and Human Services, Division of Nursing: *The registered nurse population, March 2000: findings from the national sample survey of registered nurses,* Washington, DC, 2001, Government Printing Office, p 9.)

To participate fully in the celebration of diversity and the multicultural society we live in, individual nurses need to develop a sensitivity to and appreciation of the differences among cultures. More than ever before in the history of the profession, today's nurses must integrate knowledge, attitudes, and skills that enhance cross-cultural communication and appropriate interactions with others (Southern Regional Education Board, 1999). This is known as **cultural competence.** Attention to the development of culturally competent nurses has become an integral part of all progressive nursing education programs and is likely to become an even stronger influence in the future. A more thorough discussion of the influence of culture on the family and nursing is found in Chapter 17.

In addition to individual nurses attaining cultural competence, schools of nursing, professional nursing organizations, corporations, and the federal government are seeking to address diversity issues in nursing. Prominent among these efforts is "Nursing's Agenda for the Future," a document published in April 2002 by a steering committee consisting of 19 major nursing organizations. Funded by the American Nurses Foundation, Nursing's Agenda focused on 10 domains or areas that must be addressed by the profession before 2010 to achieve particular goals. The domain related to diversity includes a vision statement and five strategies identified to achieve the vision. It also identifies the organizations that will take the lead in implementing the strategies (the entire document is accessible in .pdf format online at *http://www.nursingworld.org/naf*).

A comprehensive governmental assessment of racial/ethnic diversity within nursing was set forth in a report to the Secretary of Health and Human Services and Congress in 2000 by the National Advisory Council on Nurse Education and Practice (NACNEP). Titled "A National Agenda for Nursing Workforce Racial/Ethnic Diversity," this document presented challenges to achieving diversity and recommended goals and actions that could serve as a national action agenda to address those challenges. The report is available at no charge from The Health Resources and Services Administration *(http://www.ask.hrsa.gov/detail.cfm?id= BHP0008)*. An executive summary of the document can also be accessed online *(http://www.bhpr.hrsa.gov/nursing/nacnep/divrepex.htm)*.

Technological Advances

Advances in biomedical technology and information technology have had a major impact on the practice of nursing. Since the early 1950s, health care has been increasingly supported by advances in technology, and the hospital business has become a major technologically based industry.

Types of technology

Thompson and colleagues (1994) grouped health care technology into three major categories: biomedical, information, and knowledge.

Biomedical technology involves complex machines or implantable devices used in patient care settings—for example pacemakers, insulin pumps, artificial organs, and various monitoring systems. This form of technology affects nursing practice because nurses often assume responsibility for monitoring the data generated from these machines and for assessing the safety and effectiveness of implantable equipment in relation to patient well-being.

Information technology (**IT**) refers to a variety of computer-based applications used to communicate, store, manage, retrieve, and process information. Nurses assumed much of the responsibility for data entry and retrieval with the advent of this technology. Simpson described a **nursing information system** as a:

> [s]oftware system that automates the nursing process, from assessment to evaluation, including patient care documentation. It also includes a means to manage the data necessary for the delivery of patient care, e.g., patient classification, staffing, scheduling and costs. The system can be either a stand-alone system or a sub-system of a larger hospital information system (1992, p. 28).

Increasingly in major medical centers and health care organizations, nursing information systems have become handheld. This means that nurses can enter and access data about the patient directly from the patient's side, whether in an inpatient, outpatient, or home setting. Some of the advantages of this **point of care technology** include (1) improvement in data accuracy and timeliness of documentation, (2) increase in nursing productivity because an electronic chart is always available for ready access, and (3) easy retrieval of patient clinical information (Happ, 1994).

The privacy and confidentiality of patient information is both an ethical and a legal issue. The proliferation of information technologies in health care increases the opportunities for patient confidentiality to be violated. Nurses must use every available mechanism (always signing off properly, protecting passwords, taking care with written materials, telephoning in private) to safeguard patient information when using any form of communication device.

Knowledge technology is described as "technology of the mind." It involves the use of computer systems to transform information into knowledge and to generate new knowledge. Through the creation of "expert systems," this form of technology will assist nurses with clinical judgments about patient management problems in the future. Deciding what expert knowledge to enter in these systems for clinical decision making, however, remains a question that only experienced clinical nurses can answer (Thompson, Amos, and Graves, 1994).

High-tech versus high-touch nursing care

With the proliferation of various types of technology, one might wonder, "Where is the patient?" One of the most widely debated issues is "high-tech" versus "high-touch" nursing. Technological advances now allow nurses to monitor their patients' conditions on computer screens at remote sites. Without even seeing the patient, nurses can gather large amounts of information and make nursing decisions based on that information. The high-technology environment encountered in hospitals has moved into the home as health care has become more community-based. This trend is expected to continue.

It may seem to patients and their families that nurses pay more attention to machines than to patients themselves. Indeed, there is a very real risk that the "effectiveness of a nurse's practice may be diminished if the nurse cannot integrate the information technology into his or her practice in a seamless fashion. A high degree of comfort will lessen the amount of attention that must be given to the technology and will keep it as a tool to facilitate the practice of nursing" (Milholland, 1998, p. 14), as opposed to allowing it to become a distraction. It cannot be overemphasized that nurses must actively guard against ignoring patients' needs for human interaction as a result of attention to technology (Figure 3-6). It is important for nurses to see themselves as liaisons between machines and patients, never forgetting the human being behind the machines.

Nurses' comfort in using technology, regardless of its sophistication, is imperative. But are nurses aware of the many opportunities being opened by the explosion of technologies? Do nurses passively accept technology or actively shape it? Do they "react" to the transfer of technology or do they "act" to ensure that technology and medical device use is "appropriate"? (McConnell and Murphy, 1990, p. 334).

These are questions that bear thoughtful consideration. In 1995, Locsin described a model of **caring technology.** Technology and caring coexist in nursing practice, and Locsin's model was an attempt to explain the interconnectedness of technology and nursing that is still relevant today. Successfully combining technology and caring requires sensitivity to patients' physical, emotional, and spiritual needs. This has always been a part of nursing's skills set. This type of emotional connectivity has been termed **emotional intelligence** (Simpson and Keegan, 2003).

Technology can be viewed either as a strategic opportunity or a strategic threat to nurses, according to Simpson (2003). Box 3-4 describes how one nurse, Patricia Brennan, found the strategic opportunity in a new technology, turning that innovative technological intervention into a caring opportunity.

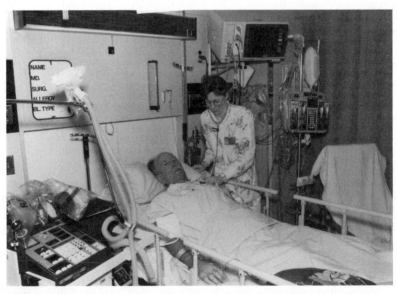

Figure 3-6
Nurses in high-tech environments such as this coronary care unit must remember that the patient also needs human touch. (Photo by Kelly Whalen.)

Box **3-4** Combining Technology and Caring

Over 350,000 Americans undergo coronary artery bypass graft (CABG) surgery each year. It takes up to 6 months for these individuals to recover, and they often experience adverse psychological and physical functioning during that time. Complicating the picture is the fact that hospital stays are shorter than ever, but patients undergoing the procedure are sicker and older than ever. It has become a major challenge for nurses to prepare these patients adequately for discharge and home recovery.

Patricia Brennan, PhD, RN, FAAN, Moehlman Bascan Professor of Nursing and Engineering, University of Wisconsin-Madison, led a research team that developed a system to help bridge the gap between hospitalization and recovery. HeartCare is a "computerized, Internet-based information and support system that provides continuation and enhancement of traditional nursing services" (p. 702) after patients return home. HeartCare includes "patient-centered, individualized and time-relevant information, as well as both peer and professional support to patients recovering from CABG in their homes" (p. 702).

Education about what to expect during recovery and information about self-care are vitally important to patients and can reduce their stress and speed healing. To meet patients' information needs, the research team developed about 200 web pages and selected 360 existing pages that, when combined, addressed most of the information CABG patients seek. They divided the pages into categories of information needed during four time periods during recovery: weeks 1-2, weeks 3-6, weeks 7-12, and weeks 13-26. Information in each period focuses on the tasks of recovery during that period—for example, wound management immediately following discharge or making long-term lifestyle changes during weeks 13-26. In addition to this information, each patient can access e-mail-based peer and professional support.

To deliver the information and support, the team chose a simple-to-operate device, called a WebTV, with preprogrammed functions for ease of access and navigation of the HeartCare website. Patients were trained in the use of the device during hospitalization and it was delivered to each home within 1-2 days of discharge.

The next step in this multiphased research project is to evaluate HeartCare's effect on patient outcomes. A study is being conducted to compare HeartCare with two other cardiac recovery systems. The team concluded that:

"Whilst there will always be a role for nurses in preparing patients for discharge and managing their recovery, well-designed and validated technologies can be of great assistance to nurses in extending and supplementing nursing services from hospital to home" (p. 706).

Brennan PF, Moore SM, Bjornsdottir G, et al: HeartCare: an Internet-based information and support system for patient home recovery after coronary artery bypass graft (CABG) surgery, *J Adv Nurs* 35(5):699-708, 2001.

Violence in America

Nurses are increasingly affected, both personally and professionally, by the prevalence of violence in this country. Despite overwhelming media attention to the problem and congressional debates about gun control, violence continues to be an ugly reality in the lives of many Americans. Perhaps this is because the root causes of violence are complex, multiple, and not readily changeable.

The Surgeon General's Workshop: 1985

Official concerns about violence in America were brought to the attention of the public as early as 1985 when the Surgeon General of the United States identified violence as a major public health issue (Cron, 1986). The resulting Surgeon General's Workshop on Violence and Public Health, held in 1985, brought together more than 100 health professionals to discuss violence-related issues. Since then, thousands of research studies have been done and millions of dollars have been spent in attempts to understand violent behavior, its causes and effects, and effective interventions. Little progress has been made. We *have* learned that the roots of violence extend deep into the historical, social, economic, and cultural soil of our society (Fairly, 1988).

Causes and types of societal violence

Violence has been linked with poverty, family breakdown, racism, poor education, substance abuse, ready availability of weapons, the media, and a culture of tolerance for violence. Intervening in these problems has proved to be politically, economically, and strategically overwhelming; thus the violence continues. In this section we will discuss three major types of violence: sexual assault, domestic abuse, and other assaults with weapons, such as knives and guns. All three of these types of crime are significantly correlated with poverty. The untold physical and emotional damage wrought by these crimes has a profound effect not only on victims but also on the nursing practice.

Sexual assault. The National Institute of Justice estimates that there are more than a million sexual assaults each year, two-thirds of which go unreported. Sexual assault rates have risen four times as fast as the total crime rate in the last decade (American Medical Association, 1996). Victims of sexual assault are usually, but not always, women, with men comprising only 5 percent of the victims. A relatively new nursing role, the **Sexual Assault Nurse Examiner (SANE),** has been created to prepare nurses to interview sexual assault victims in a sensitive manner while treating their injuries and collecting forensic evidence needed to prosecute perpetrators successfully. Children and the elderly are also increasingly victims of sexual assault. The needs of child victims of sexual assault are extraordinary; sexual violence against children can be life-threatening as well as psychologically devastating.

Domestic abuse. It is estimated that between 850,000 and 1.5 million women are assaulted by their domestic partners annually (Bureau of Justice, 1999; Centers for Disease Control, 2000). Domestic abuse is believed to account for more injuries than rape, automobile accidents, and muggings combined. Typically, victims of domestic abuse are vulnerable—most often young women, children, and the elderly. The rate of children dying as a result of maltreatment in the home in 2000 was 1.71 percent per 100,000 children (U.S. Department of Health and Human Services, 2000). Many others are neglected, physically or sexually abused, or psychologically abused. A National Elder Abuse Incidence Study conducted in 1996 found that 551,011 elders, defined as those age 60 or older, were victims of abuse, neglect, and/or self-neglect (National Center on Elder Abuse, 2003). Dealing with battered women (and men) creates the need for nurses to be aware of the sometimes subtle signs of abuse that victims are often unwilling to report for fear of reprisal. Nurses must be able to determine whether the injuries seen could in fact have been caused by the "accident" reported. This requires careful physical assessment and interviewing when abuse is suspected. Failure to report suspected abuse can result in legal action against the nurse.

Assaults with weapons. Assaults with weapons are chiefly perpetrated by young men on other young men. These assaults are the leading cause of spinal cord injuries and emergency ostomy procedures in emergency departments in large cities. Trauma units nationwide are filled with victims of gunshot wounds. Not only are more trauma nurses needed to deal with this type of violence, but additional rehabilitation nursing care, including ostomy nursing care, is also needed, especially in cases of firearm assaults.

Nursing's response to violent crime

In addition to becoming clinically proficient in caring for the physical needs of victims of violence, nurses must meet the emotional and psychiatric needs of these patients. Victims of violence often experience **posttraumatic stress disorder (PTSD)**. This entity was initially identified in Vietnam veterans but has since been diagnosed in victims of rape, incest, domestic violence, and other violence and even in witnesses to violence, including fire, police, and emergency personnel who respond to these crimes. Battered women's syndrome is another disorder created by violence in our culture; unfortunately, there are many others. School nurses must be alert to signs of abuse, as well as potentially violent behavior in students themselves. Gerontology nurses, too, must be alert to signs of abuse. Sadly, there is hardly a group of nurses today whose practices have not been affected by the increase in violent behavior in our society.

How has nursing responded? The Nursing Network on Violence and Abuse International (NNVAI) advocates including spouse abuse content in nursing curricula and educating practicing nurses through continuing education. Individual nurses have qualified to become sexual assault nurse examiners, expert witnesses, trauma nurses, spinal cord rehabilitation specialists, and nurses in other violence-related specialty areas; however, much more can be done. A short list of ideas follows. (You and your classmates can probably think of other ways nurses can be activists in preventing violence.)

- Nurses can become politically active in advocating for health policies that promote nursing research into violence, nursing interventions, and effective violence prevention strategies.
- Nurses can take leadership positions in ensuring that their communities have adequate shelters, rape crisis centers, prevention programs, and coalitions of people concerned with these issues.
- Nurses can advocate for gun control by writing, calling, faxing, e-mailing, and visiting their representatives and senators to support pending legislation.
- Nurses can contribute time and money to initiatives designed to reduce or prevent violence, whoever the victims may be.

Violence against nurses

"The violence that permeates society at large does not stop at the hospital walls" (Archer-Gift, 2003). Violence in the health care workplace is on the rise and becoming a worldwide problem. A 1998 survey by the Colorado Nurses Association found that more than 30 percent of the responding nurses in the seven-state survey had been victims of violence during the past year (Archer-Gift, 2003). In a similar survey in the United Kingdom, an alarming 97 percent of nurses who responded knew a nurse who had been physically assaulted within the past year.

The National Institute for Occupational Safety and Health (NIOSH) has defined workplace violence as any physical assault, threatening behavior, or verbal abuse occurring in the work setting: "It includes but is not limited to beatings, stabbings, suicides, shootings, rapes, near homicides, psychological trauma such as threats, obscene phone calls, an intimidating presence, and harassment of any nature such as being followed, sworn at or shouted at" (OSHA, 1996, p. 1). Workplace violence may be committed by strangers, patients, co-workers, or the victim's personal acquaintances.

Incidents of nurses being injured or killed have occurred in emergency departments, psychiatric facilities, waiting rooms, geriatric units, schools of nursing, and on home visits, among other settings. The type of assaults ranged from threats, slaps, kicks, and shoves to injuries from weapons; many of these assaults have resulted in death.

Although it is not always the case, violence against nurses tends to follow a pattern of nonverbal threatening behavior that escalates to verbal threats or harassment and continues on to actual physical violence. A classic case of escalating levels of violent behavior can, in retrospect, be seen in the behavior of Robert Flores, the University of Arizona College of Nursing student who killed three nursing faculty members and then himself in October 2002. Fellow students and other faculty later reported that his behavior had followed a pattern of increasing threat (Gassen, 2002) as he experienced difficulty passing nursing courses.

Most incidents of workplace violence against nurses do not end as tragically as the Flores case in Arizona, but clearly, violence toward nurses in the workplace is a cause for concern for individual nurses as well as the profession as a whole.

IMBALANCE IN SUPPLY AND DEMAND FOR NURSES

There is nothing new about periodic imbalances between the number of nurses working and available nursing positions. Over the past three decades, there have been infrequent and brief periods of *oversupply* of nurses, at least in urban areas, and more frequent and longer-lasting nursing *shortages*. By far the more common concern is an inadequate supply of registered nurses to meet the health care needs of the nation.

External and Internal Causes of Nursing Shortages

The generic term *nursing shortage* is misleading because actual shortages are usually confined to institutional settings such as hospitals and nursing homes. Causes of shortages may be seen as either external or internal. Internal causes include salary issues, long hours, increased responsibility for unlicensed workers, and significant responsibility with little authority. External causes include changes in demand for nursing services, the increasing age of the American population, greater **patient acuity** (degree of illness) of hospitalized individuals, public perceptions of nursing as a profession, and ever-widening career options for women.

Historical efforts to manage nursing shortages

In the past, each time a shortage of registered nurses became acute, two solutions were tried: (1) increase the supply of nurses and (2) create a less trained worker to supplement the number of nurses. Practical nursing programs, which produce graduates in only 1 year, were created to meet civilian and military needs of the United States during World War II. The nursing shortage of the 1950s stimulated a desire to shorten basic RN programs, and 2-year associate degree programs were the result. In the 1960s, shortages led to the creation of the position of unit manager; this manager was expected to take over certain tasks to relieve nurses, who could then concentrate on providing patient care. The 1970s produced other new positions, such as emergency medical technicians (EMTs), physician's assistants, respiratory therapists, and others who took on various aspects of patient care formerly performed by nurses. The shortage of nurses in the late 1980s resulted in a proposal by the American Medical Association to create yet another "nurse extender" called the registered care technician. (Tired of seeing "solutions" to nursing shortages that entailed substituting unlicensed personnel for nurses, nurses responded quickly and negatively, and the idea of the registered care technician was dropped. This is an example of the collective power nurses have when they unite to act as a group.)

Another method of increasing the supply of nurses is to import them from other English-speaking countries. Nurses from the United Kingdom, Australia, New Zealand, certain Caribbean islands, South Africa, and the Philippines are targeted for recruitment. Companies have been established to prepare them to take the NCLEX-RN successfully in order to practice in this country. Regardless of what American nurses think of this practice, it is widespread, profitable for companies, and continues today.

As mentioned earlier, shortages are often limited to certain geographic areas or specialties. In those cases, redistributing already-licensed RNs can be seen as a solution. Many agencies specialize in providing nurses for short-term assignments, often called "traveling nurses." The American Hospital Association reported in 2003 that 56 percent of hospitals surveyed were using traveling or agency nurses—at great expense—to fill vacancies (Joint Commission on Accreditation of Healthcare Organizations, 2003).

The current shortage

The current nursing shortage, which began in some areas in 2000, is deepening and will continue to do so for the foreseeable future (Figure 3-7). This results from a combination of external and internal factors. A major external factor is an increased demand for nurses because of the growth in total population and especially in the aging population. The major internal factor is the aging of the RN workforce itself. According to the National Sample Survey of Registered Nurses (U.S. Department of Health and Human Services, 2001), there are three aspects contributing to the aging of the RN workforce:

- A decline in the total number of nursing school graduates
- The higher average age of recent graduates
- The aging of the entire existing pool of licensed nurses

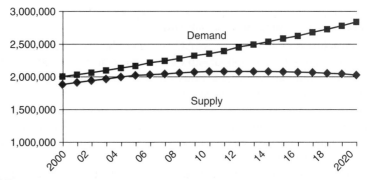

Figure **3-7**

National supply and demand projections for FTE registered nurses, 2000-2020. In 2000, the national supply of FTE (full-time equivalent) registered nurses was estimated at 1.89 million, whereas the demand was estimated at 2 million, a shortage of 110,000, or 6 percent. Based on what is known about trends in the supply of RNs and their anticipated demand, the shortage is expected to grow relatively slowly until 2010, by which time it will have reached 12 percent. At that point, demand will begin to exceed supply at an accelerated rate, and by 2015 the shortage will have almost quadrupled to 20 percent. If not addressed, and if current trends continue, the shortage is projected to grow to 29 percent by 2020. Factors driving the growth in demand include an 18 percent increase in population, a larger proportion of elderly persons, and medical advances that heighten the need for nurses. (From U.S. Department of Health and Human Services, Health Resources and Services Administration: *Projected supply, demand, and shortages of registered nurses: 2000-2020,* Washington, DC, 2002, Government Printing Office, pp 2-3.)

In 2000, the average age of registered nurses was 45.2 years compared with 44.3 years in 1996. As these nurses approach retirement and withdraw from the profession for various reasons, there are not enough younger nurses "in the pipeline" to replace them. This numbers crunch will occur gradually but will peak at a time when the demand for nursing care is at an all-time high because of the fast growing elderly population, the members of which generally use health care at a higher rate than younger people.

Another external factor in the current shortage involves more affluent, well-educated consumers who demand better quality and quantity of health care. In addition, because nurses are identified as the ideal health care workers to provide care in a variety of settings, they are increasingly employed outside hospitals, for example, in ambulatory care clinics, extended care facilities, and in community/home health.

Shortages are sometimes blamed on the phenomenon of nurses leaving hospital work for nonhospital nursing positions, such as in the insurance industry or in pharmaceutical sales. In spite of the fact that in 2000 nearly half a million licensed nurses were employed in fields outside nursing, the fact remains that hospitals employ nearly the same proportion of the total pool of registered nurses, 59 percent, as they did in 1980, when they employed 66 percent. The total number of RNs working in hospitals has increased by nearly one-half million during the same period (U.S. Department of Health and Human Services, 2001). This apparent paradox is accounted for by the fact that today's ratio of nurses to hospitalized patients is higher. This is due to several factors.

- More nursing care hours per capita are being provided to hospitalized patients today because they have illnesses and needs that demand greater attention.
- Patients are discharged to home care as soon as possible to control costs, so there are fewer patients recuperating in the hospital.
- Technological advances, such as open-heart surgery, organ transplants, and the like, have created the need for special care units, staffed with specialized nurses. In these units, because patients are critically ill, one nurse can safely care for only one or two patients.
- Advances in technology prolong lives of chronically ill patients, which in turn creates more need for long-term nursing care.
- Cost-containment measures have caused hospital consolidations, downsizing, and reengineering. The result is more patients in fewer hospitals staffed with reduced numbers of personnel.

Initiatives to provide a stable supply of RNs

Recognizing that dramatic swings in the supply of and demand for registered nurses harm the profession, jeopardize patient care, and are costly to nurses and their employers, organizations inside and outside of nursing have called for mechanisms to ensure more even distribution of the work force. Here are four major initiatives making an impact:

- The Robert Wood Johnson Foundation (RWJF), a private foundation that funds innovative health care initiatives, has committed tens of millions of dollars to pursuing programs that help nursing schools, hospitals, and other health care agencies create regional work force development systems. This initiative is named "Colleagues in Caring."
- Johnson & Johnson, the health care corporation, has funded an initiative called "The Campaign for Nursing's Future" and has contributed over $20 million toward the four-part project. They are working in partnership with the National Student Nurses Association (NSNA), the National League for Nursing (NLN), the American Nurses Association (ANA), the Association of Nurse Executives (AONE), and Sigma Theta Tau International Honor Society of Nursing.
- The federal government is also involved in the effort. On August 1, 2002, President Bush signed into law the Nurse Reinvestment Act, which provided for a number of meaningful incentives to bring more nurses into the profession.
- The American Nurses Credentialing Center (ANCC) Magnet Recognition Program is a model for employers to earn the designation "employer of choice" by implementing a model program designed to attract and retain nurses in acute hospital settings.

Numerous other initiatives by nursing associations, colleges of nursing, and states are also underway. To learn more about the four efforts described above, visit Evolve for WebLinks related to the content of this chapter: **http://evolve.elsevier.com/ Chitty/professional/.**

To date there are no clear-cut solutions to the problem of periodic imbalances in the supply of and demand for nurses. It should be kept in mind that periods of oversupply may actually reflect poor distribution of nurses. Nurses who are willing to relocate away from major population centers have usually been able to find work easily. With dramatic demographic and health care system changes on the horizon, however, periodic shortages and oversupplies of nurses are likely to remain a recurring theme for the immediate future.

Summary of Key Points

- Women have traditionally been socialized to seek security and avoid risk and conflict.
- Because nursing is a female-dominated profession, the development of nursing has been affected by the traditional socialization of women in Western society.
- In the past, nurses themselves have unwittingly contributed to the stereotype by looking outside the profession for solutions rather than dealing with them responsibly within nursing.
- Social trends that have affected nursing include feminism, the women's movement, the consumer movement, the "graying of America," cultural diversity, men in nursing, violence, and technological advances in health care and information management.
- Powerful social influences, such as the media, project an image of nursing that is often distorted. This has led the public to develop misconceptions about nursing and nurses themselves.
- Individual nurses must take direct action when nursing is presented in an unfavorable light in any medium.
- The number of men in nursing is gradually increasing.
- Consumers, aided by information available on the Internet, are becoming more aware and demanding that they be treated as equal members of the health care team.
- Nurses are expected to become culturally competent in order to meet the needs of an increasingly diverse population.
- With the dizzying array of technology in use today, nurses must be always mindful of meeting the human needs of patients.
- Imbalances in the supply of and demand for nurses arise periodically because of changes in society and in health care itself. A number of ongoing initiatives have been designed to ensure an adequate supply of registered nurses.

CRITICAL THINKING QUESTIONS

1. Explain how being a female-dominated profession has affected the development of the nursing profession.
2. Analyze the social influences that affected your decision to enter the nursing profession. Did the media image of nursing and nurses play a positive or negative role? What other influences can you recall?
3. Describe your ideal nurse. What social stereotypes does your description reveal? Does your "ideal nurse" belong to a particular gender, race, or ethnic group?
4. What positive and negative impacts has the consumer movement had on health care in the United States? How do you yourself reflect consumerism when using the health care system?
5. Using the principles of adult learning found in Box 17-8, a copy of the old Patient's Bill of Rights from an earlier edition of this book, and the new brochure being disseminated by the American Hospital Association

(www.hospitalconnect.com:80/aha/ptcommunication/index.html), assess whether and how the new brochure is an improvement.

6. List three social factors that have the potential to stimulate or diminish interest in nursing as a profession and explain their impact. Recommend ways the profession can capitalize on or combat each factor you listed.

7. Describe three actions you personally can take to improve the public's image of nursing in your community.

REFERENCES

Aber CS, Hawkins JW: Portrayal of nurses in advertisements in medical and nursing journals, *IMAGE: J Nurs Sch* 24(4):289-293, 1992.

American Association of Colleges of Nursing: Annual state of the schools, Online, 2002 (*http://www.aacn.nche.edu/Media/annualreport02.pdf*).

American Assembly of Men in Nursing: Purpose and objectives, Online, 2003 (*http://www.aamn.org*).

American Medical Association: Facts about sexual abuse, Online, 1996 (*http://www.acep.org/2,614,0.html*).

Archer-Gift C: Violence towards the caregiver: a growing crisis for professional nursing, Part I. *Michigan Nurse* 76(1):11-12, 2003.

Black VL, Germaine-Warner C: Image of nursing. In Deloughery GL, editor: *Issues and trends in nursing,* St. Louis, 1995, Mosby, pp 455-473.

Boughn S: Why do men choose nursing? *Nurs & Health Care* 15(8):406-411, 1994.

Boughn S: Why women and men choose nursing, *Nurs Health Care Perspect* 22(1):14-19, 2001.

Buerhaus PI, Auerbach D: Slow growth in the United States of the number of minorities in the RN workforce, *IMAGE: J Nurs Sch* 31(2):179-183, 1999.

Bunting S, Campbell JC: Feminism and nursing: historical perspectives. In Chinn PL, editor: *Developing the discipline: critical studies in nursing history and professional issues,* Gaithersburg, MD, 1990, Aspen Publishers, pp 181-195.

Bureau of Justice: Intimate partner violence and age of victim, 1993-1999, Online, 1999 (*http://www.ojp.usdoj.gov/bjs/abstract/ipva99.htm*).

Buresh B, Gordon S: Taking on the TV shows, *Am J Nurs* 95(11):18-20, 1995.

Campbell-Heider N, Hart CA, Bergren MD: Conveying professionalism: working against the old stereotypes. In Bullough B, Bullough V, editors: *Nursing issues for the nineties and beyond,* New York, 1994, Springer, pp 212-231.

Centers for Disease Control and Prevention: Intimate partner violence fact sheet, Online, 2000 (*http://www.cdc.giv/ncipc/dvp/dvam/htm*).

Cron T: The Surgeon General's workshop on violence and public health: review of recommendations, *Pub Health Rep* 101:8-14, 1986.

Cummings SH: Attila the Hun versus Attila the hen: gender socialization of the American nurse, *Nurs Admin Quart* 19(2):19-29, 1995.

Cyr J: Males in nursing, *Nurs Management* 23(7):54-55, 1992.

Evans J: Men in nursing: issues of gender segregation and hidden advantage, *J Adv Nurs* 26: 226-231, 1997.

Fairly A: Family violence: a contemporary social phenomenon, *Proceedings: family violence: public health social work's role in prevention,* Washington, DC, 1988, Department of Health Services Administration.

Farley S: *Developing community partnerships: shifting power from health professionals to citizens.* In McCloskey JC, Grace HK, editors: Current issues in nursing, St. Louis, 1994, Mosby, pp 226-232.

Gary F, Sigsby LM, Campbell D: Feminism: a perspective for the 21st century, *Issues in Mental Health Nursing* 19:139-152, 1998.

Gassen SG: Flores on the edge for years, Arizona Daily Star, Online, November 26, 2002 (*http://www.azstarnet.com/specialreports/21126FLORES.html*).

Gray DP: Feminism and nursing. In Strickland OL, Fishman DJ, editors: *Nursing issues in the 1990s,* Albany, NY, 1994, Delmar, pp 505-527.

Happ B: Point of care technology: Does it improve the quality of patient care? In Strickland OL, Fishman DJ, editors: *Nursing issues in the 1990s,* Albany, NY, 1994, Delmar, pp 254-266.

Hilton L: Why are there so few male nurses? Online, 2002 (*http://www.medzilla.com/press61102.html*).

Hood PR: Life as a male nurse, *RN* 65(2):37-38, 2002.

Huffstutler SY, Stevenson SS, Mullins IL, et al: The public's image of nursing as described to baccalaureate prenursing students, *J Prof Nurs* 14(1):7-13, 1998.

Joint Commission on Accreditation of Healthcare Organizations: Quick statistics on the nursing shortage, Online, 2003 (*http://www.jcaho.org/News+Room/Press+Kits/quick+statistics+on+the+nursing+shortage.htm*).

Kalisch PA, Kalisch BJ: A comparative analysis of nurse and physician characters in the entertainment media, *J Adv Nurs* 11(2):179-195, 1986.

Kalisch PA, Kalisch BJ: *The changing image of the nurse,* Reading, MA, 1987, Addison-Wesley.

Kane D, Thomas B: Nursing and the "F" word, *Nurs Forum* 35(2):17-24, 2000.

Kelly NR, Shoemaker M, Steele T: The experience of being a male student nurse, *J Nurs Ed* 35(4):170-174, 1996.

Ketter J: Sex discrimination targets men in some hospitals, *Am Nurse* 94(1):24, 1994.

Leininger M: Transcultural nursing: the study and practice field, *Imprint* 38(2):55-66, 1991.

Locsin RC: Technology and caring in nursing. In Boykin A, editor: *Power, politics, and public policy: a matter of caring,* New York, 1995, NLN Press, pp 24-36.

McConnell EA, Murphy EK: Nurses' use of technology: an international concern, *Internat Nurs Rev* 37(5):331-334, 1990.

Mikulencak M: Fact or fiction? Nursing and realism on TV's newest medical dramas, *Am Nurse* 95(3):31, 1995.

Milholland DK: Information systems technologies: rewards and risks. In Shinn LJ, editor: *Take control: a guide to risk management* (Tab III), Chicago, 1998, Kirke-VanOrsdale, Inc.

Moss MT: Developing glass-breaking skills, *Nurs Admin Quart* 19(2):41-47, 1995.

Muff J: *Women's issues in nursing: socialization, sexism, and stereotyping,* Prospect Height, IL, 1988a, Waveland Press.

Muff J: Of images and ideals: a look at socialization and sexism in nursing. In Jones AH, editor: *Images of nurses: perspectives from history, art, and literature,* Philadelphia, 1988b, University of Pennsylvania Press, pp 197-220.

National Advisory Council on Nurse Education and Practice: A national agenda for nursing workforce racial/ethnic diversity, Online, 2000 (*http://www.bhpr.hrsa.gov/nursing/nacnep/divrepex.htm*).

National Center on Elder Abuse: The basics: major types of elder abuse, Online, 2003 (*http://www.elderabusecenter.org/basic/index.html*).

National Center for Victims of Crime: Elder victimization, Online, 2002 (*http://www.ncvc.org/resources/statistics/eldervictimization/*).

Nurses of America: *Who counts and who doesn't in news coverage of health care: a project of the Tri-Council of Nursing Organizations,* Washington, DC, 1991, Nurses of America.

Nurses of America: *Summary report and recommendations,* Washington, DC, 1991, Nurses of America.

Nursing's Agenda for the Future, Online, 2002 (*http://www.nursingworld.org/naf*).

Occupational Safety and Health Administration: *Protecting community workers against violence,* Fact sheet No. OSHA 96-53. Washington, DC, 1996, Government Printing Office.

Powell KA, Abels L: Sex-role stereotypes in TV programs aimed at the preschool audience: an analysis of Teletubbies and Barney & Friends, *Women & Language* 25(2):14-22, 2002.

Seabrook J: The white dress: What should nurses wear? *The New Yorker* 78(4):122-128, 2002.

Sex discrimination in the RN labor market? *Nurs Econ* 20(4):155, 2002.

Shea CA: Feminism: the new look in nursing. In McCloskey JC, Grace HK, editors: *Current issues in nursing,* St. Louis, 1994, Mosby, pp 572-579.

Sigma Theta Tau International: *The Woodhull Study on nursing and the media: health care's invisible partner,* Indianapolis, IN, 1998, Sigma Theta Tau International's Center Nursing Press.

Simpson RL: What nursing leaders are saying about technology, *Nurs Management* 23(7): 28-30, 1992.

Simpson RL: It takes a village: improving health care in the 21st century, *Nurs Admin Quart* 27(2):180-183, 2003.

Simpson RL, Keegan AJ: How connected are you? Emotional intelligence in a high-tech world, *Nurs Admin Quart* 26(2):80-86, 2003.

Solchalski J: Nursing shortage redux: turning the corner on an enduring problem, *Health Affairs* 21(5):157, 2002.

Southern Regional Education Board, Council on Collegiate Education for Nursing: *Preparing graduates to meet the needs of diverse populations,* Atlanta, 1999, Southern Regional Education Board.

Sowell R: Personal communication, 1999.

Thompson CB, Amos LK, Graves JR: Knowledge technology: Costs, benefits, and ethical considerations. In McCloskey JC, Grace HK, editors: *Current issues in nursing,* St. Louis, 1994, Mosby, pp 746-751.

Ulmer BC: The image of nursing, *AORN Journal* 71(6):26-27, 2000.

Ulrich B: A matter of trust, *NurseWeek,* Online, 2003 (*http://www.nurseweek.com/ednote/03/121803_ca_sc_print.html*).

U.S. Bureau of the Census: *Statistical abstract of the United States: 2002,* ed 122, Washington, DC, 2002, Government Printing Office.

U.S. Department of Health and Human Services, Children's Bureau: *Child maltreatment 2000,* Chapter 1, Online, 2000 (*http://www.acf.hhs.gov/programs/cb/publications/cm00/chapterone.htm*).

U.S. Department of Health and Human Services, Division of Nursing: *Notes from the national sample survey of RNs, March 1996,* Washington, DC, 1996, Government Printing Office.

U.S. Department of Health and Human Services, Division of Nursing: *The registered nurse population, March 2000: findings from the national sample survey of registered nurses,* Washington, DC, 2001, Government Printing Office.

U.S. Department of Health and Human Services, Health Resources and Services Administration: *Projected supply, demand, and shortages of registered nurses: 2000-2020,* Washington, DC, 2002, Government Printing Office.

Villeneuve MJ: Recruiting and retaining men in nursing: a review of the literature, *J Prof Nurs* 10(4):217-228, 1994.

Williams CL: *Gender differences at work: women and men in nontraditional occupations,* Berkeley, 1989, University of California Press.

Williams CL: Hidden advantages for men in nursing, *Nurs Admin Quart* 19(2):63-70, 1995.

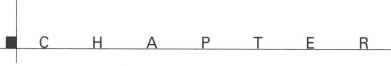

CHAPTER 4

Professional Associations

Diane J. Mancino*

Key Terms

American Association of
  Colleges of Nursing (AACN)
American Nurses
  Association (ANA)
American Organization of
  Nurse Executives (AONE)
Associations
Certification
*Code of Academic and Clinical
  Conduct*
Code of Ethics for Nurses
Collective Action
Collective Bargaining

Constituent Member
  Associations (CMAs)
Contracts
Delegates
Economic and General
  Welfare
Grassroots Activism
International Council of
  Nurses (ICN)
Lobby
Mission
National League for Nursing
  (NLN)

National Student Nurses
  Association (NSNA)
Network
Professional Association
Resolution
Shared Governance
Sigma Theta Tau International
  (STTI)
Unlicensed Assistive
  Personnel
Whistle-blower
Workplace Advocacy

Learning Outcomes

After studying this chapter, students will be able to:

- Explain why professions have associations.
- Demonstrate an understanding of the complex role that associations play in the profession and in society.
- Analyze professional association management of select issues and the political stances or strategies used.
- Recognize the opportunities that associations offer to increase the leadership capacity of nursing students and registered nurses.

*The author wishes to acknowledge the contribution of the following organizations in the preparation of this chapter: American Association of Colleges of Nursing, American Nurses Association, American Organization of Nurse Executives, National League for Nursing, National Student Nurses Association, and Sigma Theta Tau International.

Associations are organizations of members with common interests. Merton defined a **professional association** as "an organization of practitioners who judge one another as professionally competent and have banded together to perform social functions which they cannot perform in their separate capacity as individuals" (1958, p. 50). Associations exist in all professions and in all parts of the world. Although state governments have legal control of nursing licensure, associations provide professional standards of practice and ethical conduct for their members to ensure the public of the availability of high-quality services. Associations also serve their individual members through a variety of services and leadership development opportunities.

WORK OF NURSING ASSOCIATIONS

Major nursing associations in Great Britain, Canada, and the United States all formed at about the same time in the late 1890s. Chapter 1 described the instrumental role played by Isabel Hampton Robb in establishing the forerunners of the **American Nurses Association (ANA)** and the **National League for Nursing (NLN)**. Also mentioned was Lillian Wald's early leadership role in establishing the National Organization of Public Health Nurses.

Nursing association founders had two major concerns: (1) the need for laws to assure the public of a standard of quality nursing care and protection from poorly prepared nurses and (2) lack of standardization in nursing education. The newly formed associations have dealt with these concerns first by successfully lobbying for the establishment of state licensure laws and later by promoting accreditation of schools of nursing.

As society evolves, the nursing profession must change so that it continues to meet its responsibilities to the public. Professional associations provide a vehicle for nurses to meet present and future challenges and work toward positive, profession-wide changes that keep pace with society's complex health needs.

Whom Do Professional Associations Serve?

Nursing associations have three major constituents: the public, the nursing profession, and individual nurses. Associations serve each constituent group in different ways.

They serve the public by establishing codes of ethics and standards of practice, socializing new members to these codes and standards, and enforcing codes and standards in practice. These measures, when combined with state licensure laws, assure the public that nurses are competent professionals with safe standards of practice and appropriate ethical principles.

Associations serve the nursing profession by being the organization through which the interests of its members are pressed collectively and focused politically (Aydelotte, 1990). **Collective action** is a frequently misunderstood term. It simply means that activities are undertaken on behalf of a group of people who have common interests. Professional associations help nurses use collective action to advocate for political responses to benefit recipients of health care and members of the profession.

Associations serve individual members by providing continuing education, recognizing skills in practice by offering certification, and ensuring mechanisms for a professional workplace.

Associations address all these interests by advocating for adequate numbers of well-prepared registered nurses to serve the public, by forming partnerships with the public and other professions, and by ensuring that the profession's work is properly understood and supported by the public, government officials, and other health care professionals. Associations also provide an unparalleled influential national **network** of professionals at all levels and in all specialties who support one another. Belonging to a professional association helps to broaden and enhance professional knowledge and build leadership skills. Members are given the opportunity to work with, learn from, and become leaders. For new graduates, networking opportunities in professional organizations can facilitate the transition from new graduate to professional nurse.

Examples of Professional Association Activities

One of the most important activities of professional associations is communication. Most nursing associations have newsletters, journals, and websites—some have all of these. Publications carry news stories, editorials, and articles of interest to members, information about pending legislation and political issues affecting nursing and health care, and notices of continuing education offerings.

The official newspaper of the American Nurses Association is *The American Nurse*, published six times each year. The *American Journal of Nursing* is the official journal of the ANA. Other associations' publications include *Nursing and Health Care Perspectives*, published bimonthly by the National League for Nursing; *Imprint*, published quarterly by the National Student Nurses Association; *NurseLeader*, published bimonthly by the American Organization of Nurse Executives; *Journal of Professional Nursing*, published bimonthly by the American Association of Colleges of Nursing; and *Journal of Nursing Scholarship*, published quarterly by Sigma Theta Tau International. There are many others. Subscriptions to some journals, such as the National Student Nurses Association's *Imprint* magazine, are included in the association's dues, whereas others must be subscribed to separately. Most publications have reduced student fees—for example, students can subscribe to *The American Nurse* for a nominal fee.

In addition to communicating with members, professional associations engage in many other activities. The following examples offer greater insight into how collective action by association members addresses the needs of members and influences policy development.

Example A

Nursing students who were members of a school chapter of the **National Student Nurses Association (NSNA)** were concerned about attaining adequate educational preparation to practice in complex health care delivery systems before they graduated from nursing school. A group of students became aware that in the practice setting registered nurses are expected to know the basics of intravenous administration, including, for example, starting infusions, knowing the proper vein placement, assessing patients during therapy, and knowing the advantages and disadvantages of different delivery methods.

After researching the problem, they discovered that not all programs preparing students for registered nurse licensure included this competency in their undergraduate curricula. They decided to take collective action by writing a **resolution** to encourage all schools of nursing to incorporate or increase levels of instruction on the concepts of intravenous insertion and therapy in their curricula. As members of the NSNA, they first brought the resolution to their state association convention, where it was presented to the voting members. The resolution passed and was then brought to the NSNA House of Delegates to be presented to more than 500 voting **delegates** (Figure 4-1). During the debate, delegates expressed concerns about insufficient safety devices, fear of becoming infected with blood-borne pathogens, and lack of workers' compensation coverage if infection did occur. Following a lively debate, the resolution was adopted by the House of Delegates and is now part of the NSNA's policies. As a result of this policy, the NSNA works with other organizations, such as the NLN, the AACN, and the Infusion Nurses Society to encourage nursing schools to prepare students with basic intravenous insertion and maintenance theory and skills. In addition, the NSNA will continue to use its communication tools and educational programs to raise awareness about this issue.

By participating in collaborative decision making, students can take important actions on issues critical to them as students and to their future as professional nurses.

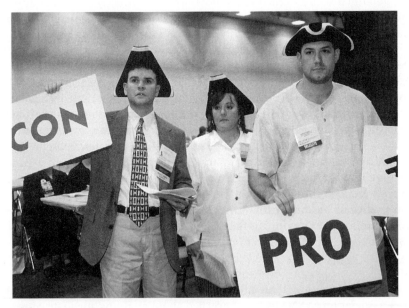

Figure 4-1
Students serving as delegates to the National Student Nurses Association House of Delegates learn leadership and political skills while having fun and meeting others from around the United States, Puerto Rico, and Guam. In this photo, students voice their views about resolutions being considered by the delegates. (Courtesy National Student Nurses Association.)

A powerful synergy results when students from different nursing programs, cultural backgrounds, and perspectives get together to share ideas, analyze issues, make informed decisions, and take collective action.

Example B

Nurses working in a hospital were concerned about inadequate staffing and feared for the well-being of patients. Caring for older, more acutely ill patients with shortened hospital stays was complicated by having fewer staff registered nurses, many of whom were working mandatory overtime hours, and using **unlicensed assistive personnel,** whose skill level was inadequate to meet patient care needs. When registered nurses tried to work within the hospital chain of command to solve staffing problems and to address concerns about quality of care, they found their issues were unresolved. In some cases, those registered nurses raising concerns even became targeted as troublemakers. Many nurses wanted to report unsafe staffing to the appropriate state agency or to the Joint Commission on Accreditation of Healthcare Organizations (JCAHO) but feared reprisal if their employer found out.

Nurses such as these need abundant support, strategies, and resources to tackle issues that obstruct their ability to meet a primary professional imperative: ensuring that patients receive safe and appropriate care. For some, union **contracts** are in place that include provisions giving staff nurses control over scheduling decisions; these contracts may also prohibit or limit mandatory overtime. The majority of nurses, however, do not have contracts. All nurses need to know their rights and responsibilities and to understand the potential consequences of actions and available recourse. In short, they need an organization that can provide this type of information and support.

Working at the state level with their ANA **constituent member associations (CMAs),** as well as with other nurses, registered nurses can shape legislative and regulatory strategies. They can create public education and communication campaigns to ensure that quality of care is monitored and reported in a standardized manner and that nurses advocating for patient well-being are protected in the process. Additional resources come from the ANA to support and augment the work of CMAs and to share strategies and accomplishments with the membership. The ANA and the CMAs are working on protections for nurses who speak out against unsafe patient care practices. Several states have already secured **whistleblower** protections through legislation, and many more are seeking similar protective measures. At the federal level, the ANA has advocated for inclusion of whistleblower protections in the Registered Nurse Safe Staffing Act, which also addresses the development of staffing systems. Further, the ANA also worked with lawmakers to introduce the Safe Nursing and Patient Care Act of 2003, which proposed to limit the use of mandatory overtime scheduling for nurses. Both federal measures are under consideration by the 108th Congress.

Example C

While caring for others, registered nurses routinely faced the risk for a needlestick or sharps injury and exposure to potentially lethal blood-borne pathogens such as human immunodeficiency virus (HIV) and hepatitis C. Although the technology existed to protect health care workers from needlesticks for years, some U.S. hospitals failed to make available safe needle devices, such as retractable needles, to their nursing staff. As a result, registered nurses and other health care workers were sustaining between 600,000 and 1 million needlestick and sharps injuries every year, resulting in at least 1,000 new cases of HIV infection, hepatitis C, or hepatitis B annually. To prevent these workplace injuries, the ANA worked with Congress to craft the Needlestick Safety and Prevention Act, a federal law that became effective in April 2001 and that followed on the heels of several states' actions. This federal law requires health care facility employers to have in place safer needle devices to prevent needlestick and sharps injuries. Among other provisions, the law mandates health care facilities to solicit the input of frontline nurses in selecting and evaluating devices. The ANA continues to work with CMAs to advance legislation to protect nurses not covered by the federal law.

Although these achievements have significantly contributed to reducing the incidence of needlestick and sharps injuries, the ANA is continuing to collaborate with its CMAs to further reduce the risk for occupational exposure to disease through such activities as training workshops, legislative campaigns, and informational support.

Example D

Technologies such as ventilators keep many comatose people alive, even though their quality of life is no longer what they would have desired. Lifetime savings and emotional resources of families may be exhausted by maintaining a family member in a persistent vegetative state.

Nurses frequently face situations in which patients or their families no longer want to continue this kind of existence; yet in the health care system there are not adequate legal and decision mechanisms to deal with end-of-life issues. In 1985, in response to the need for guidance on this and other ethical issues, a special task force of the ANA created a document entitled the *Code for Nurses.* Periodically revised and now known as *The **Code of Ethics for Nurses,*** this document helps nurses clarify their responsibilities. (The 2001 version of *The Code of Ethics for Nurses with Interpretive Statements* can be purchased from *www.nursesbooks.org* or viewed online at *www.nursingworld.org/ethics/code/ethicscode150.htm*).

Although the *Code of Ethics for Nurses* provides broad direction, the ANA also provides specific guidance on a broad range of ethical issues of concern to nurses. A number of ANA position statements have been published, including such diverse topics as:

- Privacy and confidentiality
- HIV-infected nurses, ethical obligations, and disclosure
- HIV infection and nursing students
- Tuberculosis and public health nursing
- Use of placebos for pain management in patients with cancer
- Violence against women

A brief summary of the ANA position statement on assisted suicide can be found in Box 4-1. A comprehensive listing of ANA's position statements and the full text of the statements themselves can be found online *(www.nursingworld.org/readroom/position/index.htm).*

Box **4-1** Summary of the American Nurses Association's Position Statement on Assisted Suicide

The American Nurses Association believes that the nurse should not participate in assisted suicide. Such an act is in violation of the *Code for Nurses with Interpretive Statements (Code for Nurses)* and the ethical traditions of the profession. Nurses, individually and collectively, have an obligation to provide comprehensive and compassionate end-of-life care, which includes the promotion of comfort and the relief of pain, at times forgoing life-sustaining treatments.

There is a continuum of end-of-life choices that encompasses a broad spectrum of interventions ranging from the alleviation of suffering, adequate pain control, do-not-resuscitate orders, and withdrawing/withholding of artificially provided nutrition and hydration, to requests for assisted suicide and active euthanasia. Throughout this continuum nurses can respond to patients with compassion, faithfulness, and support; yet nurses must understand the subtleties and distinctions of these issues in order to respond in a reasoned and ethically permissible manner.

Reprinted with permission of the American Nurses Association: *Position statement on assisted suicide,* Washington, DC, 1994, American Nurses Association.

The NSNA's *Code of Academic and Clinical Conduct* (Box 4-2) provides guidance for nursing students in the personal and professional development of an ethical foundation for nursing practice. In addition, the Code of Professional Conduct offers guidelines for students participating in professional nursing organizations. The NSNA *Student Bill of Rights and Responsibilities* includes grievance procedure guidelines to assist students in understanding due process when situations call for such action. All of these documents are available online *(www.nsna.org/pubs/index.asp)*.

Example E

Schools of nursing are feeling the pressure to expand student capacity in response to the nursing shortage. Although enrollments in entry-level baccalaureate programs were up in both 2001 and 2002, efforts to further increase enrollments are hampered by a shortage of nurse faculty. In fact, over 5,000 qualified nursing school applicants were turned away in both 2000 and 2002, largely as a result of an insufficient number of faculty.

As the representative of baccalaureate and graduate nursing education programs, AACN is working to minimize the impact of the nurse faculty shortage and identify strategies to bridge this gap. AACN leverages its resources to secure federal funding for faculty development programs, collect data on faculty vacancy rates, identify possible solutions, and focus media attention on this issue. The association, along with the ANA, was instrumental in establishing a provision within the Nurse Reinvestment Act of 2002, which created a new Faculty Loan Program to remove financial barriers to careers as nurse faculty.

In May 2003, AACN's Task Force on Future Faculty released a comprehensive white paper titled *Faculty Shortages in Baccalaureate and Graduate Nursing Programs: Scope of the Problem and Strategies for Expanding Supply* to bring attention to this issue. The publication describes the growing faculty shortage, identifies contributing factors, and advances strategies for expanding the future pool of nurse faculty. This paper can be read online *(www.aacn.nche.edu/Publications/WhitePapers/FacultyShortages.htm)*.

Box 4-2 **National Student Nurses Association's Code of Academic and Clinical Conduct**

Preamble

Students of nursing have a responsibility to society in learning the academic theory and clinical skills needed to provide nursing care. The clinical setting presents unique challenges and responsibilities while caring for human beings in a variety of health care environments.

The *Code of Academic and Clinical Conduct* is based on an understanding that to practice nursing as a student is an agreement to uphold the trust which society has placed in us. The statements of the Code provide guidance for the nursing student in the personal development of an ethical foundation and need not be limited strictly to the academic or clinical environment but can assist in the holistic development of the person.

A Code for Nursing Students

As students are involved in the clinical and academic environments, we believe that ethical principles are a necessary guide to professional development. Therefore within these environments we:

1. Advocate for the rights of all clients.
2. Maintain client confidentiality.
3. Take appropriate action to ensure the safety of clients, self, and others.
4. Provide care for the client in a timely, compassionate, and professional manner.
5. Communicate client care in a truthful, timely, and accurate manner.
6. Actively promote the highest level of moral and ethical principles and accept responsibility for our actions.
7. Promote excellence in nursing by encouraging lifelong learning and professional development.
8. Treat others with respect and promote an environment that respects human rights, values, and choice of cultural and spiritual beliefs.
9. Collaborate in every reasonable manner with the academic faculty and clinical staff to ensure the highest quality of client care.
10. Use every opportunity to improve faculty and clinical staff understanding of the learning needs of nursing students.
11. Encourage faculty, clinical staff, and peers to mentor nursing students.
12. Refrain from performing any technique or procedure for which the student has not been adequately trained.
13. Refrain from any deliberate action or omission of care in the academic or clinical setting that creates unnecessary risk for injury to the client, self, or others.
14. Assist the staff nurse or preceptor in ensuring that there is full disclosure and that proper authorizations are obtained from clients regarding any form of treatment or research.
15. Abstain from the use of alcoholic beverages or any substances that impair judgment in the academic and clinical setting.
16. Strive to achieve and maintain an optimal level of personal health.
17. Support access to treatment and rehabilitation for students who are experiencing impairments related to substance abuse and mental or physical health issues.
18. Uphold school policies and regulations related to academic and clinical performance, reserving the right to challenge and critique rules and regulations according to school grievance policy.

Adopted by the NSNA House of Delegates, Nashville, TN, on April 6, 2001.

Example F

Nurse managers and nurse executives in acute care hospitals must deal with the critical issue of the nursing shortage. In previous nursing shortages, great gains were made by concentrating on recruitment efforts. However, that is no longer an effective strategy if it is not combined with efforts directed at retention of the staff who are being recruited and, as important, retention of the staff who are already employed. AONE recognized that this was a significant challenge for nurse leaders and initiated a strategic effort to assist nurse managers and executives in addressing this important issue. AONE members were contacted to identify success stories in both recruitment and retention. These examples were published in several AONE monographs. The monographs listed the initiatives, how they were developed and implemented, and the results. Contact information was also provided so that leaders could talk to one another to explore strategies and results. Several of the best examples were featured in audio-web conferences. In these conferences, dialogue was exchanged among the presenters and the participants so that questions and ideas could be explored. Multiple efforts were directed at disseminating the good practices to other leaders in the field.

Retention programs are vital to any nursing department. These programs are aimed at creating a work environment that is professionally satisfying for the nurses who work there. Key factors in retention of nurses are autonomy for professional practice issues, shared decision making about unit operations and practice, collaborative relationships with other professional colleagues, and support and respect from the nursing leadership. AONE promotes these goals and strategies through publications, education, and advocacy work. The ability to recruit and retain qualified nurses is the first step for any hospital to be able to offer and deliver safe and effective care to patients.

Joining and Using Professional Associations in Nursing

The previous six examples of the range of activities and issues addressed by professional associations demonstrate how associations work on behalf of the profession and ultimately benefit the public by helping nurses to provide high-quality nursing care.

Nurses have a responsibility to belong to one or more nursing associations, both as an extension of their interest in nursing and to support their fellow nurses. A strong professional organization is a characteristic of mature professions (as discussed in Chapter 6). Below is a discussion of how nurses can make effective decisions about which nursing associations to join and how they can learn to use these groups to meet their needs for professional growth and to stimulate activities on behalf of members of the group (otherwise known as collective action).

TYPES OF ASSOCIATIONS

The names of nursing associations and their Internet addresses are provided in Box 4-3. This list dramatically demonstrates the number and variety of associations nurses can join. Understandably, individual nurses often express confusion about

Box **4-3** **Nursing Organizations**

Go to *www.nsna.org* **and click on "Links/Resources" for direct links to the following organizations:**

- Academy of Medical-Surgical Nurses: *www.amsn.inurse.com/*
- Academy of Neonatal Nurses: *www.academyonline.org/*
- Alliance for Psychosocial Nursing: *www.psychnurse.org/*
- Alpha Tau Delta: *www.atdnursing.org/*
- American Academy of Ambulatory Nursing: *www.aaacn.org/*
- American Academy of Nurse Practitioners: *www.aanp.org/*
- American Academy of Nursing: *www.nursingworld.org/aan/*
- American Assembly for Men in Nursing: *www.people.delphiforums.com/brucewilson/*
- American Association for Continuity of Care: *www.continuityofcare.com/*
- American Association for the History of Nursing: *www.aahn.org/*
- American Association of Colleges of Nursing: *www.aacn.nche.edu/*
- American Association of Critical-Care Nurses: *www.aacn.org/*
- American Association of Diabetes Educators: *www.aadenet.org/*
- American Association of Legal Nurse Consultants: *www.aalnc.org/*
- American Association of Neuroscience Nurses: *www.aann.org/*
- American Association of Nurse Anesthetists: *www.aana.com/*
- American Association of Nurse Attorneys: *www.taana.org/*
- American Association of Nurse Life Care Planners: *www.aanlcp.org/*
- American Association of Managed Care Nurses: *www.aamcn.org/*
- American Association of Occupational Health Nurses: *www.aaohn.org/*
- American Association of Office Nurses: *www.aaon.org/*
- American Association of Spinal Cord Injury Nurses: *www.aascin.org/*
- American College of Nurse-Midwives: *www.acnm.org/*
- American College of Nurse Practitioners: *www.nurse.org/acnp/index.shtml*
- American Holistic Nurses Association: *www.ahna.org/*
- American Nephrology Nurses Association: *www.anna.inurse.com/*
- American Nurses Association: *www.nursingworld.org/*
- American Nursing Informatics Association: *www.ania.org/*
- American Organization of Nurse Executives: *www.hospitalconnect.com/DesktopServlet*
- American Psychiatric Nurses Association: *www.apna.org/*
- American Public Health Association—Public Health Nursing Section: *www.csuchico.edu/~horst/*
- American Radiological Nurses Association: *www.arna.net/*
- American Society of Pain Management Nursing: *www.aspmn.org/*
- American Society of Plastic and Reconstructive Surgical Nurses: *www.aspsn.org/*
- American Society of PeriAnesthesia Nurses: *www.aspan.org/*
- Association for Practitioners in Infection Control: *www.apic.org/*
- Association of Black Nursing Faculty: *www.abnfinc.org/index.shtml*
- Association of Camp Nurses: *www.campnurse.org/*
- Association of Child and Adolescent Psychiatric Nursing: *www.ispn-psych.org/html/acapn.html*
- Association of Community Health Nursing Educators: *www.uncc.edu/achne/*
- Association of Nurses in AIDS Care: *www.anacnet.org/*
- Association of periOperative Registered Nurses: *www.aorn.org/*

Box 4-3 **Nursing Organizations—cont'd**

- Association of Pediatric Oncology Nurses: *www.apon.org/*
- Association of Rehabilitation Nurses: *www.rehabnurse.org/*
- Association of Women's Health, Obstetric, and Neonatal Nurses: *www.awhonn.org/*
- Baromedical Nurses Association: *www.hyperbaricnurses.org/*
- Chi Eta Phi: *www.chietaphi.com/*
- Commission on Graduates of Foreign Nursing Schools: *www.cgfns.org/*
- Dermatology Nurses Association: *www.dna.inurse.com/*
- Developmental Disabilities Nurses Association: *www.ddna.org/*
- Emergency Nurses Association: *www.ena.org/*
- Hospice Nurses Association: *www.hpna.org/*
- Infusion Nurses Society: *www.ins1.org/*
- International Association of Forensic Nurses: *www.forensicnurse.org/*
- International Council of Nurses: *www.icn.ch/*
- International Organization of Multiple Sclerosis Nurses: *www.iomsn.org/*
- International Society of Nurses in Cancer Care: *www.isncc.org/*
- International Society of Nurses in Genetics: *www.globalreferrals.com/*
- International Society of Psychiatric–Mental Health Nurses: *www.ispn-psych.org/*
- NANDA International: *www.nanda.org/*
- National Association of Clinical Nurse Specialists: *www.nacns.org/*
- National Association of Directors of Nursing Administration in Long-Term Care: *www.nadona.org/*
- National Association of Hispanic Nurses: *www.thehispanicnurses.org/*
- National Association of Neonatal Nurses: *www.nann.org/*
- National Association of Nurse Massage Therapists: *www.nanmt.org/*
- National Association of Orthopaedic Nurses: *www.orthonurse.org/*
- National Association of Pediatric Nurse Practitioners and Associates: *www.napnap.org/*
- National Association of School Nurses: *www.nasn.org/*
- National Black Nurses Association: *www.nbna.org/*
- National Council of State Boards of Nursing: *www.ncsbn.org/*
- National Flight Nurses Association: *www.astna.org/*
- National Gerontological Nurses Association: *www.ngna.org/*
- National League for Nursing: *www.nln.org/*
- National Nurses in Business Association: *www.nnba.net/*
- National Nursing Staff Development Organization: *www.nnsdo.org/*
- National Organization for the Advancement of Associate Degree Nursing: *www.noadn.org/*
- National Student Nurses Association: *www.nsna.org*
- Nurses Christian Fellowship: *www.intervarsity.org/ncf/ncfindex.html*
- Nurses Society on Addictions: *www.intnsa.org/*
- Nurse Healers Professional Associates International: *www.therapeutic-touch.org/*
- Nurse Practitioners in Women's Health: *www.npwh.org/*
- Nursing Network on Violence Against Women International: *www.nnvawi.org/*
- Nursing Organization of Veterans Affairs: *www.vanurse.org/*
- Nursing Organizations Alliance: *www.nursing-alliance.org/*
- Oncology Nursing Society: *www.ons.org/*

Continued

Box **4-3** Nursing Organizations—cont'd

- Philippine Nurses Association of America: *www.pna-america.org/*
- Sigma Theta Tau International: *www.nursingsociety.org/*
- Society for Vascular Nursing: *www.svnnet.org/html/aboutsvn.htm*
- Society of Gastroenterology Nurses and Associates: *www.sgna.org/*
- Society of Otorhinolaryngology and Head-Neck Nurses: *www.sohnnurse.com/*
- Society of Pediatric Nurses: *www.pedsnurses.org/*
- Society of Trauma Nurses: *www.traumanursesoc.org/*
- Society of Urologic Nurses and Associates: *www.suna.org/*
- Space Nursing Society: *www.geocities.com/spacenursingsociety/*
- Transcultural Nursing Society: *www.tcns.org/*
- Uniformed Nurse Practitioner Association: *www.unpa.org/*
- Wound, Ostomy, and Continence Nurses Society: *www.wocn.org/*

which associations to join. In general, associations can be classified as one of three main types:

1. Broad purpose professional associations
2. Specialty practice associations
3. Special interest associations

An example of a broad purpose association in nursing is the ANA. Individual nurses can belong directly to the ANA or to one of its 54 state and territorial nurses associations known as CMAs. The purposes of the ANA are threefold:

1. To work for the improvement of health standards and the availability of health care services for all people
2. To foster high standards for nursing
3. To stimulate and promote the professional development of nurses and advance their **economic and general welfare**

As the nursing profession's body of knowledge and research grows and diversifies, many nurses limit their practices to specialty practice areas, such as maternal/infant care, school or community health, critical care, or perioperative or emergency/trauma nursing. Members of specialty practice nursing associations frequently choose also to belong to the ANA or one of its CMAs because specialty associations focus only on standards of practice or professional needs of the particular specialty or group.

Examples of special interest organizations include Sigma Theta Tau International (the Honor Society of Nursing, which one must be invited to join) and the American Association for the History of Nursing, which focuses on a particular area of study in nursing. Comprehensive and frequently updated lists of nursing organizations are available online *(www.nurse.org/orgs.shtml* and *www.nursing-world.org/affil/index.htm)*.

Nurses are also connected internationally through the **International Council of Nurses (ICN).** The ICN is a federation of national nurse associations (NNAs), representing nurses in 118 countries. The ANA represents U.S. registered nurses in the ICN, and the NSNA represents U.S. nursing students in the ICN.

Founded in 1899, the ICN is the world's first and widest-reaching international organization for health professionals. Operated by nurses for nurses, the ICN works to ensure quality nursing care for all, sound health policies globally, the advancement of nursing knowledge, the presence worldwide of a respected nursing profession, and a competent and satisfied nursing workforce. For additional details about the ICN's activities in professional nursing practice, nursing regulation, and the socioeconomic welfare of nurses, visit the ICN home page *(www.icn.ch)*.

BENEFITS OF BELONGING TO PROFESSIONAL ASSOCIATIONS

A variety of benefits result from membership in professional associations. Most nurses are drawn to their profession because it exemplifies caring for others, it makes a difference in others' lives, and it demands full use of their intellectual, interpersonal, and emotional talents. Once in nursing, however, both students and practicing nurses have many unique needs.

Developing Leadership Skills

Students have opportunities to learn from and socialize with their peers in school and at the state and national levels of the NSNA. As NSNA members, they benefit from developing leadership and organizational skills to help them in many phases of their professional career and personal lives. Students need to learn how associations function and how to participate as active, effective members. The NSNA, which has local and state chapters in addition to the national organization, provides all of these opportunities and more.

Through a new program, the NSNA Leadership University, the NSNA recognizes students for their leadership and management competencies with a certificate presented at the annual NSNA convention. The NSNA Leadership University provides an opportunity for nursing students to earn academic credit for their participation in NSNA's many leadership activities. From the school chapter level to the state and national levels, nursing students learn how to work in **shared governance** and cooperative relationships with peers, faculty, students in other disciplines, community service organizations, and the public. In addition to preparing students to participate in professional organizations, practicing shared governance also prepares students to work in health care delivery settings that incorporate unit-based decision making, such as magnet hospitals. By participating in the NSNA Leadership University, students learn and practice the skills needed for future leadership. A list of those skills and competencies is provided in Box 4-4. For complete details about the NSNA Leadership University and all of the NSNA's programs, visit their websites *(www.nsna.org* and *www.nsnaleadershipu.org)*.

Nurses have multiple opportunities to exercise leadership. Leadership is not limited to the definition of a formal role. Nurses must be able to lead at the bedside, in clinical teams, and in management teams. Nurses who aspire to formal leadership roles require additional preparation to move into the administrative arenas. In addition to the clinical knowledge and skills, there are business, human resource, organizational behavior, and health care system issues that must be mastered. Leadership is a rewarding and challenging lifelong learning commitment.

Box 4-4 Attributes and Competencies Needed by Future Nurse Leaders and Managers*

- Demonstrates intellectual and analytical capacity
- Develops critical thinking ability
- Develops systems thinking
- Comprehends interdisciplinary models
- Communicates effectively
- Demonstrates effective interpersonal skills
- Listens empathetically and actively
- Adapts quickly to new situations
- Identifies global, national, and local trends
- Accepts high moral and ethical standards
- Manages conflict and masters conflict resolution
- Facilitates collaboration and group process
- Motivates others to participate in decision making
- Demonstrates capacity to interchange leadership/followership roles
- Mentors future leaders
- Empowers others
- Functions as a team player
- Understands strategic/tactical planning, implementation, and outcome evaluation
- Treats all human beings with respect and acceptance
- Strives for an inclusive society
- Balances professional responsibilities and personal life
- Accepts responsibility and accountability for decisions
- Demonstrates a commitment to lifelong learning
- Practices the spirit of cooperation
- Balances "high tech" with "high touch"
- Solves problems creatively
- Demonstrates the capacity for deep introspection and reflection
- Demonstrates the capacity to connect with the spiritual nature of human beings

Compiled by Dr. Diane J. Mancino, Executive Director, NSNA.
*These competencies and attributes are developed during participation in NSNA's leadership activities at the school, state, and national levels of the association. Visit *www.nsnaleadershipu.org* for more details.

Leadership skills are foundation blocks for nursing professional practice. Professional associations offer a supportive environment, in which members can experiment and practice the acquisition of important behavioral skills. Public speaking, project planning, management of resources, and developing resolutions and position papers are opportunities to practice skills essential to formal leadership roles. It is no accident that nurses who are active in associations also tend to be recognized leaders in their work settings.

Professional Association Recognition Through Certification

Practicing nurses want to be recognized, through both compensation and position, for their level of professional expertise. Toward those ends, they may pursue **certification** in a specialty area. Certification is granted through professional associations. As discussed in Chapter 2, certification is a formal but voluntary process of demonstrating expertise in a particular area of nursing. Certified nurses may receive salary supplements and special opportunities. For information about credentials in nursing, visit the website of the ANA's subsidary, the American Nurses Credentialing Center (ANCC), which offers a range of certification credentials *(www.nursingworld.org/ancc)*. Links to additional websites of specialty nursing organizations that offer certification can also be found online *(www.nsna.org/resources/index.asp)*.

Legislative Lobbying Power

As their careers develop, nurses may obtain master's-level and doctoral-level preparation or become nurse practitioners and practice independently outside an institution. These nurses desire and deserve direct reimbursement for their work, and they need state laws that mandate direct reimbursement of nurses. Others work in settings in which there are not enough registered nurses available to provide the quality of care the residents need. These nurses need laws that ensure appropriate RN staffing and control educational requirements for unlicensed assistive personnel.

Some nurses work in settings in which they have little voice in the quality of care, are inadequately compensated for their level of education and responsibility, and are required to "float" to cover specialized units for which they have not been trained. Although nurses may choose to address these issues through union representation, others may decide to improve salary, working conditions, and improve patient care through workplace advocacy strategies, such as initiatives aimed at influencing policymakers.

In each of these instances, nursing's general purpose association, the ANA, is involved in vital work supporting nurses as they fulfill their roles as professionals. The ANA's constituent member associations **lobby** state representatives to support laws affecting nursing, such as those mandating insurance companies to reimburse nurse practitioners for the services they provide. State-level associations also influence debate on laws determining how many registered nurses are required to staff nursing homes and educational requirements for unlicensed assistive personnel, for whom nurses are legally responsible. Many CMAs assist nurses in dealing with workplace issues, such as salaries, working conditions, and appropriate staffing systems, through either **collective bargaining** or workplace advocacy strategies.

Nursing organizations also work collaboratively as coalitions, focusing on specific legislative and regulatory efforts that affect the profession and the delivery of health care. For example, the mission of the Americans for Nursing Shortage Relief (ANSR) coalition is to ensure quality health care for the United States by supporting nurse education and training and building and sustaining an adequate supply of nurses. ANSR works with members of Congress to influence funding for nursing education, to establish loan repayment programs, to create nurse retention strategies, and to advocate for quality patient care. Nurses can become involved at the grassroots level by contacting their representatives in Congress to support these legislative initiatives.

Other Benefits

These examples—developing leadership skills, achieving recognition through certification, and banding together for legislative lobbying and other forms of activism—represent major benefits of association membership. There are many other benefits, such as access to publications, eligibility for group health and life insurance, networking with peers, continuing education opportunities, and discounts on products and services.

DECIDING WHICH ASSOCIATIONS TO JOIN

Once you have decided to belong to an association, visit the group's website to find out more about its activities. Then ask yourself the following questions:

1. What is the **mission** and what are the purposes of this association?
2. Are the association's purposes compatible with my own?
3. How many members are there nationally, statewide, and locally?
4. What activities does the association undertake?
5. How active is the local chapter?
6. What opportunities does the association offer for involvement and leadership development?
7. What are the benefits of membership?
8. Does the association offer continuing education programs?
9. Does this organization lobby for improved health care legislation? How successful is it?
10. Is membership in this association cost-effective?
11. Even if I am not active, what benefit will I derive from the legislative agenda and other activities that the association undertakes to advocate for nurses and patients?

Answering these questions and speaking with current association members should provide nurses with adequate information to make reasoned decisions.

BECOMING AN INVOLVED ASSOCIATION MEMBER

Members get involved with a nursing association by attending meetings, volunteering for leadership and committee involvement, and participating in the association's activities. Members directly influence the association's priorities and, in the absence of association staff, provide the volunteer labor that makes the association function. By becoming active participants in professional associations, nurses become part of something larger than their personal work situation, an organization central to their professional role, and a way through which they can make a difference throughout their professional lives. By adding their voices to those of other nurses, nursing concerns are heard, with a difference in the lives of patients and nurses resulting.

PERSPECTIVES OF NURSING LEADERS ABOUT PROFESSIONAL ASSOCIATIONS

To present readers with a personal view of what organizations do and mean to nurses, the leaders of major nursing associations were asked to describe their organization, the benefits members receive, and what they personally have gained through involvement with their own organizations.

National Student Nurses Association, Matthew Arant, President

The NSNA mission is to organize, represent, and mentor students preparing for initial licensure as registered nurses, as well as those enrolled in baccalaureate completion programs; convey the standards and ethics of the nursing profession; promote development of the skills that students will need as responsible and accountable members of the nursing profession; advocate for high-quality health care; advocate for and contribute to advances in nursing education.

The formation of the National Student Nurses Association was initiated by nursing students while attending the 1952 American Nurses Association Convention. The idea of an independent student nurses association had been in the "making" for a few years before this, but the proposal to finally develop an independent association came to fruition during this convention in Atlantic City (Mancino, 2002).

I would like to break down the NSNA mission to show readers how the NSNA represents and advances the interests of nursing students. The NSNA mission is to ...

"... organize, represent, and mentor students preparing for initial licensure as registered nurses ... "

Just as the nursing profession is dynamic, the NSNA has changed as well. NSNA's current mission statement provides the direction that student nurses need today. The opportunities offered by professional organizations are numerous. As health care advances are made, the need for professionals prepared to make immediate impact is crucial. Active membership in a preprofessional association modeled after professional associations introduces nursing students to an invaluable training ground for success in their future careers.

"... convey the standards and ethics of the nursing profession ... "

To meet the mission statement, the NSNA has developed documents to train and prepare members. The NSNA Code of Ethics is composed of two parts: the Code of Professional Conduct and the Code of Academic and Clinical Conduct (see Box 4-2). These codes, established by NSNA delegates, delineate the expectations in all stages of clinical and academic preparation.

"... promote development of the skills that students will need as responsible and accountable members of the nursing profession ... "

NSNA's bylaws and policies provide structural integrity and continuity for the association and help members to learn and understand what components are beneficial to the success of the professional organizations they will join. Participation in the Annual House of Delegates allows members to bring resolutions before the delegates for consideration. This opportunity provides an arena to debate issues affecting health care and the nursing profession. Members are given the opportunity to express concerns, support, and opposition along with rationales in efforts to persuade delegates to vote for or against a particular resolution.

"... advocate for high-quality health care ... "

As the largest health care force in America, nurses have a responsibility and commitment to provide and advocate for the best care possible for each patient. Understanding how to represent patient needs and encourage progressive changes in health care are vital elements in the role nursing occupies in today's health care setting. The NSNA is instrumental in providing leadership opportunities in which members can participate in and influence this process.

"… advocate for and contribute to advances in nursing education."

Finally, continual progress in nursing education will serve to strengthen health care. Scientifically proven methods and models provide recognized data and support for evidence-based nursing practice. Advanced technology and treatment modalities challenge all nurses to become "lifelong learners."

Each opportunity provided by the NSNA prepares students to operate effectively within the scope of nursing, contribute to the profession of nursing, and further develop personal and professional skills and knowledge as a professional nurse.

In short, the NSNA's mission is to develop nurses who seek to contribute to the advancement of the profession. Energy, idealism, and high hopes mark the faces and hearts of many of our members. Our goal is to help fine-tune and encourage the gifts and talents of each member to carry the tradition and integrity of this profession during his or her lifetime. As the NSNA president, I have learned that it is more important to give one's time and talents to benefit an organization rather than to seek benefit from what the organization provides to the individual member. I encourage all students to begin their journey to becoming a professional nurse by joining NSNA. Please visit *www.nsna.org* and discover how you can contribute right now, as a nursing student, to advance the profession of nursing (Arant, 2003).

American Nurses Association, Barbara A. Blakeney, President

For more than 100 years, the American Nurses Association has represented the nation's registered nurses as the only professional organization that addresses ethics, clinical standards, public policy, and the economic and general welfare of nurses. Through the ANA's constituent member associations, including the federal nurses association (FedNA), as well as associate organizational members (AOMs) and organizational affiliates (specialty nursing organizations), ANA unites nurses' voices for a common cause: to protect patients, support individual nurses, and advance the nursing profession.

ANA has made unprecedented strides at securing a seat for nursing in the national health care policy arena (Figure 4-2). On the international level, the ANA represents U.S. nurses in the ICN.

Under a new structure approved in 2003, ANA will continue to focus on the core issues of the profession, including the nursing shortage, appropriate staffing, workplace rights, workplace health and safety, patient safety/advocacy, and its cornerstone work, ethics and standards.

Concerned with great gaps in the health care system, delegates at ANA's 2003 House of Delegates (HOD) passed a motion calling for ANA to commit itself as an active force in shaping the current debate on health care system reform, ensuring access to care for all. Delegates also requested that ANA investigate and evaluate

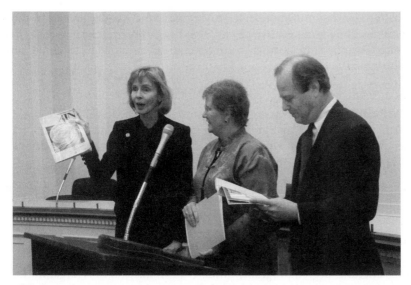

Figure **4-2**
This photograph was taken at a March 2003 press conference announcing the formation of a Congressional Nursing Caucus in the U.S. House of Representatives. ANA President Barbara Blakeney *(center)* looks on as Congresswoman Lois Capps (D-CA) holds a magazine featuring an article on the topic. Founded by Representatives Capps and Ed Whitfield (R-KY, *right*), the purpose of the bipartisan caucus is to educate Congress on all aspects of the nursing profession and how nursing issues affect the delivery of safe, quality care. The caucus was formed after consultation between congressional leaders and ANA. (Courtesy American Nurses Association.)

current proposals for universal health care and the validity of claims regarding cost-containment and the effect on nursing practice and its workforce.

Recently, ANA has advocated for acknowledging, protecting, and strengthening the role of public health nurses and the infrastructure of the public health system, both of which are under increased demands as a result of preparedness requirements for anthrax, smallpox, and other biological threats. As part of this initiative, ANA has developed quality indicators that capture public health nursing functions while advocating for information systems technology and training to strengthen the public health infrastructure. Greater federal funding for public health nursing has also been recommended.

As rich old traditions are blended with the exciting potential of the new, nurses have much to gain from ANA membership. *The American Nurse* and the ANA's Nursing World website *(www.nursingworld.org)* give members unparalleled access to crucial information. Other association benefits include discounts on books and continuing education, as well as certification through the American Nurses Credentialing Center. Through local and state meetings, publications, and vigorous advocacy efforts, CMAs enhance collegiality and enable members to influence state legislation, policy, and workplace concerns. Membership in the American Nurses Association, one or more of its constituent member associations, and an associated organization demonstrates true professionalism on the part of the individual nurse. The ANA, as the voice and advocate of the profession, needs a robust, committed membership in order to continue to advance the profession as a whole (Blakeney, 2003).

National League for Nursing, Dr. Ruth Corcoran, Chief Executive Officer

The National League for Nursing was established in 1893 at the Chicago World's Fair as the Association of School Superintendents of the United States and Canada. As such, it is the oldest organization for nursing in this country. The mission of the NLN is as follows:

> The National League for Nursing advances quality nursing education that prepares the nursing work force to meet the needs of diverse populations in an ever-changing health care environment.

The NLN is the national organization concerned with quality nursing for all types of nursing education programs, from licensed practical nurse programs through doctoral degree programs; until 1998 it was the only organization that accredited schools of nursing as a mechanism for ensuring quality. In 2001, the NLN created a separate corporation, the NLN Accrediting Commission, to fulfill the function of accreditation.

In addition to the very visible activity of accreditation, the NLN is concerned with activities and programs related more broadly to quality education; for example, the NLN is a leader in curriculum development and serves as a resource for cutting-edge knowledge of teaching/learning strategies, particularly relevant for nursing education. NLN provides a testing service that schools of nursing and health care providers use to assist them in assessing student knowledge comprehensively and in various subject areas.

The membership of the NLN is both unique and visionary. It consists of individuals and organizations, such as schools of nursing and other organizations with an interest in nursing education. Individual members include nurses from nursing education and practice settings. Furthermore, there are nonnurse members, which makes the NLN unique among professional associations, in that it is the only professional nursing association that welcomes individuals other than members of the profession. These public members clarify the perspective of people beyond the profession. This inclusiveness of membership is the reason that the name of the organization is the National League *for* Nursing rather than the National League *of* Nursing.

My advice to students is to be active in the NSNA and to become a member of the ANA and a specialty organization *the day you graduate*. Then, within a few years, as you begin to see and understand more fully the benefits and responsibilities of a professional to support our collective vision and voice and begin to reflect on your own education and how education should be shaped to prepare nurses for the future, add the NLN to your membership commitments. These three memberships will keep you connected to the state of science in your practice and to the profession, including its future. For more information about the NLN, visit our website at *www.nln.org* (Corcoran, 2003).

American Association of Colleges of Nursing, Dr. Kathleen Ann Long, President

The **American Association of Colleges of Nursing (AACN)** was established in 1969 to advance nursing education at the baccalaureate and graduate levels, and it remains the only national organization dedicated exclusively to achieving this goal. With more than 570 institutional members, AACN represents the interests of the entire academic unit, including 10,000 nursing school deans and faculty members and more than 150,000 students enrolled in baccalaureate, master's, and doctoral programs in nursing. The association's mission extends to assisting nurse educators in preparing a workforce well equipped to meet the demand for innovative and expanded nursing care.

Although representing a variety of constituent groups, AACN's programming is focused on four key areas:

- Establishing quality standards for nursing education at the baccalaureate and graduate levels
- Assisting deans, directors, and faculty to implement those standards
- Influencing the nursing profession to improve health care
- Promoting public support of baccalaureate and graduate education, research, and practice in nursing

Since its inception, AACN has helped schools of nursing to remain as adaptable and attuned to change as the health care environment itself. AACN's curriculum standards, position statements, issue bulletins, and other educational tools serve as rich resources for nurse educators and students wishing to stay abreast of emerging issues and curricular innovations. The association's website—*www.aacn.nche.edu*—serves as the portal to this information, which may be accessed and circulated to augment both student and faculty learning. AACN encourages nursing school faculty members to continue their professional development and encourages students to embrace education as a means of developing strong competencies in nursing care delivery and exploring new horizons within the nursing profession.

AACN also strives to generate interest in academia as a career option for nurses. The association identifies and shares best practices related to promoting the faculty role to diverse nursing populations. To support faculty development, AACN hosts conferences each year for faculty and advanced practice nursing students. AACN conferences give educators and students personal contact with key decision makers in health care, higher education, and government. Association meetings offer a stimulating source of continuing education and professional development that builds leadership and administrative skill. AACN's role in sparking interest in faculty careers is gaining in importance in light of the intensifying nursing faculty shortage.

Personally, my association with AACN has enriched my leadership development and provided a platform from which to help shape the future of the nursing profession. Through networking opportunities and regular meetings, the association has created a community of scholars interested in improving patient care, building nursing's science base, and steering the profession. I encourage all students and faculty to take advantage of your institution's association with AACN and avail yourself of the information resources and training opportunities available through this organization (Long, 2003).

American Organization of Nurse Executives, Rita Turley, President

The **American Organization of Nurse Executives (AONE)** is an organization for nursing leaders in all areas of nursing practice. Founded in 1966, the organization is 37 years old. AONE is focused on developing and empowering nursing leaders to improve the health care delivery system. The organization is a subsidiary of the American Hospital Association and is the voice of nursing for the American Hospital Association.

AONE offers membership to nursing leaders both nationally and internationally. The goals of AONE are to promote nursing leadership, to advocate for nursing and nursing leadership at the political level, to represent nursing leadership in a variety of settings, and to prepare and educate future nursing leaders. The AONE has taken a national leadership role in developing and disseminating new research on the nursing work environment. Its most recent work is focused on addressing the nursing shortage and foreign nurse recruitment, improving diversity in nursing, and establishing criteria for new models of nursing care delivery. The work of the organization is dynamic, challenging, and complex, just as health care is today.

The AONE offers its members information resources, educational programs, political advocacy, mentoring relationships, and the most current knowledge on nursing leadership available. These offerings are available through face-to-face opportunities, as well as through a robust web-based e-news and e-learning format. Members have the opportunity for active involvement in the organization locally, nationally, and internationally through committees, taskforces, and elected involvement (Turley, 2003).

Sigma Theta Tau International, Dr. Daniel J. Pesut, President

Sigma Theta Tau International (STTI), Honor Society of Nursing, provides leadership and scholarship in practice, education, and research to enhance the health of all people. We support the learning and professional development of our members, who strive to improve nursing care worldwide. The vision of STTI is to create a global community of nurses who lead by using scholarship, technology, and knowledge to improve the health of the world's people.

The honor society is organized into chapters within accredited schools of nursing that grant baccalaureate and higher degrees. Currently, 424 chapters on over 523 college and university campuses provide professional activities and opportunities for approximately 120,000 members residing in 90 different countries and territories. As members of STTI, inductees connect with a global community of leaders and scholars who use their knowledge to influence practice. Participation in the society provides members with opportunities and resources for individualized career development, mentoring, education, publishing, leadership skill development, research, and knowledge building and use.

STTI nurtures the leadership and scholarship skills of members through four primary initiatives:

- Research, including electronic knowledge generation and sharing through the Virginia Henderson International Nursing Library
- Leadership

- Evidence-based nursing
- Programming, publication, and public relations

Research opportunities include funding, paper and poster presentations at international assemblies, and sponsorship for attendance at local, regional, and international research conferences. The Virginia Henderson International Nursing Library provides members with the services of the Registry of Nursing Research, an individualized literature and book review service, clinical knowledge base indexes, and conference abstracts. Leadership opportunities include individually designed mentoring, skills workshops and online resources in clinical leadership and management, publishing, career planning and advising, a job registry, and organizational board leadership. Evidence-based nursing resources include clinically based online case studies, tools and guidelines for practice and the publication, and access to *Worldviews on Evidence-Based Nursing,* a peer-reviewed journal focused on informing practice through knowledge and evidence. Programming opportunities on timely clinical issues are available through local, regional, international, and online offerings. The society's research journal, *Journal of Nursing Scholarship,* and news magazine, *Reflections on Nursing Leadership,* provide opportunities for publishing and showcase nursing knowledge in action. Public relations opportunities include media training and conferences linking media, nursing, and public information officers, as well as opportunities to connect with influential members of other disciplines.

Membership in STTI is an honor that creates new beginnings for professional development in scholarship and leadership. It is a springboard for placing members in the forefront of the profession and is highly regarded by employers and other leaders in the profession and in health care. In summary, STTI provides many avenues globally to connect, develop, and showcase nursing excellence. Please visit our website at *www.nursingsociety.org* for more information about our programs (Pesut, 2003).

ANALYSIS OF SELECTED ISSUES ADDRESSED BY NURSING ASSOCIATIONS

Through the work of associations, practicing nurses and nurse educators can address issues of critical importance to themselves, their students, their patients, and the future of the profession. The NLN, for example, strives to maintain high-quality nursing education programs at all levels of nursing education (associate degree, diploma, baccalaureate, and advanced degree). In another example, the ANA works to unify nurses through its CMAs to benefit nurses and patients through advocacy in work situations and a comprehensive federal legislative agenda. Each of these issues will be described briefly.

Nursing Education Issues

High-quality nursing education is important to nursing students, nurse educators, registered nurses, and the recipients of nursing care. The NLN helps to advance the quality of nursing education, which prepares the nursing workforce to meet the needs of diverse populations in an ever-changing health care environment. For more than 100 years, the NLN has helped to shape the development of nursing curricula and educational models that anticipate, reflect, and respond to the changing health care needs of diverse student and patient populations. The dynamic nature of nursing education and the need to examine priorities continually is reflected in the NLN's Priorities for Nursing Education Research. These priorities suggest areas of research that are important to nursing students, including:

1. Nursing students should understand the changing role of the student in learning. New learning structures will demand that the nursing student take a more active role in the education process. This new model will focus more on the participation of the student, as opposed to the student simply attending lectures.

2. Nursing students should understand the coming changes in nursing education that focus on bridging the gap between education and practice.

3. Nursing students should expect not only to be engaged in the health care of their communities for educational purposes but also to play an integral role in the delivery of the health care in that community.

By encouraging nursing education scholars to address these priorities, the NLN ensures that nursing education remains relevant to a dynamic health care system and society.

AACN's curriculum standards provide a framework for positioning baccalaureate and graduate-degree nursing programs to meet today's health care challenges. Nursing deans and faculty nationwide have implemented the association's guidelines in curricula used to prepare professional nurses to thrive in a system marked by continual change. AACN produced the first national guidelines to define the essential knowledge, skills, and values expected of new baccalaureate-prepared nurses, the first comprehensive standards for master's degree education of advanced practice nurses, and the first indicators of quality for doctoral nursing programs. To ensure program quality, AACN also established the Commission on Collegiate Nursing Education, the nation's only agency focused exclusively on accrediting baccalaureate and graduate-degree nursing education programs.

Throughout its history, AACN has worked collaboratively with the nursing community to produce specialized sets of guidelines that influence how nurses are educated across the country. AACN's most recent work in setting curriculum standards extends to several emerging areas of nursing education and practice. These include developing competencies for nurses to respond to bioterrorism and other mass casualty events through affiliation with the International Nursing Coalition for Mass Casualty Education, partnering with the National Organization of Nurse Practitioner Faculties to release primary care competencies for nurse practitioners, and working with The John A. Hartford Foundation of New York to strengthen geriatric content in entry-level nursing programs. Together with an expert panel from the practice community, AACN is currently developing a curriculum to prepare nurse graduates for a new practice role, the Clinical Nurse Leader.

The transition from being a student to becoming a professional nurse in the workplace is a journey that all nurses must take. Students face significant challenge as they move into the current environment as graduate nurses, and there is growing recognition that this transition period is critical. New models such as residency programs are creating bridges for students so that they can be successful in their first clinical roles. It is also critical that once safely across that bridge, graduate nurses continue to reach out to those following them and help those students to cross over successfully as well.

Advocacy in Work Situations

Nursing advocacy embraces activities including education, lobbying, and individual and collective advocacy in order to advance nursing's agenda. Individual nurses may use the tools of collective bargaining or **workplace advocacy** to achieve their objectives.

As mentioned earlier, in 2003, the ANA's policy-setting body, the House of Delegates, passed historic bylaws changes aimed at better meeting the needs of the nation's 2.7 million nurses through the creation of independent yet affiliated collective bargaining and workplace advocacy "arms" of the association. The United American Nurses (UAN), AFL-CIO, is a national labor union focusing on broad-reaching workplace issues and supporting CMAs in organizing and collective bargaining efforts. The UAN is the largest, most effective union for registered nurses in the country, representing nearly 100,000 RNs nationwide. It uses organizing and collective bargaining to help members reach their goals, such as ending mandatory overtime and improving staffing levels through legally binding, negotiated contract language.

The other arm of the ANA, the Center for American Nurses (CAN), works to strengthen the voice of individual nurses not represented by collective bargaining. It uses advocacy strategies, such as educational campaigns, that seek to provide skills for nurses to use in their individual work settings. Both the UAN and CAN are associate organizational members of the ANA, a new membership category created by the 2003 changes in the ANA bylaws. The ANA also uses advocacy strategies, from federal lobbying to media campaigns, to support its core issues: nursing shortage, appropriate staffing, patient safety and advocacy, workplace health and safety, and workplace rights.

Federal Lobbying Efforts by Professional Associations

All professional associations have an interest in shaping federal legislation favorable to their constituents and the publics they serve. Some examples of these efforts are reviewed below.

American Nurses Association legislative initiatives

The ANA has achieved many important and historic advances at the federal level in recent years. Its strength on Capitol Hill is a direct result of the collaboration and coordination of three critical components of its federal legislative program: lobbying, grassroots activities, and political action. The backbone of nursing's power in the U.S. Congress is the political and **grassroots activism** of thousands of nurses across the country. As that participation continues to increase, so will the voices and victories of nursing in the federal legislative arena.

Legislative agendas are constantly changing as new congressional sessions occur. Some examples of the ANA's legislative agenda for the first session of the 108th Congress (2003) were:

- Registered Nurse Safe Staffing Act. The ANA wants to ensure that patients receive safe, quality nursing care in hospitals and other health care institutions. That means having sufficient registered nursing staff to provide care.

This legislation mandates the development of staffing systems that require the input of direct-care registered nurses. It also provides protections for registered nurses who speak out about patient care issues.

■ Safe Nursing and Patient Care Act. The ANA has been working aggressively on several fronts to stop health care employers from mandating nurses to work overtime, a practice that puts the health of nurses and patients in jeopardy. This legislation would prohibit health care facilities that receive Medicare funding from requiring nurses to work beyond their regularly scheduled shift. Furthermore, nurses could not be forced to work more than 12 hours in a 24-hour period or for more than 80 hours in a 2-week period.

■ Medicaid reimbursement. The ANA continues to support measures that expand patient access to quality health care. These measures include requiring states to offer Medicaid coverage for primary health care services provided by advanced practice registered nurses (APRNs). One of the measures, the Medicaid Nursing Incentive Act, addresses APRN coverage limitations by requiring Medicaid managed care plans to include nurse practitioners, clinical nurse specialists, and certified nurse-midwives on their provider panels.

■ Nurse Education Act. Every year, the ANA must garner support from Congress and the White House to include sufficient funds in the federal budget for programs under the Nurse Education Act. Those programs include the awarding of grants and scholarships to nurses who want to pursue advanced degrees, as well as to persons from underrepresented populations who want to attend nursing programs. During the 108th Congress, the ANA called on its grassroots network—Nurses Strategic Action Team (N-STAT)—to urge their senators and representatives to appropriate at least $175 million for fiscal year 2004 for the Nurse Education Act, which the ANA believes is vital to stemming the growing nursing shortage.

■ Medicare. The ANA has continued to lobby Congress and health care policy-makers for reforms in the Medicare system to ensure seniors have access to the multifaceted care they need. One of the largest issues of debate has been prescription drug coverage. In 2003, as the House and Senate began ironing out differences in their Medicare modernization and drug prescription bills, the ANA voiced its concerns about gaps that would force beneficiaries to continue to pay prohibitively high costs for the medications they need. The American Nurses Association has also proposed to reform the ailing Medicare program, reaffirming a long-standing commitment to strengthening the program. Recommending that much of Medicare's framework remain the same, the ANA also advocated strong measures to simplify and improve the program to better meet the diverse health care needs of the growing population of older Americans. A fundamental underpinning of the ANA's proposal involved refocusing the Medicare program on primary health care services, prevention, wellness, and early intervention. This is in contrast to the "medical model of care" in which the emphasis is on treatment of disease and in which coordination of care among health care providers is negligible. The ANA was the first health professional association to support Medicare when it was introduced as legislation and has been an ardent supporter of the Medicare program since its inception in 1965. The ANA will remain actively involved in the public policy debate surrounding Medicare reform.

- Workplace Rights. The ANA and its members scored a major victory when the U.S. House of Representatives dropped a proposed bill that would have allowed employers to substitute compensatory time off for time-and-a-half overtime pay. The ANA sent a letter to every member of Congress and also urged nurses to call on their lawmakers to defeat this measure. For many nurses, overtime pay is essential to meeting their financial needs. Furthermore, the ANA vehemently opposed the idea that employers would "pay" workers with a promise of time off in the future when the employer—not the worker—deemed it convenient.
- Health and Safety. In a world of bioterrorist threats and emerging diseases, the ANA has worked to ensure that the health and well-being of Americans and nurses are safeguarded. In one effort, the ANA worked with White House and key congressional leaders to protect health care providers who might be harmed by the smallpox vaccine. The ANA also pushed for adequate funding of public health departments to ensure they can provide routine services, such as well baby care, in addition to meeting bioterrorism preparedness demands. Among other activities, in August 2003, the ANA participated in a national forum looking at the state of health in America.

Visit the American Nurses Association website at *www.nursingworld.org/gov* for the latest ANA legislative initiatives.

American Association of Colleges of Nursing legislative initiatives

Although sharing many of ANA's legislative priorities, AACN focuses its advocacy efforts on issues specifically related to nursing education. AACN works closely with Congress and federal agencies to ensure funding and regulatory policies that provide stable and sufficient support for nursing education. The association has been effective in securing sustained federal funding for nursing education and research, in shaping legislative and regulatory policy affecting nursing school programming, and in ensuring continuing financial assistance for nursing students.

AACN played a pivotal role in the creation of a new Nurse Faculty Loan Program contained in the Nurse Reinvestment Act of 2002. Through this program, nurses prepared at the graduate level are entitled to educational loan forgiveness in exchange for a commitment to serve as nursing faculty. Beyond this important initiative, AACN's governmental affairs staff members work to increase funding for Title VII and Title VIII nursing education programs, support funding for the National Institute of Nursing Research, and encourage legislation to alleviate the growing shortage of registered nurses.

AACN staff members actively monitor legislation and regulations to identify emerging issues that may have an impact on nursing education and research. New issues of importance to the association include bioterrorism preparedness, changes to Medicare and Medicaid reimbursements, and initiatives to ensure patient safety. When necessary, AACN mobilizes the nursing education community and launches grassroots campaigns to rally support for programs that advance professional nursing practice.

Visit the AACN's website at *www.aacn.nche.edu/Government/index.htm* for details on the association's government advocacy efforts.

Summary of Key Points

- Professional associations are the vehicle through which nursing takes collective action to improve both the nursing profession and health care delivery.
- There are many nursing associations from which to choose, and they offer a variety of benefits to the public, to the nursing profession as a whole, and to individual members.
- Membership in professional associations is essential for professionals, but selecting which associations to join can be a challenge. Prospective members should ask several key questions to help them select wisely.
- The National Student Nurses Association develops leaders whose future membership in their states constituent member associations will strengthen the profession.
- The American Nurses Association, which represents all nurses, is at the forefront in addressing issues of importance to all nurses, including nurse staffing, occupational health and safety, as well as the enactment of legislative proposals that address protections for nurses in the workplace and patients' rights.
- The National League for Nursing ensures quality of nursing education through accreditation of schools of nursing, consultation in curriculum construction and teaching-learning strategies, and standardized aptitude and achievement testing.
- The American Association of Colleges of Nursing advocates on behalf of baccalaureate and higher-degree nursing programs and serves as an accrediting body for those programs.
- The American Organization of Nurse Executives focuses on developing and empowering nursing leaders to improve the health care delivery system.
- Sigma Theta Tau International is the Honor Society for Nursing. Membership is by invitation. STTI encourages scholarship, research, evidence-based practice, and leadership skills in its members.
- All professional nursing organizations work to improve the profession through legislative initiatives.

CRITICAL THINKING QUESTIONS

1. Look in a local newspaper for articles about federal legislation that support nursing's concerns, such as the Nurse Education Act, or other nursing- or patient-related legislation pending in your state. Write a letter to the editor of your local paper about these bills, taking a stand on the issues.
2. Find out whether there is a student nurses association on your campus. If there is, learn all you can about it and consider joining. If there isn't one, consider establishing one. (Resources: go to *www.nsna.org;* click on "Program Activities.")
3. As a student, attend a local or state nurses association meeting to gain a better sense of the issues in the profession, so that you can be prepared for what lies ahead when you graduate. How is the association addressing these issues? Do they interest you? How can you get involved?
   Consider the following hypothetical situations:
4. You read in a local newspaper that students at your university have a high rate of drug and alcohol use. The following week, a story appears about a senior university student who died following a car crash. The student was driving under the influence of alcohol. How can nursing students address the need for education

about drug and alcohol use? What collective action can you initiate to address this or another issue of importance to your college or university community? (Resource: go to *www.nsna.org;* click on "Publications" to download Guidelines for Planning Community Health Projects.)

5. The demand for nursing services is increasing, but the availability of registered nurses will not meet this demand. The student nurses association chapter has formed a recruitment committee to address this issue and answer the following questions: Why are students not considering nursing as a career? Why are students considering nursing as a career? How many registered nurses will be needed in the future? Why do many nursing programs have waiting lists to enter the program? Plan a collective action project that can be implemented by the student nurses association to increase interest in the nursing profession. (Resource: go to *www.nsna.org;* click on "Publications" to download Guidelines for Planning Breakthrough to Nursing Projects.)

6. Students at your school must struggle to pay tuition. Many students work part-time while attending school full-time. They have taken out student loans and have applied for scholarships to help pay for tuition, books, and other school-related expenses. A faculty member announces in class that the Nurse Reinvestment Act is going before Congress for funding authorization. What collective actions can the student nurses association take to ask Congress to increase funding for undergraduate nursing education and for student loan repayment programs? (Resources: go to *www.nsna.org;* click on "Publications" to download Guidelines for Planning Legislative Activities.)

7. A classmate asks you to share a paper you prepared for a leadership course she is now taking so that she can see how you handled the assignment. You willingly give her a copy of your "A" paper. At the end of the semester, the faculty member who teaches the leadership course calls you into her office. She shows you the paper you wrote for her course last semester, but it now has your classmate's name on it instead of yours! What collective action can the student nurses association take to prevent plagiarism and cheating? (Resources: go to *www.nsna.org;* click on "Publications" to download the NSNA Bill of Rights and Responsibilities for Students of Nursing and the NSNA Code of Academic and Clinical Professional Conduct.)

8. As emerging members of the profession, nursing students should be familiar with issues affecting nursing education, research, and practice. "Hot issues" in nursing are often detailed in white papers produced by professional associations like AACN. These papers generally include a detailed analysis of a particular topic and recommendations for action. Read an AACN white paper of your choice (see *www.aacn.nche.edu*), summarize the issue, and outline the action steps needed to influence the national agenda related to this concern.

REFERENCES

American Nurses Association: *Position statement on assisted suicide,* Washington, DC, 1994, American Nurses Association.

American Nurses Association: *Code of ethics for nurses with interpretive statements,* Washington, DC, 2001, American Nurses Publishing.

Arant M: Personal communication, 2003.

Aydelotte MK: The evolving profession: The role of the professional organization. In Chaska NL, editor: *The nursing profession: turning points,* St. Louis, 1990, Mosby.

Blakeney B: Personal communication, 2003.

Corcoran R: Personal communication, 2003.

Long KA: Personal communication, 2003.

Mancino D: *50 years of the National Student Nurses Association,* New York, 2002, National Student Nurses Association.

Merton RK: The functions of the professional association, *Am J Nurs* 58(1):50-54, 1958.

National Student Nurses Association: *Mission statement,* New York, 2002, National Student Nurses Association.

Pesut DJ: Personal communication, 2003.

Turley R: Personal communication, 2003.

5

Nursing Today

Kay Kittrell Chitty

Learning Outcomes

After studying this chapter, students will be able to:

- Describe the "average" registered nurse of today.
- Identify the broad range of settings in which today's registered nurses practice.
- Discuss emerging practice opportunities for nurses.
- Cite similarities and differences among nursing roles in various practice settings.
- Explain the roles of advanced practice nurses and the preparation required to assume these roles.

Far-reaching economic and social changes in the United States have profoundly affected the way health care is provided. Many of the changes outlined in Chapter 3 have opened avenues to new and exciting employment opportunities for nurses. This chapter provides an overview of the registered nurse (RN) population in the United States and briefly presents a selection of employment options available to nurses today in hospital and community settings. Integrated into this chapter are interviews with several nurses who describe their work and the rewards and challenges of their positions.

CURRENT STATUS OF NURSING IN THE UNITED STATES

What are the profiles of typical nurses today? Is there an "average" registered nurse? Where do nurses work? What incomes do they earn in today's market? Are there enough opportunities to provide employment for all nurses? How have health care technologies affected nurses and nursing practice? As health care changes and nursing evolves to meet new challenges, the answers to these questions also change.

Characteristics of Registered Nurses

To provide current information about practicing nurses, the federal government conducts a national survey of actively licensed registered nurses in the United States every 4 years. The most recent survey was conducted in March 2000. Data from this survey were published in 2001 by the U.S. Department of Health and Human Services, Division of Nursing, in a document entitled *The Registered Nurse Population: March 2000.* This document and information provided by the American Nurses Association (ANA) and the National League for Nursing (NLN) provide a comprehensive look at the characteristics of registered nurses today.

Numbers

Registered nurses represent the largest group of health care providers in the United States. Nearly 2.7 million individuals held licenses as registered nurses in 2000, with over 2.2 million (81.77 percent) of that number actively working in nursing. The remainder of the registered nurse population (18.3 percent) was either not working at all or working in fields other than nursing. Figures also indicated that fewer than three quarters (71.6 percent) of employed registered nurses worked full-time, whereas more than a quarter (28.4 percent) worked part-time. The total number of licensed RNs working full-time within nursing, therefore, is not nearly as great as the total population indicates.

Gender

Not surprisingly, the Division of Nursing's 2000 survey also showed that most registered nurses were women. Among employed RNs, only 5.4 percent were men. This figure indicates a leveling off of the proportion of men in nursing, since the 1996 percentage was also 5.4 percent. Even though the percentage of men in nursing has stabilized for the time being, the number of men is still growing at a rate faster than that for the total registered nurse population. This is partially due to the fact that approximately 88 percent of male RNs were employed in nursing, compared with 81 percent of female RNs.

In terms of absolute numbers, there was a 226 percent increase in the number of male RNs between 1980 (when there were only 45,060) and 2000 (when there were 146,902). In addition, anecdotal reports from nursing faculty indicate that larger numbers of men are currently in the educational pipeline. The historic status of nursing as a female-dominated profession will slowly change as male graduates of basic nursing programs enter the workforce.

Race and ethnicity

As of 2000, the total registered nurse population was overwhelmingly composed of white, non-Hispanic individuals (86.6 percent). The 2000 survey showed that distribution by ethnic/racial backgrounds of the 12.3 percent employed nonwhite registered nurses included African-American, 4.9 percent; Asian/Pacific Islander, 3.7 percent; Hispanic, 2.0 percent; and Native American/Alaskan Native, 0.5 percent. The remaining percentage (1.2 percent) was of unknown race/ethnicity, since more than 32,334 registered nurses either did not indicate their racial/ethnic background or reported two races.

Although the number of nonwhites in the registered nurse population is growing at a rate higher than that of the total population, the need exists both to recruit and to retain nonwhite members in the practice of nursing. Nursing has a long way to go before the racial/ethnic composition of the profession more accurately reflects that of American society as a whole, which the 2000 survey found was 69.1 percent white and 30.9 percent nonwhite.

Age

In respect to age, the registered nurse population is similar to the rest of American society: It is getting older. This "graying" of the workforce can be illustrated by comparing 1980 statistics with those from 2000. In 1980, the average age of all registered nurses was 40.3 years. This figure had risen to 45.2 years by 2000. With new nurses entering practice each year, the average age might be expected to remain the same or decline. Many new nurses are beginning second careers, however, and are significantly older than the typical college graduate. Only 9.1 percent of newly licensed registered nurses in 2000 were under age 30 (Figure 5-1).

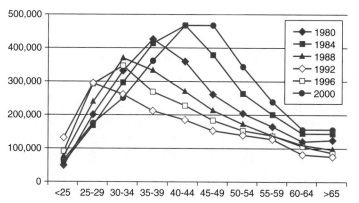

Figure 5-1

Age distribution of the registered nurse population, 1980-2000. (Data from U.S. Department of Health and Human Services, Health Resources and Services Administration: *The registered nurse population, March 2000: findings from the national sample survey of registered nurses,* Washington, DC, 2001, Government Printing Office, p 8.)

Marital status

The marital status of nurses has also been studied. In 2000, 71.5 percent of nurses were married, 17.9 percent were widowed/divorced/separated, and 9.9 percent had never been married. Only 52 percent of employed nurses had children at home, with 8 percent of those children reportedly under 6 years of age. Registered nurses who were part of a two-parent family with children under 6 years were more likely to work part-time than any other group.

Education

Nursing has more levels of preparation than most professions, because of the variety of educational pathways that one can take to become a registered nurse. In 2000, of the 2,696,540 licensed registered nurses, 22.3 percent had diplomas as their highest nursing-related educational preparation; 34.3 percent held associate degrees; 32.7 percent had baccalaureate degrees; 9.6 percent held master's degrees in nursing; and 0.6 percent were prepared at the doctoral level (U.S. Department of Health and Human Services, 2001). Figure 5-2 illustrates trends in the educational preparation of registered nurses in the United States from 1980 to 2000 (U.S. Department of Health and Human Services, 2001).

Employment Opportunities for Nurses

As members of the largest health care profession in the United States, nurses serve in diverse settings such as hospitals, clinics, offices, homes, schools, work places, extended care facilities, the military, community centers, nursing homes, children's camps, and homeless shelters, among others. Increasingly, as state nurse practice acts are revised to cover advanced practice roles, registered nurses also work in

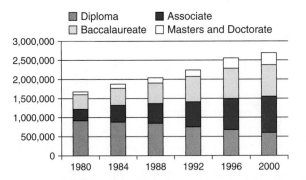

Figure 5-2

Distribution of the RN population by highest nursing educational preparation, 1980-2000. (Data from U.S. Department of Health and Human Services, Health Resources and Services Administration: *The registered nurse population, March 2000: findings from the national sample survey of registered nurses,* Washington, DC, 2001, Government Printing Office, p 7.)

private practice. Nurses in private practice must have advanced degrees or specialized education, training, and certification.

In 2000, hospitals were the primary work site for registered nurses (reported by 59.1 percent of those employed). Community settings showed the largest increase in employment from 1996 to 2000, with 18.2 percent of registered nurses working in community health/public health settings such as state or local health departments, home health services, community health centers, student health, occupational health, and parish nursing. **Ambulatory care** settings, such as physician-based practices, nurse-based practices, telenursing, or health maintenance organizations (HMOs), accounted for 9.5 percent. An additional 6.9 percent worked in nursing homes or **extended care** facilities. The remainder of the registered nurses worked in settings such as schools of nursing; nursing associations; local, state, or federal governmental agencies; state boards of nursing; or insurance companies (U.S. Department of Health and Human Services, 2001).

Not all nurses provide direct patient care as the primary part of their roles. A small but important group of nurses spend the majority of their time conducting research, teaching undergraduate and graduate students, managing companies as chief executives, and consulting with health care organizations. Nurses who have advanced levels of education, such as master's and doctoral degrees, are prepared to become researchers, educators, administrators, and advanced practice nurses, including nurse practitioners, clinical nurse specialists, certified nurse-midwives, and certified registered nurse anesthetists. These advanced practice roles are discussed in greater detail later in this chapter.

In deciding which of the many available practice options to select, nurses should consider several salient points: educational preparation required; their special talents, likes, and dislikes; and whether their preparation, talents, and preferences are a good match with the employment opportunities under consideration. Although a majority of nurses are employed in hospitals, many others are pursuing challenges elsewhere. Numerous new opportunities and roles are being developed that use nurses' skills in different and exciting ways. What follows are descriptions of a sampling of the broad range of settings in which nurses now practice. In some instances, nurses are interviewed. It must be stressed that these areas represent only a sampling of the growing variety of opportunities available.

Hospital-based nursing

Nursing care originated in home and community settings and moved into hospitals only within the last century. Hospitals vary widely in size, comprehensiveness of services offered, and geographic location. In general, nurses in hospitals work with patients who have medical or surgical conditions, with children, with women and their newborns, with cancer patients, and with people who have had severe traumas or burns.

Nurses work in various units, such as operating suites or emergency departments, coronary and other special care units, on step-down or progressive care units, and in many other capacities. In addition to providing direct patient care, they serve as educators, managers, and administrators who teach or supervise others and establish the direction of nursing hospital-wide. A number of generalist and specialist certification opportunities are appropriate for hospital-based nurses, including medical-surgical nurse, pediatric nurse, perinatal nurse, acute care nurse practitioner, gerontological nurse, psychiatric and mental health nurse, nursing administration, nursing administration–advanced, nursing continuing education or staff development nurse, and informatics nurse. There is perhaps no other single work setting that offers so much variety to nurses as do hospitals.

The educational credentials required of registered nurses practicing in hospitals can range from associate degrees and diplomas to doctoral degrees. Generally, entry-level positions require only an RN license. Many hospitals require nurses to hold baccalaureate degrees to advance on the clinical ladder or to assume management positions. A **clinical coordinator,** who is responsible for the management of more than one unit, is generally expected to have a master's degree.

Most new nurses choose to work in acute care hospitals initially to gain experience in organizing and delivering patient care. For many, staff nursing is extremely gratifying, and they continue in this role for their entire careers. Others pursue additional education, often provided by the hospital, in order to work in specialty units such as coronary care. Although specialty units usually require clinical experience and advanced training, some hospitals do allow exceptional new graduates to work in these units.

Some nurses find that management is their strength. **Nurse managers,** formerly called head nurses, are in charge of all activities on their units, including patient care, continuous quality improvement, personnel selection and evaluation, and resource management. Being a nurse manager in a hospital today is somewhat like running a business, and nurses need an entrepreneurial spirit and some business savvy to be most effective in this role.

Most nurses in hospitals provide direct patient care. In the past, it was necessary for nurses to assume administrative or management roles to be promoted or receive salary increases. Such positions removed them from bedside care. Today, in hospitals with clinical ladder programs, nurses no longer must make that choice; clinical ladder programs allow nurses to progress while staying in direct patient care roles.

A **clinical ladder** is a multiple-step program that begins with entry-level staff nurse positions. As nurses gain experience, participate in continuing education, demonstrate clinical competence, pursue formal education, and become certified, they are eligible to move up the rungs of the ladder.

At the top of most clinical ladders are clinical nurse specialists, who are nurses with master's degrees in specialized areas of nursing, such as oncology. The role varies but generally includes responsibility for serving as a clinical mentor and role model for other nurses, as well as setting standards for nursing care on one or more particular units. The oncology clinical specialist, for example, works with the nurses on the oncology unit to help them stay informed of the latest research and skills useful in the care of patients with cancer. The clinical specialist is a resource person for the unit and often provides direct care to patients or families with particularly difficult or complex problems, establishes nursing protocols, and is responsible for seeing that nurses adhere to high standards of care.

Salaries and responsibilities increase at the upper levels of clinical ladders. The clinical ladder concept benefits nurses by allowing them to advance while still working directly with patients. Hospitals also benefit by retaining experienced clinical nurses in direct patient care, thus improving the quality of nursing care throughout the hospital. And patients benefit from having mature, experienced nurses who have chosen direct patient care because it is most gratifying to them.

One of the greatest drawbacks to hospital nursing in the past was the necessity for nurses to work rigid schedules, which usually included evenings, nights, and weekends. Although hospital nurses still must work a fair share of undesirable times, **flexible staffing** is becoming the norm. Sometimes nurses on a particular unit negotiate with one another and establish their own schedules to meet personal needs while still ensuring that appropriate patient care is provided.

Each hospital nursing role has its own unique characteristics. In the following profile, a registered nurse discusses his role as a bedside nurse in a burn unit:

> A burn nurse has to be gentle, strong, and patient enough to go slow. You must be confident enough to work alone; you must believe that what you're doing is in the patient's best interest because some of the procedures hurt far worse than anyone can imagine. Every burn is unique and a challenge. Fifteen years ago, the prognosis for surviving an extensive burn was not good, but with today's techniques for fluid replacement and the development of effective antibiotics, many patients are surviving the first few critical days. During the long hours of one-on-one care you really get to know your patient. There is nothing more rewarding.

When the "fit" between nurses and their role requirements is good, nursing is a gratifying profession, as an oncology nurse demonstrates in discussing her role:

> Being an oncology nurse and working with people with potentially terminal illnesses brings you close to patients and their families. The family room for our patients and their families is very homelike. Families bring food in and have dinner with their loved one right here. Working with dying patients is a tall order. You must be able to support the family and the patient through many stages of the dying process, including anger and depression. Experiencing cancer is always traumatic, with the diagnosis, the treatment, and the struggle to cope. But today's statistics show that more people experience cancer and live. Because of research and early detection, being diagnosed with cancer is no longer the automatic death sentence it used to be. I love getting involved with patients and their families and feel that I can contribute to their positive mental attitude, which can impact their disease process, or hold their hand and help them to die with dignity. They cry, I cry—it is part of my nursing, and I would have it no other way.

These are only two of the many possible roles nurses in hospital settings may choose. Although brief, these descriptions convey a flavor of the responsibility, complexity, and fulfillment to be found in hospital-based nursing (Figure 5-3).

Community health nursing

Lillian Wald is credited with initiating community health nursing when she established the Henry Street Settlement in New York City (see Chapter 1). **Community health nursing** today is a broad field encompassing what were formerly known as public health nursing and home health nursing. Community health nurses work in ambulatory clinics, health departments, hospices, and a variety of other community-based settings, including homes, where they provide nursing care to home-bound patients.

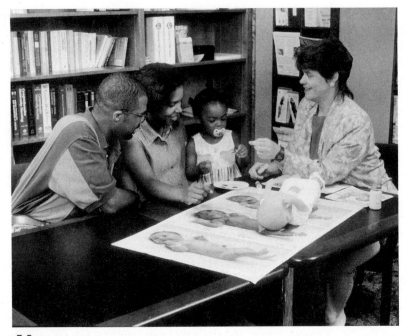

Figure **5-3**
Hospital nurses work closely with the families of patients, as well as with the patients themselves. (Courtesy Memorial Hospital, Chattanooga, Tennessee.)

Community health nurses may work for either government or private agencies. Those working for public health departments provide care in clinics, schools, retirement communities, and other community settings. They focus on improving the overall health of communities by planning and implementing health programs, as well as delivering care. These community health nurses provide educational programs in health maintenance, disease prevention, nutrition, and child care, among others. They conduct immunization clinics and health screenings and work with teachers, parents, physicians, and community leaders toward a healthier community.

Many health departments also have a home health component. Since 1980, there has been a tremendous increase in the number of public and private agencies providing home health services, a form of community health nursing. In fact, home health care is a fast-growing segment of the health care industry (Figure 5-4). Many home health nurses predict that most health care services in the future will be provided in the home.

Home health care has traditionally been, and will continue to be, nursing's "turf." Home health nurses across the United States provide quality care in the most cost-effective and, for patients, comfortable setting possible—the home. Patients cared for at home today tend to be more seriously ill than ever; this is largely due to early hospital discharges in efforts to control costs. As a result, more high-technology equipment is being used in the home. Equipment and procedures formerly unheard

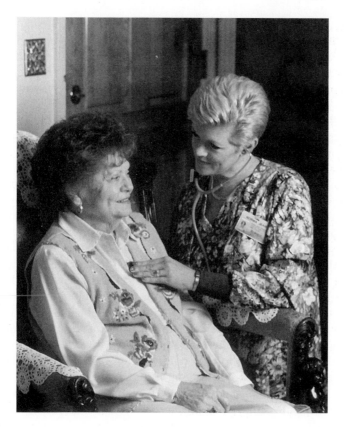

Figure **5-4**
Home health nursing is a fast-growing segment of the health care industry. (Courtesy Memorial Hospital, Chattanooga, Tennessee.)

of outside of hospital settings, such as ventilators, intravenous pumps, and chemotherapy setups, are routinely encountered in home care today.

Home health nurses must possess up-to-date nursing knowledge and be secure in their own nursing skills, since they do not have the backup of physicians or more experienced nurses as they might in a hospital setting. These nurses must have strong assessment and communication skills. They must make independent judgments and be able to recognize patients' and families' teaching needs. Home health nurses must also know their limits and seek help when the patient's needs are beyond the scope of their abilities. A registered nurse working in home health relates her experience:

> I have always found a tremendous reward in working with the terminally ill and the elderly, and I get a great deal of contact with this particular population working in home health. One patient I cared for developed a pressure ulcer while at home. I was able to assess the patient's physiological needs as well as teach the family how to care for their loved one to prevent future skin breakdown. Within a few weeks the skin looked good, and the family felt important and involved. To me this is real nursing.

Community health nursing is growing as more and more nursing care is delivered outside the walls of hospitals. The American Nurses Credentialing Center offers certification in both community health and home health nursing at the generalist and clinical specialist levels. The increase in demand for nurses to work in a variety of community settings is expected to increase for the foreseeable future.

Nurse entrepreneurship

Some nurses are creative, energetic people who like the idea of finding new forms of expression and are challenged by the risks of starting a new enterprise. Such nurses make good candidates for nurse entrepreneurship.

Similar to an entrepreneur in any field, a **nurse entrepreneur** identifies a need and creates a service to meet the identified need. Nurse entrepreneurs enjoy the **autonomy** that is derived from owning and operating their own health-related businesses. Groups of nurses, some of whom are faculty members in schools of nursing, have opened nurse-managed centers to provide direct care to clients. Nurse entrepreneurs are self-employed as consultants to hospitals, nursing homes, and schools of nursing. Others have started **nurse-based practices** and carry their own caseloads of patients with physical or emotional needs. They are sometimes involved in presenting educational workshops and seminars. Some nurses establish their own creative apparel businesses, which provide articles of clothing for premature babies or physically challenged individuals. Others own and operate their own health equipment companies, health insurance agencies, and home health agencies. In today's burgeoning health care environment, there is no limit to the opportunities available to nurses with the entrepreneurial spirit. Here are a few comments from one such entrepreneur, the chief executive officer of a privately owned home health agency:

> I enjoy working for myself. I know that my success or failure in my business is up to me. Having your own home health agency is a lot of work. You have to be very organized, manage other people effectively, and have excellent communication skills. You cannot be afraid to say no to the people. There is nothing better than the feeling I get when a family calls to say our nurses have made a difference in their loved one's life, but I also have to take the calls of complaint about my agency. Those are tough.

Increasingly, nurses are taking the business of health care into their own hands. They seem to agree that the opportunity to create their own companies has never been better. One such company offers nursing care for mothers, babies, and children. This company's emphasis is the care of women whose pregnancies may be complicated by diabetes, hypertension, or multiple births. The registered nurse founder described the services offered by her company:

> Our main specialty is managing high-risk pregnancies and high-risk newborns. Home care for these individuals is a boon not only to the patients themselves, but also to hospitals, insurance companies, and doctors. With the trend toward shorter hospital stays, risks are minimized if skilled maternity nurses are on hand to provide patients with specialty care in their homes.

As with almost any endeavor, disadvantages come with owning a small business. There is the risk of losing your investment if the business is unsuccessful.

Fluctuations in income are common, especially in the early months, and regular paychecks may become a memory, at least at first. A certain amount of pressure is created because of the total responsibility for meeting deadlines and paying bills, salaries, and taxes. But there is great opportunity, too. Aspiring entrepreneurs can eliminate much of the risk involved in small business ownership by completing four preliminary steps:

1. Conduct a thorough needs assessment to determine whether the service or product you wish to provide is needed and wanted by consumers in your community.
2. Develop a detailed business plan complete with short-term and long-term goals, marketing plans, and schedules for business development, taking competition into consideration.
3. Have enough capital to carry the business for at least a year, even if there is no profit, and keep overhead low. Rent or borrow equipment and space and postpone capital purchases until the business is established.
4. Prepare appropriately by learning about effective business practices—for example, budgeting, accounting, personnel policies, and legal aspects of small business. The Chamber of Commerce's Service Core of Retired Executives (SCORE) will provide free consultation and advice on these and other business matters.

In addition to financial incentives, there are intangible rewards in entrepreneurship. For some people, the autonomy and freedom to control their own practice are more than enough to compensate them for increased pressure and initial uncertainty.

With rapid changes occurring daily in the health care system, new and exciting possibilities abound. Alert nurses who possess creativity, initiative, and business savvy have tremendous opportunities as entrepreneurs. The Research Note on p. 146 describes the work of one such nurse.

Office-based nursing

Nurses who are employed in medical office settings work in tandem with physicians or nurse practitioners and their patients. Office-based nursing activities include performing health assessments, drawing blood, giving immunizations, administering medications, and providing health teaching. Nurses in office settings also act as liaisons between patients and physicians or NPs. They amplify and clarify orders for patients, as well as provide emotional support to anxious patients. They may visit hospitalized patients, and some assist in surgery. Often, these nurses supervise other office workers, such as practical nurses, nurse aides, scheduling clerks, and record clerks. Educational requirements, hours of work, and specific responsibilities vary, depending on the preferences of the employer.

A registered nurse who works for a group of three nephrologists describes a typical day:

> I first make rounds independently on patients in the dialysis center, making sure that they are tolerating the dialysis procedure and answering questions regarding their treatments and diets. I then make rounds with one of the physicians in the hospital as he visits patients and orders new treatments. The afternoon is spent in the office assessing patients as they come for their physician's visit. I may draw blood for a diagnostic test on one patient and do patient teaching regarding diet to another. No 2 days are alike, and that is what I love about this position. I have a sense of independence but still have daily patient contact.

RESEARCH note

Kathleen Vollman is a master's prepared critical care nurse practicing in Detroit, Michigan. In the early 1980s she observed that about 60 to 70 percent of her patients with acute respiratory distress syndrome (ARDS) died from a lack of oxygen. Attempts to oxygenate them with ventilators often further injured their lungs. Inspired by an article on animal research left in the break room by a pulmonologist, Kathleen began to think about positioning patients for maximum oxygenation.

First, she tried turning her patients with ARDS from side to back to side every 30 minutes, as had been done in the animal study. She took blood gas readings in each position and developed a schedule for each patient based on that person's unique responses. Patients seemed to do better when she used this simple, noninvasive, independent nursing function of positioning.

Encouraged by her patients' responses, she read more research studies and found two articles dealing with the beneficial effect of prone (face down) positioning on gas exchange. She tried this with positive results but encountered problems turning very ill patients into the prone position. Solving this problem became the subject of her master's research.

Kathleen and a relative who is a mechanical engineer developed a turning frame and tested it on healthy people in a simulated critical care environment. After testing, the device was modified twice and then tested with ARDS patients. Data were collected for over 10 months and showed the usefulness of the frame in improving oxygenation of these critically ill patients. Kathleen has since won several research awards and has patented her device. She licensed the device to a major manufacturer of hospital beds, and now the Vollman Prone Positioner is marketed internationally. The device costs $2,000 and can be reused after disinfecting. Kathleen serves as a consultant to the company on the marketing of the device and the education of those who will use it.

Kathleen Vollman's story is an example of how a practicing nurse, making an observation and thinking creatively through possible solutions, became a researcher, an inventor, and ultimately, an entrepreneur. This is not an overnight success story, however; it has been nearly 20 years since Kathleen made her initial observations. She continues her research in prone positioning science today. You can read more about Kathleen Vollman's entrepreneurial spirit online *(www.vollman.com/index.html)*.

From Vollman KM: My search to help patients breathe, *Reflections* 25(2):16-18, 1999, and Vollman KM, Bander JL: Improved oxygenation utilizing a prone positioner in patients with acute respiratory distress syndrome, *Intensive Care Med* 22:1105-1111, 1996.

Registered nurses considering employment in office settings need good communication skills, because a large part of their responsibilities includes communicating with patients, families, employers, pharmacists, and hospital admitting clerks. They should be careful to inquire about the specifics of the position because office practice nursing roles may range from routine task performance to the challenging, multi-faceted functions described by the nurse interviewed above.

Occupational health nursing

Many large companies today employ **occupational health nurses** to provide basic health care services, health education, screenings, and emergency treatment to company employees at the workplace. Corporate executives have long known that good employee health reduces absenteeism, insurance costs, and worker errors, thereby improving company profitability. Occupational health nurses represent an important investment by companies. They are often asked to serve as consultants on health matters within the company. These nurses may participate in health-related policy development, such as policies governing employee smoking or family leaves (formerly limited to maternity leaves). Depending on the size of the company, the occupational health nurse may be the only health professional employed in a company and therefore may have a good deal of autonomy.

The usual educational requirement for nurses in occupational health roles is licensure. Some positions call for a baccalaureate degree in nursing. These nurses must possess knowledge and skills that enable them to perform routine physical assessments, including vision and hearing screenings for all employees. Good interpersonal skills to provide counseling and referrals for lifestyle problems, such as stress or substance abuse, are a plus for these nurses. They must also know first aid and cardiopulmonary resuscitation (CPR). If employed in a heavy manufacturing setting where burns or traumas are a risk, they must have special training in those medical emergencies.

Occupational health nurses also have responsibilities for identifying health risks in the entire work environment. They must be able to assess the environment for potential safety hazards and work with management to eliminate or reduce them. They need a working knowledge of governmental regulations, such as the requirements of the Occupational Safety and Health Administration (OSHA), and must ensure that the company is complying with them. These nurses also need to understand workers' compensation regulations and coordinate the care of injured workers with the treating physician.

Nurses in occupational settings have to be confident in their nursing skills, be effective communicators with both employees and managers, motivate employees to adopt healthier habits, and be able to function independently in providing care. Certification for occupational health nurses is available through the American Board for Occupational Health Nurses (ABOHN).

School nursing

A **school nurse** should enjoy working with children, their families, teachers, and school administrators. The purpose of school nursing is to enhance the educational process by improving the "well-being, academic success, and life-long achievement" (NASN, 2003, homepage) of the target population, children and adolescents. Although many states have well-developed school nurse programs, others do not. Very few states achieve the recommended ratio of 1:750 (a recommended minimum number of one school nurse for every 750 students). In fact, a number of states have up to 10,000 students under the care of one school nurse (U.S. Department of Health and Human Services, 2001). With such high ratios, it is difficult to imagine how children in these states can be deriving substantial health benefits from the school nurse program.

Health care futurists believe that school nursing is the wave of the future. In medically underserved areas, the role of school nurse may even be expanded to include members of the school child's immediate family. Obviously, this will require many more school nurses—along with willingness by state and local school boards to pay them. Without adequate qualified staffing, the nation's children cannot enjoy the full potential of school nurse programs.

Most school systems require nurses to have a minimum of a baccalaureate degree in nursing, whereas some school districts have higher educational requirements. Prior experience working with children is also usually required. School health has become a specialty in its own right, and in states where school health is a priority, graduate programs in school health nursing have been established. The National Board for Certification of School Nurses (NBCSN) is now the official certifying body for school nurses.

School nurses need a working knowledge of human growth and development to detect developmental problems early. Counseling skills are important because many children turn to the school nurse as counselor. School nurses keep records of children's required immunizations and are responsible for seeing that immunizations are current. When an outbreak of a childhood communicable disease occurs, school nurses educate parents, teachers, and students about treatment and prevention of transmission.

Although the essentially well child is the focus of the school nurse's work, the practice of mainstreaming has brought many chronically ill, injured, developmentally delayed, and physically challenged students into regular school classrooms. School nurses must work closely with families, teachers, and the community to provide these children with the special care they need while at school—and these needs can be significant.

School nurses work closely with teachers to incorporate health concepts into the curriculum. They conduct vision and hearing screenings. Parents may expect school nurses to make referrals to qualified physicians and other health care providers when routine screenings identify problems outside the nurses' scope of practice.

School nurses must be prepared to handle both routine illnesses of children and adolescents and emergencies. One of their major concerns is safety. Accidents are the leading cause of death in children of all ages, yet accidents are preventable. First aid for minor injuries and emergency care for more severe ones are additional skills school nurses use.

Preventive aspects of child health are a major focus of school health nurses. In terms of safety, prevention requires both protection from obvious hazards and education of teachers, parents, and students about how to avoid accidents. School nurses practice safety, are alert to safety needs in the school and surrounding environment, and recognize the need for safety education in contributing to accident reduction. Preventing the spread of infections is also a major focus of this nursing role.

School nursing is a complex and multifaceted field that is constantly expanding. It represents a challenge for those nurses who choose it as a career.

Hospice and palliative care nursing

Hospice and palliative care nursing is a rapidly developing specialty in nursing dedicated to improving the experience of seriously ill and dying patients and their families. It was initiated as a result of a $28 million study by the Robert Wood Johnson Foundation in the mid-1990s. This study found that there were significant problems associated with the care of seriously ill and dying patients. The problems reported included poor communication, continued aggressive treatment after treatment was no longer effective, and high levels of pain. The study pointed out the "overriding need to change the kind of care dying Americans receive" (Last Acts Task Force, 1998, p. 109).

According to the ANA document *Scope and Standards of Hospice and Palliative Care Nursing Practice*, "Hospice and palliative care nursing reflects a holistic philosophy of care implemented across the life span and across diverse health settings. ... The goal of hospice and palliative nursing is to promote the patient's quality of life through the relief of suffering along the illness trajectory, through the death of the patient, and into the bereavement period of the family" (ANA, 2002, p. 5). The ANA (2002) identified three major precepts underlying hospice and end-of-life care:

- Persons are living until the moment of death.
- Coordinated care should be offered by a variety of professionals, with attention to the physical, psychological, social, and spiritual needs of patients and their families.
- Care should be sensitive to patient/family diversity or cultural beliefs.

Nursing curricula traditionally have not included extensive content to prepare nurses to deal effectively with dying patients and their families. The American Association of Colleges of Nursing (AACN) used the three precepts identified above to develop a document entitled "Peaceful Death." This document identifies the competencies needed by baccalaureate nurses for palliative/hospice care and outlines where these competencies can fit into nursing curricula. You can review this document and other resources online *(www.aacn.nche.edu/Publications/deathfin.htm)*.

End-of-life care is largely the responsibility of nurses. In recognition of this fact, the ANA formulated a position statement "regarding the promotion of comfort and relief of pain of dying patients, reinforcing the nurse's obligation to promote comfort and ensure aggressive efforts to relieve pain and suffering" (ANA, 2002, p. 3). This position statement can also be found online *(www.nursingworld.org/readroom/position/ethics/etpain.htm)*.

Hospice and palliative care nurses work in a variety of settings, including inpatient palliative/hospice units, community-based or home hospice programs, ambulatory palliative care programs, teams of consultants in palliative care, and skilled nursing facilities. Both generalist and advanced practice nurses work in palliative care. The certifying agency is the National Board for the Certification of Hospice and Palliative Nurses (NBCHPN). By 2004, over 7,400 registered nurses had become certified hospice and palliative nurses.

With the aging population, end-of-life needs are expected to increase. Every nurse, not just specialists in hospice and palliative care, should be familiar with the precepts of palliative and end-of-life nursing care.

Case management nursing

Case management is a dynamic, challenging, and relatively new field in nursing, having evolved in the mid-1980s as a way of managing patient **length of stay (LOS).** It involves systematic collaboration with patients, their significant others, and their health care providers to coordinate high-quality health care services in a cost-effective manner with positive patient outcomes. Another aspect of nursing case management includes decreasing fragmentation and duplication of care (Huber, 2002). The case manager is the person responsible for this process, and although registered nurses are not the only professionals who act as case managers, they are uniquely prepared for this role. Because of their broad educational backgrounds, skill in arranging and providing patient education and referrals, orientation toward holistic care and health promotion, and communication and interpersonal skills, nurses are particularly well suited for case management.

Depending on the case management model being used—and there are many—the nursing case manager may follow the patient from the diagnostic phase through hospitalization, rehabilitation, and back to home care. Through careful planning, every step of the patient's care can be coordinated in a timely manner.

One key to making case management work is the use of critical paths that include specific time lines and standard treatment protocols. A **critical path** is an abbreviated version of the case management plan and is used for daily decision making about patient care. It lists key nursing and medical interventions that should occur within a certain time line to ensure positive patient outcomes. Case management is considered successful if the patient is well enough for discharge within the length of stay directed by the diagnostic-related grouping. A sample critical path can be found on the Evolve website (**www.evolve.elsevier.com/Chitty/professional/**).

Both patient and nurse satisfaction are high with the one-on-one relationship fostered with case management. Patients like the security of having one familiar person managing their care, and a nursing case manager has the satisfaction of coordinating a patient's care from beginning to end (McKenzie, Torkelson, and Holt, 1989). Certification in nursing case management is offered by the American Nurses Credentialing Center. You may also hear case management nursing referred to as "care management nursing," a name more consistent with nursing's values.

Telehealth nursing

Telehealth nursing is generally not a separate nursing role. Few nurses use telehealth exclusively in their practices. Rather, it is most often found as a part of almost every other nursing role. Nurses have always used the telephone to communicate with physicians, patients, and other health care providers. Today's technologies have evolved far beyond the telephone to include computers, interactive audio and video linkages, teleconferencing, real-time transmission of patients' diagnostic and clinical data, and more. Telehealth is defined as "the removal of time and distance barriers for the delivery of health care services and related health care activities through telecommunication technology" (American Nurses Association, 1999, p. 1).

The use of telehealth expands access to health care for underserved populations and individuals in both urban and rural areas. It also serves to reduce the sense of professional isolation experienced by those who work in such areas and may assist in attracting and retaining health care professionals in remote areas (American Nurses Association, 1999).

Practical uses of telehealth technology include faxing a change in a patient's drug order; consulting by telephone with other care providers; accessing a lab report from a remote site with a wireless, handheld computer; or participating in interactive video sessions such as an interdisciplinary team consultation about a complex patient issue. Although the fundamentals of basic nursing practice do not change because nurses use telehealth technologies, its use may require adaptation or modification of usual procedures. In addition, telenurses must develop competence in the use of each new type of telehealth technology, and they may change rapidly. The American Nurses Association identified "Competencies for Telehealth Technologies in Nursing" (1999) to assist nurses to evaluate and guide their practice.

Numerous legal and regulatory issues surround nursing care delivered through telehealth technologies. The Online Journal of Nursing Issues has posted a comprehensive article enumerating these *(www.nursingworld.org/ojin/topic16/tpc16_3.htm)*.

You can learn more about telehealth, an area of growing interest in nursing and other health professions, from the Association of Telemedicine Service Providers *(www.atsp.org)* and from the American Telemedicine Association *(www.atmeda.org)*.

Parish nursing

Interest in spirituality and its relation to wellness and healing has prompted an emerging practice area known as **parish nursing.** This area of nursing takes a holistic approach to healing that involves partnerships between congregations, their pastoral staffs, and health care providers. Since its development in the Chicago area in the mid-1980s by a hospital chaplain, Dr. Granger E. Westberg, parish nursing has spread rapidly and now includes more than 5,000 nurses in paid and volunteer positions across the country (Abuelouf, 1998). According to the American Nurses Association definition,

> Parish nursing is a unique, specialized practice of professional nursing that focuses on health promotion and disease prevention within the context of the values, beliefs, and practices of a faith community, such as a church, synagogue, or mosque, and its mission and ministry to its members (families and individuals), and the community it serves (American Nurses Association, 1998, p. 1).

The spiritual dimension is central to parish nursing practice. The nurse's own spiritual journey is an essential aspect of this nursing role. Parish nursing is based on the belief that spiritual health is central to well-being and influences a person's entire being.

Parish nurses serve as members of the ministry staff or clergy of a church or other faith community. They practice independently, within the legal scope of the individual state's nurse practice act. Roles of the parish nurse include health educator and counselor, advocate for health services, referral agent, coordinator of volunteer health ministers, developer of support groups, and integrator of spiritual practices and health. Interview on p. 152 provides a discussion with a parish nurse who describes her calling and her practice.

interv i e w *with Amy L. Corder, RN, MSN, CRRN*

Interviewer: Describe a typical day in your practice.

Corder: There is no "typical" day. Every day is different, which is what I love about parish nursing. There are many aspects of my work, a number of which are not usually thought of as nursing. I help the congregation understand the interaction and connection between body, mind, and spirit. This is important because unhealthy behaviors or emotions often affect us physically in harmful ways.

Interviewer: What is the focus of your practice?

Corder: One aspect is health maintenance, such as teaching nutrition and diet, dental health, medication management, blood pressure screenings, and the like. I also visit parishioners in their homes, mostly older adults. Recently I visited a lady with a stasis ulcer on her leg. After my assessment and much discussion, she agreed to let me make a referral to a wound specialist. I don't do invasive procedures like a home health nurse might do. My focus is in the role of teaching, counseling, supporting, and often just encouraging people about how to improve their lives physically, mentally, and spiritually both within the congregation and the community.

Interviewer: What has surprised you about parish nursing?

Corder: It surprised me how much writing I do. I am frequently asked to write an article for a newsletter or a small local paper about my current programs or about what I do as a parish nurse. I also make a lot of presentations, which takes some research. I sure didn't appreciate writing all of those papers in school, but now I'm glad because it gave me confidence in my writing and research skills.

Interviewer: How did you prepare yourself to be a parish nurse?

Corder: By searching and establishing my own spiritual foundation and having an open mind and heart, in order to hear God's calling. Parish nursing is a calling by God. I do not believe you can be totally effective in assisting others in discovering and improving their spirituality for better health unless you have achieved a certain amount of spiritual awareness within your own life. Education-wise, I have a BSN and a master's degree in gerontological nursing. I have primarily worked in the areas of rehabilitation nursing and long-term care, which has prepared me well for what I do.

Interviewer: What is the most challenging part of your work?

Corder: The most challenging part of my work is learning about the philosophy of health ministry and parish nursing and applying it to my practice. Although parish nursing has been around for 12 to 15 years, it is still a relatively new field. I am the first parish nurse for my congregation, and there are fewer than a dozen other parish nurses in our community, although that number is growing. This is an exciting time for our congregation as we explore the role of health ministry and parish nursing together.

Although there is no standardized educational requirement for parish nurses, a number of hospitals and colleges of nursing offer certificate courses designed to prepare nurses for the unique role of parish nurse. Taught by clinical pastoral educators (CPE), these courses typically last for about 20 weeks and involve a variety of classroom and clinical experiences. To date, no organization is yet offering certification for parish nurses.

In a unique partnership, the American Nurses Association and the Health Ministries Association, Inc., an interfaith organization supporting wellness within places of worship, jointly published the *Scope and Standards of Parish Nursing Practice* in 1998. This document, which sets forth the responsibilities for which parish nurses are accountable and reflects the values and priorities of the specialty, can be obtained from the American Nurses Association.

Informatics nursing

Another new and exciting specialty area evolving in nursing is nursing informatics (NI). The **informatics nurse** combines nursing science with information management science and computer science to manage information nurses need and to make that information accessible. This field encompasses the full range of activities that focus on information handling in nursing (American Nurses Association, 2001) and assists nurses to do the work of nursing efficiently and effectively. Since it "has been estimated that nurses spend as much as 50 percent of their time gathering, coordinating, and documenting information" (Meadows, 2002), it is easy to understand the potential benefits of streamlining this process. Benefits of clinical information systems include improved patient safety, reduction in variability of care, improved communication, improved clinical decision making, and increased efficiency of staff.

In contrast to computer science systems analysts, informatics nurses must clearly understand the information they handle and how other nurses will use it. Nursing knowledge is specialized and must be accessible by nurse users; otherwise, it is useless in improving patient care. Complex information systems are more likely to fail when end-users are not consulted during the planning and design process (American Nurses Association, 2001). Because they are nurses themselves, informatics nurses are best able to understand the needs of nurses who use the systems and can design them with the needs, skills, and time constraints of those nurses in mind.

Informatics nurses may work in clinical areas, ensuring that the direct caregiver nurse is provided with complete and accurate information about patients' health needs and nursing care requirements. They may also practice in nonclinical areas such as nursing education or administration, where they design ways to make information needed by teachers, students, and managers easily accessible. In addition to practicing in hospitals and universities, informatics nurses also work in the military, health maintenance organizations, and research settings.

Information technology can help nurses deliver more effective care in a number of ways. Some examples of the practice of nursing informatics include computerizing a nursing document or system; writing a program to support nursing care of patients; developing an interactive video disc system for educational purposes; helping nurse managers develop systems to use nursing resources effectively (people, money, supplies); or designing systems to collect and aggregate clinical data so they can be analyzed to assess the cost and outcomes of nursing care.

As a minimum, informatics nurses should have a bachelor's degree in nursing and additional knowledge and experience in the field of informatics. Advanced practice in nursing informatics requires preparation at the graduate level in nursing (American Nurses Association, 2001). Certification for informatics nurses is available through the American Nurses Credentialing Center.

NURSING OPPORTUNITIES REQUIRING HIGHER DEGREES

Many registered nurses choose to pursue roles that require a master's degree, doctoral degree, or specialized education in a specific area. These roles include clinical nurse specialists, nurse managers, nurse executives in hospital settings, nurse educators (whether in clinical or academic settings), nurse anesthetists, nurse midwives, and other advanced practice nurses.

Nurse Educators

About 2.1 percent of registered nurses (46,655) work in nursing education (U.S. Department of Health and Human Services, 2001). These nurses teach in LPN/LVN programs, diploma programs, associate degree programs, baccalaureate and higher-degree programs, and programs preparing nursing assistants. Nurse educators in accredited schools of nursing offering a baccalaureate or higher degree must hold a minimum of master's degree in nursing; in 2002, 49.4 percent had doctoral degrees in nursing or other fields. This is a significant increase from 1992, when 21.4 percent of nursing faculty were doctorally prepared, and even more favorable when compared with only 10.6 percent in 1984 and 3 percent in 1972 (American Association of Colleges of Nursing, 2003).

Most nursing faculty (96.3 percent) are women, and 9.2 percent are members of minority groups (American Association of Colleges of Nursing, 2003). In 2002-2003, only 3.5 percent of master's students chose nursing education to prepare for a teaching role, compared with 8.3 percent in 1995. This downward trend contributes to continued concerns about a critical shortage of nursing faculty in the future.

Advanced Practice Nursing (APN)

Advanced practice nursing is growing rapidly, with approximately 196,279 of registered nurses (7.3 percent) in 2000 having the education and credentials to work as advanced practice nurses, up from 161,712 in 1996. This growth is spurred by several factors, including increased demand for primary care coupled with increased specialization of physicians and heightened demand for efficient and cost-effective treatment. **Advanced practice nurse (APN)** is an umbrella term applied to a registered nurse who has met advanced educational and clinical practice requirements beyond the 2 to 4 years of basic nursing education demanded of all registered nurses.

Patient acceptance of advanced practice nurses is high. A growing body of evidence is accumulating that confirms that advanced practice nurses deliver high-quality care, exceeding that delivered by physicians on several measures. It is estimated

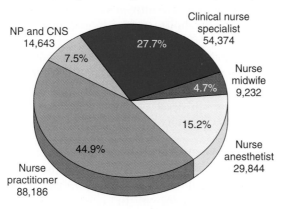

Total: 196,279 (7.3% of Registered Nurse Population)

Clinical nurse specialist
54,374

NP and CNS
14,643

27.7%

7.5%

Nurse midwife
9,232

4.7%

15.2%

44.9%

Nurse anesthetist
29,844

Nurse practitioner
88,186

Figure 5-5
Numbers of advanced practice nurses by areas of specialty. (Data from U.S. Department of Health and Human Services, Health Resources and Services Administration: *The registered nurse population, March 2000: findings from the national sample survey of registered nurses,* Washington, DC, 2001, Government Printing Office, p 21.)

that 60 to 80 percent of primary and preventive care traditionally performed by physicians can be safely done by advanced practices nurses.

There are four categories of advanced practice nurses: nurse practitioner, clinical nurse specialist, certified nurse-midwife, and certified registered nurse anesthetist. Figure 5-5 shows the breakdown of advanced practice nurses by area of specialty in 2000.

Nurse practitioner (NP)

Opportunities for nurses in expanded roles in health care has created a boom in **nurse practitioner** (**NP**) education. There were 150 nurse practitioner education programs in 1992. By 2003, this number had risen to 328 (AACN, 2003). These programs grant master's degrees or postmaster's certificates and prepare nurses to sit for national certification examinations as nurse practitioners. The length of the programs varies, depending on prior education of the students. In 2000, there were 102,829 nurse practitioners in the United States. This figure includes the 14,643 who are also clinical nurse specialists (U.S. Department of Health and Human Services, 2001).

States also vary in the amount of practice autonomy accorded to nurse practitioners. According to the annual survey conducted by *The Nurse Practitioner: The American Journal of Primary Health Care* (Pearson, 2003), there are 26 states in which the board of nursing has sole authority in NP scope of practice. In those states there are no statutory or regulatory requirements for physician collaboration, direction, or supervision. An additional 14 states require physician collaboration. Physician supervision is required in 6 states. In 5 states, the scope of NP practice is determined jointly by the board of nursing and the board of medicine (Pearson, 2003).

Nurse practitioners beginning practice should check on the status of the advanced practice laws before making firm commitments.

Nurse practitioners work in clinics, nursing homes, their own offices, or physicians' offices. Others work for hospitals, health maintenance organizations (HMOs), or private industry. Most nurse practitioners choose a specialty area such as adult, family, or pediatric health care. They are qualified to handle a wide range of basic health problems. These nurses can perform physical examinations, take medical histories, diagnose and treat common acute and chronic illnesses and injuries, order and interpret laboratory tests and x-ray films, and counsel and educate clients (Figure 5-6).

In 2003, nurse practitioners could legally write prescriptions in 38 states with some physician supervision, whereas in 13 states and the District of Columbia, nurse practitioners could prescribe independent of physician involvement (Pearson, 2003). Many NPs are independent practitioners and can be reimbursed by Medicare, Medicaid, and military and private insurers for their work.

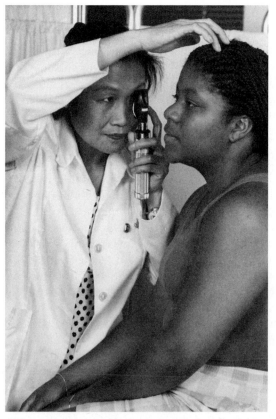

Figure 5-6
A nurse practitioner examines her patient. (Photo by Fielding Freed.)

Clinical nurse specialist (CNS)

Similar to a nurse practitioner, a **clinical nurse specialist (CNS)** works in a variety of settings, including hospitals, clinics, nursing homes, their own offices, private industry, home care, and health maintenance organizations. These nurses hold advanced nursing degrees—master's or doctoral—and are qualified to handle a wide range of physical and mental health problems. They are experts in a particular field of clinical practice, such as mental health, gerontology, cardiac care, cancer care, community health, or neonatal health, and they perform health assessments, make diagnoses, deliver treatment, and develop quality control methods. Additionally, clinical nurse specialists work in consultation, research, education, and administration. Direct reimbursement to some clinical nurse specialists is possible through Medicare, Medicaid, and military and private insurers. In 2000, there were 69,017 clinical nurse specialists in the United States, including 14,643 who were both nurse practitioners and clinical nurse specialists (U.S. Department of Health and Human Services, 2001).

Certified nurse-midwife (CNM)

In 2000, there were an estimated 9,232 certified nurse-midwives in the United States (U.S. Department of Health and Human Services, 2001). **Certified nurse-midwives (CNMs)** provide well-woman care and attend to or assist in childbirth in various settings, including hospitals, birthing centers, and homes. They are prepared in formal nurse-midwife courses of at least 9 months in length. Most of the 47 nurse-midwife programs accredited by the American College of Nurse-Midwives offer a master's degree, accounting for an average of 1.5 years of specialized education beyond basic nursing education. Virtually all practicing nurse-midwives are nationally certified.

Births attended by nurse-midwives are among the safest. According to the National Center for Health Statistics, certified nurse-midwives attended 297,902 births in 2000. This represented about 9.5 percent of all U.S. vaginal births that year (American College of Nurse-Midwives, 2002). Historically, births attended by nurse-midwives have resulted in half the national cesarean section rate and nearly triple the national rate of successful vaginal births after a previous cesarean (American Journal of Nursing, 1996).

A 1998 study examining birth certificate data found that the infant mortality rate for nurse-midwives was 4.1 per 1000, whereas the national average for physicians in the study year was 8.6 per 1,000 (National Center for Health Statistics, 1998). A study published in the June 2003 edition of *American Journal of Public Health* documents that "low-risk patients receiving collaborative midwifery care had birth success rates comparable to those who saw only physicians, with fewer interventions, more options, and lower cost to the health care system" (Jackson, Lang, Swartz, et al., 2003, p. 1003).

Certified nurse-midwives have the widest prescriptive rights of all advanced practice nurses. As of 2002, certified nurse-midwives were able to prescribe medication in 48 states and 3 jurisdictions, including the District of Columbia (American College of Nurse-Midwives, 2002).

Because of patient acceptance and a good safety record, deliveries attended by nurse-midwives are expected to increase in the future.

Certified registered nurse anesthetist (CRNA)

There were 29,844 **certified registered nurse anesthetists (CRNAs)** in the United States in 2000 (U.S. Department of Health and Human Services, 2001). Nurse anesthetists administer more than 65 percent of the 26 million anesthetics given to patients each year and are the only anesthesia providers in nearly one third of U.S. hospitals. Collaborating with physician anesthesiologists or often working independently, they are found in a variety of settings, including operating suites; obstetrical delivery rooms; the offices of dentists, podiatrists, ophthalmologists, and plastic surgeons; and ambulatory surgical facilities (American Association of Nurse Anesthetists, 2003).

To become a certified registered nurse anesthetist, nurses must complete 2 to 3 years of specialized education in a master's program beyond the required 4-year bachelor's degree. There are 88 accredited nurse anesthesia programs in the United States, ranging from 24 to 36 months in length. Nurse anesthetists must also meet national certification and recertification requirements. According to the American Association of Nurse Anesthetists, 45 percent of the nation's CRNAs are men, as compared with only 5.4 percent in all nursing fields.

The safety of care delivered by CRNAs is well established. According to a 1999 report from the Institute of Medicine, anesthesia care today is nearly 50 times safer than it was 20 years ago. Reinforcing that finding is the fact that since 1988, nurse anesthetist professional liability premiums have decreased across the country (American Association of Nurse Anesthetists, 2003).

Issues in advanced practice nursing

Each year in January, the journal *Nurse Practitioner* publishes an update on legislation affecting advanced practice nursing. Over the years, advances have been made toward removing the barriers to autonomous practice for advanced practice nurses in many, but not all, states.

In the past, substantial barriers to APN autonomy existed because of the overlap between traditional medical and nursing functions. A decade ago, the picture was considerably less optimistic than it now is. The issue of APNs practicing autonomously was a politically charged arena, with organized medicine positioned firmly against all efforts of nurses to be recognized as independent health care providers receiving direct reimbursement for their services. Organized nursing, however, persevered. Nurses, through their professional associations, continued their efforts to change laws that limit the scope of nursing practice. Their efforts were aided by the fact that numerous published studies validated the safety, cost-efficiency, and high patient acceptance of APN care.

According to the 2003 *Nurse Practitioner* update (Pearson, 2003), by 2005 there will be as many nurse practitioners as family physicians in this country. Both the public and legislators at state and national levels have begun to appreciate the role that advanced practice nurses have played in increasing the efficiency and availability of primary health care delivery while reducing costs. However, opposition to APN autonomy persists: "The remaining roadblocks to full practice autonomy continue, primarily because of the resistance of organized physician groups to relinquish control over the health care dollar. This sad reality reinforces the need for all APNs to continue the struggle" (Pearson, 2003, p. 3). Until the U.S. Congress approves legislation to provide primary health care for all citizens and makes provisions for advanced practice nurses to share fully in the provision of that care, the practice parameters of advanced practice nurses are at the mercy of the various state legislatures.

EMPLOYMENT OUTLOOK IN NURSING

The Bureau of Labor Statistics, a division of the U.S. Department of Labor, is confident about nursing's overall employment prospects in the near and distant future. According to the Bureau, nurses can expect their employment opportunities to grow "faster than the average" (meaning a 21 to 35 percent increase) through the year 2010 (U.S. Department of Labor, 2003). Registered nurses topped the Bureau's list of the 10 occupations with the largest projected job growth in the years 2002-2012 (Horrigan, 2004). Several factors are fueling this growth, including technological advances and the increasing emphasis on primary care. The aging of the nation's population also has an impact, since older people are more likely to require medical care. And as aging nurses retire, many additional job openings will result.

Opportunities in hospitals, traditionally the largest employers of nurses, will grow more slowly than those in community-based sectors. The most rapid hospital-based growth is projected to occur in outpatient facilities, such as same-day surgery departments, rehabilitation programs, and outpatient cancer centers.

Home health care positions are expected to increase the fastest of all. This is in response to the expanding elderly population's needs and preference for home care. Furthermore, technological advances are making it possible to bring increasingly complex treatments into the home.

Another expected area of high growth will occur in nursing home care; this is primarily in response to the larger number of frail elderly in their 80s and 90s requiring long-term care. As hospitals come under greater pressure to decrease the average patient length of stay (LOS), nursing home admissions will increase, as will growth in long-term rehabilitation units.

An additional factor influencing employment patterns for registered nurses is the tendency for sophisticated medical procedures to be performed in physicians' offices, clinics, ambulatory surgical centers, and other outpatient settings. Registered nurses' expertise will be needed to care for patients undergoing procedures formerly performed only in hospital settings (U.S. Department of Labor, 2003).

Advanced practice nurses can also expect to find themselves in higher demand for the foreseeable future. The evolution of integrated health care networks focusing on primary care and health maintenance are ideal settings for advanced nursing practice.

Nursing Salaries

Salaries in the nursing profession vary widely according to practice setting, level of preparation and credentials, experience, and region of the country. The latest survey of *The Registered Nurse Population: March 2000* (U.S. Department of Health and Human Services, 2001) shows positive signs in terms of salaries for registered nurses. The 2000 average annual salary of a full-time registered nurse in a staff position was

$42,133, up from $38,567 in 1996. This represents an increase of 8.8 percent in 4 years (U.S. Department of Health and Human Services, 2001).

Although salaries have increased nationwide, discussing salary trends from a national perspective is often misleading. For instance, salaries in urban areas are much higher than those in rural communities. Readers should bear this in mind when reviewing these figures. Regional salaries tend to be more realistic measures. Figure 5-7 shows the average annual salaries of staff nurses in each geographical area of the United States. Regional variations are apparent. It should be noted that these figures do not include salaries of advanced practice nurses, whose earnings are higher than the averages shown for staff nurses.

Nationwide in 2000, the average salary of nurse practitioners was $60,126. For certified nurse-midwives, the average was $64,940. The average salary of clinical nurse specialists was lower, at $50,800, whereas certified registered nurse anesthetists averaged $93,787, the highest of any advanced practice specialty group (U.S. Department of Health and Human Services, 2001). Clearly, additional preparation and responsibility increase earning potential.

Most of the wage growth for nurses appears early in their careers and tapers off in time. In 2000, staff RNs employed full-time in nursing who had been working for

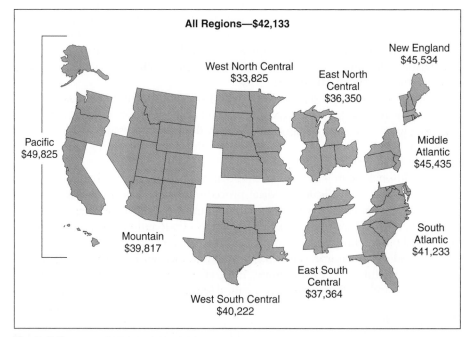

Figure 5-7

Average annual salaries of full-time registered nurses in staff positions by geographic region, March 2000. (Data from U.S. Department of Health and Human Services, Health Resources and Services Administration: *The registered nurse population, March 2000: findings from the national sample survey of registered nurses,* Washington, DC, 2001, Government Printing Office.)

5 years typically earned salaries 15 to 17 percent higher than those newly entering the field. But these same nurses earned only 1 to 3 percent less than nurses who graduated 15 to 20 years earlier (U.S. Department of Health and Human Services, 2001). This decreased potential for salary improvements may account for nurses leaving patient care for additional education and/or other careers in nursing or outside the profession, an issue that must be addressed to improve retention in the profession.

Summary of Key Points
- There are more than 2.7 million registered nurses in the United States, and over 2.2 million are actively practicing. Fewer than 75 percent work full-time.
- Approximately 59.1 percent of working nurses are employed in hospitals, a traditional setting for nursing practice, but one that will see dramatic changes as health care in the United States continues to become more community-based.
- An exciting trend is the growth of opportunities for nurses in practice settings outside the traditional hospital.
- Increased use of advanced practice nurses may be part of the solution to the U.S. health care crisis being brought on by the aging of the baby boom generation, the fast-growing group of frail elderly, technological advances, and cost-containment measures in the health care sector.
- Advanced practice nurses are capable of delivering high-quality care to many segments of the population not currently receiving health care or receiving substandard care.
- If the nation is to benefit from the services of advanced practice nurses, legal barriers to their practice must be removed through political action of organized nursing and politically active nurses.
- Although opinions are mixed, government projections are for the demand for nurses, particularly advanced practice nurses, to increase through the year 2012 and beyond.

CRITICAL THINKING QUESTIONS
1. What characteristics do nurses of today have in common, and in what ways do they differ?
2. Think of the areas of nursing that interest you most. How do your personal and professional qualifications compare with the characteristics needed in the roles discussed in this chapter?
3. Interview nurses in various practice settings, especially those not covered in this chapter. Find out how they prepared for their positions, what their daily activities are, and what they find most challenging and rewarding about their work.
4. Call the nurse recruiter or personnel office of a nearby hospital and inquire about salaries and other benefits for entry-level and advanced practice nursing positions. How do they compare with those listed in this chapter?
5. Interview an advanced practice nurse working in your community. What does he or she see as the major barriers to practice?
6. Contact your state nurses association to find out what legislative initiatives are being undertaken to remove these barriers in your state.

REFERENCES

Abuelouf A: Community health ministry: meeting many needs, *Tennessee Nurse* 61(6):22, 31, 1998.

American Association of Colleges of Nursing: *Enrollment and graduations in baccalaureate and graduate programs in nursing, 2002-2003,* Washington, DC, 2003, American Association of Colleges of Nursing.

American Association of Nurse Anesthetists: Nurse anesthetists at a glance, Online, 2003 *(http://www.aana.com/crna/ataglance.asp).*

American College of Nurse-Midwives: Basic facts about certified nurse-midwives, Online, 2002 *(http://www.midwife.org/prof/display.cfm?id=6).*

American Nurses Association: *Scope and standards of nursing informatics practice,* Washington, DC, 2001, American Nurses Association.

American Nurses Association: *Scope and standards of hospice and palliative nursing practice,* Washington, DC, 2002, American Nurses Publishing.

American Nurses Association and Health Ministries Association: *Scope and standards of parish nursing practice,* Washington, DC, 1998, American Nurses Association and Health Ministries Association.

Horrigan MW: Employment projections to 2012: concepts and context, *Mo Labor Rev* 127(2):3-22, 2004.

Huber DL: The diversity of case management models, *Lippincott's Case Management* 7(6): 212-220, 2002.

Jackson DJ, Lang JM, Swartz WH, et al: Outcomes, safety, and resource utilization in a collaborative care birth center program, *Am J Public Health* 98(6):999-1006, 2004.

Last Acts Task Force: National policy statements on end of life care: precepts of palliative care, *J Palliative Med* 1(2):109-112, 1998.

McKenzie CB, Torkelson NG, Holt MA: Care and cost: nursing case management improves both, *Nurs Management* 20(10):30-34, 1989.

Meadows G: Nursing informatics: an evolving specialty, *Nurs Econ* 20(6):300-301, 2002.

National Association of School Nurses: Definition of school nursing, Online, 2003 *(www.nasn.org).*

Pearson LJ: Fifteenth annual legislative update: how each state stands on legislative issues affecting advanced nursing practice, *The Nurse Practitioner: The Am J Prim Health Care* 28(1):26-32, 2003.

U.S. Department of Health and Human Services, Health Resources and Services Administration: *The registered nurse population, March 2000: findings from the national sample survey of registered nurses,* Washington, DC, 2001, Government Printing Office.

U.S. Department of Health and Human Services, Health Resources and Services Administration: *Projected supply, demand, and shortages of registered nurses: 2000-2020,* Washington, DC, 2002, Government Printing Office.

U.S. Department of Labor, Bureau of Labor Statistics: *Occupational outlook handbook, 2002-2003,* Washington, DC, 2003, Government Printing Office, Available online *(http://www.bls.gov/oco/ocos083.htm).*

Vollman KM: My search to help patients breathe, *Reflections* 25(2):16-18, 1999.

Vollman KM, Bander JL: Improved oxygenation utilizing a prone positioner in patients with acute respiratory distress syndrome, *Intensive Care Med* 22:1105-1111, 1996.

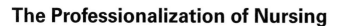

CHAPTER 6

The Professionalization of Nursing

Kay Kittrell Chitty

Key Terms

Accountability	Collective Identity	Occupation
Altruism	Collegiality	Profession
Autonomy	Evidence-Based Practice	Professional
Code of Ethics	Flexner Report	Professionalism
Cognitive	Nursing Process	Professionalization

Learning Outcomes

After studying this chapter, students will be able to:

- Identify the characteristics of a profession.
- Distinguish between the characteristics of professions and occupations.
- Describe how professions evolve.
- Evaluate nursing's position on the professionalism continuum.
- Explain the elements of nursing's contract with society.
- Recognize characteristic behaviors of professional nurses.

What is a profession, and who can be called a professional? These terms are used loosely in everyday conversation. Historically, only medicine, law, and the ministry were accepted as professions. Today, however, **professional** is a term commonly used to identify many types of people, ranging from plumbers to pharmacists. Are all these individuals professionals? Or is the value of the term *professional* diminished when it is used indiscriminately to describe any work done by any group? The answers to these questions are explored in this chapter.

One method of defining a profession is to identify specific criteria that must be met by professionals. For example, in sports a professional is distinguished from an amateur by being paid. So in sports, making money is one characteristic of being a professional. Professionals are generally better at what they do than are others.

Therefore, knowledge, skills, and expertise are also part of being a professional. As you will see in this chapter, there are many other criteria to be examined in a discussion of what contributes to **professionalism**.

HISTORICAL REVIEW: CHARACTERISTICS OF A PROFESSION

For nearly a century scholars have grappled with the meaning of profession. They have generally agreed that a **profession** is an occupational group with a set of attitudes, behaviors, or both. In this section we will briefly review several definitions by scholars through the years and identify major similarities.

Abraham Flexner

Every serious study of professions must begin with a tribute to Abraham Flexner. In the early 1900s, the Carnegie Foundation issued a series of papers about professional schools. The first of these reports was based on sociologist Abraham Flexner's 1910 study of medical education (Flexner, 1910). The **Flexner Report,** as it became known, is a classic piece of educational literature that provided the impetus for the much-needed reform of medical education.

Flexner went on to study other disciplines and later, in a paper about social work, published a list of criteria that he believed were characteristic of all true professions (Flexner, 1915). Flexner's work has stood the test of time. Since his original criteria were published, they have been widely used as a benchmark for determining the status of various occupations in terms of professionalism and have had a profound influence on professional education in several disciplines, including nursing (see Critical Thinking Exercise 6-1).

Flexner's criteria stipulate that a profession:

1. Is basically intellectual (as opposed to physical) and is accompanied by a high degree of individual responsibility.
2. Is based on a body of knowledge that can be learned and is refreshed and refined through research.
3. Is practical, in addition to being theoretical.
4. Can be taught through a process of highly specialized professional education.
5. Has a strong internal organization of members and a well-developed group consciousness.

CRITICAL THINKING *Exercise 6-1*

Is Nursing a Profession or Semiprofession?

Feminists in nursing have expressed concern that traditional definitions of profession, such as Flexner's, are incomplete because they embody only the masculine worldview. They believe that adhering to traditional criteria for professions has had the effect of relegating nursing, teaching, social work, and other female-dominated fields to the status of "semiprofessions." Explore this idea in a class or small group discussion, remembering to respect different viewpoints from your own.

6. Has practitioners who are motivated by altruism (the desire to help others) and who are responsive to public interests (Figure 6-1).

Since 1915, other authorities have identified criteria for professions, building on but varying slightly from Flexner's.

Richard H. Hall

Another sociologist, Richard H. Hall, published a seminal work on professionalism in 1968. Hall described a professional model that classified attributes such as educational qualifications, professional organizations, and sense of calling. He identified five indicators of an individual's attitude toward professionalism (1968):

1. Use of a professional organization as a primary point of reference.
2. Belief in the value of public service.
3. Belief in self-regulation.
4. Commitment to profession that goes beyond economic incentives.
5. A sense of autonomy in practice.

Hall recommended that each profession needed to develop its own methods of measuring professionalism that recognize the uniqueness of that discipline.

Hybrid Conceptualizations of Profession

A pharmacy profession task force recently spent 5 years studying and promoting pharmacy student professionalism (Task Force on Professionalism, 2000). In the process the task force reviewed the history of professional development in the broad sense, reviewing the work of numerous scholars. From this review they

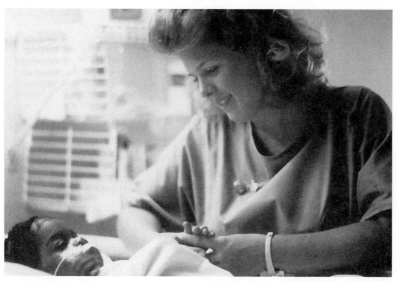

Figure **6-1**
According to Flexner, professionals are motivated by altruism, a desire to help others. (Courtesy Medical University of South Carolina.)

distilled a list of 10 common characteristics of the members of a profession:

1. Prolonged specialized training in a body of abstract knowledge
2. A service orientation
3. An ideology based on the original faith professed by members
4. An ethic that is binding on the practitioners
5. A body of knowledge unique to the members
6. A set of skills that forms the technique of the profession
7. A guild of those entitled to practice the profession
8. Authority granted by society in the form of licensure or certification
9. A recognized setting in which the profession is practiced
10. A theory of societal benefits derived from the ideology

Major Similarities

As you see, authorities have disagreed about the number of criteria and the types of behaviors and characteristics of professions. A review of a variety of publications on this topic, however, reveals that there are three criteria that consistently appear: service/altruism, specialized knowledge, and autonomy/ethics (Flexner, 1915; Hall, 1968, 1982; Carr-Saunders and Wilson, 1933; Adams, Miller, and Beck, 1996; Huber, 2000).

1. Service implies a sense of calling to the discipline, a sense of mission, and a responsibility to the public.
2. Knowledge implies specialized education, including both theoretical knowledge and techniques or skills.
3. Practice autonomy implies having control over one's own practice. It also implies having a code of ethics governing standards of conduct within the profession (Huber, 2000).

After nearly a century of study, contemplation, and deliberation, there is still no clear-cut consensus about what constitutes a profession, nor is there likely to be. Occupational groups are constantly pushing to become more professional and to receive public acknowledgement of their professional status. As they do so, conceptions of profession change. Next, we will explore how an occupational group evolves into a profession.

THE EVOLUTION FROM OCCUPATION TO PROFESSION

Professions usually evolve from occupations that originally consisted of tasks but developed more specialized educational pathways and publicly legitimized status. The established professions, such as law, medicine, and the ministry, generally followed a typical developmental pattern of stages that occurred sequentially. First, practitioners performed full-time work in the discipline. They then determined work standards, identified a body of knowledge, and established educational programs in institutions of higher learning. Next, they promoted organization into effective occupational associations. Then they worked toward legal protection that limited practice of their unique skills by outsiders. Finally, they established codes of ethics (Carr-Saunders and Wilson, 1933). This process can be termed **professionalization.**

Another analysis of the evolution from occupation to profession was done by Houle (1980). He identified a number of characteristics that indicate an occupational group is moving along the continuum toward professional status. First is the definition of the group's mission and foundations of practice. Then comes mastery of theoretical knowledge, development of the capacity to solve problems, the use of practical knowledge, and self-enhancement (continued learning and development). Finally, Houle identified nine characteristics that indicate than an occupation is developing a **collective identity** or group identification, which is necessary for professions. These include formal training, credentialing, creation of a subculture, legal right to practice, public acceptance, ethical practice, discipline of incompetent/ unethical practitioners, relationship to other practitioners, and relationship to users of services.

The term *occupation* is often used interchangeably with *profession,* but their definitions differ. *Webster's New World Dictionary* (1996) defines **occupation** as "what occupies, or engages, one's time; business; employment." In this discussion we define profession as "a calling, vocation, or form of employment that provides a needed service to society and possesses characteristics of expertise, autonomy, long academic preparation, commitment, and responsibility" (Huber, 2000, p. 34).

There is widespread, overall agreement that a profession is different from an occupation in at least two major ways—preparation and commitment.

Professional Preparation

Professional preparation usually takes place in a college or university setting. Preparation is prolonged to include instruction in the specialized body of knowledge and techniques of the profession. Professional preparation includes more than knowledge and skills, however. It also includes orientation to the beliefs, values, and attitudes expected of the members of the profession. Standards of practice and ethical considerations are also included. These components of professional education are part of the process of socialization into a profession and are discussed in Chapter 8. According to Miller (1985), preparation enables professional practitioners to act in a logical, rational manner rather than relying on intuition and speculation. Notice that this gives no credence to intuition, long considered a feminine attribute, as an important consequence of preparation. An ever-expanding base of knowledge in all disciplines complicates the challenges of professional preparation. The Research Note on p. 168 describes a study that examined nursing students' beliefs about what it means to be a professional.

Professional Commitment

Professionals' commitment to their profession is strong. They derive much of their personal identification from their work and consider it an integral part of their lives. People engaging in a profession often consider it their "calling." Historically, professionals' commitment to their profession has transcended their expectation of material reward. Although people may readily change occupations, it is less common for people to change professions. Several critical differences between occupations and professions are summarized in Table 6-1.

RESEARCH note

Three professors at a Tennessee university sought to understand how students develop professional identity. They conducted a qualitative, existential-phenomenological study of baccalaureate students to determine their ideas of what it means to be a professional. Sixty-nine nursing students at various levels of education were asked to describe specific experiences in which they "felt professional." The researchers analyzed these figural (outstanding) experiences for common patterns or themes. Three interrelated themes were identified: belonging, knowing, and affirmation.

- An example of *belonging*: "I knew ... that I had acted as a professional and knowledgeable nurse and even though that man died, the team did everything they could to keep him alive and I was a team member. It was a satisfying moment."
- An example of *knowing*: "For myself, my nursing knowledge and actions make me a professional. However, when this nursing knowledge is applied and the client and family express their appreciation of my nursing efforts, then I feel professional."
- An example of *affirmation*: "I had one family who just couldn't believe I was in nursing school. They stated that I was so 'professional and caring' and that I was a 'great nurse.' Then I said, 'Well, I'm not a nurse yet; I'll be graduating in one year.' That made me feel like I was actually a nurse."

The researchers suggested that courses encouraging students to reflect on the meaning of the profession and being a professional should be offered early in the curriculum. They stated their belief that "developing a sense of professionalism is equally important as knowledge and skills."

From Secrest J, Norwood BR, Keatley VM: "I was actually a nurse": the meaning of professionalism for baccalaureate nursing students, *J Nurs Ed* 42(2):77-82, 2003.

BARRIERS TO PROFESSIONALISM IN NURSING

As a group, nurses must strive to reduce the barriers to professionalization. The first step in that process is developing an awareness of those barriers. Several major barriers will be discussed here.

Variability in Educational Preparation

The most obvious barrier to nursing's achievement of professional status is the variability of educational backgrounds of its practitioners. There is no other profession that allows entry into practice at less than the baccalaureate level. Quite the contrary, many professions, such as law, medicine, and physical therapy require postgraduate preparation for professional practice. Because professional status and power increase with education, a legitimate question is "How can nursing take its place as a peer among the professions when most nurses currently in practice hold less than a baccalaureate degree?" The differentiation between professional nursing and technical nursing is a challenging issue that has not yet been resolved.

Table 6-1 COMPARISON OF CHARACTERISTICS OF OCCUPATIONS AND
PROFESSIONS

Occupation	Profession
Training may occur on the job.	Education takes place in a college or university.
Length of training varies.	Education is prolonged.
Work is largely manual.	Work involves mental creativity.
Decision making is guided largely by experience or by trial and error.	Decision making is based largely on science or theoretical constructs.
Values, beliefs, and ethics are not prominent features of preparation.	Values, beliefs, and ethics are an integral part of preparation.
Commitment and personal identification vary.	Commitment and personal identification are strong.
Workers are supervised.	Workers are autonomous.
People often change jobs.	People are unlikely to change professions.
Material reward is main motivation.	Commitment transcends material reward.
Accountability rests primarily with employer.	Accountability rests with individual.

Educational diversity within nursing has slowed the progress toward acceptance of the baccalaureate or higher degree as the prerequisite for professional practice. Lack of resolution of these differences threatens to undermine nursing's continued steady development as a profession (Christman, 1998). This is a painful issue for nurses, creating division and anger whenever it is discussed. For the profession as a whole to progress, we must move beyond personal feelings to look objectively at how nursing stacks up when compared with other groups—groups to whom we wish to be compared—and adjust our aims accordingly.

Gender Issues

Although gender was not identified as a criterion by any of the scholars of professionalism, it plays a major role in the perceived value of female-dominated professions such as teaching, social work, and nursing. Although the number of men in nursing is gradually increasing, a gender balance may never be achieved. This will continue to be a hindrance, because of the persistent prevalence of outmoded thinking and the resultant devaluing of "women's work" in our society.

Historical Influences

Nursing's historical connections with religious orders and the military continue to have influence, both positive and negative, today. Aspects that have become liabilities with the passage of time include unquestioning obedience, which runs counter to the professional values of autonomy and self-determination, and altruism, which mitigates against the fair economic valuation of the work of nursing. Nurses should be aware that unquestioning obedience stifles the creative thinking and problem solving required for professional practice. Similar to other helping professionals, nurses must resist pressures to feel guilty or greedy for expecting to be paid well for their complex and demanding work.

External Conflicts

As nurses have become more highly educated and able to provide services that were formerly part of medical practice, conflicts with medicine have inevitably arisen. Much of the power, influence, and resources of organized nursing has gone toward lobbying efforts in state legislatures to ensure that the scope of nursing practice is protected and appropriately enhanced. These efforts should and will continue on the professional association level. On the personal level, however, nurses must strive for collaboration, not competition, with physicians and other health personnel with whom they work. Nurses must demonstrate their unique knowledge, expertise, and skills so that professional autonomy can be exercised within the various bureaucratic organizations in which they work.

Internal Conflicts

Professional nursing's power is fragmented by subgroups and dissension. Rivalry among diploma-educated, associate degree–educated, and baccalaureate-educated nurses saps the vitality of the profession. The proliferation of nursing organizations (see Box 4-3 for a partial list) and competition among them for members also diminish nursing's potential. Only 6 percent of the 2.7 million registered nurses in the United States are members of the ANA (American Nurses Association, 2003). The fact that most nurses are not members of any professional organization impairs nursing's ability to lobby effectively. These are major challenges for nursing if it is to realize its potential collective professional power and autonomy.

NURSING'S PATHWAY TO PROFESSIONALISM

Nursing's pathway to professionalism has not been smooth. For decades an ongoing subject for discussion in nursing circles has been the question "Is nursing a profession?" Much has been spoken and written on both sides of this issue over the years. Nursing sociologists do not all agree that nursing is a profession. Some believe that it is, at best, an *emerging* profession. Others cite the progress nursing has made toward meeting the commonly accepted criteria for full-fledged professional status. Still others believe that nursing leaders, by embracing the masculine orientation to professionalism embodied in the work of Flexner and others, have supported the existing patriarchal order, thereby prolonging the subordination of nursing to male-dominated professions such as medicine (Wuest, 1994). Let's look critically now at various criteria and nursing's status in relation to them.

Bixler and Bixler's Criteria

Genevieve and Roy Bixler, a husband and wife team of nonnurses who were nevertheless advocates and supporters of nursing, first wrote about the status of nursing as a profession in 1945. In 1959, they again appraised nursing according to their original seven criteria, noting the progress made (Bixler and Bixler, 1959).

Their criteria included the following:

1. "A profession utilizes in its practice a well-defined and well-organized body of specialized knowledge which is on the intellectual level of the higher learning" (p. 1142).
2. "A profession constantly enlarges the body of knowledge it uses and improves its techniques of education and service by the use of the scientific method" (p. 1143).
3. "A profession entrusts the education of its practitioners to institutions of higher education" (p. 1144).
4. "A profession applies its body of knowledge in practical services which are vital to human and social welfare" (p. 1145).
5. "A profession functions autonomously in the formulation of professional policy and in the control of professional activity thereby" (p. 1145).
6. "A profession attracts individuals of intellectual and personal qualities who exalt service above personal gain and who recognize their chosen occupation as a life work" (p. 1146).
7. "A profession strives to compensate its practitioners by providing freedom of action, opportunity for continuous professional growth, and economic security" (p. 1146).

Kelly's Criteria

Lucie Kelly, RN, PhD, FAAN, is an outstanding nurse writer, teacher, and influential leader. She was editor of the journal *Nursing Outlook* and president of Sigma Theta Tau International Honor Society of Nursing, among many career highlights. Dr. Kelly has spent much of her nursing career exploring the dimensions of professional nursing. She compiled the following set of eight characteristics of a profession many years ago (1981, p. 157), but they remain relevant today:

1. The services provided are vital to humanity and the welfare of society.
2. There is a special body of knowledge that is continually enlarged through research.
3. The services involve intellectual activities; individual responsibility (**accountability**) is a strong feature.
4. Practitioners are educated in institutions of higher learning.
5. Practitioners are relatively independent and control their own policies and activities (autonomy).
6. Practitioners are motivated by service (altruism) and consider their work an important component of their lives.
7. There is a code of ethics to guide the decisions and conduct of practitioners.
8. There is an organization (association) that encourages and supports high standards of practice.

Let us examine how well contemporary nursing fulfills these eight characteristics.

"The services provided are vital to humanity and the welfare of society"

If random students were asked why they chose nursing, most would reply, "To help people." Certainly nursing is a service that is essential to the well-being of people and to society as a whole. Nursing promotes the maintenance and restoration of health of individuals, groups, and communities. The goal of nursing is to assist others to attain the highest level of wellness of which they are capable. Caring—meaning nurturing and helping others—is a basic component of professional nursing.

"There is a special body of knowledge that is continually enlarged through research"

In the past, nursing was based on principles borrowed from the physical and social sciences and other disciplines. Today, however, there is a body of knowledge that is uniquely nursing's own. Although this was not always so, the amount of investigation and analysis of nursing care has expanded rapidly in the past 30 years. Nursing theory development is also proceeding swiftly. Nursing is no longer based on trial and error but increasingly relies on theory development and research as a basis for practice. We call the reliance on research as a basis for nursing practice **evidence-based practice.** You will learn more about theory, research, and evidence-based practice later in this book.

"The services involve intellectual activities; individual responsibility (accountability) is a strong feature"

Nursing developed and refined its own unique approach to practice, called the **nursing process.** The nursing process is essentially a **cognitive** (mental) activity that requires both critical and creative thinking and serves as the basis for providing nursing care. The profession is now engaged in an ongoing effort to identify and standardize nursing diagnoses, interventions, and outcomes, all of which are parts of the nursing process.

Individual accountability in nursing has become the hallmark of practice. Accountability, according to the American Nurses Association's (ANA) *Code of Ethics for Nurses* (2001), is being answerable to someone for something one has done. Provision 4 of the new (2001) Code states, "The nurse is responsible and accountable for individual nursing practice and determines the appropriate delegation of tasks consistent with the nurse's obligation to provide optimum patient care" (p. 5). Through legal opinions and court cases, society has demonstrated that it, too, holds nurses individually responsible for their actions as well as for those of unlicensed personnel under their supervision.

"Practitioners are educated in institutions of higher learning"

As presented in Chapter 2, the first university-based nursing program began in 1909 at the University of Minnesota. Several studies, including Esther Lucille Brown's 1948 report, *Nursing for the Future,* called for nursing education to be based in universities and colleges. Recall that another milestone was the 1965 position paper of the ANA, which called for all nursing education to take place in institutions of higher education (American Nurses Association, 1965).

The majority of programs offering basic nursing education are now associate degree and baccalaureate programs located in colleges and universities. There are growing numbers of master's and doctoral programs in nursing, although the number of graduates is small compared with other health professions.

"Practitioners are relatively independent and control their own policies and activities (autonomy)"

Autonomy, or control over one's practice, is another controversial area for nursing. Although many nursing actions are independent, most nurses are employed in hospitals, where authority resides in one's position. One's place in the hierarchy, rather than expertise, confers or denies power and status. Physicians are widely regarded as gatekeepers, and their authorization or supervision is required before many activities can occur. Nurse practice acts in most states reinforce nursing's arguable self-determination by requiring that nurses perform certain actions only when authorized by supervising physicians or hospital protocols.

There are at least three groups that have historically attempted to control nursing practice: organized medicine, health service administration, and organized nursing. Both the medical profession and health service administration have attempted to maintain control of nursing because they believe it is in their best interest to keep nurses dependent on them. Both are well organized and have powerful lobbies at state and national levels.

"Practitioners are motivated by service (altruism) and consider their work an important component of their lives"

As a group, nurses are dedicated to the ideal of service to others, which is also known as **altruism.** This ideal has sometimes become intertwined with economic issues and historically has been exploited by employers of nurses. No one questions the right of other professionals to charge reasonable fees for the services they render; when nurses want higher salaries, however, others sometimes call their altruism into question. Nurses must take responsibility for their own financial well-being and for the health of the profession. This will, in turn, ensure its continued attractiveness to those who might choose nursing as a career. If there are to be adequate numbers of nurses to meet society's needs, salaries must be comparable with those in competing disciplines. Being concerned with salary issues does nothing to diminish a nurse's altruism or professionalism.

Another issue, consideration of work as a primary component of life, has been a thornier problem for nurses. Commitment to a career is not a value equally shared by all nurses. Some still regard nursing as a job and drop in and out of practice depending on economic and family needs. This approach, although appealing to many nurses and conducive to traditional family management, has retarded the development of professional attitudes and behaviors for the profession as a whole.

"There is a code of ethics to guide the decisions and conduct of practitioners"

An ethical code does not stipulate how an individual should act in a specific situation; rather, it provides professional standards and a framework for decision making. The trust placed in the nursing profession by the public requires that nurses act with integrity. To aid them in doing so, both the International Council of Nurses (ICN) and the ANA, among others, have established codes of nursing ethics through which profession-wide standards of practice are established, promoted, and refined. The *Code of Ethics for Nurses,* which will be discussed later in the chapter, can be found on the inside back cover of this text.

In 1893, long before these codes were written, "The Florence Nightingale Pledge" (Box 6-1) was created by a committee headed by Lystra Eggert Gretter and presented to the Farrand Training School for Nurses located at Harper Hospital in Detroit, Michigan (Dock and Stewart, 1920). Its similarities to the medical profession's

Box **6-1** The Florence Nightingale Pledge

> I solemnly pledge myself before God and in the presence of this assembly to pass my life in purity and to practice my profession faithfully.
>
> I will abstain from whatever is deleterious and mischievous, and will not take or knowingly administer any harmful drug. I will do all in my power to maintain and elevate the standard of my profession, and will hold in confidence all personal matters committed to my keeping and all family affairs coming to my knowledge in the practice of my calling.
>
> With loyalty will I endeavor to aid the physician in his work and devote myself to the welfare of those committed to my care.

From Dock LL, Stewart IM: *A short history of nursing,* New York, 1920, Putnam.

Hippocratic Oath are obvious. The Nightingale Pledge can be considered nursing's first code of ethics. It is presented here not only for its historic value but also because it established the roots for our current Code.

"There is an organization (association) that encourages and supports high standards of practice"

As discussed in Chapter 4, a number of professional associations have been formed to promote the improvement of the nursing profession. Among these is the ANA, which all registered nurses are eligible to join. According to its bylaws, the purposes of the ANA are to work for the improvement of health standards and the availability of health care services for all people, to foster high standards of nursing, and to stimulate and promote the professional development of nurses and advance their economic and general welfare (Figure 6-2; American Nurses Association, 1997). The ANA is also the official voice of nursing and therefore is the primary advocate for nursing interests in general. Unfortunately, fewer than 1 of 10 nurses belongs to this official professional organization. The political power that could be derived from the unified efforts of 2.7 million registered nurses nationwide would be impressive; sadly, that goal has not yet been realized.

Miller's Wheel of Professionalism in Nursing

Using commonalities she detected in the work of sociologists and nursing leaders, as well as statements from *Nursing's Social Policy Statement* and Code for Nurses, Miller (1985, 2001) created a model (or visual expression) to conceptualize nursing professionalism. She titled this model the Wheel of Professionalism (Figure 6-3).

In Miller's wheel, the center represents the essential foundation of nursing education in an institution of higher learning. According to Adams and Miller (1996), "Each of the eight spokes represents other behaviors deemed necessary in maintaining or increasing nurses' professionalism. They are competence and continuing education; adherence to the code of ethics; participation in the primary and referent professional organization, i.e., ANA and state constituent member association;

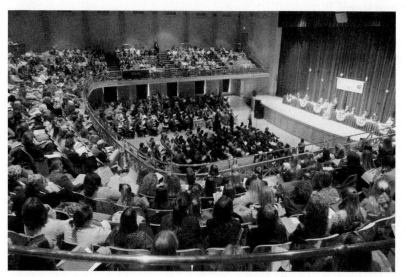

Figure 6-2
Professionals belong to associations that encourage and support ethical standards of practice.
(Courtesy Tennessee Nurses Association.)

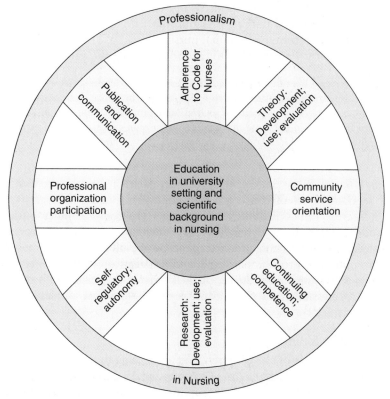

Figure 6-3
The Wheel of Professionalism in nursing. (Copyright 1984 Barbara Kemp Miller.)

publication and communication; orientation toward community services; theory and research development and utilization; and self-regulation and autonomy" (p. 79). To test the wheel model, Adams and Miller devised their own instrument, Professionalism in Nursing Behaviors Inventory, which was revised and tested. Research continues to refine this instrument, which is to be used by nurses themselves to evaluate their professional growth.

Standards Established by the Profession Itself

Any exploration of nursing's development as a profession would be incomplete without a discussion of two major documents that guide all nurses in their professional commitments. These are *Nursing's Social Policy Statement* (2003) and the *Code of Ethics for Nurses with Interpretive Statements* (American Nurses Association, 2001).

Nursing's Social Policy Statement: a contract with society

Although criteria for professions vary, all professions have one criterion in common: an obligation to the recipients of their services. Nursing, therefore, has an obligation to those who receive nursing care. The nature of the social contract between the members of the nursing profession and society is summarized in *Nursing's Social Policy Statement.* This document, last revised in 2003, is the result of several years of work by literally hundreds of nurses. It serves "as a framework for understanding professional nursing's relationship with society and nursing's obligation to those who receive professional nursing care" (p. 1). Here is part of what *Nursing's Social Policy Statement* has to say about nursing as a profession:

> Professional nursing, like other professions, is an essential part of the society from which it grew and within which it continues to evolve. Professional nursing is dynamic, rather than static, reflecting the changing nature of societal need. Professional nursing can be said to be "owned by society in the sense that a profession acquires recognition, relevance, and even meaning in terms of its relationship to that society, its culture and institutions, and its other members" (American Nurses Association, 2003, pp. 1-2).

Nursing's Social Policy Statement is only 15 pages in length; yet it addresses a broad array of topics of concern that occur when nursing intersects with the society it serves. Topics include the following: the social context of nursing; values and assumptions undergirding the Statement; a definition of nursing; the knowledge base for nursing practice; the scope of both basic and advanced nursing practice; and the professional, legal, and self-regulation of nursing practice. A careful reading of this brief document will provide the reader with the essence of nursing's professionalism. (It is available from American Nurses Publishing; see References.)

The code of ethics for nurses

As you will recall, most of the early scholars attempting to define *profession* mentioned ethical behavior as a hallmark of a profession. In fact, a code of ethics is generally considered a tool that guides a group toward professional self-definition and provides evidence of professional legitimacy.

A **code of ethics** is a written, public document that reminds practitioners and the public they serve of the specific responsibilities and obligations accepted by the profession's practitioners. Since the inception of formalized education for nurses, the practice of nursing has been guided by ethical standards promoted first by Florence Nightingale and thereafter by nursing groups. The *Code of Ethics for Nurses* has been modified over the years as nursing and its social context have evolved. It is intended to guide the practice of registered nurses in all practice settings with all types of clients. The most recent version, *Code of Ethics for Nurses with Interpretive Statements,* was approved in 2001.

There are nine provisions in the 2001 Code, each of which is accompanied by interpretive statements intended to clarify the provision. The first three provisions describe "the fundamental values and commitments of the nurse; the next three address boundaries of duty and loyalty; and the last three address aspects of duties beyond individual patient encounters" (p. 2). Read the provisions of the *Code of Ethics for Nurses* on the inside back cover of this text. The entire document, including interpretive statements, is available for review online *(www.nursingworld.org/ ethics/code/ethicscode150.htm)*.

Today's health care environment often presents challenges to nurses' ethics. Cost-conscious hospitals, managed care plans, staffing insufficiencies created by both economic factors and nursing shortages are just a few of the many strains on nursing practice (Hook, 2001). The Code exists to strengthen and guide nurses' decision making as they navigate the troubled waters that now exist in many practice settings. The Code empowers nurses to maintain their focus on the patient as the center of health care.

COLLEGIALITY AS AN ATTRIBUTE OF THE PROFESSIONAL NURSE

A sometimes overlooked but increasingly important aspect of professionalism in nursing is collegiality. The promotion of collaboration, cooperation, and recognition of interdependence among members of the nursing profession is the essence of **collegiality.** Professional nurses demonstrate collegiality by sharing with, supporting, assisting, and counseling other nurses and nursing students. These behaviors can be seen when nurses, for example, take part in professional organizations, mentor less experienced nurses, willingly serve as role models for nursing students, welcome learners and their instructors in the practice setting, assist researchers with data gathering, publish in professional literature, and support peer-assistance programs for impaired nurses.

The value placed on collegiality as a professional attribute can be seen in the ANA's 2004 publication, *Nursing: Scope and Standards of Practice,* which includes collegiality as one of only nine standards of professional performance. The practice of nursing would be enhanced if the commitment nurses feel toward their patients was equaled by their commitment to one another and to nurturing the next generation of professional nurses.

An article entitled "Being Good and Doing Good" by Bruhn (2001) outlines twelve points on professionalism, a number of which serve as reminders of the value of collegiality (Box 6-2).

Box 6-2 Twelve Points on Professionalism

- Be civil—Treat people with respect. You do not have to like or agree with a person to treat him or her as you would want to be treated.
- Be ethical—Stand up for personal and professional standards. Do what is right, not what is expected.
- Be honest—Be forthright; do not participate in gossip and rumor.
- Be the best—Strive to be better than good.
- Be consistent—Behavior should coincide with values and beliefs.
- Be a communicator—Invite ideas, opinions, and feedback from patients and colleagues.
- Be accountable—Do what you say you will do. Take responsibility for your own actions.
- Be collaborative—Work in partnership with others for the benefit of patients.
- Be forgiving—Everyone makes mistakes; give people a fair chance.
- Be current—Keep knowledge and skills up to date.
- Be involved—Be active at local, state, and national levels.
- Be a model—What a person says and does reflects on his or her profession.

From Bruhn J G: Being good and doing good: the culture of professionalism in the health professions, *Health Care Manag* 19(4):47-58, 2001.

NEED FOR A NEW PARADIGM

As society and health care have become more complex, perhaps the time has come to shift away from a rigid conceptualization of profession toward viewing the achievement of professional status as a dynamic, ongoing process. Huber (2000) recommends that we view professionalization as a continuum from nonprofessional to semiprofessional to professional, related to the degree to which an occupational group is characterized by the achievement of identified professional criteria. Instead of asking, "Is nursing a profession?" it may be more fruitful to ask, "How is nursing progressing in the dynamic process of professionalization?" or "Where on the professional continuum is nursing right now?" Although barriers remain, some of which were identified earlier in this chapter, nursing has made a great deal of progress in the past few decades and is poised to continue that progress in the future.

To summarize this discussion of professionalism in nursing, read Critical Thinking Exercise 6-2 and identify the professional behaviors exhibited in the case study presented.

Summary of Key Points
- Commitment to a profession is different from having a job or an occupation.
- A review of scholarly writing about professions reveals that there are several characteristics that all professions have in common.
- A body of knowledge, specialized education, service to society, accountability, autonomy, and ethical standards are a few of the hallmarks of professions.

CRITICAL THINKING *Exercise 6-2*

Identifying Professional Nursing Behaviors

Instructions: If being a *professional* nurse is different from practicing the *occupation* of nursing, there must be certain behaviors that differentiate the two. Read the case study below; then, using various criteria for professions presented in this chapter and the *Code of Ethics for Nurses*, identify professional behaviors exhibited by Joan. For each behavior you identify, state which source or document promotes that behavior.

Joan is a 32-year-old married mother of two. She graduated from River City College of Nursing at the age of 26 and has been practicing since her graduation. Her first position was as a staff nurse at Providence Hospital, a 300-bed private hospital. Nursing administration at Providence encourages nurses to provide individualized nursing care while protecting the dignity and autonomy of each patient and family. She chose Providence because the philosophy of nursing there paralleled her own. Another reason Joan selected this hospital was that she wanted to practice oncology (cancer) nursing, and there is an oncology unit at Providence.

Each day Joan uses the nursing process in caring for her patients and in dealing with their families. That means she assesses their condition, plans and implements their care, and evaluates the care she has given. Then she enters what she has done in each patient's database in the accepted format. She communicates clearly to the other members of the nursing staff and to the other health care professionals involved in the care of the patients on her unit but refuses to discuss them with others not involved in their direct care.

After 2 years as a staff nurse, Joan accepted a position as a team leader. This means that now she takes responsibility not only for her own practice but also for that of licensed practical nurses and nursing assistants on her team. To do this effectively, she stays abreast of changes in her state's nursing practice act and Providence Hospital's policies and procedures. In addition, she updates her knowledge by reading current journals and research periodicals. She makes it a policy to attend at least two nursing conferences each year to stay on top of trends. She belongs to her professional organization and participates as an active member. She finds that this is another source of the latest information on professional issues.

Joan looks forward to working with the nursing students at Providence Hospital. She remembers when she was a student and how a word from a practicing nurse could make or break her day. Of course, students do mean extra work, but she sees this as a part of her role and patiently provides the guidance they need, even when she is busy.

In the course of her daily work, Joan sometimes has a question about certain procedures. She is not embarrassed to seek help from more experienced nurses, from textbooks, or from other health professionals. Sometimes she offers suggestions to the head nurse and the oncology clinical nurse specialist about possible research questions and participates in gathering data when the unit takes on a research study.

Providence Hospital uses a shared governance model, which means nurses serve on committees that develop and interpret nursing policies and procedures. Joan serves on two committees and chairs another. Right now the hospital is preparing a self-study for an upcoming accreditation, so the meetings are frequent. Instead of complaining about the meetings, Joan prepares and organizes her portion of the meeting so that everyone's time is

Continued

CRITICAL THINKING *Exercise 6-2*

Identifying Professional Nursing Behaviors—cont'd

used most effectively. She has to delegate some of her patient care responsibilities to others while she is attending meetings. Because she has taken the time to know the other workers' skills and abilities, she does not worry about what happens while she is gone.

At the end of the day when Joan goes home, she occasionally gets a call from a friend with a health-related question or a request to give a neighbor's child an allergy injection. Although she is tired, she recognizes that in the eyes of others, she represents the nursing profession. She is proud to be trusted and respected for her knowledge, skills, and dedication. Helping others through nursing care is something Joan has wanted to do since she was small, and she finds it very fulfilling.

Lately, Joan has recognized in herself some troubling signs: She has been irritable and impatient with family and co-workers and generally out of sorts. She has gained weight and is exercising less than usual. She wonders whether working with terminally ill patients and their families is the source of her stress. Joan's husband has suggested that she take "a break" from nursing and stay home with the children, but after talking it over with her nurse manager, she has decided to ask for assignment to different nursing responsibilities for a while. She knows that she needs to be her own advocate and take care of herself. Next week she will begin a 3-month stint in outpatient surgery, where she believes the emotional intensity will be a bit lower.

- The feminist perspective includes the belief that the emphasis on professionalism has not helped nursing and has prevented nurses from appreciating, valuing, exploring, and refining the feminine caring experience (Wuest, 1994).
- Although nursing has a briefer history than some traditional professions and is still dealing with autonomy, preparation, and commitment issues, great progress has been made in moving nursing along the professionalization continuum.
- An awareness of the characteristics of professions and professional behavior helps nurses assume leadership in continuing progress toward professionalism.
- *Nursing's Social Policy Statement* is considered nursing's contract with society.
- Being a professional is a dynamic process, not a condition or state of being.
- Professional growth evolves throughout the different stages of nurses' careers.

CRITICAL THINKING QUESTIONS
1. How might nursing be different today if all its practitioners viewed it as their profession rather than a job?
2. What impact might the traditional male orientation toward work as a lifelong career commitment have on the potential for success of men in nursing? On their earning potential?
3. What is the relationship between training and education?
4. On a scale of 1 to 10, rate nursing on each of the criteria for professions identified by Flexner, Hall, Bixler and Bixler, and Kelly.

5. Identify at least two concerns about traditional views of professionalism expressed by nurses with a feminist perspective.
6. Describe at least five characteristic behaviors of professional nurses.
7. Discuss the Nightingale Pledge (see Box 6-1) as a historical document, as an ethical statement, and as a reflection of Florence Nightingale's social and cultural environment. What value does this document have for today's nurse?
8. Using Miller's Wheel of Professionalism, identify specific activities that fit under each of the "spokes." How might a novice nurse's behaviors in relation to each spoke differ from those of a seasoned practitioner?

REFERENCES

Adams D, Miller BK: Professionalism in nursing behaviors of nurse practitioners, *J Prof Nurs* 17(4):203-210, 2001.

Adams D, Miller, BK, Beck L: Professionalism behaviors of hospital nurse executives and middle managers in 10 western states, *West J Nurs Res* 18(1):77-89, 1996.

American Nurses Association: *Educational preparation for nurse practitioners and assistants to nurses: a position paper,* Kansas City, MO, 1965, American Nurses Association.

American Nurses Association: *Association bylaws,* Kansas City, MO, 1997, American Nurses Association.

American Nurses Association: *Code of ethics for nurses with interpretive statements,* Washington, DC, 2001, American Nurses Publishing.

American Nurses Association: House of delegates votes on "new" ANA, *Am J Nurs* 103(8):22-23, 2003.

American Nurses Association: *Nursing: scope and standards of practice,* Washington, DC, 2004, nursesbooks.org.

American Nurses Association: *Nursing's social policy statement,* ed 2, Washington, DC, 2004, nursesbooks.org.

Bixler GK, Bixler RW: The professional status of nursing, *Am J Nurs* 59(8):1142-1147, 1959.

Brown EL: *Nursing for the future,* New York, 1948, Russell Sage Foundation.

Bruhn JG.: Being good and doing good: the culture of professionalism in the health professions, *Health Care Manag* 19(4):47-58, 2001.

Carr-Saunders AM, Wilson PA: *The professions,* Oxford, 1933, Clarendon Press.

Christman L: Who is a nurse? *Image: J Nurs Scholar* 30(3):211-214, 1998.

Dock LL, Stewart IM: *A short history of nursing,* New York, 1920, Putnam.

Flexner A: *Medical education in the United States and Canada: a report to the Carnegie Foundation for the advancement of teaching,* Bethesda, MD, 1910, Science & Health Publications.

Flexner A: Is social work a profession? *School Soc* 1(26):901, 1915.

Hall RH: Professionalization and bureaucratization, *Am Sociol Rev* 33:92-104, 1968.

Hall RH: The professionals, employed professionals, and the professional association. In *Professionalism and the Empowerment of Nursing,* Kansas City, MO, 1982, American Nurses Association.

Hook K: Empowered caring and the code of ethics, *ANA Ethics & Human Rights Issues Update* 1(2), Online, 2001 *(www.nursingworld.org/ethics/update/vol1no2a.htm).*

Houle C: *Continuing learning in the professions,* San Francisco, CA, 1980, Jossey-Bass.

Huber D: *Leadership and nursing care management,* Philadelphia, 2000, WB Saunders.

Kelly L: *Dimensions of professional nursing,* ed 4, New York, 1981, Macmillan.

Miller BK: Just what is a professional? *Nurs Success Today* 2(4):21-27, 1985.

Nativio D: Professionalism revisited, *Nurs Outlook* 48(2):71-72, 2001.

Secrest J, Norwood BR, Keatley VM: "I was actually a nurse": the meaning of professionalism for baccalaureate nursing students, *J Nurs Ed* 42(2):77-82, 2003.

Task Force on Professionalism: White paper on pharmacy student professionalism, *J Am Pharm Assoc* 40(1):96-100, 2000.

Webster's new world dictionary, New York, 1996, Simon & Schuster.

Wuest J: Professionalism and the evolution of nursing as a discipline: a feminist perspective, *J Prof Nurs* 19(6):357-367, 1994.

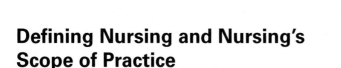

CHAPTER 7

Defining Nursing and Nursing's Scope of Practice

Kay Kittrell Chitty

Key Terms

Active Collaborator	Health Promotion	Milieu
Caring	Holistic Values	Nurse Practice Act
Educative Instrument	Humanistic Nursing Values	Scope of Practice
Health Maintenance	Maximum Health Potential	Standards of Practice

Learning Outcomes

After studying this chapter, students will be able to:

- Describe the benefits of defining nursing and nursing's scope of practice.
- Recognize the evolutionary nature of definitions.
- Compare early definitions of nursing with contemporary ones.
- Recognize the impact of historical, social, economic, and political events on definitions of nursing and scope and standards of practice.
- Identify commonalities in existing definitions of nursing.
- Develop personal definitions of nursing.
- Name four documents every professional nurse should possess and tell why they are important.

Definitions of nursing and nursing's scope of practice seek to describe who nurses are and what they do. They answer questions such as "What is nursing?" "What is the role of the nurse?" "What is unique about nursing?" and "What are the boundaries of nursing practice?" The answers to these questions are far from simple.

In this chapter we will first examine definitions of nursing and then discuss definitions of the scope of nursing practice.

DEFINING NURSING: HARDER THAN IT SEEMS

It may be surprising to learn that finding a universally acceptable definition of nursing has been an elusive goal. It seems that even nurses themselves have been unable to agree on one definition. For more than 150 years, individuals, including the venerable Florence Nightingale, and organizations around the world, such as the International Council of Nurses (ICN), the United Kingdom's Royal College of Nursing, and the American Nurses Association (ANA), and others have made attempts to achieve a consensus on a definition of nursing. Some efforts have been more successful than others.

Most of the definitions reviewed in this chapter have commonalities. Considering the variations in knowledge and technology during the different points in history when these definitions were written, the similarities are remarkable. All the definitions are rooted in history and were affected by significant political, economic, and social events that shaped the form of nursing as it is now known.

Why Define Nursing?

Why is it important to spend time trying to define nursing? Having an accepted definition of nursing is helpful in a variety of ways and provides a framework for nursing practice. It establishes the parameters (or boundaries) of the profession, clarifies the purposes and functions of the work, guides the educational preparation of aspiring practitioners, guides nursing research and theory development, and makes the work of nursing visible and valuable to the public and to policy makers who determine when, where, and how nurses can practice. Norma Lang, an influential contemporary nursing leader put it succinctly by stating, "If we cannot name it, we cannot control it, finance it, research it, teach it, or put it into public policy. It's just that blunt!" (Styles, 1991).

Definitions clarify purposes and functions

Nursing is a complex enterprise that is often confusing to its own practitioners, as well as to the public. Defining nursing assists people to grasp its nuances, many of which are not readily observable. Nursing benefits when people such as journalists, public policy makers, insurers, other health care professionals, and the public understand what it is that nurses do.

Definitions differentiate nursing from other health occupations

The proliferation of various types of health care workers in the past several decades has led to the development of over 200 different allied health occupations. Each new advance in technology bred a new "technician" who needed to be educated, hired, oriented, and paid with limited health care dollars (a trend that continues today). The resulting cost was a major factor leading to significant redesign of the health care system during the 1990s. This was accompanied by a period of redefining roles within the system. In light of these changes, defining the essence of nursing care has become even more important in order to manage the overlap of nursing with other fields without losing the core identity of nursing.

Definitions influence health policy at local, state, and national levels

Policy makers, such as legislators and regulators, need to understand the role and scope of nursing. Without that understanding, they cannot effect good health care policy that fully uses nurses' unique skill set to improve the health of citizens. Another important reason to define nursing is that nursing practice is regulated by the states. Nurse practice acts of each state need to reflect the increasing expertise and autonomy of nurses. When the role of nurses and advanced practice nurses are well defined, legislators can appreciate the need to pass progressive laws regulating nursing practice. Otherwise, nurse practice acts will restrict nursing practice and inhibit professional growth.

Definitions aid in developing educational curricula and research agendas

When nursing faculty members sit together to plan the curriculum of a school of nursing, one of the major determinants of the design is how they define nursing. Without the foundation of a definition, it would be impossible to know what to include and how to prioritize the incredible array of information nurses today need to know. In much the same way, researchers cannot easily determine areas of concern for nursing unless they are clear about the boundaries and purposes of nursing actions.

Evolution of Definitions of Nursing

In the last century and a half since nursing became a progressively formal area of study and practice, many have attempted to distill the essence of nursing into one definition. Let's review a selection of definitions that have evolved over the years.

Nightingale defines nursing

Florence Nightingale was the first person to recognize that the complex and multifaceted nature of nursing led to difficulty in defining it. Considering how relatively undeveloped nursing was during her time, Nightingale's definitions contain surprisingly contemporary concepts. Remember that during Nightingale's day, formal schooling in nursing was just beginning. In *Notes on Nursing: What It Is and What It Is Not* (originally published in 1859), she became the first person to attempt a written definition of nursing, stating, "And what nursing has to do … is put the patient in the best condition for nature to act upon him" (Nightingale, 1946, p. 75). She also wrote:

> I use the word nursing for want of a better. It has been limited to signify little more than the administration of medicines and the application of poultices. It ought to signify the proper use of fresh air, light, warmth, cleanliness, quiet, and the proper selection and administration of diet—all at the least expense of vital power to the patient (Nightingale, 1946, p. 6).

Although Nightingale lived in a time when little was known about disease processes and available treatments were extremely limited, these definitions foreshadowed contemporary nursing's focus on the therapeutic **milieu** (environment), as well as the modern emphasis on **health promotion** and **health maintenance.** She accurately observed that although simply possessing observational skills does not make someone a good nurse, without these skills a nurse is ineffective. Indeed, observation has always been an integral part of the process of nursing. Nightingale was also the first person to differentiate between nursing provided by a professional nurse using a unique body of knowledge and nursing care provided by a layperson such as a mother caring for a sick child.

Early twentieth-century definitions

Fifty years after Nightingale wrote *Notes on Nursing,* the search for a definition began in earnest. Following the English model, many schools of nursing had been established in the United States, and numbers of "trained nurses" were in practice. These nurses sought to develop a professional identity for their rapidly expanding discipline. Shaw's *Textbook of Nursing* (1907) defined nursing as an art: "It properly includes, as well as the execution of specific orders, the administration of food and medicine, the personal care of the patient" (pp. 1-2). Harmer's *Textbook of the Principles and Practice of Nursing* (1922) elaborated on Shaw's bare-bones definition: "The object of nursing is not only to cure the sick … but to bring health and ease, rest and comfort to mind and body. Its object is to prevent disease and to preserve health" (p. 3). The fourth edition of the Harmer text, which showed the influence of coauthor and nursing notable Virginia Henderson, redefined nursing: "Nursing may be defined as that service to an individual that helps him to attain or maintain a healthy state of mind or body" (Harmer and Henderson, 1939, p. 2). Henderson's perceptions represented the emergence of contemporary nursing and were so inclusive that they remained useful for many years. We will see her influence again in the next section.

Post–World War II definitions

World War II helped advance the technologies available to treat people, which, in turn, influenced nursing. The war also made nurses aware of the influential role emotions play in health, illness, and nursing care. Hildegard Peplau (1952), widely regarded as a pioneer among contemporary nursing theorists and herself a psychiatric nurse, defined nursing in interpersonal terms: "Nursing is a significant, therapeutic, interpersonal process. … Nursing is an **educative instrument** … that aims to promote forward movement of personality in the direction of creative, constructive, productive, personal and community living" (p. 16). Peplau reinforced the idea of the patient as an **active collaborator** in his or her own care.

During the late 1950s and early 1960s, the number of master's programs in nursing increased. As more nurses were educated at the graduate level and learned about the research process, they were anxious to test new ideas about nursing. Nursing theory was born. (See Chapter 11 for an in-depth discussion of nursing theory.)

One of the theorists who began work during this early period of theory development was Dorothea Orem. Her 1959 definition captures the flavor of her later, more completely elaborated self-care theory of nursing: "Nursing is perhaps best described as the giving of direct assistance to a person, as required, because of the person's specific inabilities in self-care resulting from a situation of personal health" (Orem, 1959, p. 5). Orem's belief that nurses should do for a person only those things the person cannot do without assistance also emphasized the patient's active role.

By 1960, Henderson's earlier definition had evolved into a statement that had such universal appeal that it was adopted by the International Council of Nurses:

> The unique function of the nurse is to assist the individual, sick or well, in the performance of those activities contributing to health or its recovery (or to a peaceful death) that he would perform unaided if he had the necessary strength, will or knowledge. And to do this in such a way as to help him gain independence as rapidly as possible (Henderson, 1960, p. 3).

Never before or since has one definition of nursing been so widely accepted both in the United States and throughout the world. Many believe it is still the most comprehensive and appropriate definition of nursing in existence.

Another pioneer nursing theorist, Martha Rogers, included the concept of the nursing process in her definition: "Nursing aims to assist people in achieving their **maximum health potential.** Maintenance and promotion of health, prevention of disease, nursing diagnosis, intervention, and rehabilitation encompass the scope of nursing's goals" (Rogers, 1961, p. 86).

Professional association definitions

Nursing organizations worldwide have also struggled with defining nursing. Definitions to be reviewed here include those of the American Nurses Association, the Royal College of Nursing, and the International Council of Nursing. As you read these definitions, notice that some new concepts and terms are introduced in the more recent American definitions. In the United States, nursing defines itself as the health discipline that "cares."

A **caring** professional is one who watches over, attends to, and provides for the needs of others. Modern nursing stresses **humanistic nursing values,** that is, viewing professional relationships as human-to-human experiences rather than nurse-to-patient. The meaning of the patient's experience is an important aspect of humanistic nursing. **Holistic values** are also receiving emphasis in modern definitions of nursing. Holism is a system of comprehensive care that takes the physical, emotional, social, economic, and spiritual needs of the person into consideration (Figure 7-1).

American Nurses Association. The American Nurses Association (ANA) has published several definitions of nursing over the years. The second edition of *Nursing's Social Policy Statement* defined nursing comprehensively. This definition included six essential features of contemporary nursing practice (American Nurses Association, 2003, p. 5):

- Provision of a caring relationship that facilitates health and healing
- Attention to the range of human experiences and responses to health and illness within the physical and social environments
- Integration of objective data with knowledge gained from an appreciation of the patient or group's subjective experience
- Application of scientific knowledge to the processes of diagnosis and treatment through the use of judgment and critical thinking
- Advancement of professional nursing knowledge through scholarly inquiry
- Influence on social and public policy to promote social justice

A more succinct definition also put forth by the ANA is found in the preface to the *Code of Ethics for Nurses* (2001): "Nursing encompasses the prevention of illness,

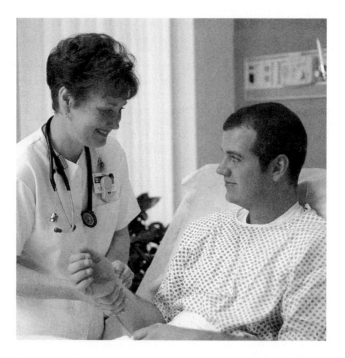

Figure **7-1**
Holistic nursing practice takes the physical, emotional, social, economic, and spiritual needs of the person into consideration. (Courtesy Hamilton Medical Center, Dalton, Georgia.)

the alleviation of suffering, and the protection, promotion, and restoration of health in the care of individuals, families, groups, and communities" (p. 4).

Royal College of Nursing. The Royal College of Nursing (RCN) is the United Kingdom's voice of nursing and is the largest professional union of nurses in the world. This organization embarked upon an 18-month-long initiative to define nursing, culminating in the April 2003 publication of the document *Defining Nursing* (Royal College of Nursing, 2003).

The RCN definition of nursing has a core statement supported by six defining characteristics. The core statement is this: "Nursing is the use of clinical judgment in the provision of care to enable people to improve, maintain, or recover health, to cope with health problems, and to achieve the best possible quality of life, whatever their disease or disability, until death."

The six defining characteristics are too lengthy to reprint here; however, the entire document is worthy of examination and reflection because of its comprehensiveness and thoughtfulness. You can find it online *(www.rcn.org.uk/downloads/definingnursing/definingnursing-a5.pdf)*.

International Council of Nurses. The International Council of Nurses (ICN) is a federation of national nurses associations representing nurses in more than 120 countries. Because ICNs membership is very diverse, their definition of nursing might be expected to differ from those of single-nation organizations such as the ANA and RCN. It is, however, quite similar in both tone and content.

According to the ICN:

> Nursing encompasses autonomous and collaborative care of individuals of all ages, families, groups, and communities, sick or well, and in all settings. Nursing includes the promotion of health, prevention of illness, and the care of ill, disabled, and dying people. Advocacy, promotion of a safe environment, research, participation in shaping health policy and in patient and health systems management, and education are also key nursing roles (International Council of Nurses, 2003, homepage).

Much more can be learned about ICN online *(www.icn.ch)*.

Box 7-1 summarizes our brief review of selected definitions of nursing generated during the past 150 years.

Box 7-1 **The Evolution of Definitions of Nursing, 1859-2003**

Nightingale, 1859 (1946)

"I use the word nursing for want of a better. ... It ought to signify the proper use of fresh air, light, warmth, cleanliness, quiet, and the proper selection and administration of diet—all at the least expense of vital power to the patient.

"It has been said and written scores of times, that every woman makes a good nurse. I believe, on the contrary, that the very elements of nursing are all but unknown" (p. 6).

"And what nursing has to do ... is put the patient in the best condition for nature to act upon him" (p. 75).

- The nurse's center of concern is the patient.
- Nature and a healthful, restful environment are the nurse's allies.
- Health maintenance and restoration are the nurse's goals.

Shaw, 1907

"Nursing is an art. ... It properly includes as well as the execution of specific orders, the administration of food and medicine, the personal care of the patient. ... To fill such a position requires certain physical and mental attributes as well as special training" (pp. 1-2).

- More than knowledge and skills are needed by nurses. The attribute of personal caring is also required.

Harmer, 1922

"Nursing is rooted in the needs of humanity. ... Its object is not only to cure the sick ... but to bring health and ease, rest and comfort to mind and body. Its object is to prevent disease and to preserve health" (p. 3).

- Disease prevention and health promotion are the focus.
- Nursing is based on human needs.

Harmer and Henderson, 1939

"Nursing may be defined as that service to an individual that helps him to attain or maintain a healthy state of mind or body" (p. 2).

- Nursing deals with the health of both psyche (mind) and soma (body).

Continued

| Box **7-1** | The Evolution of Definitions of Nursing, 1859-2003 — cont'd |

Peplau, 1952

"Nursing is a significant, therapeutic, interpersonal process. ... Nursing is an educative instrument ... that aims to promote forward movement of personality in the direction of creative, constructive, productive, personal and community living" (p. 16).

- Effective nursing results from a therapeutic relationship between nurse and patient.

Orem, 1959

"Nursing is ... described as the giving of direct assistance to a person, as required, because of the person's specific inabilities in self-care resulting from a situation of personal health" (p. 5).

- Nursing is doing for a person what he cannot do at this time because of health-related limitations. Return to self-care is the goal.

Henderson, 1960

"The unique function of the nurse is to assist the individual, sick or well, in the performance of those activities contributing to health or its recovery (or to a peaceful death) that he would perform unaided if he had the necessary strength, will or knowledge. And to do this in such a way as to help him gain independence as rapidly as possible" (p. 3).

- Both well and ill people are the focus of nursing.
- Responsibility for care is shared by nurse and patient.
- The goal is independence of the patient.

Rogers, 1961

"Nursing aims to assist people in achieving their maximum health potential. Maintenance and promotion of health, prevention of disease, nursing diagnosis, intervention, and rehabilitation encompass the scope of nursing's goals" (p. 86).

- Each person has a personal maximum health potential. Nursing seeks to strengthen each human being's capacity to achieve that potential.

Watson, 1979

"Nursing is both scientific and artistic. I seek to combine science with humanism. ... Nursing is a therapeutic interpersonal process. ... Nursing is a scientific discipline that derives. ... its practice base from scientific research" (p. xvii).

- Nursing represents a balance between science and humanism.
- The interpersonal features of nursing are paramount.
- Nurses care for people with a holistic approach even while using the scientific approach.

American Nurses Association, 1980

"Nursing is the diagnosis and treatment of human responses to actual and potential health problems" (p. 9).

- Nursing focuses on human responses to illness or the threat of illness.

American Nurses Association, 1995

"Attention to the full range of human experiences and responses to health and illness without restriction to a problem-focused orientation; integration of objective data with knowledge gained from an understanding

Continued

Box **7-1** The Evolution of Definitions of Nursing, 1859-2003—cont'd

of the patient or group's subjective experience; application of scientific knowledge to the processes of diagnosis and treatment; and provision of a caring relationship that facilitates health and healing" (p. 6).

- Reflects the multifaceted, complex nature of nursing.
- Integrates the science of caring with traditional knowledge.
- Retains the commitment to care of both healthy and ill people, individually or in groups and communities.
- Reflects a commitment to holism.

Royal College of Nursing, 2003

"Nursing is the use of clinical judgment in the provision of care to enable people to improve, maintain, or recover health, to cope with health problems, and to achieve the best possible quality of life, whatever their disease or disability, until death."

- Health is the focus.
- Quality of life, even in the presence of chronic illness or disability, is a goal.
- Reflects holistic values.

International Council of Nurses, 2003

"Nursing encompasses autonomous and collaborative care of individuals of all ages, families, groups and communities, sick or well and in all settings. Nursing includes the promotion of health, prevention of illness, and the care of ill, disabled and dying people. Advocacy, promotion of a safe environment, research, participation in shaping health policy and in patient and health systems management, and education are also key nursing roles."

- Emphasizes both autonomy and collaboration.
- Focus is broad: all people wherever found.
- Promotes activist roles in advocacy, health policy, and health systems.

Developing Definitions of Nursing

Since the profession of nursing is ever evolving and is influenced by changing social, economic, and political forces, so too will definitions of nursing continue to evolve. From time to time, all parties who have an interest in nursing—faculties of schools of nursing, leaders in agencies and institutions providing nursing care, individuals, and state legislatures—attempt to define it. We will review some of their efforts.

Definitions developed by schools of nursing

Students may not realize that faculties of accredited schools of nursing are encouraged to develop definitions of nursing as part of the school's statement of philosophy. Some of the most spirited discussions during faculty meetings center around what various faculty members believe nursing really is. A description of nursing that combines humanistic and holistic values can be found in the University of Rochester, New York, School of Nursing's comprehensive philosophy statement:

We believe that the profession of nursing has as its essence, assisting people to attain and maintain optimal health and to cope with illness and disability. Nursing derives its rights and responsibilities from society and is, therefore, accountable to society as well as to the individuals who comprise it. The nurse functions as a caring professional in both autonomous and collaborative professional roles, using critical thinking, ethical principles, effective communication, and deliberative action to render holistic care, facilitate access to health care, and aid consumers in making decisions about their health (University of Rochester School of Nursing, 2003, p. 1).

Another thoughtful and somewhat more specific definition comes from the University of Akron (Ohio) College of Nursing faculty, who wrote:

Nursing is an art and a science. The discipline of nursing is concerned with individual, family, and community, and their responses to health within the context of the changing health care environment. Professional nursing includes the appraisal and the enhancement of health. Personal meanings of health are understood in the nursing situation within the context of familial, societal, and cultural meanings. The professional nurse uses knowledge from theories and research in nursing and other disciplines in providing nursing care. The role of the nurse involves the exercise of social, cultural, and political responsibilities, including accountability for professional actions, provision of quality nursing care, and community involvement (University of Akron College of Nursing, 2003, p. 4).

Although these two definitions are quite different, commonalities are evident.

Definitions developed by hospitals

Most hospitals have developed definitions of nursing to guide practice in that institution. Accreditation guidelines for hospitals require that much consideration be given to defining the nursing care provided. The following definition was developed by the Division of Nursing at St. Vincent's Medical Center in Jacksonville, Florida:

The practice of nursing is the caring and competent application of a specialized body of knowledge and judgment within the framework of the nursing process. This process encompasses the assessment, planning, intervention, and evaluation of actual and potential health care needs. Nursing Practice is further based on the core values of Baptist St. Vincent's, the philosophy of the Division of Nursing, and the Nurse Practice Act of the State of Florida (St. Vincent's Medical Center Division of Nursing, 2003, p. 1).

Most hospital definitions of nursing make reference to the nurse practice act of the state in which the hospital is located, and many simply adopt the practice act's definition as their own. This prevents any conflict between the legal scope of practice and practices sanctioned by the institution. Approximately two thirds of the hospitals surveyed for this chapter used nurse practice act definitions as their own. For example, Hamilton Medical Center in Dalton, Georgia, simply recognizes the definition of nursing as defined by the Georgia Board of Nursing:

[Nursing is] … the performance for compensation of any act in the care and counsel of the ill, injured, or infirm, and in the promotion and maintenance of health with individuals, groups, or both throughout the life span. It requires substantial specialized knowledge of the humanities, natural sciences, social sciences and nursing theory as a basis for assessment, nursing diagnosis, planning, intervention, and evaluation. It includes, but is not limited to, provision of nursing care; administration, supervision, evaluation, or any combination thereof, of nursing practice; teaching; counseling; the administration of medications and treatments as prescribed by a physician practicing medicine in accordance with Article 2 of Chapter 34 of this title, or a dentist practicing dentistry in accordance with Chapter 11 of this title, or a podiatrist practicing podiatry in accordance with Chapter 35 of this title (Hamilton Medical Center, 2003, p. 1).

Definitions developed by state legislatures

It is important to keep in mind that one of the most significant definitions of nursing is contained in the **nurse practice act** of the state in which a nurse practices. Regardless of how restrictive or permissive it may be, this definition constitutes the legal definition of nursing in a particular state, and the wise nurse maintains familiarity with the latest version of the act. Ohio's nurse practice act contains wording typical of many states' act (Ohio Board of Nursing, 2003):

> "Practice of nursing as a registered nurse" means providing to individuals and groups nursing care requiring specialized knowledge, judgment, and skill derived from the principles of biological, physical, behavioral, social, and nursing sciences. Such nursing care includes:
>
> 1. Identifying patterns of human responses to actual or potential health problems amenable to a nursing regimen;
> 2. Executing a nursing regimen through the selection, performance, management, and evaluation of nursing actions;
> 3. Assessing health status for the purpose of providing nursing care;
> 4. Providing health counseling and health teaching;
> 5. Administering medications, treatments, and executing regimens prescribed by licensed physicians, dentists, optometrists, and podiatrists; or until January 1, 2010, advanced practice nurses authorized to prescribe under section 4723.56 of the Revised Code;
> 6. Teaching, administering, supervising, delegating, and evaluating nursing practice.

If the language in these nurse practice acts sound like familiar nursing language, that is not accidental. State nurses associations and boards of nursing are actively involved with legislators to assist them in drafting laws that accurately reflect the nature and scope of nursing. The current nurse practice act in each state can be obtained by calling or writing the state board of nursing. The addresses of the boards of nursing can be found on the Evolve website (**www.evolve.elsevier.com/ Chitty/professional/**).

Before moving on to the next discussion, take time to look at the accompanying Critical Thinking Exercise. How would you define nursing?

CRITICAL THINKING *Exercise*

Nursing is ...

Instructions: Using your thoughts, as well as elements of others' definitions, write your own definition of nursing. Explain it to a classmate, giving your rationale for what you included and excluded. Keep it among your professional papers to refer to in later years. See how it evolves over time.

DEFINING NURSING'S SCOPE OF PRACTICE

The **scope of practice** for the nursing profession establishes boundaries of practice for all nurses. Since there is potential for harm, scope of practice is established by law to protect the public from nurses who exceed their education and competence. The scope may be narrowed for nurses within particular settings, but it may not be broadened without legal and ethical ramifications.

Defining nursing's scope of practice is important for many of the same reasons definitions of nursing are important. Having a defined scope of practice:

- Forms the basis from which policy makers and governing bodies determine laws and regulations governing nursing practice.
- Guides educational institutions in the preparation of nursing students.
- Enables employers of nurses to prepare job descriptions that accurately reflect nursing practice.
- Allows the public to know who is qualified to provide various nursing services.
- Assists practicing nurses to reexamine practice roles in a time of rapid changes in health care.
- Enables other health professionals, such as nursing assistants, LPN/LVNs, physicians, and social workers to clarify boundary issues and resolve potential conflicts.
- Allows governments to ensure that the most cost-effective mix of providers is available.

As discussed in Chapter 3, a number of forces in society at large are altering the way nursing is practiced. Among them are the aging population, technological advances, cultural diversity, the rise in consumerism, and violence. These changes create opportunities for nurses to develop more independent roles outside traditional hospital settings. Practicing more autonomously can create role strain. Even within traditional settings, insufficient staffing creates ethical dilemmas daily. As more nurses achieve advanced degrees, specialization increases, contributing to pressure to revise definitions of scope of practice. Entrepreneurial nursing practice also challenges the boundaries of traditional practice roles. Nurses need guidance in knowing how far outside the core of traditional nursing practice they can expand. Definitions of scope of practice provide needed guidance.

In the United States, the scope of nursing is legally defined by the states. In the past, simple lists of tasks and procedures nurses were authorized to perform sufficed. With the increasing complexity of health care and educational advances within nursing, this is no longer sufficient. We are now moving toward the goal of providing broad, enabling principles that provide maximum scope and flexibility for nurses practicing in a rapidly changing environment. We will explore the aspects of a model nurse practice act in Chapter 20.

The American Nurses Association has taken the position that attempts to define the scope of nursing practice should flow from the nursing process. The ANA publishes scope and standards statements for more than 24 nursing specialty areas in addition to the broad document, *Nursing: Scope and Standards of Practice,* which covers all clinical practice. These are not legal documents but statements by the profession of the accountability of nurses. They, in conjunction with other documents, are therefore widely used in legal cases to determine whether a particular nurse has met the "standard of care."

FOUR DOCUMENTS YOU SHOULD POSSESS

All the efforts that have gone into defining nursing and nursing's scope and **standards of practice** are fruitless unless nurses use these documents to guide practice. As a professional nurse, you should have the latest versions of the following four documents in your libraries and refer to them regularly:

- The Nurse Practice Act of the state(s) in which you practice; your state's board of nursing can be found on the Evolve website (**www.evolve.elsevier.com/ Chitty/professional/**)
- *Nursing's Social Policy Statement* (ANA)
- The *Code of Ethics for Nurses* (ANA)
- Scope and Standards of Clinical Practice for the area in which you practice—if not available, substitute *Nursing: Scope and Standards of Practice* (ANA)

Summary of Key Points

- Although attempts to define nursing have been under way since the days of Nightingale, all attempts have fallen short of capturing the diversity and richness that constitutes nursing.
- Definitions reviewed in this chapter have more commonalities than differences.
- Definitions change over time as society and nursing change and as each individual's perceptions about, and experiences in, nursing change.
- The dynamic nature of the nursing profession, society, and health care will likely prevent us from ever developing one eternal, universally accepted definition of nursing.
- In the United States, nursing's scope of practice is defined by each state in its nurse practice act.
- Understanding nursing's scope of practice, as determined by the relevant nurse practice act and other documents, is the obligation of every professional nurse.

CRITICAL THINKING QUESTIONS

1. Obtain your school's definition of nursing. How is it similar to or different from definitions in this chapter?
2. From the definitions of nursing presented in this chapter, select the one you most prefer and explain your choice.
3. How might new technologies, economic factors, social trends, and new practice options for nurses affect future definitions of nursing? How might these factors affect the scope of nursing?
4. If you are already a practicing nurse, how has your personal definition of nursing changed over time? How have you seen the scope of nursing change since you entered practice?
5. Using the appropriate address, obtain a copy of the nurse practice act for your state. Find the legal definition of nursing and compare it with other definitions found in this chapter. How are they alike, and how are they different? How does your state define the scope of nursing practice?

REFERENCES

American Nurses Association: *Code of ethics for nurses,* Washington, DC, 2001, American Nurses Publishing.

American Nurses Association: *Nursing: a social policy statement,* Kansas City, MO, American Nurses Association.

American Nurses Association: *Nursing: scope and standards of practice,* Washington, DC, 2004, nursebooks.org.

American Nurses Association: *Nursing's social policy statement,* Washington, DC, 1995, American Nurses Association.

American Nurses Association: *Nursing's social policy statement,* ed 2, Washington, DC, 2004, nursebooks.org.

Hamilton Medical Center: *Definition of nursing,* Dalton, GA, 2003, Hamilton Medical Center.

Harmer B: *Textbook of the principles and practice of nursing,* New York, 1922, Macmillan.

Harmer B, Henderson V: *Textbook of the principles and practice of nursing,* ed 4, New York, 1939, Macmillan.

Henderson V: *Basic principles of nursing care,* London, 1960, International Council of Nurses.

International Council for Nurses: The ICN definition of nursing, Online, 2003 *(www.icn.ch/definition.htm).*

Nightingale F: *Notes on nursing: what it is and what it is not,* Philadelphia, 1946, JB Lippincott, Reprint (originally published in 1859).

Orem D: *Guidelines for developing curricula for the education of practical nurses,* Washington, DC, 1959, Government Printing Office.

Peplau H: *Interpersonal relations in nursing: a conceptual frame of reference for psychodynamic nursing,* New York, 1952, GP Putnam's Sons.

Rogers M: *Educational revolution in nursing,* New York, 1961, Macmillan.

Royal College of Nursing, Defining nursing, Online, 2003 *(www.rcn.org.uk/downloads/definingnursing/definingnursing-a5.pdf).*

St. Vincent's Medical Center Division of Nursing: Definition of nursing, Jacksonville, FL, 2003, St. Vincent's Medical Center Division of Nursing.

Shaw CW: *Textbook of nursing,* ed 3, New York, 1907, Appleton.

State of Ohio Board of Nursing: Law and rule information, Online, 2003 *(www5.state.oh.us/nur/Law_and_Rule.htm).*

Styles MM: Bridging the gap between competence and excellence, *ANNA J* 18(4):353-366, 1991.

University of Akron College of Nursing: *Philosophy of the College of Nursing,* Akron, OH, 2003, University of Akron College of Nursing.

University of Rochester School of Nursing: *Philosophy of the School of Nursing,* Rochester, NY, 2003, University of Rochester School of Nursing.

Watson J: *The philosophy and science of caring,* Boston, 1979, Little, Brown.

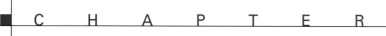

CHAPTER 8

Professional Socialization

Kay Kittrell Chitty

Key Terms

Biculturalism
Burnout
Cognitive Rebellion
Conceptual Model
Culture of Nursing
Dissonance
Distance Learning

Formal Socialization
Inertia
Informal Socialization
Internalize
Internship
"Job Hopping"
Mentor

Modeling
Mutuality
Preceptor
Professional Socialization
Reality Shock
Resocialization
Work Ethic

Learning Outcomes

After studying this chapter, students will be able to:

- Discuss how students' initial images of nursing are transformed through professional education and experiences.
- Differentiate between formal and informal socialization.
- Identify factors that influence an individual's professional socialization.
- Describe developmental models of professional socialization and how they can be used.
- Explain similarities and differences in basic and RN students' stresses during role transitions.
- Differentiate between the elements of professional socialization that are the responsibility of nursing programs and those that are the individual's responsibility.
- Describe strategies to ease the transition from student to professional nurse.
- Discuss employer expectations of the new nurse.
- Describe the advantages of effective time management, preceptors, and mentors in easing the transition from student to practicing nurse.

All students are in a process of transition, whether just beginning nursing education or returning to school as RNs seeking baccalaureate degrees. All arrive with preconceived ideas of what nursing is about, acquired through observation of media images, contact with friends or family members who are nurses, personal experiences as patients, or actual practice as RNs. Although the attitudes and behaviors that characterize professional nurses cannot all be learned from a book, the complex process of perspective transformation begins during formal schooling.

This process requires that students **internalize,** or take in, new knowledge, skills, attitudes, behaviors, values, and ethical standards and make these a part of their own professional identity. For the RN, a modification of an already-forming professional identity occurs. This process of internalization and development or modification of an occupational identity is known as **professional socialization.** Professional socialization in nursing begins during the period students are in formal nursing programs and continues as they practice in "the real world."

The goal of professional socialization is the development of professionalism. Serious negative outcomes result from inadequate socialization. These include turnover, attrition, and decreased productivity (Boyle, Popkess-Vawter, and Taunton, 1996). In this chapter, the effects of both educational and clinical experiences on nurses' professional socialization are examined.

EDUCATION AND PROFESSIONAL SOCIALIZATION

What kinds of educational experiences are needed to make the transition from student to professional nurse? How does a student make the transition from novice to initiate, a person who thinks and feels like a nurse? Learning any new role is derived from a mixture of formal and informal socialization. Little boys, for example, learn how to assume the father role by what their own fathers purposely teach them (formal socialization) and by observing their own and other fathers' behavior (informal socialization). In nursing, **formal socialization** includes lessons the faculty intends to teach, such as how to plan nursing care, write a paper on professional ethics, perform a physical examination on a healthy child, start an IV, or practice communication with a psychiatric patient (Figure 8-1). **Informal socialization** includes lessons that occur incidentally, such as the unplanned observation of a nurse teaching a young mother how to care for her premature infant, participating in a student nurse association, or hearing nurses discuss patient care in the nurses' lounge. Part of professional socialization is simply absorbing the **culture of nursing,** that is, the rites, rituals, and valued behaviors of the profession. This requires that students spend enough time with nurses in work settings for adequate exposure to the nursing culture to occur. Most nurses agree that informal socialization experiences were often more powerful and memorable than formal socialization in their own development.

Learning a new vocabulary is also part of professional socialization. Each profession has its own jargon, which generally is not well understood by outsiders. Professional students in any field usually enjoy acquiring the new vocabulary and practicing it among themselves. Students of nursing certainly do, as eavesdropping on lunchroom conversations will confirm.

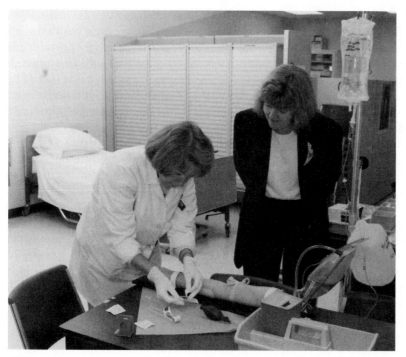

Figure 8-1
During formal socialization, students internalize the knowledge, skills, and beliefs of nursing in planned, educational experiences and interactions with faculty and other nurses. (Courtesy University of Akron.)

Learning any new role creates some degree of anxiety. Disappointment and frustration sometimes occur when students' learning expectations come into conflict with educational realities. Students' ideas of what they need to learn, when they need to learn it, and what might be the best way to learn it may differ from how their education actually unfolds. They sometimes become disillusioned when they observe nurses behaving in ways that are in contrast to their ideas about how nurses should behave. Knowing in advance that these things may happen can help students accurately assess the sources of their anxiety and manage it more effectively.

Factors Influencing Socialization

As students progress through nursing programs, a variety of factors challenge their customary ways of thinking. These include personal feelings and beliefs, some of which may conflict with professional values. For example, if students have strong religious beliefs, they may be uncomfortable working with patients who have no such belief or whose beliefs are different from their own. Yet the very first statement in the *Code of Ethics for Nurses* (American Nurses Association, 2001) requires that nurses work with all patients regardless of their beliefs.

Growing children are first influenced by the values, beliefs, and behaviors of the significant adults around them and later by peers. Ideas about health, health care, and nursing are also shaped through this process. If a nurse's family valued fitness, for example, it may be difficult for that nurse to empathize with an overweight cardiac patient who refuses to exercise. In this example, a family value (fitness) comes into conflict with a professional value (nonjudgmental acceptance of patients). Other patient issues that sometimes challenge students' values are substance abuse; self-destructive behaviors; abortion; issues related to sexuality, such as sexual identity, infertility, and genetic manipulation; and end-of-life issues.

All people have biases. Unexamined biases are more apt to influence behavior than examined ones. Nurses need to be aware of their biases and discuss them with peers, instructors, and professional role models. Failure to do so may adversely affect the nursing care provided to certain patients. Professional nurses make every effort to avoid imposing their personal beliefs on others (see Chapter 18 for further discussion of self-awareness and nonjudgmental acceptance as necessary attributes of professional nurses). Becoming a professional nurse requires learning how to deal with values conflicts such as these while respecting patients' differing viewpoints. This cannot be taught but is the responsibility of each aspiring professional.

As seen from this brief overview, socialization is much more than the transmission of knowledge and skills. It serves to develop a common nursing consciousness and is the key to keeping the profession vital and dynamic.

A New Factor Influencing Socialization—Distance Learning

Distance education in nursing is a fast-growing phenomenon. More nursing schools are utilizing technology to deliver education to nurses who do not have access to traditional on-campus programs. Initially, single courses or continuing education short courses were offered by distance education. Today entire nursing curricula are offered by **distance learning** and the amount of on-campus time may be very limited. Programs vary, using a variety of methods from traditional printed correspondence courses to video teleconferencing to online methods. This trend is expected to increase as demand and technological developments continue.

Questions about whether students could achieve educational outcomes through distance learning have been answered: they can and do pass their courses, some with distinction, using these methodologies (Cragg, Plotnikoff, Hugo, et al., 2001). Questions then arose about whether professional attitudes and values—in other words, professional socialization—could be effectively achieved through distance education. Although more study is needed, initial indicators have been positive (Cragg, Plotnikoff, Hugo, et al., 2001; Nesler, Hanner, Melburg, et al., 2001). The Research Note on p. 201 describes a study comparing traditional students with distance learning students, resulting in some surprising findings.

MODELS OF PROFESSIONAL SOCIALIZATION

In thinking about professional socialization, it is helpful to have theoretical models to consider. During the 1970s and 1980s, a number of models of professional socialization of basic and RN students were developed. Cohen (1981) and Hinshaw (1976)

RESEARCH note

A group of nursing researchers, noting the rise in the number of distance learning nursing programs, wondered whether students in these programs might have difficulty becoming socialized into the profession as a result of limited face-to-face interactions with faculty. Because these researchers recognized that lack of professional socialization of graduates would represent significant weakness and accreditation concerns for distance learning programs, they decided to conduct a quantitative study to answer their question. The research hypothesis was this: "Senior BSN students enrolled in distance education nursing programs will not differ on measures of professional socialization from campus-based senior BSN student, and both groups will score significantly higher in socialization than nonnursing students" (p. 296).

The research subjects consisted of a sample of 1,194 students from 26 traditional campus-based programs, three distance learning programs, and one nonnursing program (i.e., psychology majors). All geographic regions of the United States and all regional accrediting agencies were represented by these institutions. The three distance learning programs varied in the amount of on-campus time required of students, but contact with faculty was limited in all three programs. All required less than campus-based programs (p. 297).

Two instruments were selected to measure professional socialization, both of which had been used before but neither of which was standardized or nationally normed. These instruments were the Stone Health Care Professional Attitude (STONE) Inventory and the Nursing Care Role Orientation Survey (NCROS).

The results surprised the researchers. Students nearing completion of distance learning programs in nursing scored significantly higher on two measures of socialization than the campus-based students, even when the results were controlled for age and RN status. Not surprisingly, both groups scored higher than the nonnursing student group. The researchers speculated that differences were due to demographic factors: the distance education students were older, more experienced in health care overall, and 62.4% were already RNs. Even though statistical analyses should have controlled for these differences, the strength of greater experience in health care settings seemed to have prevailed. More research in this area was recommended.

Abstracted from Nesler MS, Hanner MB, Melburg V, et al: Professional socialization of baccalaureate nursing students: can students in distance nursing programs become socialized? *J Nurs Ed* 40(7):293-302, 2001.

described developmental models appropriate for beginning nursing students. Bandura (1977) described a type of socialization he called *modeling*, which is useful when learning any new behavior. Benner (1984) identified five stages nurses pass through in the transition from "novice to expert." Throwe and Fought (1987) described a developmental model of professional socialization of registered nurse (RN) students.

Recently, work in this area of concern has focused on specific aspects of socialization, such as stresses or coping skills, but this has not resulted in development of new models of the overall process. Each of the older models is considered briefly below. As they are reviewed, students should bear in mind that they rely on observation and anecdotal reports. Unless so stated, they are not based on empirical data. Therefore they are **conceptual models,** which are useful as a springboard for discussion or further research, but should not be taken literally.

Cohen's Model of Basic Student Socialization

Cohen (1981) proposed a model of professional socialization consisting of four stages. Basing her work on developmental theories and studies of basic students' attitudes toward nursing, she asserted, "Students must experience each stage in sequence to feel comfortable in the professional role" (p. 16). She believed that a positive outcome in all four stages is necessary for satisfactory socialization to occur.

Cohen identified the first stage in her model, stage I, as unilateral dependence. Owing to inexperience and lack of knowledge, students at this stage rely on external limits and controls established by authority figures such as teachers. During stage I, students are unlikely to question or analyze critically the concepts teachers present because they lack the necessary background to do so.

In stage II—negativity/independence—students' critical thinking abilities and knowledge bases expand. They begin to question authority figures. Cohen called this occurrence **cognitive rebellion.** Much as young children learn that they can say no, students at this level begin to free themselves from external controls and to rely more on their own judgment. They think critically about what they are being taught.

Stage III—dependence/mutuality—is characterized by what Cohen described as students' more reasoned evaluation of others' ideas. They develop an increasingly realistic appraisal process and learn to test concepts, facts, ideas, and models objectively. Students at this stage are more impartial; they accept some ideas and reject others.

In stage IV—interdependence—students' needs for both independence and **mutuality** (sharing jointly with others) come together. Students develop the capacity to make decisions in collaboration with others. The successfully socialized student completes stage IV with a self-concept that includes a professional role identity that is personally and professionally acceptable and compatible with other life roles. Table 8-1 summarizes the key behaviors associated with each of Cohen's stages.

Readers may wish to compare themselves and nursing classmates against these four stages. A reminder, however: although it is interesting and potentially useful, this model has not been subjected to rigorous testing or validated (confirmed).

Hinshaw-Davis Model of Basic Student Socialization

Another potentially useful model describing the educational aspects of professional socialization was discussed by Ada Sue Hinshaw in a 1976 publication for the National League for Nursing. Hinshaw, a nurse, based her model on work done 10 years earlier by Davis, a sociologist who described his findings in the classic paper "Professional Socialization as Subjective Experience: The Process of Doctrinal Conversion Among Student Nurses" (Davis, 1966).

Table 8-1   Cohen's Model of Basic Student Socialization

Stage	Key Behaviors
I: Unilateral dependence	Reliant on external authority; limited questioning or critical analysis
II: Negativity/independence	Cognitive rebellion; diminished reliance on external authority
III: Dependence/mutuality	Reasoned appraisal; begins integration of facts and opinions following objective testing
IV: Interdependence	Collaborative decision making; commitment to professional role; self-concept now includes professional role identity

Data from Cohen HA: *The nurse's quest for professional identity,* Menlo Park, CA, 1981, Addison-Wesley.

In the Hinshaw-Davis model, stage I—initial innocence—is characterized by idealized images and expectations of nursing. Students have gained these images from the media and from their own experiences with nurses. For example, they may expect that as nursing students they will immediately begin to work with ill patients, that nurses are always treated with respect by other health care workers, or that they will always be able to make things better for their patients.

In stage II—incongruities—students realize that their innocent images of nursing differ from the real structure and challenges of a nursing program. For example, they discover that they must complete anatomy, physiology, nutrition, and a host of other courses before working with patients. Or they discover that students are expected to defer to more experienced nurses and instructors. Or they encounter patients with chronic, intractable pain. This **dissonance** (lack of harmony) between their expectations and the real situation produces tension and frustration. During the dissonant stage, differences are sufficiently well formulated to discuss with others. Students at this stage may overtly question whether or not they should continue in the program and some may choose not to do so.

In stage III—identification—students select and carefully observe role models. These role models may be particularly admired instructors or nurses observed in clinical settings. This stage is closely followed by stage IV—role simulation—in which they practice the role behaviors they have observed. At first, the new behaviors may feel strange or phony, which sometimes causes confusion and self-doubt. Students learning therapeutic communication techniques, for example, often feel awkward and obvious when they first try out these techniques in conversation.

Stage V—vacillation—is characterized by the student's desire to cling to the old ideas and images about nursing while recognizing that new ideas and images are based on life experiences. Evidence of this stage can be seen in new graduates who feel guilty when they are unable to provide intense, individualized care for every patient because of patient load and time constraints.

The last stage, stage VI—internalization—occurs when there is stable and reliable use of the internalized professional model. This stage can be seen in nurses

Table 8-2 Hinshaw-Davis Model of Basic Student Socialization

Stage	Key Behaviors
I: Initial innocence	Initial image of nursing unaffected by reality
II: Incongruities	Initial expectations and reality collide; questions career choice; may drop out
III: Identification	Observes behaviors of experienced nurses
IV: Role simulation	Practices observed behaviors; may feel unnatural in role
V: Vacillation	Old images emerge and conflict with new professional image
VI: Internalization	Acceptance and comfort with new role

Data from Hinshaw AS: *Socialization and resocialization of nurses for professional nursing practice,* New York, 1976, National League for Nursing; and Davis F: *Professional socialization as subjective experience: the process of doctrinal conversion among student nurses,* Paper presented at the Sixth World Congress of Sociology, Evian, France, September 1966.

who, after practicing for some time, have developed a balance between their expectations of themselves as professionals, employers' expectations, and their other life role expectations. Again, remember that the Hinshaw-Davis model has not been validated through extensive research. Table 8-2 contains the stages of socialization described in this model.

Bandura's Concept of Modeling (Both Basic and RN Socialization)

Another method of professional socialization is modeling, as discussed by Bandura (1977), a social psychologist. In **modeling,** students learn by observing role models. Bandura believed that there are two requirements for successful modeling: models must be seen as competent, and students must have an opportunity to practice the behaviors they see modeled. This is different from the informal socialization process described earlier, because modeling involves a *conscious decision* on the part of learners to model themselves after the selected role model. This is an important distinction.

Bandura's concepts can apply to any profession and can be adapted to use in nursing. Students who wish to try modeling should identify nurses or instructors who share their values and attitudes and observe them closely. The next step is to "try out" the behaviors they most admire. Because people are not equally talented in all areas, students may choose to observe several models, each of whom excels in a different area. The basis of modeling as a method of professional socialization is careful observation and intentional simulation of the admired behaviors or characteristics. This is a legitimate method of acquiring desirable professional behaviors that can be useful to both basic and RN students interested in being more active in their own socialization.

Benner's Stages of Nursing Proficiency (Basic Student Socialization)

Patricia Benner, a nurse, wondered how nurses made the transition from inexpert beginners to highly expert practitioners. She described a process of five stages of nursing practice, on which she based her 1984 book, *From Novice to Expert.* The stages Benner described are "novice," "advanced beginner," "competent practitioner," "proficient practitioner," and "expert practitioner." Advancing from stage to stage occurs gradually as nurses gain more experience in patient care. Clinical judgment is stimulated when the nurse's "preconceived notions and expectations" (p. 3) collide with, or are confirmed by, the realities of everyday practice.

In 2000, many years after she generated this model, Benner's work was one of several theories presented to a group attempting to demonstrate how learning theories apply to adult skill acquisition. They tested and confirmed that Benner's model was valid, and they suggested that her stages apply to any adult learning situation (Hom, 2003).

Benner's novice stage, or stage I, begins with students entering nursing school. Because they generally have little background on which to base their clinical behavior, they must depend rather rigidly on rules and expectations established for them. Their practical skills are limited.

By the time learners enter the advanced beginner period, or stage II, they have discerned that a particular order exists in clinical settings (Benner, Tanner, and Chesla, 1996). Their performance is marginally competent. They can base their actions on both theory and principles but tend to experience difficulty formulating priorities, viewing many nursing actions as equally important.

Competent practitioners, or stage III learners, usually have 2 to 3 years' experience in a setting. As a result, they feel competent, organized, and efficient most of the time. These feelings of mastery are due to planning and goal-setting skills and the ability to think abstractly and analytically. These learners can coordinate several complex demands simultaneously.

It generally takes 3 to 5 years of practice to reach Benner's level of proficient practitioner, represented by stage IV. These nurses are able to see patient situations holistically rather than in parts, to recognize and interpret subtleties of meaning, and to recognize easily priorities for care. They can focus on long-term goals and desired outcomes.

Expert practitioner, or stage V, status is reached only after extensive practice experience. These nurses perform intuitively, without conscious thought, automatically grasping the significance of the patient's complete experience. They move fluidly through nursing interventions, acting on the basis of their feeling of "rightness" of nursing action. They may find it difficult to express verbally why they selected certain actions, so integrated are their responses. Their expertise seems, both to themselves and to observers, to "come naturally." Table 8-3 summarizes Benner's stages from novice to expert.

Throwe and Fought's Model for Socialization of Registered Nurse Students

When registered nurses return to school for their baccalaureate degrees, their needs are different from those of basic nursing students. They may experience feelings of frustration and anxiety in returning to the student role. Often these nurses have practiced for years and wonder what anyone can teach them about nursing. Some may even feel insulted when they are placed in classes with students who are just beginning in nursing education. What needs to be recognized is that these registered nurses are not being socialized into nursing; they are in the process of **resocialization,** a process that often creates uncomfortable tension.

Table 8-3 BENNER'S STAGES OF NURSING PROFICIENCY
(BASIC STUDENT SOCIALIZATION)

Stage	Nurse Behaviors
I: Novice	Has little background and limited practical skills; relies on rules and expectations of others for direction
II: Advanced beginner	Has marginally competent skills; uses theory and principles much of the time; experiences difficulty establishing priorities
III: Competent practitioner	Feels competent, organized; plans and sets goals; thinks abstractly and analytically; coordinates several tasks simultaneously
IV: Proficient practitioner	Views patients holistically; recognizes subtle changes; sets priorities with ease; focuses on long-term goals
V: Expert practitioner	Performs fluidly; grasps patient needs automatically; responses are integrated; expertise comes naturally

Data from Benner P: *From novice to expert: excellence and power in clinical nursing practice,*
Menlo Park, CA, 1984, Addison-Wesley.

Throwe and Fought (1987) developed a conceptual (unvalidated) model of RN socialization. They believed that the stages registered nurses must master during resocialization could be assessed using the theories of Erikson (1950), who described eight developmental stages individuals master as they progress from infancy to old age. Throwe and Fought designed a framework for registered nurses in BSN programs to assess their own growth as they progress through school. The framework can also be used by faculty and non-RN students to help them appreciate and support registered nurses' experiences. Table 8-4 contains Throwe and Fought's assessment tool. Students are encouraged to examine this tool critically, assessing each task and behavior carefully, comparing it with their own experiences.

Table 8-4 THROWE AND FOUGHT'S MODEL FOR SOCIALIZATION OF REGISTERED NURSE STUDENTS

Developmental Task	Role-Resisting Behaviors Observed	Role-Accepting Behaviors Observed
Trust/mistrust: Learns to trust the worlds of education and work through consistency and repetitive experiences	Physically isolated from peers both in class and clinicals; does not initiate interactions with others; responds only if called on	Involved with classmates; readily and quickly forms/joins groups when directed; initiates discussions with others; asks for clarification
Autonomy/doubt: Begins to develop independence while under supervision	Delays joining groups for unstructured activities; does not contribute equally; forgets or suppresses assignment dates; does not meet target dates; self-conscious about being evaluated by others	Joins groups for unstructured activities (study groups); shares information with group; prepares for activities; meets target dates; able to interact in the teaching/learning environment; begins to develop independence with guidance

Table 8-4   THROWE AND FOUGHT'S MODEL FOR SOCIALIZATION OF REGISTERED NURSE STUDENTS—CONT'D

Developmental Task	Role-Resisting Behaviors Observed	Role-Accepting Behaviors Observed
Initiative/guilt: Can independently identify, plan, and implement skills/assignments	Perceives objectives and assignments as not worthwhile; stress-related symptoms increase; has difficulty setting priorities; waits for instructor to initiate priority setting; lacks initiative to deal with conflicts; is unaware of available resources	Objectives and assignments take on meaning; applies new skills, content to other work settings; effective in time management; renegotiates deadline extensions when appropriate; takes initiative in resolving conflict situations; is aware of and uses available resources
Industry/inferiority: Behavior is dominated by performance of tasks and curiosity—individuals need encouragement to attempt and master skills	Elicits performance rewards and feedback from others; needs direct encouragement, especially when performing affective and cognitive skills; last to volunteer to demonstrate new behaviors; seeks rewards by performing old familiar skills rather than those in new dimensions; demonstrates disengaging behaviors (late, uninterested, resistant to learning opportunities)	Able to reward self; confidence thrives; eager to try out new skills; takes risks; volunteers to demonstrate new behaviors; profits from guidance and direction of others; applies self beyond family/work settings; curiosity channeled through educational system
Identity/role confusion: Individual searches for continuity and structure; is concerned with how he or she is accepted by others; is concerned how he or she is accepted by self; each individual struggles to shape or formulate own identity	Needs a structured clinical setting to develop ego identity further; sees old job as ideal and denies need for change; serious about learning (content and clinical practice); frustrated with nursing as a career choice; too ideological or overly critical of others	Searches for continuity and structure but can adapt to unstructured clinical settings; identifies role models in clinical setting; articulates need for change or for modification of job-related roles and procedures; appears to enjoy learning and performing in clinical settings; realistic about own achievements and progress in educational system
Intimacy/isolation: Seeks to combine identity with other self-selected individuals	Participates as a member, but resists group leader role; does not participate in professional meetings; unsupportive of others' educational advancement; feels no increased esteem in performing new role behaviors; meets minimal requirements and sees instructor only in evaluative role; resists using newly developed skills, more comfortable with previous level of performance; avoids giving feedback to agency personnel	Volunteers to lead work/study groups; participates in professional organizations; recruits others and and represents school; demonstrates pride in new role behaviors and shares with others in work settings; seeks out instructor for additional learning, information, and professional growth opportunities; values symbols of profession (using assessment tools, RN name tags); evaluates ability of clinical agencies to facilitate meeting learner objectives; provides feedback to agency personnel

Continued

Table 8-4   THROWE AND FOUGHT'S MODEL FOR SOCIALIZATION OF REGISTERED NURSE STUDENTS—CONT'D

Developmental Task	Role-Resisting Behaviors Observed	Role-Accepting Behaviors Observed
Generativity/stagnation: Efforts are made to guide and direct incoming students; assists others	Avoids social interaction and sharing information with incoming students; provides minimal care; unconcerned about continuity of patient care; selects patients with common, familiar clinical disorders; no increased ease of learning or improved test-taking abilities; does not elect to test out of course requirements; stagnates in same job setting	Guides and directs incoming students; provides quality nursing care to patient, family, and community; takes calculated risks (questions level of care, seeks multiple learning opportunities, shares level of expertise, elects to test out of required/elective courses); demonstrates critical problem-solving skills; attains mastery of test-taking skills; is a self-directed learner; demonstrates clinical problem solving in own work setting; uses holistic approach to delivery of health care
Ego integrity/despair: Acceptance of one's own progress, achievement, and goals through realistic self-appraisal	Frustrated with progress and achievement, stagnated in developing new goals; crisis-prone when changing roles; self-appraisal unrealistic; does not participate in structured educational opportunities; returns to old job and does not modify role performance; sees no reward in risk taking; high risk for dissatisfaction with profession	Accepts progress, achievement, and goal attainment; realistic in self-appraisal; resets professional goals (graduate school, participation in continuing education, certification); joins new perspectives on old job by use of critical thinking; takes risks (new jobs, different clinical setting, and leadership roles)

Recent Studies of Socialization

As mentioned earlier, much of the work on stages and phases of socialization was completed decades ago. More recently researchers have focused on the RN to baccalaureate students' attitudes, concerns, and priorities. Typical of these are Davidhizar, Gigen, and Reed's 1993 review of the literature and Zuzelo's 2001 study of concerns of RNs returning to school. The major concerns identified in these two studies were remarkably consistent and included the following:

- Meeting multiple role demands (role strain); juggling family/school/work responsibilities
- Time constraints; difficulty scheduling classes and clinicals
- Tuition costs and the resulting drain on family finances
- Difficulty documenting prior learning
- Fears of possible inability to complete course requirements

- Lack of faculty availability and support
- Difficulty adapting back into the student role
- Questions about the degree providing desired mobility

So far in this discussion, professional socialization has sounded like something that happens *to* students. Although much is out of their control, students do not have to be passive recipients of socialization. On the contrary, as active participants, they can influence the socialization process. Let us now turn our attention to ways students can effectively adapt to the socialization process.

Actively Participating in One's Own Professional Socialization

Davidhizar, Gigen, and Reed (1993) recommended strategies for RNs to decrease the stress they experience upon returning to school. These strategies could apply to all students.

- Actively involve yourself in the learning process.
- Keep your eye on the prize. You are temporarily uncomfortable but will ultimately get something you want (certification, promotion, sense of self-confidence, personal growth, graduate school, etc.).
- Keep your perspective. You are in school by choice. No one is doing this to you.
- Set aside preconceived ideas, prejudices, and habits. Give yourself and the school experience a chance.
- Open up your creative side, your abstract thinking, and willingness to engage in hypothetical thinking. Everything need not be immediately applicable in the work setting to be of value.
- Be receptive to feedback, even if it is critical. If you were perfect, you would not need to be here.
- Develop your time management skills. Learn to use bits of time, such as listening to tapes while driving.
- Get a mentor for emotional support—another nurse, older friend, relative or faculty member.
- Use faculty members as resources. They want to be helpful but cannot read your mind.

For other ideas about how to become an active participant in your own socialization process, use the checklist in Box 8-1.

As part of being active participants and consumers of educational services, students need to know what to expect of their nursing programs in terms of professional socialization. Schools are responsible for some activities, whereas the individual is responsible for others. The checklist in Box 8-2 provides ideas about what takes place in nursing programs around the United States to enhance students' professional socialization. Students can compare their experiences with those in this guide.

POSTGRADUATE RESOCIALIZATION TO THE WORK SETTING

When nurses graduate, is their professional socialization over? Most authorities believe that socialization, similar to learning, is a lifelong activity. The transition from student to professional is just another of life's challenges and, similar to most challenges, is one that helps people grow.

| Box **8-1** | **A Do-It-Yourself Guide to Professional Socialization** |

Listed below are 20 possible behaviors demonstrated by students who take responsibility for their own professional socialization. Place a check next to the behaviors you regularly exhibit. Be honest with yourself.

1. I interact with other students in and out of class.
2. I participate in class by asking intelligent questions and initiating discussion occasionally.
3. I have formed or joined a study group.
4. I use the library, labs, and teachers as resources.
5. I organize my work so that I can meet deadlines.
6. If I have a conflict with another student or a teacher, I take the initiative to resolve it.
7. I don't let minor personality problems distract me from my goals.
8. I seek out new learning experiences and sometimes volunteer to demonstrate new skills to others.
9. I have chosen professional role models.
10. I am realistic about my performance.
11. I try to accept constructive criticism without becoming defensive.
12. I recognize that *trying* to do good work is not the same as *doing* good work.
13. I recognize that each teacher has different expectations, and it is my responsibility to learn what is expected by each.
14. I demonstrate respect for my teachers' time by making appointments whenever possible.
15. I demonstrate respect for my classmates, patients, and teachers by never coming to class or clinical unprepared.
16. I recognize my responsibility to help create a dynamic learning environment and am not satisfied to be merely an academic spectator.
17. I participate in the student nurse association and encourage others to do the same.
18. I represent my school with pride.
19. I project a professional appearance.
20. One of my goals is to become a self-directed, lifelong learner.

Scoring: 1 to 10 checks—You need to examine your behavior and think about taking more responsibility for your own socialization; 11 to 15 checks—You are active in your own behalf. Try to begin using some of the remaining behaviors on the list or come up with your own; more than 15 checks—You are a role model of positive action in your own professional socialization process.

It can seem that just as students become well socialized to the culture of the educational setting, they graduate and must become resocialized to a work setting. Most new nursing graduates feel somewhat unprepared and overwhelmed with the responsibilities of their first positions. Although agencies that employ new graduates realize that the orientation period will take time, graduates may have unrealistic expectations of themselves and others.

During the early days of practice, most graduate nurses quickly realize that the ideals taught in school are not always possible to achieve in everyday practice. This is largely due to time constraints and produces feelings of conflict and even guilt. In school, students are taught to spend time with patients and to consider their emotional as well as physical needs. In practice, the emphasis may seem to be on finishing tasks, completing checklists and flow sheets, and the like. Talking with patients, engaging in patient teaching, or counseling family members may be viewed as an

Box **8-2** **A Consumer's Guide to Professional Socialization**

The following statements indicate some positive socialization attitudes and behaviors students should expect in their nursing programs. Check the ones that apply to your program.

1. My teachers are interested in students' learning.
2. My teachers can tolerate ideas that are different from their own.
3. My program offers me the opportunity to explore different values.
4. Considering the size of the community, my program offers me rich clinical opportunities.
5. My program emphasizes knowledge and techniques, as well as values, ethics, and social behaviors of the nursing profession.
6. My teachers provide regular, direct, constructive feedback on my performance.
7. The program's philosophy and curriculum have been explained to me.
8. The faculty members take pride in the school and actively work to improve it.
9. Faculty members model healthy personal behaviors.
10. Faculty members model professional behavior and project a positive nursing image on campus and in the community. They are active in professional nursing associations.
11. My teachers model respect for one another and for nurses in agencies where we have clinical experiences.
12. Faculty members respect students and avoid authoritarianism ("big me/little you").
13. My program makes every effort to accept students who have the potential to succeed.
14. My teachers maintain school standards.
15. My teachers help students cope with anxiety.
16. My program encourages students to participate in extracurricular activities available in the institution and to participate in student nurse association activities.
17. My teachers avoid favoritism.
18. My teachers keep on top of new developments in nursing and health care and are clinically competent.
19. My teachers value teaching as much as they value their other academic interests.
20. My teachers view me as a consumer of educational services.

Scoring: Compare your responses with other students' scores and identify commonly agreed-on areas of strength and weakness. Discuss both strengths and weaknesses in class. With your teacher as a resource, decide how to use the information in a positive way.

unproductive use of time. In the early days of professional practice, having time to do comprehensive, individualized nursing care planning, such a staple of life for nursing students, may seem like an unrealistic luxury.

New nurses also must adapt to collaborating with other nursing care personnel, such as nursing assistants, patient care technicians, and other unlicensed assistive personnel who help them in caring for patients. This is a difficult adjustment for some nurses who are unaccustomed to delegating, are unsure of the abilities of others, or believe only they can provide quality care.

An overlooked aspect of stress in new graduates is the sheer physical fatigue caused by 8- to 12-hour shifts accompanied by the standing, walking, lifting, bending, and stooping that are necessitated by patient care. Many new graduates have never spent an entire shift on a unit during schooling. When physical fatigue combines with the mental and emotional stress of decision making, efforts to become integrated into a peer group, uncertainty about policies or procedures, and lack of role clarity, sensory overload is almost certain to occur.

If you would like to follow the experiences of new RNs as they "navigate their first steps into the working world" (Ulrich and Paolucci, 2003), you can do so online at websites entitled "Finding Their Way: 2002 RN Graduates Share Their Hopes, Fears During First Year of Nursing" *(www.nurseweek.com/news/features/02-07/graduates_print.html)* and "Into the Fire" *(www.nurseweek.com/news/features/03-01/odyssey_print.html)*.

Reality shock

Although it has been 30 years since the term **reality shock** was used to describe the feelings of powerlessness and ineffectiveness experienced by new graduates (Kramer, 1974), the term is still relevant. Kramer's studies demonstrated that psychological stresses generated by reality shock decrease the ability of individuals to cope effectively with the demands of the new role. Causes of reality shock include the following:

- Absence of positive reinforcement (such as coaching) and frequent communication
- Lack of support, such as faculty availability
- The gap between the ideals taught in school and the actual work setting
- The inability to implement desired nursing care because of circumstances such as a heavy case load or time constraints

Unfortunately, some new nurses "drop out" at this point, rather than taking steps to resolve reality shock. Kramer identified several ways nurses may drop out:

- Disengaging mentally and emotionally
- Driving oneself and others to the breaking point by trying to do it all
- **"Job hopping"**—looking for the perfect, nonstressful job that is completely compatible with professional values
- Prematurely returning to school
- Burning out
- Leaving the nursing profession entirely, which neither nursing nor society can afford

Burnout

Burnout is a result of unresolved reality shock. It is a state of emotional exhaustion due to cumulative stress. Burnout is more common in people with idealistic and perfectionistic personalities, which are not at all unusual in nursing. Symptoms of burnout include irritability, cynicism, impatience, loss of concentration, tendency to be late or to take frequent sick days, excessive drinking and/or eating, being indifferent or uncaring toward patients, carelessness, and guilt (Hom, 2003).

Preventing Burnout and Minimizing Reality Shock

Being aware that there are stages most new graduates go through before settling comfortably into their professional roles can help reduce anxiety, increase coping, and avoid burnout. Kramer (1974) identified a model for resolving reality shock that consists of four stages.

1. *Mastery of skills and routines.* In busy acute care settings, which most new nurses choose for their first jobs, certain activities must be accomplished each day, and

specific behaviors are required to accomplish them. During this stage, nurses focus on the mastery of essential skills and routines. They may temporarily lose sight of the bigger picture and may have to be reminded not to focus so much on the technical aspects of care that they fail to see patients' emotional needs.

2. *Social integration.* In this stage, which overlaps with the first stage, new nurses face the challenge of fitting into the work group. Issues of getting along and being accepted surface. Most people have a desire for peer recognition and approval. It is sometimes a challenge to retain the goodwill of co-workers while keeping high ideals and standards. Learning that they may have to sacrifice the esteem of some workers to maintain their professional values can be a painful, but necessary, lesson for nurses in this stage.

3. *Moral outrage.* Once they realize that they cannot do it all because their commitments to the needs of the organization, to the profession, and to patients often conflict, frustration and anger result. For instance, is it more important to attend a staff meeting or to talk to Mr. Jameson's daughter, who needs to discuss home care versus nursing home placement for her father? Managing these sorts of priorities is a challenge even for experienced nurses.

4. *Conflict resolution.* Kramer (1974) identified several possible resolutions of these problems:

    a. Change behavior while retaining values. For example, find a new work setting that is more compatible with beliefs or, if that is impossible, leave nursing altogether.

    b. Give up professional values (attending to patients' emotional needs) and accept the values of the work organization (get work done quickly) and just try to fit into the employer's existing system.

    c. Give up both sets of values; for example, adopt a "go-with-the-flow" attitude; survival becomes the goal.

    d. Become a "bicultural nurse" (p. 162), who learns to use the values of both the nursing profession and the work organization to influence positive change in the employment setting.

Adopting biculturalism is the most effective of these four options for resolving the conflict between the ideal and reality. **Biculturalism** is the term Kramer used to describe nurses who learn to balance both cultures—the ideal nursing culture they learned about in school and the real one they experience in practice—and to use the best of both of them.

How do bicultural nurses behave? First, they are realists. They recognize that there is no perfect work situation. They also recognize that if they are able to establish credibility and gain respect, they can later be leaders in making improvements.

Next, they accept the fact that newcomers have to demonstrate competence before they can become genuine leaders. They know that people follow only those whom they respect. So they invest time in proving themselves before they start trying to make changes in the system. During this time, they demonstrate, through their own work, the approach to nursing care they value. They do this quietly and without fanfare, however, seeking support from like-minded peers.

Bicultural nurses observe the political system around them. Who are the real opinion makers? Who are the formal and informal leaders? Are they the same? When changes are made, who is involved, and how is it done? Who can be counted on to react to new ideas positively, and who is always negative and complaining? Is there anything that "turns on" the complainers? Are there some people who are so chronically underfunctioning that they just cannot or will not change? Answering these questions provides an appraisal of some of the political realities in the system.

Bicultural nurses willingly serve on committees to demonstrate their ability to address institution-wide issues and to meet others within the system who may share their values. They limit their committee service, however, to those committees that they believe are useful and constructive.

Bicultural nurses work at having rewarding personal lives. These nurses realize that when people meet most of their emotional needs at work, they are vulnerable and they want to fit in so badly that they tend to sacrifice their own professional values if they conflict with those of the work system or with the values of others.

Bicultural nurses take care of themselves. They negotiate for a position and do not just accept what is offered. They expect reasonable compensation and schedules most of the time, although they work their fair share of undesirable shifts. They do not routinely allow their employer to take advantage of them and set them up for physical and emotional exhaustion, or burnout, but they are also cooperative. They demonstrate commitment and loyalty to the organization and show that nursing is more than just a job to them.

Bicultural nurses demonstrate many of the professional behaviors discussed in Chapter 6. In the final analysis, biculturalism and professionalism have many of the same attributes.

Other strategies for minimizing reality shock

Much can be done to reduce reality shock in the transition from student to professional. Students must recognize that schools cannot provide enough clinical experience to make graduates comfortable on their first day as new nurses. They can take responsibility for obtaining as much practical experience as possible outside of school. Working in a health care setting during summers, on school breaks, and on weekends is helpful. They should avoid work during the school week, if at all possible, or keep it to an absolute minimum because academic responsibilities take priority during that time, and exhausted students make poor learners.

Some schools offer programs in which students are paired with practicing nurses (**preceptors**) and work closely with them to experience life as registered nurses do. If your school offers such a program, take advantage of it. If not, seek out information about similar programs at area hospitals. Many agencies, including hospitals and the military, are now providing excellent opportunities for students nearing graduation to function in expanded roles.

Knowing employers' expectations. New nurses approaching graduation should realistically appraise their strengths, weaknesses, and preferences. To reduce reality shock, nurses must ensure that there is a good "match" between their abilities and employers' expectations. Ellis and Hartley (1998) suggest that nurses examine themselves in seven areas in which employers of new graduates have expectations.

1. *Theoretical knowledge* should be adequate to provide basic patient care and to make clinical judgments. Employers expect new nurses to be able to recognize the early signs and symptoms of patient problems, such as an allergic reaction to

a blood transfusion, and take the appropriate nursing action, that is, discontinue the transfusion. They are expected to know potential problems related to various patient conditions, such as postoperative status, and what nursing actions to take to prevent complications.

2. The ability to use the *nursing process* systematically as a means of planning nursing care is important. Employers evaluate nurses' understanding of the phases of the process: assessment, analysis, nursing diagnosis/outcome identification, planning, intervention, and evaluation. They expect nurses to ensure that all elements of a nursing care plan are used in delivering nursing care and that there is documentation in the patient's record to that effect. The ability to follow critical paths or other already-developed plans of care is also expected.

3. *Self-awareness* is critically important. Employers ask prospective employees to identify their own strengths and weaknesses. They need to know that new nurses are willing to ask for help and recognize their limitations. New graduates who are unable or unwilling to request help pose a risk to patients—a risk that employers are unwilling to accept.

4. *Documentation ability* is an increasingly important skill that employers value. Although patient documentation systems differ from facility to facility, employers expect new graduates to recognize what patient data should be charted and to know that all nursing care should be entered in patient records. Accuracy, legibility, spelling, and use of correct grammar and approved abbreviations are minimal expectations. The increasing use of bedside computers for patient record keeping places another demand on new graduates. Employers increasingly expect graduates to adapt their computer skills to the agency's systems in a reasonable time.

5. *Work ethic* is another area in which employers are vitally interested. **Work ethic** means that prospective employees understand what is expected of them and are committed to providing it. Nursing is not, and never has been, a 9-to-5 profession. Although work schedules are more flexible today than ever before, patient care still goes on around the clock, on weekends, and on holidays. Employers expect new graduates to recognize that the most desirable positions and work hours do not usually go to entry-level workers in any field. Nursing is no different in this respect from accounting, broadcasting, or investment banking. In the nursing profession, a nurse cannot leave work until patient care responsibilities have been turned over to a qualified replacement; therefore, being late to work or "calling in sick" when not genuinely incapacitated are luxuries professional nurses cannot afford. Tardy nurses quickly lose credibility with their peers. Employers expect new nurses to recognize and accept that employment means some sacrifices in personal convenience—as in every other profession.

6. *Skill proficiency* of new graduates varies widely, and employers are aware of this. Most large facilities now provide fairly lengthy orientation periods, during which each nurse's skills are appraised and opportunities are provided to practice new procedures. In general, smaller and rural facilities have less formalized orientation programs, and earlier independent functioning is expected. It is useful to keep a log of nursing procedures learned during school. Many schools provide a skills checklist that is helpful in identifying areas in which students need more practice. Students can then be assertive in seeking specific types of patient assignments.

7. *Speed of functioning* is another area in which new nurses vary widely. By the end of a well-planned orientation period, the new graduate should be able to manage the average patient load without too much difficulty. Time management is a skill that is closely related to speed of functioning. Managing your time well means managing yourself well and requires self-discipline. The ability to organize and prioritize nursing care for a group of patients is the key to good time management. Box 8-3 and Figure 8-2 provide guidelines on how to keep poor

---

Box 8-3 Time Management Self-Assessment

Effective time management is a skill that can be developed. Listed are principles reflecting good time management. For each of statements A through J, circle the answer that most closely characterizes how you manage your time.

A. I spend some time each day planning how to accomplish school and other responsibilities.
   0. Rarely
   1. Sometimes
   2. Frequently
B. I set specific goals and dates for accomplishing tasks.
   0. Rarely
   1. Sometimes
   2. Frequently
C. Each day I make a "to do" list and prioritize it. I complete the most important tasks first.
   0. Rarely
   1. Sometimes
   2. Frequently
D. I plan time in my schedule for unexpected problems and unanticipated delays.
   0. Rarely
   1. Sometimes
   2. Frequently
E. I ask others for help when needed.
   0. Rarely
   1. Sometimes
   2. Frequently
F. I take advantage of short but regular breaks to refresh myself and stay alert.
   0. Rarely
   1. Sometimes
   2. Frequently
G. When I really need to concentrate, I work in a specific area that is free from distractions and interruptions.
   0. Rarely
   1. Sometimes
   2. Frequently
H. When working, I turn down other people's requests that interfere with completing my priority tasks.
   0. Rarely
   1. Sometimes
   2. Frequently
I. I avoid unproductive and prolonged socializing with fellow students or employees during my workday.
   0. Rarely
   1. Sometimes
   2. Frequently
J. I keep a calendar of important meetings, dates, and deadlines and carry it with me.
   0. Rarely
   1. Sometimes
   2. Frequently

Scoring: Give yourself 2 points for each "Frequently," 1 point for each "Sometimes," and 0 points for each "Rarely." If your score is 0-10, you need to improve your time management skills; 11-15, you are doing fine but can still improve; 16-18, you have very good time management skills; and 19-20, your time management skills are too good to be true!

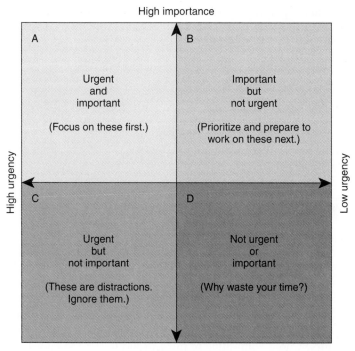

High importance

| A | B |

Urgent
and
important

(Focus on these first.)

Important
but
not urgent

(Prioritize and prepare to
work on these next.)

High urgency | | Low urgency

| C | D |

Urgent
but
not important

(These are distractions.
Ignore them.)

Not urgent
or
important

(Why waste your time?)

Low importance

Figure **8-2**
Setting priorities is an important aspect of time management. Use this grid to determine whether a task should go to the top, middle, or bottom of your daily list or whether it is a time-waster and should be ignored.

time management from becoming a problem while you are a student. Once you have established good time management skills, they will carry over to the work setting.

8. *Collaboration skills,* including communication with patients, families, co-workers, and other health professionals, are increasingly important. The delivery of high-quality nursing care is related to how well the care delivery team works together. Nurses are expected to take the lead in establishing a tone of mutual respect within the team. This requires the effective application of the communication and collaboration skills discussed in Chapter 18.

Orientations, internships, preceptors, and mentors. Other measures to reduce reality shock include seeking an employment situation with an **internship** or long orientation period. Inquire about these during the pre-employment interview. Ask about **preceptor** opportunities, that is, working alongside an experienced nurse, and assess the level of professional development activities offered in each facility under consideration by talking to nurses who actually work in the position you are seeking. Box 8-4 lists preceptor qualities to look for (Hom, 2003).

Recognize that all large systems include a certain amount of **inertia** (disinclination to change), and as good as a new nurse's ideas are, they may not be welcomed.

Box **8-4** Characteristics of a Good Preceptor

- Has at least 2 to 3 years of experience
- Clinically proficient
- Interested in teaching
- Has good communication skills
- Self-confident
- Patient
- Demonstrates knowledge of standards of care
- Applies the nursing process
- Thinks critically and creatively
- Values the preceptor process

Hom EM: Coaching and mentoring new graduates entering perinatal nursing practice, *J Perinat/Neonat Nurs* 17(1):35-49, 2003.

Learning how change is accomplished in the institution is an important first step in becoming a positive influence on its system of operation. Identifying which battles to fight and which to ignore is a key learning process for all new professionals.

Talking with other new graduates about feelings is one of the best ways to combat reality shock. Take the initiative to form a group for mutual support—others need it too! Another interpersonal strategy is to seek a professional mentor. A **mentor** is an experienced nurse who is committed to nursing and to sharing knowledge with less experienced nurses to help advance their careers. A mentor can be a great source of all types of knowledge, as well as another source of support. Having a mentor is different from having a preceptor. It involves forming a long-term relationship through which ideas, experiences, and successful behavior patterns are transmitted.

Ask a nurse whose work you admire to be your mentor and identify what he or she can offer. Some inexperienced nurses are fearful of approaching potential mentors with this request. They should remember that this process is not a one-way street; it has benefits to both parties because it complements and validates the mentor's knowledge and self-esteem, as well as providing important information and support to the nurse being mentored.

In preparing for a relationship with a mentor, you must first do the following (Hagenow and McCrea, 1994):

1. Complete a self-assessment to identify your professional and personal needs and skills.
2. Select a mentor who seems to share your nursing values and beliefs.
3. Ask for an appointment to share your needs and values and determine the areas of mutual interest in the mentoring process.
4. Be prepared to communicate openly with your mentoring experience. Be aware that to grow you must be willing to identify your vulnerabilities and needs.

Box 8-5 lists six essential attributes of a mentoring experience (Stewart and Krueger, 1996).

An exciting opportunity to pair with a mentor is now possible through the World Wide Web. If you would like to establish a mentoring relationship online, go to *www.nursingnet.org* and learn about NursingNet's mentoring project. This website

Box **8-5** **Six Essential Attributes of a Mentoring Experience**

1. A teaching-learning process
2. A reciprocal role
3. A career-development relationship
4. A knowledge differential between mentor and mentee
5. A resonating phenomenon
6. An extended duration

Reprinted with permission of Stewart BM, Krueger LE: An evolutionary concept analysis of mentoring in nursing, *J Prof Nurs* 12(5):311-321, 1996.

was created and is maintained by practicing nurses who seek to improve professionalization in nursing.

In the final analysis, you—and only you—are responsible for your own lifelong professional socialization. Where you choose to work can, however, either facilitate or retard your development. Be sure to find out about orientation experiences and opportunities for continuing education in the agencies you are considering and factor that information into your decision-making process.

Summary of Key Points
- Professional socialization is a critical process that turns novices into fully functioning professionals.
- Two major components of socialization to professional nursing are socialization through education and socialization in the workplace.
- Several thought-provoking conceptual models of professional socialization are applicable for both basic students and RNs. These models identify stages in the process and key behaviors occurring at each stage.
- Individuals have responsibility for actively participating in their own professional socialization. They should identify needed learning experiences and seek opportunities that provide them.
- Reality shock has been identified as a stressful period new nurses may experience when entering nursing practice. Understanding the stages of reality shock and how to resolve them can assist new graduates through this transition.
- Knowing what employers expect can help students plan more effectively and help them be more assertive in seeking experiences they need.
- Good time management skills are invaluable to students and practicing nurses.
- Preceptors and mentors can be valuable resources in enhancing and enriching the professional socialization experience.

CRITICAL THINKING QUESTIONS
1. Describe how both formal and informal socialization experiences in school are modifying your image of nursing.
2. Select one model of socialization discussed in this chapter and place yourself in one of the stages. Give your rationale for that placement. If none of the models or stages fits your experience, create your own model (or stage) and share it with the class.

3. List five things you can do to take active responsibility for your own professional socialization.

4. Interview a new nurse and discuss his or her experience with reality shock. How is this individual handling the transition from student to practicing nurse? What can you learn from his or her experience?

5. Identify several personal and professional areas in which a mentor might be helpful to you. Select a potential mentor and talk with him or her about your needs. If possible, establish a relationship with a mentor using guidelines in this chapter.

6. Using the time management grid in Figure 8-2, review your day and see where each of your activities belongs on the grid—A, B, C, or D. How well did you manage your priorities? What can you do differently tomorrow?

REFERENCES

American Nurses Association: *Code of ethics for nurses with interpretive statements,* Washington, DC, 2001, American Nurses Publishing.

Bandura A: *Social learning theory,* Englewood Cliffs, NJ, 1977, Prentice-Hall.

Benner P: *From novice to expert: excellence and power in clinical nursing practice,* Menlo Park, CA, 1984, Addison-Wesley.

Benner P, Tanner CA, Chesla CA: *Expertise in nursing practice: caring, clinical judgment, and ethics,* New York, 1996, Springer.

Boyle DK, Popkess-Vawter S, Taunton RL: Socialization of new graduates in critical care, *Heart & Lung,* 25:141-154, 1996.

Cohen HA: *The nurse's quest for professional identity,* Menlo Park, CA, 1981, Addison-Wesley.

Cragg CE, Plotnikoff RC, Hugo K, et al: Perspective transformation in RN-to BSN distance education, *J Nurs Ed* 40(7):317-322, 2001.

Davidhizar R, Gigen JN, Reed C: RN to BSN: avoiding the pitfalls, *Health Care Supervisor* 12(1):48-56, 1993.

Davis F: *Professional socialization as subjective experience: the process of doctrinal conversion among student nurses,* Paper presented at the Sixth World Congress of Sociology, Evian, France, September 1966.

Ellis JR, Hartley CL: *Nursing in today's world: challenges, issues, trends,* ed 6, Philadelphia, 1998, JB Lippincott.

Erikson E: *Childhood and society,* New York, 1950, WW Norton.

Hagenow NR, McCrea MA: A mentoring relationship: two viewpoints, *Nurs Management* 25(12):42-43, 1994.

Hinshaw AS: *Socialization and resocialization of nurses for professional nursing practice.* New York, 1976, National League for Nursing.

Hom EM: Coaching and mentoring new graduates entering perinatal nursing practice, *J Perinat/Neonat Nurs* 17(1):35-49, 2003.

Kramer M: *Reality shock: why nurses leave nursing,* St. Louis, 1974, Mosby.

Nesler MS, Hanner MB, Melburg V, et al: Professional socialization of baccalaureate nursing students: can students in distance nursing programs become socialized? *J Nurs Ed* 40(7):293-302, 2001.

Stewart BM, Krueger LE: An evolutionary concept analysis of mentoring in nursing, *J Prof Nurs* 12(5):311-321, 1996.

Throwe AN, Fought SG: Landmarks in the socialization process from RN to BSN, *Nurse Educator* 12(6):15-18, 1987.

Ulrich B, Paolucci M: Into the fire, Online, 2003 *(www.nurseweek.com/news/features/03-01/odyssey_print.html)*.

Ulrich, B, Paolucci, M: Finding their way: 2002 RN graduates share their hopes, fears during first year of nursing. Online, 2003 *(www.nurseweek.com/news/features/02-07/graduates_print.html)*.

Zuzelo PR: Describing the RN-BSN learner perspective, *J Prof Nurs* 17(1):55-65, 2001.

Philosophies of Nursing

Kay Kittrell Chitty

Key Terms

Aesthetics	Epistemology	Nonjudgmental
Belief	Ethics	Philosophy
Belief System	Logic	Politics
Bioethics	Metaphysics	Values

Learning Outcomes

After studying this chapter, students will be able to:

- Define and give examples of beliefs.
- Define and give examples of values.
- Cite examples of nursing philosophies.
- Discuss the impact of beliefs and values on nurses' professional behaviors.
- Explain why nurses and organizations educating and employing nurses need a philosophy of nursing.
- Identify personal beliefs, values, and philosophies as they relate to nursing.

U p to now, this book has focused on describing and defining nursing from the outside. We have examined the historical milestones of the profession, how its practitioners are educated, the social context in which nursing has evolved, the organizations nurses belong to, how nursing measures up as a profession, how nurses define their profession, and how new nurses are socialized. Now we will begin to examine what nurses themselves think, believe, and value, and how their care of patients is influenced by these thoughts, beliefs, and values. In other words, nursing will be explored from the inside.

Certain beliefs have evolved during the development of professional nursing. Specific statements of beliefs were generated by the members of the American Nurses Association (ANA) and published in the *Code of Ethics for Nurses with*

Interpretive Statements (2001). Statements such as the Code exist to affirm the beliefs of the profession and to guide the practice of nursing.

Beliefs about nursing and values pertaining to nursing are at the core of philosophies of nursing. This chapter examines the relationship of attitudes, beliefs, values, and philosophies to the practice of nursing; reviews several philosophies of nursing that were developed by an individual, two hospitals, and three schools of nursing; and assists readers in beginning to develop their own philosophies of nursing.

BELIEFS

A **belief** represents the intellectual acceptance of something as true or correct. Beliefs can also be described as convictions. Groupings of beliefs form codes and creeds. Beliefs are opinions that may be, in reality, true or false. They are based on attitudes that have been acquired and verified by experience. Beliefs are generally transmitted from generation to generation, are stable, and are resistant to change.

Beliefs are organized into **belief systems** that serve as roadmaps for thinking and decision making (Grube, Mayton, Ball-Rokeach, 1994). Individuals are not necessarily aware of how their beliefs interrelate or how their beliefs affect their behavior.

Although all people have beliefs, relatively few have spent much time examining their beliefs. In nursing, it is important to know and understand one's beliefs because the practice of nursing frequently challenges a nurse's beliefs. Although this conflict may create temporary discomfort, it is ultimately good because it forces nurses to consider their beliefs carefully. They have to answer the question: "Is this something I really believe, or have I accepted it because some influential person [such as a parent or teacher] said it?" Abortion, advance directives, the right to die, the right to refuse treatment, alternative lifestyles, and similar issues confront all members of contemporary society. Professional nurses must develop and refine their beliefs about these and many other issues. This is often difficult to do, but it pays dividends in self-awareness.

Beliefs are exhibited through attitudes and behaviors. Simply observing how nurses relate to patients, their families, and nursing peers reveals something about those nurses' beliefs. Every day nurses meet people whose beliefs are different from, or even diametrically opposed to, their own. Effective nurses recognize that they need to adopt **nonjudgmental** attitudes toward patients' beliefs. A nurse with a nonjudgmental attitude makes every effort to convey neither approval nor disapproval of patients' beliefs and respects each person's right to his or her beliefs (Figure 9-1).

An example of differences in beliefs that directly affect nursing is the position taken by some religious groups that all healing should be left to a divine power. For members of such groups, seeking medical treatment, even lifesaving measures such as blood transfusions or chemotherapy for cancer, is not condoned. From time to time, there have been news reports of parents who are charged with criminal acts because they did not take a sick child to a physician. Typical of such incidents was the one reported in Georgia when the parents of a 19-year-old severely injured in an automobile accident refused to give permission for their unconscious Jehovah's Witness son to continue receiving blood transfusions. He died 2 days later (Eustis, 2002).

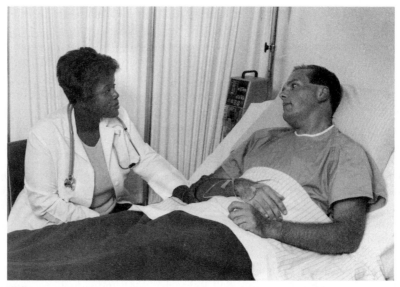

Figure **9-1**
Professional nurses make every effort to maintain a nonjudgmental attitude toward patients. A nonjudgmental attitude is one of nursing's values. (Photo by Fielding Freed.)

The courts were involved, but the issue has not been resolved. You can read more about this case online (*www.rickross.com/reference/jw/jw90.html*).

Because you are in a health profession, you clearly have beliefs about the value of modern medicine. Think about how your health care beliefs differ from those of the family just described. What feelings might you have if assigned to work with a family with these beliefs? From this brief consideration, you may be able to appreciate how difficult it can be to maintain a nonjudgmental attitude toward the beliefs of patients. Nevertheless, it is essential.

Three Categories of Beliefs

People often use the terms *beliefs* and *values* interchangeably. Even experts disagree about whether they differ or are the same. Although they are related, beliefs and values are differentiated in this chapter and discussed separately.

Theorists studying belief systems have identified three main categories of beliefs:

1. Descriptive or existential beliefs are those that can be shown to be true or false. An example of a descriptive belief is "The sun will come up tomorrow morning."
2. Evaluative beliefs are those in which there is a judgment about good or bad. The belief "Dancing is immoral" is an example of an evaluative belief.
3. Prescriptive (encouraged) and proscriptive (prohibited) beliefs are those in which certain actions are judged to be desirable or undesirable. The belief "Every citizen of voting age should vote in every election" is a prescriptive belief, whereas the belief "People should not engage in sexual intercourse outside of marriage" is a proscriptive belief. Prescriptive and proscriptive beliefs are closely related to values (Rokeach, 1973, pp. 6-7).

VALUES

Values are the freely chosen principles, ideals, or standards held by an individual, class, or group that give meaning and direction to life. A value is an abstract representation of what is right, worthwhile, or desirable. Values define ideal modes of conduct and reflect what the individual or group endorse and try to live up to. Values, like beliefs, are relatively stable and resistant to change.

Although many people are unaware of it, values help them make small, day-to-day choices, as well as important life decisions. Just as beliefs influence nursing practice, values also influence how nurses practice their profession, often without their conscious awareness. Diann B. Uustal (1985), a contemporary nurse who has written and spoken extensively about values, said, "Everything we do, every decision we make and course of action we take is based on our consciously and unconsciously chosen beliefs, attitudes and values" (p. 100). Uustal also asserts, "Nursing is a behavioral manifestation of the nurse's value system. It is not merely a career, a job, an assignment; it is a ministry" (1993, p. 10). She believes that nurses must give "caring attentiveness and presence" to their patients and to do otherwise "is equivalent to psychological and spiritual abandonment" (Uustal, 1993, p. 10). Do you agree or disagree with these statements?

Nature of Human Values

Values evolve as people mature. An individual's values today are undoubtedly different from those of 10, or even 5, years ago. Rokeach (1973, p. 3) made several assertions about the nature of human values:

1. Each person has a relatively small number of values.
2. All human beings, regardless of location or culture, possess basically the same values to differing degrees.
3. People organize their values into value systems.
4. People develop values in response to culture, society, and even individual personality traits.
5. Most observable human behaviors are manifestations or consequences of human values.

Authorities agree that values influence behavior and that people with unclear values lack direction, persistence, and decision-making skills (Raths, Harmin, and Simon, 1978). Because much of nursing involves having a clear sense of direction, the ability to persevere, and the ability to make sound decisions quickly and frequently, effective nurses must have a strong set of professional nursing values. A number of professional nursing values are listed in Box 9-1.

Process of Valuing

Valuing is the process by which values are determined. There are three identified steps in the process of valuing: choosing, prizing, and acting.

1. Choosing is the cognitive (intellectual) aspect of valuing. Ideally, people choose their values freely from all alternatives after considering the possible consequences of their choices.
2. Prizing is the affective (emotional) aspect of valuing. People usually feel good about their values and cherish the choices they make.

Box **9-1** Professional Nursing Values

- Accountability and responsibility for own actions
- Balancing cure and care
- Benevolence
- Caring as a foundation for relationships
- Collaborative multidisciplinary practice
- Compassion
- Competence
- Concern
- Continuous improvement of service
- Cooperative work relationships
- Courage
- Dependability
- Empathy
- Ethical conduct
- Flexibility
- Focus on patient-defined quality of life
- Health promotion
- Holistic, person-centered care
- Honesty and authenticity in communication
- Humaneness
- Humility
- Illness prevention
- Individualized patient care
- Integrity, personal and professional
- Involvement with families
- Kindness
- Knowledge

- Listening attentively
- Nonjudgmental attitude
- Objectivity
- Openness to learning
- Partnerships with patients
- Patient advocacy
- Patient education
- Presence (being fully present)
- Promotion of health
- Promotion of patient self-determination and patient preferences
- Providing care regardless of patient's ability to pay
- Quality care (physical, emotional, spiritual, social, intellectual)
- Reliability
- Respect for each person's dignity and worth
- Responsibility
- Responsiveness
- Sensitivity
- Sharing decision-making
- Sharing self through nursing interventions
- Stewardship; responsible use of resources
- Subordination of self-interest
- Support of fellow nurses
- Teamwork
- Trust in self, others, and the institution

Courtesy Diann B. Uustal, 2004.

3. Acting is the kinesthetic (behavioral) aspect of valuing. When people affirm their values publicly by acting on their choices, they make their values part of their behavior. A real value is acted upon consistently in behavior.

All three steps must be taken, or the process of valuing is incomplete. For example, a professional nurse might believe that learning is a lifelong process and that nurses have an obligation to keep up with new developments in the profession. This nurse would choose continued learning and appreciate the consequences of the choice.

He or she might even publicly affirm this choice and feel good about it. If the nurse follows through consistently with behaviors such as reading journals, attending conferences, and seeking out other learning opportunities, continued learning can be seen as a true value in his or her life.

Values Clarification

Nurses, as well as people in other helping professions, need to understand their values. This is the first step in self-awareness, which is important in maintaining a nonjudgmental approach to patients.

Considering your reactions to the following statements can help in beginning to identify some nursing values you hold:
1. Patients should always be told the truth about their diagnoses.
2. Nurses, if asked, should assist terminally ill patients to die.
3. Severely impaired infants should be kept alive, regardless of their future quality of life.
4. Nurses should never accept gifts from patients.
5. A college professor should receive a heart transplant before a homeless person does.
6. Nurses should be role models of healthy behavior.

As you react both emotionally and intellectually to these statements, something about your personal and professional values is revealed. Determining where you stand on these and other nursing issues is an important step in clarifying your values. A variety of values clarification exercises have been developed to stimulate self-reflection and help people understand their values. Box 9-2 contains a values clarification exercise you may want to complete to assist you further in understanding the valuing process.

Values Undergirding Nursing's Social Policy Statement

Professional groups, such as nursing, "have collective identities that are evidenced by their actions. These actions stem from a set of values and choices. … [B]y examining the actions of groups …, their basic values can be logically inferred" (Mohr, 1995, p. 30).

Organized nursing, through the ANA, sets forth the values that undergird the profession. This is done in a document published from time to time that is designed to explain "professional nursing's relationship with society and its obligation to those who receive nursing care" (American Nurses Association, 2003, p. 1). The most recent version, entitled *Nursing's Social Policy Statement*, was published in 2003. It set forth several underlying values and assumptions on which the Statement is based (American Nurses Association, 2003, pp. 3):
- Humans manifest an essential unity of mind, body, and spirit.
- Human experience is contextually and culturally defined.
- Health and illness are human experiences. The presence of illness does not preclude health nor does optimal health preclude illness.
- The relationship between nurse and patient involves participation of both in the process of care.
- The interaction between nurse and patient occurs within the context of the values and beliefs of the patient and the nurse.

Chapter 19 contains more about values and their relationship to nursing practice.

Box **9-2** **Clarifying Your Values**

Once you have identified a value, it is important to assess its significance to you and to clarify your willingness to act on the value. The following clarifying questions are organized based on the steps of the valuing process and can help you answer questions about what you value. First, identify a value (or values) that is (are) important to you. Write your value(s) below.

_____

_____

_____

_____

Next, use the questions below to assess the importance of a belief or attitude and to determine whether it is a value. Rephrase the questions to suit your own style of conversation.

Choosing Freely

1. Am I sure I've thought about this value and chosen to believe it myself?
2. Who first taught me this value?
3. How do I know I'm "right"?

Choosing from Among Alternatives

4. What other alternatives are possible?
5. Which alternative has the most appeal for me and why?
6. Have I thought much about this value/alternative?

Choosing After Considering the Consequences

7. What consequences do I think might occur as a result of my holding this value?
8. What "price" will I pay for my position?
9. Is this value worth the "price" I might pay?

Complement to Other Values

10. Does this value "fit" with my other values, and is it consistent with them?
11. Am I sure this value doesn't conflict with other values I deem important to me?

Prize and Cherish

12. Am I proud of my position and value? Is this something I feel good about?
13. How important is this value to me?
14. If this were not one of my values, how different would my life be?

Public Affirmation

15. Am I willing to speak out for this value?

Action

16. Am I willing to put this value into action?
17. Do I act on this value? When? How consistently?
18. Is this a value that can guide me in other situations?
19. Would I want others who are important to me to follow this value?

Box **9-2** **Clarifying Your Values—cont'd**

20. Do I think I'll always believe this? How committed to this value am I?
21. Am I willing to do anything about this value?
22. How do I know this value is "right"? Are my values ethical?

From Uustal DB: *Clinical ethics and values: issues and insights in a changing healthcare environment,* East Greenwich, RI, 1993, Educational Resources in Healthcare. Reprinted with permission.

PHILOSOPHIES

Philosophy is defined as the study of the principles underlying conduct, thought, and the nature of the universe. A simple explanation of philosophy is that it entails a search for meaning in the universe. You may have learned about philosophers such as Plato, Aristotle, Bacon, Kant, Hegel, Kierkegaard, Nietzsche, Locke, Descartes, and others in nonnursing classes. These philosophers were searching for the underlying principles of reality and truth. Nursing philosophies and theories often derive from or build upon the concepts identified by these and other philosophers.

Philosophy begins when someone contemplates, or wonders, about something. If a group of friends sometimes sits and discusses the relationship between men and women and ponders the differences in men's and women's natures and approaches to life, one might say that they were developing a philosophy about male and female ways of being. It is important to remember that philosophy is not the exclusive domain of a few erudite individuals; everyone has a personal philosophy of life that is unique.

People develop personal philosophies as they mature. These philosophies serve as blueprints or guides and incorporate each individual's value and belief systems. Nurses' personal philosophies interact directly with their philosophies of nursing and influence professional behaviors.

Branches of Philosophy

Before examining professional philosophies, we briefly explore the discipline of philosophy itself. Philosophy has been divided into specific areas of study. This section reviews six branches: epistemology, logic, aesthetics, ethics, politics, and metaphysics.

1. **Epistemology** is the branch of philosophy dealing with the theory of knowledge itself. The epistemologist attempts to answer such questions as "What can be known?" and "What constitutes knowledge?" Epistemology attempts to determine how we can know whether our beliefs about the world are true.

2. **Logic** is the study of proper and improper methods of reasoning. In logic, the nature of reasoning itself is the subject. Logic attempts to answer the question, "What should our thinking methods be in order to reach true conclusions?" Chapter 15 presents a method of logical thinking that nurses use to plan and implement effective patient care, called the nursing process.

3. **Aesthetics** is the study of what is beautiful. It attempts to answer the question, "Why do we find things beautiful?" Painting, sculpture, music, dance, and literature are all associated with beauty. Judgments about what is beautiful, however, differ from individual to individual and culture to culture. For example, Eastern music may sound discordant to the Western ear and vice versa.

4. **Ethics** is the branch of philosophy that studies standards of conduct. It attempts to answer the question, "What is the nature of good and evil?" Moral principles and values make up a system of ethics. Behavior depends on moral principles and values. Ethics, therefore, underlie the standards of behavior that govern us as individuals and as nurses. **Bioethics** is a term describing the branch of ethics that deals with biological issues. Bioethics and nursing ethics are complex areas of study that are explored in Chapter 19.

5. **Politics,** in the context of a discussion of philosophy, means the area of philosophy that deals with the regulation and control of people living in society. Political philosophers study the conditions of society and suggest recommendations for improving them. They attempt to answer the question, "What makes good governments?"

6. **Metaphysics** is the consideration of the ultimate nature of existence, reality, human experience, and the universe. Metaphysicians believe that through contemplation we can come to a more complete understanding of reality than even science can provide. They ask the question, "What is the meaning of life?" and explore the fundamental nature of all reality.

This brief review of the major branches of philosophy is presented as a backdrop for the discussion of philosophies of nursing.

Philosophies of Nursing

Philosophies of nursing are statements of beliefs about nursing and expressions of values in nursing that are used as bases for thinking and acting. Most philosophies of nursing are built on a foundation of beliefs about people, environment, health, and nursing. Each of these four foundational concepts of nursing is discussed in some detail in Chapter 10.

Individual philosophies

If asked, most nurses could list their beliefs about nursing, but it is doubtful that many have written a formal philosophy of nursing. They are influenced on a day-to-day basis, however, by their unwritten, informal philosophies. It is useful to go through the process of writing down one's own professional philosophy and revising it from time to time. Comparing recent and earlier versions can reveal professional and personal growth over time. It is also helpful to read one's philosophy of nursing from time to time to make sure daily behaviors are consistent with deeply held beliefs. Box 9-3 contains one nurse's philosophy of nursing.

Collective philosophies

Although few individuals write down their nursing philosophies, it is common for hospitals and schools of nursing to express their collective beliefs about nursing in written philosophies. In fact, both hospitals and schools of nursing are required by their accrediting bodies to develop statements of philosophy. Philosophical statements should be relevant to the setting. They are intended to guide the practice of nurses employed in that setting. Examining some of these statements clarifies what constitutes a collective philosophy of nursing.

Philosophies of nursing in two hospital settings. First, look at the philosophy of the Division of Nursing at Beth Israel Deaconess Medical Center in Boston (Box 9-4).

Box **9-3** One Nurse's Philosophy

I believe that the essence of nursing is caring about and caring for human beings who are unable to care for themselves. I believe that the central core of nursing is the nurse-patient relationship and that through that relationship I can make a difference in the lives of others at a time when they are most vulnerable.

Human beings generally do the best they can. When they are uncooperative, critical, or otherwise unpleasant, it is usually because they are frightened; therefore, I will remain pleasant and nondefensive and try to understand the patient's perception of the situation. I pledge to be trustworthy and an advocate for my patients.

I realize that my cultural background affects how I deliver nursing care and that my patients' cultural backgrounds affect how they receive my care. I try to learn as much as I can about each individual's cultural beliefs and preferences and individualize care accordingly.

My vision for myself as a nurse is that I will provide the best care I can to all patients, regardless of their financial situation, social status, lifestyle choices, or spiritual beliefs. I will collaborate with my patients, their families, and my health care colleagues and work cooperatively with them, valuing and respecting what each brings to the situation.

I am individually accountable for the care I provide, for what I fail to do and to know. Therefore, I pledge to remain a learner all my life and actively seek opportunities to learn how to be a more effective nurse.

I will strive for a balance of personal and professional responsibilities. This means I will take care of myself physically, emotionally, socially, and spiritually so I can continue to be a productive caregiver.

Box **9-4** Beth Israel Deaconess Medical Center Philosophy of Nursing

Introduction

This revised statement of philosophy and purpose has drawn on the seminal thinking of Benner, Henderson, Orlando, and Wiedenbach and on multiple documents developed by the Beth Israel Deaconess Medical Center nursing services and programs over a 20-year period, including the Statement of Philosophy first issued in 1974.

Statements such as this are meaningless unless they are translated into action. Our philosophy and purpose are perhaps most succinctly expressed in the words of one of our patients: "My primary nurse was truly a gem in the profession of nursing. She combines not only the highest level of professionalism in nursing, but also the many personal qualities which go beyond that in assisting patients to make a full recovery. She had a knack for getting me to motivate myself. Her concern was genuine, her advice sound, and her willingness to assist in my long-range rehabilitation goals ever present."

Purpose

The purpose of the Beth Israel Deaconess nursing services and programs is to ensure that each patient receives professional nursing care that is patient-centered and goal-directed and to support health care education and research in nursing and other disciplines. Beth Israel Deaconess nurses and their associates in the division of nursing carry out their activities with one focus in mind—assisting the patient to achieve optimal health outcomes.

Continued

| Box **9-4** Beth Israel Deaconess Medical Center Philosophy of Nursing—cont'd |

Philosophy

Nursing as a Professional Service

We agree with Virginia Henderson that professional nursing is a complex service that assists "… people sick or well in the performance of those activities contributing to health, or its recovery (or to a peaceful death) that they would perform unaided if they had the necessary strength, will, or knowledge. It is likewise the unique contribution of nursing to help people to be independent of such assistance as soon as possible." The activities that nurses help patients carry out (or those that nurses carry out for patients) include the therapeutic plans prescribed by physicians, by other health care providers, and by nurses themselves. In carrying out these activities, nurses practice an art through which technical, observational, analytical, and communication skills, as well as scientific knowledge and clinical judgment, are systematically applied to the health needs of others in a caring manner. Caring means being connected and having things matter. Thus by caring, the nurse creates possibilities for coping in the face of risk and vulnerability.

We believe that physical and emotional comfort is a universal health need, the provision of which is a historical and fundamental nursing responsibility. Nursing is further distinguished from other direct health care services by its tradition of continuity. For hospitalized patients, this includes 24-hour accountability for observing, recording, and reporting of the patient's condition, and for direct provision of care and comfort. For patients residing in the community, care is generally provided on an intermittent basis, incorporating the family and/or significant other in the plan to ensure continuity. The nursing care in this setting includes identifying and facilitating access to community resources and supports and encouraging patients to achieve their optimal level of functioning. Continuity of care across the spectrum of health and illness is valued and provided by all Beth Israel Deaconess nurses whatever their area of practice.

We believe that for each patient, continuity, personalization, and excellence of care is best achieved when it is planned and evaluated by a collaborative patient care team whose individual members have continuous accountability for that care. We further believe that nursing care for each patient should be planned, coordinated, and delivered by a professional registered nurse, and that direct care should be provided by a primary nurse and any designated associates. The desired endpoint of all nursing activity is to maintain or improve the patient's health status and comfort.

The art and science of professional nursing is acquired through formal higher education. It becomes refined through continuing education and training, experience, self-evaluation, evaluation by a manager, and peer review.

NOTE: The Beth Israel Deaconess nursing services philosophy also contains statements about patients, families, professional nursing, and the environment for nursing care.

Notice that this philosophy includes statements of belief about nursing services, recipients of nursing care, and professional nurses themselves. Then read Box 9-5, which contains the philosophy of nursing of Memorial Health Care System in Chattanooga, Tennessee. This philosophy describes a commitment to excellence in nursing service, practice, and leadership.

Notice differences and similarities in the two philosophies, as well as statements with which you might agree or disagree. Remember that these are both philosophies

Box **9-5** Memorial Health Care System Philosophy of Nursing

Philosophy of Nursing

Nursing Care throughout the Memorial Health Care System is committed to upholding the corporate values and the mission of Catholic Health Initiatives. We affirm that the corporate values of Reverence, Compassion, Integrity, and Excellence are in congruence with our professional values. Therefore, we believe that these principles must characterize nursing care.

Reverence

We believe …

- that each of our patients, regardless of circumstances, possesses intrinsic value from God and should be treated with dignity and respect.
- that meeting the needs of patients and other customers should always be our number-one priority.
- that nurses should collaborate with other health care team members to meet the holistic needs of our patients, which include physical, psychosocial, and spiritual aspects of care.
- that patient confidentiality and privacy should be preserved.
- that we should be sensitive to individual needs and give support, praise, and recognition to encourage professional and personal development.

Compassion

We believe …

- that each encounter with patients and families should portray compassion and concern.
- that our profession is a science and an art, the essence of which is nurturing and caring.
- that our primary duty is to restore and maintain the health of our patients in a spirit of compassion and concern.
- that compassion should be characterized in our day-to-day personal interactions, as well as being a motivating factor in management decisions.

Integrity

We believe …

- that the nursing process is an integral part of our practice as professional nurses.
- that we should aggressively promote patient and family education to allow each individual the opportunity to prevent illness and/or achieve optimal health.
- that we should encourage and support collaborative decision making by those who are closest to the situation, even at the risk of failure.
- that we are accountable to our patients, patients' families, and to each other for our professional practice.
- that we should possess an energy level and personal style that empowers and inspires enthusiasm in others.
- that justice should be applied equitably in all employment practices and personnel policies.

Excellence

We believe …

- that monitoring and evaluating nursing practice is our responsibility and is necessary to continuously improve care.

Continued

Box **9-5** **Memorial Health Care System Philosophy of Nursing—cont'd**

- that we should pursue professional growth and development through education, participating in professional organizations, and support of research.
- that we should provide a progressive environment, utilizing current technology guided by responsible stewardship, to promote the highest quality patient care and employee satisfaction.
- that we should consider suggestions and criticisms as challenges for improvement and innovation.
- that each patient should receive quality care that is cost-effective, competitive, and based on the latest technology.

From Memorial Health Care System Department of Nursing: *Memorial Health Care System philosophy of nursing*, Chattanooga, TN, 2003, Memorial Health Care System. Reprinted with permission.

of departments of nursing in hospital settings. Before taking a position in a hospital or health care agency, it is a good idea to ask for a copy of the philosophy of nursing of that institution. Read it carefully and make sure you accept the beliefs and values it contains, for it will influence nursing care in that setting.

Philosophies of three schools of nursing. Now examine philosophical statements of three schools of nursing. The philosophy of the faculty in the Department of Nursing at the University of North Florida is printed in Box 9-6. Box 9-7 contains

Box **9-6** **Philosophy of the School of Nursing, University of North Florida**

The philosophy of the School of Nursing supports the mission of the University of North Florida and the College of Health and reflects the academic goals of the greater university community. The faculty have defined a philosophy of nursing that considers two domains: the patient who is the recipient of care, and the nurse who is the caregiver. The patient domain includes beliefs about persons, environment, and health.

The faculty of the School of Nursing view patients as biopsychosocial beings with inherent dignity and worth who strive to meet a hierarchy of human needs throughout the life span. When unable to satisfy these needs, patients are at risk for alterations in health status. As risks manifest themselves in health problems, patients seek relief in the form of health care from health professionals. Nursing responds to a need for care and support and, in some cases, the need for treatments and curing techniques. Patients of nursing may be individuals, families, groups, or communities.

Patients live in an environment with an internal and external dimension. The internal environment is an open system composed of four subsystems: physical, psychological, spiritual, and cultural. The external environment is composed of groups of individuals and families, each living within their unique sociocultural milieu. These groups function in a universe influenced by political and economic forces. The dynamic relationship between internal and external environments has a profound effect on health status and on how persons adapt to physical, psychological, social, and environmental changes.

Health is viewed as a dynamic state of being on a continuum from optimal wellness to illness. Changes on this continuum are influenced and, in some cases, caused by internal and external environmental stressors. A state of health exists when a person functions as an integrated whole, living and interacting with environments in a productive manner. Movement on the health-illness continuum depends on the severity of stressors, the adaptive mechanisms of the person, and the accessibility to and quality of health care services available.

Box 9-6 **Philosophy of the School of Nursing, University of North Florida—cont'd**

The nurse/caregiver domain includes beliefs about nursing, education, and professional practice and research. Nursing is a human service that assists patients to achieve optimal wellness and cope with periods of illness and disability. The nurse uses problem-solving skills and caring behaviors to facilitate the patient's adaptive responses in an effort to maintain, promote, and/or restore an optimal state of health or facilitate a peaceful death. Specific caring behaviors are determined by the patient's individual needs and may be assistive, supportive, or facilitative in nature. The nurse assumes independent and interdependent roles at various times, based on mutually identified needs of the patient. Nurses fulfill their professional role as members of a health care team working together in the best interest of the patient.

Nursing education takes place through a planned teaching-learning process. Faculty are responsible for assisting students to achieve their full potential and are sensitive to the individual needs of students. Learning readiness, self-directed learning, recognition of the value of past experience and education, and the development of a problem-solving orientation to learning are important aspects of the teaching-learning process. Students and faculty cooperate in assuming a shared responsibility for planning and implementing learning activities within the context of the curriculum and through individual course offerings. Learning is facilitated when the educational environment provides an open, accepting atmosphere in which the faculty and students work together to achieve mutual goals. Higher education is a process through which the student is afforded opportunities to develop a liberal education, as well as a rich knowledge base on which to build a professional career.

Baccalaureate nursing education is specifically concerned with preparation for the first professional degree in nursing. This education prepares the student for professional practice and leadership roles within an ever-changing health care industry. It also serves as a foundation for graduate education and advanced nursing practice.

Graduate nursing education, at the master's level, is specifically concerned with preparing nurses with advanced practice skills. Graduates provide expert nursing care to individuals, families, and communities; contribute to nursing science; serve as mentors and teachers of nurse colleagues; and participate in planning and policy formulations for a variety of patient populations.

Professional nursing practice is based on concepts and theories from the discipline of nursing and from other fields, including the sciences and humanities. Professional nurses use the nursing process, which demands the ability to assess, analyze, plan, implement, and evaluate nursing care. The nursing process is the basis of scientific nursing practice and requires nurses to analyze data from many sources. A strong foundation from the natural sciences and the humanities assists nurses in developing the critical thinking skills essential to the nursing process. The scientific base of practice continues to be developed throughout the nursing curriculum and provides the graduate with the knowledge and skills to practice nursing in a responsible manner.

Nursing is a discipline that uses research as a process to develop a distinct body of knowledge as a basis for scientific practice. Research serves as the basis for changes that influence and improve nursing practice and patient care outcomes. The professional nurse prepared at the baccalaureate level should be an informed consumer of research findings and should be able to collaborate with others to study questions that arise from the practice of nursing and related issues. The professional nurse prepared at the master's level should function as a collaborative member of research teams, evaluate the clinical usefulness of research findings, and assume a leadership role in promoting evidence-based practice.

From University of North Florida, School of Nursing: *Philosophy of the School of Nursing,* Jacksonville, FL, 2003, University of North Florida. Reprinted with permission.

Box 9-7 Philosophy of the Department of Nursing, Central Missouri State University

The philosophy of the Department of Nursing is founded on the belief that the profession of nursing makes an essential contribution to society and that education for professional nursing and advanced practice nursing is best conducted in an institution of higher learning. For these purposes, we believe:

- Persons are the focus of nursing. Persons are moral beings endowed with individual qualities, but hold in common with others the basic need for dignity, respect, and recognition of their individual worth and uniqueness.
- Health is the actualization of inherent and acquired human potential, either as individual, aggregate, or collective humanity.
- Nursing is a human science and an art concerned with the diagnosis and treatment of human responses to actual or potential health changes (ANA).
- The professional nurse functions in an ethical manner as an independent practitioner or as a collaborator with other health team members.
- In the future the professional nurse will practice in expanded roles and, with additional formal education, will practice in advanced practice nursing roles in increasing numbers and in a variety of settings, many of which will be outside acute care institutions.
- Teaching is an interactive, interpersonal activity whereby the teacher is a learner, facilitator, and collaborator. The role of the teacher is to provide structure, climate, and dialogue so that the student can explore and discover self.
- Learning is a process whereby the student begins to view wholes, develop insights into situations, find meanings, evaluate rules and values, project consequences, and predict from knowns to unknowns using both data and intuition.
- Communicating, Nursing Reasoning, Interacting, and Professional Valuing are essential graduate outcomes.
- Formative and summative assessments are important to the development and achievement of graduate outcomes.

Through fulfillment of these beliefs, our baccalaureate degree students, upon graduation, will be prepared to practice nursing as generalists in rural and urban settings. Through their baccalaureate nursing education, our students will be provided with the foundation for further study and advancement. We feel our advanced nursing degree students, upon graduation, will be prepared to practice nursing as specialists in primarily rural areas. Through their master's level nursing education, students are provided with the foundation for advanced practice specialty practice and advanced study at the doctoral level.

From Central Missouri State University, Department of Nursing: *Philosophy of nursing,* Warrensburg, MO, 2003, Central Missouri State University. Reprinted with permission.

the philosophy of the Department of Nursing at Central Missouri State University. Box 9-8 presents the philosophy of Palm Beach Atlantic University. After reading these, identify the similarities and differences between the philosophies of nursing in hospitals and the ones in these schools of nursing. What are the differences in the state university philosophies, which are required by law to reflect a secular view, and the philosophy of a religiously affiliated school, such as Palm Beach Atlantic University?

Box **9-8** **Philosophy of the School of Nursing, Palm Beach Atlantic University**

We believe nursing is an art and a science that prepares men and women for the provision of services to individuals, families, groups, and communities designed to attain, maintain, or regain optimal wellness. The baccalaureate degree prepares the graduate for the first level of professional nursing. Nursing is a practice profession, as well as an academic discipline. For us, nursing is a ministry of Christian service to those in need that flows out of a value system based on faith in Jesus Christ and service to Him. Persons are understood to be children of God.

We believe that the professional nurse delivers wholistic care based on an organized system of nursing science. The Neuman Systems Model was selected because it presents a wholistic view of the patient/client that recognizes developmental, psychological, physiological, socioeconomic, and spiritual perspectives of the life of human beings. This model has produced evidence-based outcomes demonstrating its utility as a nursing curriculum framework for nursing of individuals, families, and communities. Therefore, our perspective of nursing provides a systematic view of persons, families, and communities in relation with their environments and the stressors or potential stressors present within those relationships that leads to comprehensive plans of care and individual artistic expressions within the nurse-patient relationship.

Nursing is designed with the patient/client in relation to stressors that may be intrapersonal, interpersonal, or extrapersonal and are identified in the mutual process of the patient and the nurse moving them toward goals for wellness for the individual patient/client/family/community. Nursing approaches are designed to include primary, secondary, and/or tertiary interventions aimed at the stressors taking into account patient/client strengths and weaknesses.

Health is understood from the patient/client's perspective; therefore their perception of their health and their stressors is vital to the provision of meaningful nursing. We understand that one person's stressor is another's zest for living, so the patient/client perception is essential for plans of care. Nurses are primary providers in health care delivery based on their consistent presence and their expert knowledge and ability for designing, providing, managing, and evaluating patient care as they collaborate with the other members of the health care team.

Teaching and learning are vital to the nurse-patient relationship and also to the student-faculty relationship. Whether with patients or students, we believe that mutual goals for teaching and learning are the most productive style for quality outcomes in the process of education.

From Palm Beach Atlantic University, School of Nursing: *Philosophy of nursing,* West Palm Beach, FL, 2003, Palm Beach Atlantic University. Reprinted with permission of Martha Alligood, RN, PhD, Dean, School of Nursing,

An important point about philosophies of nursing is that they are dynamic; they change over time. When a collective philosophy is written, it reflects the existing values and beliefs of particular group of people who wrote it. When the group members change, the philosophy may also change. Therefore, once a collective philosophy is written, it should be "revisited" regularly and modified to reflect accurately the group's current beliefs about nursing practice.

DEVELOPING A PERSONAL PHILOSOPHY OF NURSING

Your philosophy of life, whether or not you can articulate it, is the basis of your behavior. It consists of the principles that underlie your thinking and conduct.

Box **9-9** **Philosophy of Nursing Work Sheet**

Purpose: To write a beginning philosophy of nursing that reflects the beliefs and values of _____ [your name].

Today's date is _____.

I chose nursing as my profession because nursing is _____
_____.

I believe that the core of nursing is_____.

I believe that the focus of nursing is_____.

My vision for myself as a nurse is that I will _____.

To live out my philosophy of nursing, every day I must remember this about:

1. My patients: _____.
2. My patients' families: _____.
3. My fellow health care professionals: _____.
4. My own health: _____.

Therefore, developing a philosophy of nursing is not merely an academic exercise required by accrediting bodies. Having a written philosophy can help guide nurses in the daily decisions they must make in nursing practice.

Writing a philosophy is not a complex, time-consuming task. It simply involves writing down your beliefs and values about nursing. It answers the questions: "What is nursing?" and "Why do I practice nursing the way I do?" Whether individual or collective, a philosophy should provide direction and promote effectiveness.

Box 9-9 is designed to help you begin to develop your own personal philosophy of nursing. After you write a beginning philosophy, save it. As you progress through your educational program, take it out and revise it regularly, saving each version. After you graduate, look back at all the different versions and see how your values and beliefs about nursing have changed over time.

Summary of Key Points

- People develop beliefs and values that affect their attitudes and behaviors.
- Beliefs and values influence how nurses practice their profession.
- Nurses need to be aware of their beliefs and values to prevent the unintentional intrusion of personal values into nurse-patient relationships.
- A statement of beliefs can be called a philosophy.
- The purpose of developing a philosophy of nursing is to shape and guide nursing practice.
- There are numerous philosophical statements about nursing and nursing education.
- Philosophies can express either individual beliefs or the collective beliefs of a group, such as a nursing faculty.
- As nurses progress professionally, they develop ideas about the practice of nursing that they agree with and support. From these, they develop their own personal philosophies of nursing.

■ As nurses mature in the profession, they may find that their philosophies about nursing also change, even though underlying values may not.

CRITICAL THINKING QUESTIONS

1. Name two of your health-related values. How did these become your values? Describe how you expect these values to influence your nursing practice.
2. Read "One Nurse's Philosophy" in Box 9-3. Then identify at least 10 of that nurse's professional values, using the list in Box 9-1, "Professional Nursing Values." Can you identify other values that are not listed?
3. Compare the nursing philosophies of Beth Israel Deaconess Medical Center and Memorial Health Care System. What are three common elements and three differences? If you or a family member needed to be hospitalized and you had to select a hospital based on the philosophy of nursing, which of these two facilities would you choose? Why?
4. Obtain the philosophy statement of the faculty of your school of nursing. What concepts are included? Which beliefs do you agree with and disagree with? Why?
5. Using the work sheet in Box 9-9, write a beginning personal philosophy of nursing. Share your philosophy with one other person.
6. Discuss how having or not having a philosophy of nursing influences a nurse's practice.
7. Discuss how the focus on "the bottom line" affects your own and nursing's professional values.

REFERENCES

American Nurses Association: *Nursing's social policy statement,* ed 2, Washington, DC, 2003, nursesbooks.org.

Beth Israel Deaconess Medical Center Division of Nursing: *Statement of philosophy and purpose,* Boston, 2003, Beth Israel Deaconess Medical Center.

Central Missouri State University, Department of Nursing: *Philosophy of nursing,* Warrensburg, MO, 2003, Central Missouri State University.

Eustis R: Parents: Son would have chosen death over blood, Online, 2002 *(www.rickross.com/reference/jw/jw90.html).*

Grube JW, Mayton DM, Ball-Rokeach SJ: Inducing change in values, attitudes, and behaviors: belief system theory, *J Soc Iss* 50(4):153-173, 1994.

Memorial Health Care System Department of Nursing: *Memorial Health Care System philosophy of nursing,* Chattanooga, TN, 2003, Memorial Health Care System.

Mohr WK: Values, ideologies, and dilemmas: professional and occupational contradictions, *J Psych Nurs* 33(1):29-34, 1995.

Palm Beach Atlantic University, School of Nursing: *Philosophy of nursing,* West Palm Beach, FL, 2003, Palm Beach Atlantic University.

Raths L, Harmin M, Simon S: *Values and teaching,* ed 2, Columbus, OH, 1978, Charles Merrill.

Rokeach M: *The nature of human values,* New York, 1973, Free Press.

University of North Florida, School of Nursing: *Philosophy of the School of Nursing,* Jacksonville, FL, 2003, University of North Florida.

Uustal DB: *Values and ethics in nursing: from theory to practice,* East Greenwich, RI, 1985, Educational Resources in Nursing and Wholistic Health.

Uustal DB: *Clinical ethics and values: issues and insights in a changing healthcare environment,* East Greenwich, RI, 1993, Educational Resources in Healthcare.

Uustal DB: *Caring for yourself, caring for others: the ultimate balance,* East Greenwich, RI, 1998, Educational Resources in Healthcare.

Major Concepts in Nursing

Kay Kittrell Chitty

Adaptation	Health Protection	Open System
Closed System	High-Level Wellness	Output
Culture	Holism	Person
Environment	Holistic Nursing Care	Self-Actualization
Evaluation	Homeostasis	Self-Efficacy
Extended Family	Human Needs Theory	Subsystems
Family System	Individualized Nursing Care	Suprasystem
Feedback	Input	Synergy
Health	Locus of Control	System
Health Behaviors	Abraham Maslow	Throughput
Health Beliefs Model	Nuclear Family	
Health Promotion	Nursing	

L e a r n i n g   O u t c o m e s

After studying this chapter, students will be able to:

- Summarize the concepts basic to professional nursing.
- Describe the components and processes of systems.
- Explain Maslow's hierarchy of human needs and its relationship to motivation.
- Recognize how environmental factors such as family, culture, social support, the Internet, and community influence health.
- Explain the significance of a holistic approach to nursing care.
- Apply Rosenstock's health beliefs model and Bandura's theory of perceived self-efficacy to personal health behaviors and health behaviors of others.
- Devise a personal plan for achieving high-level wellness.

There are certain basic concepts, or ideas, that are essential to an understanding of professional nursing practice; they are the building blocks of nursing. These concepts are person, environment, and health. Everything professional nurses do is in some way related to one of these basic interrelated concepts.

An overview of general systems theory will assist you in understanding how the concepts relate to each other and to nursing.

SYSTEMS

General systems theory was originally developed by Ludwig von Bertalanffy in 1936. von Bertalanffy, a biologist, believed that a common framework for studying several similar disciplines would allow scientists and scholars to organize and communicate findings and more readily build upon the work of others. He described a **system** as a set of interrelated parts that come together to form a whole that performs a function. Each part is a necessary or integral component required to make a complete, meaningful whole. These parts are input, throughput, output, evaluation, and feedback.

Components of Systems

The first component of a system is **input,** which is the raw material, such as information, energy, or matter, that enters a system and is transformed by it. For a system to work well, input should contribute to achieving the purpose of the system.

A second component of a system is **throughput.** Throughput consists of the processes a system uses to convert raw materials into a form that can be used, either by the system itself or by the environment or **suprasystem. Output** is the end result or product of the system. Outputs vary widely, depending on the type and purpose of the system.

Evaluation is the fourth component of a system. Evaluation means measuring the success or failure of the output and consequently the effectiveness of the system. For evaluation to be meaningful in any system, outcome criteria, against which performance or product quality is measured, must be identified.

The process of communicating what is found in evaluation of the system is called *feedback,* the final component of a system. **Feedback** is the information given back into the system to determine whether or not the purpose, or end result, of the system has been achieved. Figure 10-1 depicts the components of systems and how they relate to one another.

Examples of Systems

It may be helpful to use a familiar example to clarify the components of systems. In a college system, *input* consists of students, faculty, ideas, the desire to learn, and knowledge. Because the purpose of the system is to educate, the students need to be ready to learn, and the faculty should be prepared to teach. The processes *(throughput)* whereby ideas, knowledge, and skills are transmitted must be clear and understandable. The *output,* or product, of the system is educated graduates. For *evaluation* of the output, a standardized examination of reading comprehension, mathematics, and analytical skills may be used. Student scores on the comprehensive examination provide *feedback* to the faculty and administrators. If students score well, the system has achieved its purpose. If not, changes need to be made in the input or in the system itself—for example, admitting brighter students, hiring more talented faculty, or designing more effective courses and curricula.

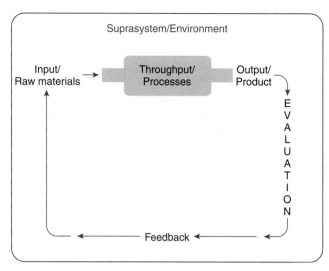

Figure **10-1**
Major components of a general systems model.

Systems are usually complex and consist of several parts called **subsystems.** Let us examine a hospital as a system. Technically, it is a system for providing health care, but the success of the system depends on the functioning of many subsystems. The subsystems include the laboratory, radiology, housekeeping, laundry, central supply, medical records, dietetics, nursing, pharmacy, and medical staffs. Each of these subsystems is a system itself. All the subsystems function collaboratively to make the health care system—the hospital—work.

Open and Closed Systems

Continuing with the example, the hospital and all its subsystems are open systems. An **open system** promotes the exchange of matter, energy, and information with other systems and the environment. The larger environment outside the hospital is called the *suprasystem*. A **closed system** does not interact with other systems or with the surrounding environment. Matter, energy, and information do not flow into or out of a closed system. There are few totally closed systems. Even a completely balanced aquarium, for example, often thought of as approaching a closed system, needs light and additional water and nutrients from time to time.

Two more points are essential to a beginning understanding of systems. First, the whole is different from and greater than the sum of its parts. Stated another way, the system is different from and greater than the sum of its subsystems. Anyone who has ever been in a hospital, for example, knows that what happens there is different from and more than the sum of the following equation: laundry + pharmacy + nurses + physicians = hospital. The second point involves synergy. **Synergy** occurs when all the various subsystems and the people who compose them collaborate to work with patients and their families.

Dynamic Nature of Systems

The final point to be made about systems is that change in one part of the system creates change in other parts. If the hospital admissions office, for example, decides to admit patients only between the hours of 8:00 AM and 10:00 AM, that decision creates changes in the nursing units, housekeeping, the business office, surgery, the laboratory, and other hospital subsystems. If that change were implemented without prior communication to the other subsystems and coordinated planning, it could create chaos in the system.

The exchange of energy and information within open systems and between open systems and their suprasystems is continuous. The dynamic balance within and between the subsystems, the system, and the suprasystems helps create and maintain **homeostasis**, or internal stability.

All living systems are open systems. The internal environment is in constant interaction with a changing environment external to the organism. As change occurs in one, the other is affected. For example, walking into a cold room (change in the external environment) affects a variety of physiological and psychological subsystems of the person's internal environment. These, in turn, affect a person's blood flow, ability to concentrate, feeling of comfort, and so on (changes in internal environment).

Application of the systems model to nursing

Why is it necessary for nurses to understand systems? Nurses work within systems every day. Using the hospital example, nurses work within the nursing department's system, a particular unit's system, and with a team system, among others. All three are open systems interacting with one another and the environment. If nurses are to work effectively in such complex systems, they need to have an understanding of how systems operate.

At the individual patient level, the openness of human systems makes nursing intervention possible. Understanding systems helps nurses assess relationships among all the factors that affect patients, including the influence of nurses themselves. Nurses who understand systems view patients holistically, including the subsystems (respiratory system, gastrointestinal system, and so on) and suprasystem (family, culture, and community). These nurses appreciate the influence of change in any part of the system. For instance, when a diabetic patient has pneumonia (change in subsystem), the infection increases the blood sugar and may result in hospitalization. Hospitalization may in turn adversely affect the patient's role in the family and community (change in suprasystem). Key concepts of systems are summarized in Box 10-1, and an excellent review of general systems theory and its relationship to nursing can be found online (*www.bsn-gn.eku.edu/BEGLEY/GSThand1.htm*). With this brief introduction to systems as a foundation, we can now examine the three basic concepts that are fundamental to the practice of professional nursing.

PERSON

The term **person** is used to describe each individual man, woman, or child. There are a number of different approaches to the study of person. This chapter briefly examines the concept of people as systems with human needs.

Box **10-1** Key Concepts About Systems

- A system is a set of interrelated parts.
- The parts form a meaningful whole.
- The whole is different from and greater than the sum of its parts.
- Systems may be open or closed.
- All living systems are open systems.
- Systems strive for homeostasis (internal stability).
- Systems are part of suprasystems.
- Systems have subsystems.

As mentioned previously, each individual is an open system with numerous subsystems that make up the whole person. For example, there are circulatory, musculoskeletal, respiratory, gastrointestinal, genitourinary, and neurological subsystems that compose the physiological subsystem. There are also psychological, social, cultural, and spiritual subsystems that combine with the physiological subsystem to make up the whole person. Each person is unique and different from all other persons. This uniqueness is determined both genetically and environmentally and is the basis for **holistic nursing care**—that is, nursing care that takes all the aspects of the person into consideration.

Certain personal characteristics are determined before birth by the genes received from one's parents. Genetically determined characteristics include eye, skin, and hair color; height; gender; and a variety of other features. Other characteristics about persons are determined by the environment. The availability of loving parents or parent substitutes, availability of nutritious foods, cultural beliefs, degree of educational opportunities, adequacy of housing, quality and quantity of parental supervision, and safety are all examples of environmental factors that influence how a person develops.

Human Needs

In addition to having personal characteristics, people have needs. A human need is a requirement for the person's well-being. In 1954, psychologist **Abraham Maslow** published *Motivation and Personality*. In this classic book, Maslow rejected earlier ideas of Freud, who believed that people are motivated by unconscious instincts, and Pavlov, who believed humans were driven by conditioned reflexes. Instead, Maslow presented his **human needs theory** and explained that human behavior is motivated by intrinsic human needs. He identified five levels of needs and organized them into a hierarchical order, as shown in Figure 10-2.

Basic needs

The most basic level of needs consists of those necessary for physiological survival: food, oxygen, rest, activity, shelter, and sexual expression. These are needs all human beings, regardless of location or culture, have in common.

Maslow identified the second level of needs as safety and security. These include physical as well as psychological safety and security needs. Psychological safety

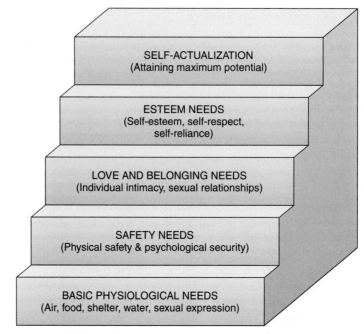

Figure 10-2
Maslow's hierarchy of needs.

and security include having a fairly predictable environment with which one has some familiarity and relative freedom from fear and chaos.

The third level of needs consists of love and belonging. To a greater or lesser extent, each person needs close, intimate relationships, social relationships, a place in the social structure, and group affiliations.

Next in Maslow's hierarchy is the need for self-esteem. This includes the need to feel self-worth, self-respect, and self-reliance.

Maslow called the highest level of needs **self-actualization.** Self-actualized people have realized their maximum potential; they use their capabilities to the fullest extent possible and are true to their own nature. People do not stay in a state of self-actualization but may have "peak experiences" during which they realize self-actualization for some period of time. Maslow believed that many people strive for self-actualization, but few consistently reach that level (Maslow, 1987).

Assumptions about needs

Maslow's hierarchy rests on several basic assumptions about human needs. One assumption is that basic needs must be at least partially satisfied before higher-order needs can become relevant to the individual. For example, a starving person can hardly be concerned with self-esteem until a life-sustaining level of nutrition is established.

A second assumption about human needs is that individuals meet their needs in different ways. One person may need 8 or 9 hours of sleep to feel rested, whereas another may require only 5 or 6 hours. Each individual's sleep needs may vary at different stages of life. Older people usually require less sleep than younger people. Individuals also eat different diets in differing quantities and at differing intervals. Some prefer to eat only twice a day, whereas others may snack six or eight times a day to meet their nutritional needs. Sexual energy also varies widely from person to person. The frequency with which normal adults desire sexual activity is determined by a broad range of individual factors.

Even though sleep, food, and sex are considered examples of basic human needs, the manner in which these needs are met, as well as the extent to which any one of them is considered a need, varies according to each individual. It is therefore extremely important to determine a person's perceptions of his or her own needs to be able to provide appropriate, individualized nursing care. If a patient is uncomfortable eating three large meals, such as those served in most hospitals, nurses can help that person by saving parts of the large meals in the refrigerator on the nursing unit and serving them to the patient between regularly scheduled meals. This is a simple example of what is meant by the term **individualized nursing care,** which recognizes each individual's unique needs and tailors the plan of nursing care to take that uniqueness into consideration.

Adaptation and human needs

Another aspect of human needs that must be considered is the nature of people to change, grow, and develop. Carl Rogers, a well-known psychologist, built a theory of personhood based on the idea that people are constantly adapting, discovering, and rediscovering themselves. His book *On Becoming a Person* (1961) is considered a classic in psychological literature. Rogers's idea that a person's needs change as the person changes is important for nurses to remember. Nurses can tap into the human potential to grow and develop to assist patients to change unhealthy behaviors and to reach the highest level of wellness possible.

The concept of **adaptation** is also helpful in understanding that people admitted to hospitals and removed from their customary, familiar environments frequently become anxious. Even the most confident person can become fearful when in an uncertain, perhaps threatening, situation. Under these circumstances, nurses have learned to expect people to regress slightly and to become more concerned with basic needs and less focused on the higher needs in Maslow's hierarchy. A "take-charge" professional person, for example, may become somewhat demanding and self-absorbed when hospitalized. As you will see in Chapter 11, several nursing theorists based their models on adaptation.

Homeostasis

When a person's needs are not met, homeostasis is threatened. Remember that homeostasis is a dynamic balance achieved by effectively functioning open systems. It is a state of equilibrium, a tendency to maintain internal stability. In humans, homeostasis is attained by coordinated responses of organ systems that automatically compensate for environmental changes. When someone goes for a brisk walk, for example, heartbeat and respiratory rates automatically increase to keep vital organs supplied with oxygen. When the individual comes home and sits down to read the newspaper, heart rate and breathing slow down. No conscious decision to speed up or slow down these physiological functions has to be made. Adjustments occur automatically to maintain homeostasis.

Individuals, as open systems, also endeavor to maintain balance between external and internal forces. When that balance is achieved, the person is healthy, or at least is resistant to disease. When environmental factors affect the homeostasis of a person, the person attempts to adapt to the change. If adaptation is unsuccessful, disequilibrium may occur, setting the stage for the development of illness or disease. How individuals respond to stress is a major factor in the development of illness. Stress and illness are discussed more fully in Chapter 17.

ENVIRONMENT/SUPRASYSTEM

The second major concept basic to professional nursing practice is environment, or the suprasystem. **Environment** includes all the circumstances, influences, and conditions that surround and affect individuals, families, and groups. The environment can be as small and controlled as a premature infant's isolette or as large and uncontrollable as the universe. Included in environment are the social and cultural attitudes that profoundly shape human experience.

The environment can either promote or interfere with homeostasis and well-being of individuals. As seen in Maslow's hierarchy of needs, there is a dynamic interaction between a person's needs, which are internal, and the satisfaction of those needs, which is often environmentally determined.

Nurses have always been aware of the influence of environment on people, beginning with Florence Nightingale, who understood well the elements of a healthful environment in which restoration and preservation of health and prevention of disease and injury were possible. Concerns about the health of the public have led governmental entities at local, state, and national levels to promulgate standards and regulations that assure citizens of the safety of their food, water, air, cosmetics, medications, workplaces, and other areas in which health hazards may occur. Environmental systems to be discussed in this section are family systems, cultural systems, social systems, and community systems.

Family Systems

The most direct environmental influence on a person is the family. The quality and amount of parenting provided to infants and growing children constitute a major determinant of health. We call this the **family system.** Children who are nurtured when young and vulnerable, who are allowed to grow in independence and self-determination, and who are taught the skills they need for social living are likely to grow into strong, productive, autonomous adults.

Factors influencing nuclear and extended families

For most of the history of humankind, immediate and extended families were relatively intact units that lived together or lived within close proximity to one another. In the **extended family,** children were nurtured by a variety of relatives, as well as by their own parents. This closeness was profoundly affected by industrialization, which fostered urbanization. When families ceased farming, which was a family endeavor, and moved to cities where fathers worked in factories, the first dilution of family influence on children began. The **nuclear family** (mother and father and their children) moved away from former sources of nurturing, as older relatives such as grandparents, aunts, and uncles, often stayed in rural areas.

During World War II, more women began to work, taking them out of the home and away from young children for hours each day. The increased geographic mobility of families since World War II has also had a destructive effect on the role of extended family in the lives of children, as nuclear families often live half a continent or more away from grandparents and other family members. The intense attention children traditionally received from adult relatives diminished, sometimes to the detriment of the child's well-being.

Factors influencing single-parent families

Today, there are more single-parent families in the United States than ever before, most of which are headed by women. As of 2000, U.S. Census data revealed that there were over 7 million single women heading households with children under 18 and no father present. In addition to single mothers, there were also 2.2 million single custodial fathers in the United States in 2000 (U.S. Census Bureau, 2000a). The average number of people per unmarried partner household was 5.2.

In 1997, the latest year for which figures are available, only 67 percent of the single custodial parents were receiving full or partial child support due from absent parents, with yearly support averaging $3,600 (U.S. Census Bureau, 2000b). These figures were only slightly improved from 1991 when Louis Sullivan, former secretary of the Department of Health and Human Services, stated, "Many of this country's societal problems can be traced back to parents not supporting their children" (Half of Single Moms, 1991).

In 2002, more than 16 percent of children under the age of 18 were living below the poverty level (U.S. Census Bureau, 2003). Lack of money often means adequate nutrition and health care are not attainable, adversely affecting the health status of all family members. Life is challenging for single parents of both sexes who must perform traditional breadwinner roles as well as traditional nurturing roles in the family. The combination of bearing multiple roles alone over long periods of time can be extremely stressful, even exhausting, to single parents.

Long-term stress affects the mental and physical health of these adults, which, in turn, affects their parenting abilities. Although many single parents manage stress well and are able to provide excellent parenting, some children's needs are neglected. The impact of this neglect can be seen in the behavior and school performance of children who have not learned the skills they need to be successful. With 26 percent of all children in the United States being born to unmarried women (U.S. Census Bureau, 1998), the trend to single parent households is likely to continue.

The examples given here represent only a few of the ways families influence the well-being of individuals. There are many others. Understanding a patient's family and home environment is part of a complete nursing assessment. Modification of the home environment may be needed, particularly when a person is returning home with a physical disability, or where there is neglect or abuse.

Nurses, social workers, and others involved in discharge planning must collaborate to ensure that needed changes occur before patients return to homes and families.

Cultural Systems

Culture is an extremely important environmental influence affecting individuals. **Culture** consists of the attitudes, beliefs, and behaviors of social and ethnic groups that have been perpetuated through generations. Patterns of language, dress, eating habits, activities of daily living, attitudes toward those outside the culture, health beliefs and values, spiritual beliefs or religious orientation, and attitudes toward children, women, men, marriage, education, work, and recreation all are influenced by culture.

According to U.S. Census Bureau estimates, there were 28.4 million foreign-born Americans in 2000, a dramatic increase from under 20 million only 8 years earlier (U.S. Census Bureau, 2001). As mentioned in Chapter 3, the United States is fast becoming the first truly multicultural society. Because basic beliefs about health and illness vary widely from culture to culture, nurses need to develop cultural competence to meet the needs of culturally diverse patients. For example, "A traditional Vietnamese folk remedy, ventouse …, involves placing a heated cup on the skin. It's believed that as the cup cools, it draws away excess energy or 'wind' causing the illness" (Grossman, 1994, p. 58). This practice can cause bruising, which can be mistaken for a sign of abuse. This is just one indication that cultural beliefs of patients have great relevance to nurses. Most cultural differences are more subtle than this and can escape the notice of nurses who have not developed cultural competence.

Effective nurses learn to be aware of and to respect cultural influences on patients. Whenever possible, they pay attention to patients' cultural preferences. They recognize that some cultural groups attribute illness to bad fortune. Individuals from cultures with these beliefs do not see themselves as active participants in their own health status. This attitude is a challenge for nurses who value the collaboration of patients in their own health care planning.

These are only two examples of the influence of cultural beliefs on the nurse-patient interaction. Wise nurses realize that integration of a patient's cultural health beliefs into the individualized treatment plan can make a strong impact on that patient's desire and ability to get well.

Understanding the relationship between culture and health is the basis for "transcultural nursing," a field of nursing practice initiated by nurse-anthropologist Madeline Leininger. Additional discussion of the influence of culture is included in Chapter 17.

Social Systems

In addition to family and cultural systems, individuals are also influenced by the social system in which they live. Social institutions such as families, neighborhoods, schools, churches, professional associations, civic groups, and recreational groups may constitute a form of social support. Social support also includes such factors as presence in the home of a spouse; proximity to neighbors, children, and other supportive individuals; access to medical care; coping abilities; educational level; and so on.

Holmes and Rahe (1967) published a study of the relationship of social change to the subsequent development of illness. People with many social changes that disrupt social support, such as death of a loved one, divorce, job changes, moving, or unemployment, were much more likely to experience illness in the following 12 months than people with few social changes. Both positive and negative changes created the need for social readjustment. In 1995 this study was updated, and the Recent Life Changes Questionnaire (Box 10-2) was devised to reflect more accurately contemporary concerns (Miller and Rahe, 1997). Numerous other researchers have found additional evidence that social support has a direct relationship to health.

Box **10-2** **Recent Life Changes Questionnaire**

The following 74 potential life changes inquire about recent events in a person's life. A 6-month total equal to or greater than 300 LCU, or a 1-year total equal to or greater than 500 LCU, is considered indicative of high recent life stress.

Life Change Event	Life Change Units
Health	
An injury or illness which:	
kept you in bed a week or more or sent you to the hospital	74
was less serious than above	44
Major dental work	26
Major change in eating habits	27
Major change in sleeping habits	26
Major change in your usual type and/or amount of recreation	28
Work	
Change to a new type of work	51
Change in your work hours or conditions	35
Change in your responsibilities at work:	
more responsibilities	29
fewer responsibilities	21
promotion	31
demotion	42
transfer	32
Troubles at work:	
with your boss	29
with coworkers	35
with persons under your supervision	35
other work troubles	28
Major business adjustment	60
Retirement	52
Loss of job:	
laid off from work	68
fired from work	79
Correspondence course to help you in your work	18

Continued

Box **10-2** Recent Life Changes Questionnaire—cont'd

Life Change Event	Life Change Units
Home and family	
Major change in living conditions	42
Change in residence:	
move within the same town or city	25
move to a different town, city, or state	47
Change in family get-togethers	25
Major change in health or behavior of family member	55
Marriage	50
Pregnancy	67
Miscarriage or abortion	65
Gain of a new family member:	
birth of a child	66
adoption of a child	65
a relative moving in with you	59
Spouse beginning or ending work	46
Child leaving home:	
to attend college	41
due to marriage	41
for other reason	45
Change in arguments with spouse	50
In-law problems	38
Change in the marital status of your parents:	
divorce	59
remarriage	50
Separation from spouse:	
due to work	53
due to marital problems	76
Divorce	96
Birth of grandchild	43
Death of spouse	119
Death of the family member:	
child	123
brother or sister	102
parent	100
Personal and social	
Change in personal habits	26
Beginning or ending school or college	38
Change of school or college	35
Change in political beliefs	24
Change in religious beliefs	29
Change in social activities	27

Box **10-2** **Recent Life Changes Questionnaire—cont'd**

Vacation	24
New, close, personal relationship	37
Engagement to marry	45
Girlfriend or boyfriend problems	39
Sexual difficulties	44
"Falling out" of a close personal relationship	47
An accident	48
Minor violation of the law	20
Being held in jail	75
Death of a close friend	70
Major decision regarding your immediate future	51
Major personal achievement	36
Financial	
Major change in finances:	
increased income	38
decreased income	60
investment and/or credit difficulties	56
Loss or damage of personal property	43
Moderate purchase	20
Major purchase	37
Foreclosure on a mortgage or loan	58

Miller MA, Rahe RH: Life changes scaling for the 1990s, *J Psychosomat Res* 43(3):279-292, 1997. Reprinted with permission.

In assessing patients, nurses need to remember that the adequacy of social support is determined by the patient, not the nurse. Individuals vary in their need and desire for social support. When it is determined that strengthening social support is desirable, nurses can encourage patients to use interest groups, parenting classes, marriage enrichment groups, religious groups, formal and informal educational groups, and self-help groups to develop stronger support from the social environment.

Increasingly, people receive support online—in chat rooms and through other computer-based forums. People with new insulin pumps, for example, can "talk" online with over 700 others who have similar pumps, ask questions, and get helpful tips to assist them. There are literally hundreds of online support groups, ranging from those for Alzheimer's caregivers to weight loss groups.

Community, National, and World Systems

The health status of people is also influenced by the larger systems in which they live. The types and availability of jobs, housing, schools, and health care, as well as the overall economic well-being, profoundly affect the citizens in a community. Although nurses may not think they have an obvious role, they can be instrumental in improving the community systems. Identifying health needs and bringing these to the attention of community planners, offering screening programs, serving on health-related committees and advisory boards, and lobbying political leaders can bring about positive change in a community. Nurses have also become politically active by running for elected offices at local, state, and national levels. They can energetically support political candidates who have sound environmental platforms. More information about political activism in nursing is provided in Chapter 21.

On a broader perspective, environment also includes the nation, the world, and the universe. A seemingly isolated incident such as an earthquake in Turkey may have worldwide health repercussions as disease epidemics occur in its aftermath. Although nothing can be done to prevent natural disasters, nurses can contribute to a healthier world environment by promoting or participating in humanitarian responses to international disasters.

Nurses' potential impact on the environment/suprasystem

Individual nurses, in the interest of world health, may choose to engage in a variety of environmentally sound practices in their personal lives and encourage others to do the same. These include recycling of household trash and hazardous materials such as batteries and paint, using pump rather than aerosol sprayers, avoiding insecticides and unnecessary use of gardening chemicals, buying energy-efficient appliances and automobiles, walking when possible instead of driving, and refusing to buy from or invest in companies that engage in environmentally unsound practices such as polluting air and water.

Professionally, nurses need to be aware that hospitals are among the highest producers of waste, including biohazardous waste. For example, hospitals are a major source of mercury pollution. This highly toxic substance, used in thermometers, blood pressure measuring devices, and other medical devices, ultimately flows into the environment, where it contaminates water. It then is concentrated in the bodies of predator fish such as tuna and swordfish, which are eventually consumed by humans. Mercury, even in small doses, poses serious health risks to pregnant women and young children. Nurses can be instrumental in encouraging their employers to avoid purchasing and using mercury-containing devices and to dispose of them properly when they are discarded.

In an effort to reduce environmental pollution, some health care facilities have committees dedicated to identifying and recommending environmentally sound products. Nurses can volunteer to serve on these committees or recommend the purchase of fewer disposable products and products with wasteful packaging. The accompanying News Note discusses the initiatives of a health-related group, Health Care Without Harm, to reduce hazardous waste emanating from health care facilities.

HEALTH

Health is the third major concept fundamental to the practice of professional nursing. Health is best viewed as a continuum rather than as an absolute state. Each individual's health status varies from day to day, depending on a variety of factors, such as rest, nutrition, and stressors. Illness is also not an absolute state. People can have chronic illnesses such as diabetes or seizure disorders and still work, take part in

news
   note

Study Shows Mercury in Tuna Threatens Developing Babies and Young Children: Hospitals Will Reduce Threat by Eliminating Mercury from Health Care

According to a report released today, some of the most commonly eaten fish contain levels of mercury that pose a risk to pregnant women and young children. In response to the problem of mercury pollution, health care providers such as Kaiser Permanente; Dartmouth-Hitchcock Medical Center in Lebanon, New Hampshire; and New York's Beth Israel Medical Centers are creating model programs for mercury elimination. By phasing out the purchase and use of mercury-containing products and devices, hospitals will eventually decrease the amount of mercury moving up the food chain until it reaches its highest concentrations in top predator fish such as tuna, swordfish, and shark.

These findings are included in the report *Protecting by Degrees,* written by the Environmental Working Group for Health Care Without Harm, a coalition of more than 170 groups dedicated to environmentally responsible health care.

Test results reported in *Protecting by Degrees* are consistent with studies done by the U.S. Food and Drug Administration (FDA) in 1993. In both instances, chunk light tuna contained levels of mercury that create serious health risks:

- A 140-pound pregnant woman risks subtle but permanent brain damage to her fetus by eating less than half of a 6-ounce can of tuna per day.
- An average 4-year-old exceeds the EPA's "safe" dose if he or she eats one 6-ounce can per week.

"Tuna fish has too much mercury to be eaten regularly by pregnant women and young children. But that's not the fault of the tuna or the people who caught or canned it," explained Charlotte Brody, RN, co-coordinator of Health Care Without Harm. "Industries that use mercury and the governments that regulate them must take responsibility for getting mercury out of our fish and out of our children's developing brains."

"Health care groups like Kaiser Permanente, Dartmouth-Hitchcock, and New York's Beth Israel Medical Center are leaders in developing a cure for the mercury problem," said Todd Hettenbach, EWG policy analyst and primary author of the report. "These hospitals are voluntarily eliminating mercury because of the threat to public health and showing other health care providers and other industries that it can be done."

Safe, cost-comparable alternatives exist for most of the mercury use in hospitals. Thermometers and blood pressure–measuring devices are two of the most commonly used mercury-containing devices. A mercury fever thermometer, such as the kind used in the home, contains enough mercury to potentially contaminate 9,000 cans of tuna fish. A desk-mounted sphygmomanometer (used for measuring blood pressure) contains enough mercury to potentially contaminate 492,000 6-ounce cans of chunk light tuna.

Continued

news note—cont'd

"As we learned with mercury instruments, some of the weapons we use to fight disease can also be weapons that compromise a healthy environment," said David Lawrence, MD, chairman and chief executive officer of Kaiser Foundation Health Plan and Kaiser Foundation Hospitals. "We need to address the long-term consequences of treatment options and challenge ourselves to devise effective alternatives that do less environmental harm."

Health Care Without Harm is an international campaign made up of health care professionals, hospitals, environmental advocates, organizations of health-impacted individuals, religious organizations, and labor unions. The campaign's mission is to transform the health care industry so it is no longer a source of environmental harm by eliminating the pollution in health care practices without compromising safety or care. The Environmental Working Group, a member organization of Health Care Without Harm, is an environmental research organization based in Washington, D. C.

HCWH press release issued Thursday, May 6, 1999. Available online *(www.noharm.org)*.

recreational activities, and maintain acceptably healthy lives. Figure 10-3 depicts the health-illness continuum.

Defining Health

There are numerous definitions of health. The World Health Organization (WHO) defined health as "a state of complete physical, mental, and social well-being and not merely the absence of disease or infirmity" (1947, p. 29). This definition was the first modern recognition of health as multidimensional. The WHO definition presented a holistic view of health that reflected the interplay between the psychological, social, spiritual, and physical aspects of human life.

A holistic view of health focuses on the interrelationship of all the parts that make up a whole person. Jan Christian Smuts (1926) first introduced the concept of **holism** in modern Western thought by emphasizing the harmony between people

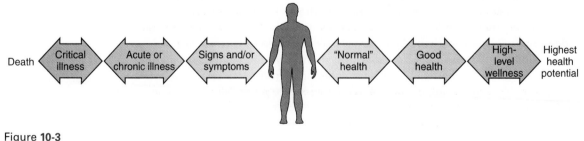

Figure **10-3**
The health-illness continuum—a holistic health model.

and nature. When viewing health holistically, individual health practices must be taken into account. Health practices are culturally determined and include nutritional habits, type and amount of exercise and rest, how one copes with stress, quality of interpersonal relationships, expression of spirituality, and numerous other lifestyle factors. As a profession, nurses value a holistic view of health.

Parsons (1959) defined health as "the state of optimum capacity of an individual for the effective performance of his roles and tasks." This definition focused on the roles individuals assume in life and the impact health or illness has on the fulfillment of those roles. A few examples of roles that are familiar may include the student role, the parent role, the breadwinner role, and the friend role. Given the activities inherent in each of these roles, it is easily seen that the state of health profoundly influences how people carry out their roles in life.

Yet another description of health is the opposite of illness (Dunn, 1959). Dunn, in his classic text, *High Level Wellness* (1961), described health as a continuum with high-level wellness at one end and death at the other. He described **high-level wellness** as functioning at maximum potential in an integrated way within the environment. A prisoner of war kept in solitary confinement and given a diet of rice for many months certainly would have difficulty maintaining health. If he keeps active, both physically and mentally, and retains a positive outlook, however, he is likely to be healthier than the prisoner who does none of these things. Using Dunn's definition and taking his environment into consideration, the prisoner may even be said to have attained high-level wellness.

Nurse-theorist Nola Pender (1987) described health promotion as "approach behavior," whereas prevention is "avoidance behavior" (p. 5). This may be a useful concept for nurses to keep in mind when seeking to help patients expand their positive potential for health.

A National Health Initiative: *Healthy People 2000/2010*

A remarkable national initiative to improve the health of the nation is now entering its third decade. The *Healthy People* initiative was an unprecedented cooperative effort that grew out of the 1979 Surgeon General's Report on health promotion and disease prevention entitled *Healthy People*. That report laid the foundation for a national prevention agenda. Federal, state, and territorial governments as well as hundreds of private, public, and nonprofit organizations and concerned individuals worked together for the first time ever. These partnerships resulted in *Healthy People 2000*, an effort designed to stimulate a national disease prevention and health promotion agenda to improve significantly the health of all Americans in the last decade of the twentieth century. On September 6, 1990, former U.S. Secretary of Health and Human Services Louis W. Sullivan released a report to the United States entitled *Healthy People 2000*.

Goals of *Healthy People 2000*

Three broad goals for health of the public in the 1990s were identified by *Healthy People 2000* (U.S. Department of Health and Human Services, 1990, p. 1):

1. Increase the span of healthy life for Americans.
2. Reduce health disparities among Americans.
3. Achieve access to preventive services for all Americans.

To meet these goals, 300 measurable objectives were identified in 22 different priority areas under the broad categories of health promotion, health protection, and preventive services. The report challenged American citizens, organizations, and communities to change behaviors and environments to support good health for all. United States public health agencies were charged with the responsibility for overseeing the initiatives in each of the 22 priority areas.

The hope of those involved in preparing this plan was that it would stimulate sustained support from a diverse base of individuals, groups, communities, associations, and governmental agencies to improve health outcomes. Particular emphasis was placed on improving access to health care by the poor, minorities, and rural populations, all of whom have borne "a disproportionate burden of suffering compared to the total population" (p. 1).

Tracking progress toward *Healthy People 2000* goals: 1995 report
Although the *Healthy People 2000* initiative stimulated much discussion and activity among those concerned about health, as of 1995, progress with respect to the health of U.S. citizens was mixed. According to McGinnis and Lee (1995), a preliminary examination of trends showed mixed results. In the area of **health promotion,** 10 of the 17 priority areas were:

> proceeding in the right direction, four are proceeding in the wrong direction, one is without change, and two have no data available on which to make comments. Particularly good progress continued for reductions in adult use of tobacco products and in alcohol-related automobile deaths. Positive but less striking gains are recorded for the proportion of adults exercising regularly, eating less fatty diets, and reporting stress-related problems (pp. 1124-1125).

Some of the gains achieved were attributed to the fact that more workplaces had health promotion programs for their workers. On the downside, the number of people with sedentary lifestyles was unchanged and a higher proportion of the population was overweight in 1995 than in 1990. The trends for youth were also mixed, with improvements in tobacco, alcohol, and marijuana use but alarming increases in the areas of homicides, other violence, and pregnancies.

Reporting on the 10 *Healthy People 2000* priorities in the area of **health protection,** McGinnis and Lee reported that 8 of the 10 were:

> proceeding in the right direction, while one is progressing in the wrong direction and one has insufficient data available on which to base a conclusion. There were fewer motor vehicle deaths, owing to reductions in drunk driving, increased use of child safety devices, increased seat belt use, speed limit enforcement, and the introduction of air bags in new cars. Air quality had improved, and reductions were noted in blood lead levels in children. Indoor air quality remained a challenge, as did the incidence of work-related injuries. Food safety had improved. Fewer old people had complete tooth loss, although children's oral health was not documented (pp. 1125-1126).

The mid-decade report also pointed out progress in reducing cholesterol levels and controlling hypertension, reductions in coronary heart disease and stroke deaths, and increasing use of recommended cancer screening services. Prenatal care during the first trimester had also improved, as had the number of children receiving childhood immunizations. Problems remained, however, for vulnerable populations, such as ethnic minorities and the chronically ill. As a result of the mixed progress, a number of midcourse corrections were recommended (McGinnis and Lee, 1995).

Tracking progress toward *Healthy People 2000* goals: 1999 report

By 1999, U.S. Secretary of Health and Human Services Donna Shalala issued a more encouraging report. She reported that 15 percent of the objectives had met their targets. "As the century draws to a close, we can be proud that we have made significant strides in improving the health of Americans. *Healthy People 2000* lets us measure the overall progress we have achieved in preventing disease and promoting health during this decade," said Secretary Shalala (U.S. Department of Health and Human Services, 1999a).

Upon closer inspection, however, the report also showed that one fifth of the original objectives were moving away from their targets, particularly in the areas of reducing obesity and increasing physical activity. A related finding was that the incidence, prevalence, complications, and mortality from diabetes were all on the rise.

Infant mortality had declined throughout the 1990s, with the death rate for children between 1 and 14 years of age down by 26 percent, surpassing the objective. Severe childhood asthma, however, was rising and was a major cause of hospitalizations.

Death rates in young people ages 15 to 24 declined substantially and met the year 2000 target of 85 deaths per 100,000. Alcohol-related vehicular deaths and suicides were lower, whereas heavy drinking among high school and college students had increased.

Mortality was also down in the 25- to 64-year-old age-group and was close to the year 2000 target. Cancer deaths were below the target, with breast and colorectal cancer deaths both down. Lung cancer deaths continued to rise but at a slower rate.

Older Americans also showed improvements in life expectancy rates, reflecting the continuing decline in heart disease and stroke-related deaths. Suicide rates for elderly white males, considered a high-risk group, were lower, but deaths from falls and vehicular accidents increased (U.S. Department of Health and Human Services, 1999b).

Next steps: *Healthy People 2010*

The next phase of the project, called *Healthy People 2010,* was launched in January 2000. It was developed by the *Healthy People* Consortium, an alliance of more than 350 national membership organizations and 250 state health, mental health, substance abuse, and environmental agencies. In addition, more than 11,000 public comments on the draft document were provided through an interactive website. *Healthy People 2010* consists of a revised set of health objectives for the nation, with two overarching goals: to increase quality and years of healthy life and to eliminate health disparities. Under these two goals are 28 focus areas that provide more specific targets. To measure the health of the nation during the decade, 10 leading health indicators will be used. Each leading health indicator reflects an important health issue and has one or more of the 28 objectives linked with it. These indicators reflect the high-priority public health concerns in this country at the beginning of the twenty-first century. Box 10-3 contains the essential elements of *Healthy People 2010.*

Box 10-3 *Healthy People 2010* **at a Glance**

Healthy People 2010 is a comprehensive set of disease prevention and health promotion objectives for the nation to achieve over the first decade of the new century. Created by scientists both inside and outside of government, it identifies a wide range of public health priorities and specific, measurable objectives.

Overarching Goals
1. Increase quality and years of healthy life
2. Eliminate health disparities

Focus Areas
- Access to Quality Health Services
- Arthritis, Osteoporosis, and Chronic Back Conditions
- Cancer
- Chronic Kidney Disease
- Diabetes
- Disability and Secondary Conditions
- Educational and Community-Based Programs
- Environmental Health
- Family Planning
- Food Safety
- Health Communication
- Heart Disease and Stroke
- HIV
- Immunization and Infectious Diseases
- Injury and Violence Prevention
- Maternal, Infant, and Child Health
- Medical Product Safety
- Mental Health and Mental Disorders
- Nutrition and Overweight
- Occupational Safety and Health
- Oral Health
- Physical Activity and Fitness
- Public Health Infrastructure
- Respiratory Diseases
- Sexually Transmitted Diseases
- Substance Abuse
- Tobacco Use
- Vision and Hearing

Box **10-3** *Healthy People 2010* **at a Glance—cont'd**

Leading Health Indicators: Ten Major Health Issues for the Nation

- Physical Activity
- Overweight and Obesity
- Tobacco Use
- Substance Abuse
- Responsible Sexual Behavior
- Mental Health
- Injury and Violence
- Environmental Quality
- Immunization
- Access to Health Care

From U.S. Department of Health and Human Services: *Healthy People 2010:* fact sheet, Online, 2002 (*www.healthypeople.gov/About/hpfact.htm*).

Healthy People 2010 offers a simple but powerful idea: provide health objectives in a format that enables diverse groups to combine their efforts and work as a team. It is a road map to better health for all and can be used by many different people, states, communities, professional organizations, and groups to improve health. The initiative has partners from all sectors (U.S. Department of Health and Human Services, 2003).

Partners are encouraged to integrate *Healthy People* objectives into their programs, special events, publications, and meetings. An example is provided by the Division of Public Health Nursing of the Los Angeles County Health Department, which has shifted its focus from providing care for individuals within families to improving the health of entire communities. Nurses in this department integrated the *Healthy People 2010's* ten leading health indicators into their public health nursing practice model. This means that these nurses consider the leading health indicators as they assess and diagnose communities with which they work. This ensures consistency within the division and with national priorities (Smith and Bazine-Barakat, 2003)—a perfect example of how the *Healthy People* initiative can be implemented at the local level.

When federal, state, and local health entities combine their efforts, improvements in the health of citizens can be made. Convincing individual Americans to change their lifestyles, however, even when to do so would result in improved health, remains a challenge. As can be seen from this review of the *Healthy People* project over more than 20 years, changing health beliefs and health behaviors is a slow process. You can learn more about *Healthy People 2010* and check progress toward its goals online (*www.healthypeople.gov*).

Health Beliefs and Health Behaviors

Health is affected by health beliefs and **health behaviors.** Health behaviors include those choices and habitual actions that promote or diminish health, such as eating

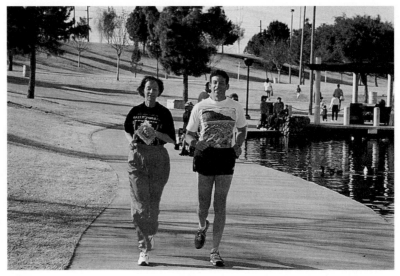

Figure 10-4
More Americans are engaging in health behaviors such as regular exercise; yet obesity is still on the rise.

habits, frequency of exercise, use of tobacco products and alcohol, sexual practices, and adequacy of rest and sleep (Figure 10-4). Much is known about health promoting behaviors, and this information is readily available to the public. Yet people do not readily change their behaviors. We will examine several theories about why people change their health behaviors—or why they do not.

Health beliefs model

Rosenstock (1966, 1990) was one of the first scholars interested in determining why some people change their health behaviors whereas others do not. For example, when the surgeon general's report on smoking first came out in 1960, some people immediately quit smoking. Over the years, evidence condemning smoking has accumulated and been widely communicated; yet many intelligent people still smoke. Rosenstock wondered why. He formulated a model of health beliefs that illustrates how people behave in relationship to health maintenance activities and has worked to refine it for three decades. Rosenstock's **health beliefs model** (HBM) included three components:

1. An evaluation of one's vulnerability to a condition and the seriousness of that condition.
2. An evaluation of how effective the health maintenance behavior might be.
3. The presence of a trigger event that precipitates the health maintenance behavior.

Using Rosenstock's model, a man chooses to participate in a stop-smoking program depending on his perception of smoking-related heart disease and his personal susceptibility to it. If, because of family history, he believes he is susceptible to heart disease and that it may cause his death prematurely and if he believes that not smoking will substantially reduce his risk, he is likely to participate in the program. If, however, the stop-smoking program is at an inconvenient location, scheduled at an inconvenient time, or not affordable, he is less likely to participate. If his sibling, who smokes, has a massive heart attack, he may be motivated to attend the stop-smoking program despite the inconvenience and cost. The illness of his sibling is what Rosenstock termed "a cue to action," or a trigger event. A trigger event propels a previously unmotivated individual into changing health behaviors.

Self-efficacy and health-related behaviors

Albert Bandura (1997), a cognitive psychologist, developed an approach designed to assist people to exercise influence over their own health-related behaviors. He observed that whether or not people considered altering detrimental health habits depended on their belief in themselves as having the ability to modify their own behavior. He called this belief in their own abilities perceived **self-efficacy.** High belief in one's self-efficacy leads to efforts to change, whereas low perceived self-efficacy leads to a fatalistic lack of change.

Bandura identified four components needed for an effective program of lifestyle change: information, skill development, skill enhancement through guided practice and feedback, and creating social supports for change (Bandura, 1992). Using Bandura's model, a man wishing to stop smoking needs knowledge of the potential dangers of smoking, guidance on how to translate concern into action, extensive practice and opportunities to perfect new, nonsmoking skills, and strong involvement in a social network supportive of nonsmoking.

Locus of control and health-related behaviors

The **locus of control** concept proposed that people tend to be influenced by either an internal or external view of control. People who believe that their health is internally controlled, that is, by what they themselves do, are said to have an internal locus of control. Those who believe their health is determined by outside factors or chance are said to have an external locus of control. A number of studies have hypothesized that internally controlled people tend to see themselves as responsible for their own health status and are therefore more amenable to change. Research findings have been inconsistent, however. Although health locus of control is a concept of general relevance to health, it requires continued attention in research aimed at better understanding behavior and health (Steptoe and Wardle, 2001).

Nurses and health beliefs models

There are numerous other models of health beliefs and health behavior ranging from simple to complex. Many are being tested through empirical studies in attempts to identify the key to motivating people to improve their health choices and behaviors. No single theory of behavior has yet fully explained the complex state called health. It is important for nurses to recognize that:

- Health is relative, ever changing, and affected by genetics, environment, personal beliefs, and cultural beliefs.
- Health affects the entire person—physically, socially, psychologically, and spiritually.

- Individuals' health beliefs are powerful and influence how they respond to efforts to change their health behaviors.
- Individuals needing or desiring change may lack knowledge, motivation, and support.
- Various models of health beliefs can be used to assess individual, family, and group readiness to change.
- The burden of action is mutually shared by patient, health care providers, and population-focused entities such as public health programs.

Influence of the Internet on Health

With more than half of adult Americans having online access, the Internet has had an impact on every aspect of life. People shop; make travel reservations; check out the latest music, movies, plays, and books; and meet potential spouses online. Is it any wonder, then, that they also seek information about health online? The World Wide Web, with its ready availability of information, ranging from the latest clinical trials and research studies to the most popular herbal remedies and diet fads, has changed the way we learn about health. Even former U.S. Surgeon General Dr. C. Everett Koop has his own website offering news and advice on a wide variety of health topics *(www.drkoop.com)*.

With the proliferation of health information sites, Americans are now armed with more information than has ever before been available to consumers. Patients are demanding to be equal partners in making health care decisions once decided only by the professionals they consulted. Health care practitioners encounter numerous patients each day who enter examining rooms with printouts of the latest research and advice, culled from the mountains of data available.

Support groups are available by the score. There is no need to dress, drive across town, or even leave the comforts of home to be in touch with dozens of people who share similar concerns or health problems. Cyberspace support groups have another advantage not shared by face-to-face groups: anonymity.

Some people are concerned about the validity of information available on the Internet (Chase, 1999). In fact, there is a lot of misinformation transmitted along with well-founded information from respected sources. The difficulty for the average citizen is telling the difference. Box 10-4 contains some helpful hints to improve the likelihood of obtaining valid health information from online sources.

Increased reliance on the World Wide Web for health information is expected to continue. This is understandable, since the Internet is readily available, day or night, whereas getting an appointment with a primary care provider can take days or weeks. Nurses have an obligation to adapt to this new influence on health by helping their patients obtain sound advice from online sources. Sharing legitimate websites and guidelines for assessing the quality of information are ways to help patients become better consumers of online health data. This means that nurses themselves must be knowledgeable and stay up to date on both helpful and unhelpful websites. Nurses also should be nondefensive when patients question traditional advice, citing the Internet as their source. Use these exchanges as opportunities to correct misinformation, if needed. Perhaps you will learn something new yourself. Visit Evolve for WebLinks related to the content of this chapter: **http://evolve.elsevier.com/Chitty/professional/.**

Box 10-4 Assessing Health-Related Sites on the World Wide Web

- Determine who sponsors the site. This should be disclosed on the site itself.
- Be skeptical. Evaluate the source to determine whether there is self-interest on the part of the sponsor.
- Make sure the author's name is clearly indicated, including credentials. Is the author qualified on this topic? Who does the author work for?
- What is the purpose of the site—to inform or to sell something?
- Is the material dated and revised frequently to ensure it is current?
- Is there editorial review of the content by a reputable authority or professional peers?
- Does the material consist of scientific information rather than testimonials?
- Determine who runs the website. University, government, and reputable medical organization sites may prove objective and less commercial than those run by companies or individuals wishing to profit.
- Is the information unbiased, and are you referred to other sources that can validate it?
- For chat rooms, go online and "lurk" before getting involved. Monitor conversations or read postings before deciding whether you want to participate.
- Find out whether the group has a moderator who can control monopolizers, commercial pitches, and inappropriate behavior by other participants.
- For interactive sites, be sure to read and understand the privacy policy.
- Until you are confident about the quality of information, cross-check it with print and electronic sources and discuss it with your health care provider.
- Use the Department of Health and Human Services' *Healthfinder* site to find online support groups *(www.healthfinder.gov)*.
- Be highly suspicious of reports of "miracle" cures. Rumors and unsupported claims are rampant on the Internet and cause untold harm. Use *Quackwatch* to check out claims that sound too good to be true *(www.quackwatch.com)*.

From Chase M: Health journal: a guide for patients who turn to the Web for solace and support, *Wall Street Journal* September 17, 1999, B1; Beyea SC: Evaluating evidence found on the Internet, *AORN J* 72(5):906-910, 2000; and Ahmann E: Supporting families' savvy use of the Internet for health research, *Pediatr Nurs* 26(4):419-423, 2000.

Devising a Personal Plan for High-Level Wellness

Each individual nurse has a personal definition of health, certain health beliefs, and individual health behaviors. How nurses view health behaviors in their own lives affects nursing practice, both directly and indirectly. The personal health practices of nurses play a direct role in their effectiveness in counseling patients on health-related matters. Patients are more likely to adopt health-related behaviors when the nurse promoting them also engages in them. Yet nurses' own health behaviors are far from exemplary. Studies have shown that in spite of nurses' knowledge, no difference exists between the health behaviors of nurses and those of the general population (Pratt, Overfield, Gill-Helton, 1994).

Nurses have a professional responsibility to model positive health behaviors in their own lives, but nurses are individuals too. Being or becoming a healthy role model may require some effort. If you are not the positive role model for health you would like to be, Box 10-5 can help you get started.

Box 10-5 **Self-Assessment: Developing a Personal Plan for High-Level Wellness**

Nurses' personal health behaviors send a powerful message to consumers of nursing care. Are you in a position to demonstrate that you practice what you preach? By answering the following questions, you can assess how well you are meeting your responsibilities in this area of nursing.

1. I weigh no more than 10 pounds over or under my ideal weight.
   T F
2. I eat a balanced diet, including breakfast, each day.
   T F
3. Of the total calories in my diet, less than 30 percent come from fat.
   T F
4. I exercise aerobically at least three times each week.
   T F
5. I get at least 7 hours of sleep each night.
   T F
6. I do not smoke or use any other form of tobacco.
   T F
7. I use alcohol in moderation (or not at all) and take mood-altering medication only when prescribed by my physician.
   T F
8. I identify and control the sources of stress in my life.
   T F
9. I have a balanced lifestyle, with work and diversional activities both playing important roles.
   T F
10. I have friends, neighbors, and/or family members who are sources of social support for me.
    T F
11. I practice responsible sex.
    T F

Directions for scoring: If you could not honestly answer "True" to all 11 questions, you need to set goals to enable you to do so.

1. On a piece of paper, begin your personal plan for high-level wellness. Write down at least two things you can do to address each "False" answer you gave to the self-assessment questions.
2. Share your health goals with one other person in your class. Make a contract with that person to serve as your "health coach."
3. Review your progress with your health coach at least once a week for the remainder of the term.
4. Begin your quest for high-level wellness today!

PUTTING IT ALL TOGETHER: NURSING

Nursing integrates concepts from person, environment, and health to form a meaningful whole. This is the holistic approach to nursing.

Holistic Nursing

Holistic nursing care nourishes the whole person, that is, the body, mind, and spirit. Not surprisingly, the root word for *nurse* and *nurture* are the same Latin word, *nutrire*, which means "to nourish." Let us look now at eight factors that contribute to a holistic approach to nursing.

1. Nursing is an example of an open system that freely interacts with, influences, and is influenced by external and internal forces.
2. Nursing is the provision of health care services that focus on assisting people in maintaining health, avoiding or minimizing disease and disability, restoring wellness, or achieving a peaceful death.
3. Nursing involves collaborating with patients and their families to help them cope and adapt to situations of disequilibrium in an effort to regain homeostasis.
4. Nursing is integrally involved with people at points along the health-illness continuum.
5. Nursing care is provided regardless of diagnosis, individual differences, age, beliefs, gender, sexual preference, or other factors. As a profession, nursing supports the value, dignity, and uniqueness of every person and takes their culture and belief system into consideration.
6. Nurses require advanced knowledge and skills; they also must care about their patients.
7. Nursing requires concern, compassion, respect, and warmth, as well as comprehensive, individualized planning of care, to facilitate patients' growth toward wellness.
8. Nursing links theory and research in an effort to answer difficult questions generated during nursing practice.

Figure 10-5 depicts the relationships among nursing's major concepts.

Summary of Key Points

- Nursing integrates three basic components—person, environment, and health—to form its focus.
- Knowledge of systems and human needs can be used to understand nursing's major concepts.
- Persons are viewed as unique open systems who are motivated by needs.
- Maslow organized human needs into a hierarchy consisting of five levels that range from basic physiological needs, which are common to all people, to self-actualization, which is attained by few.
- Environment consists of all the circumstances, influences, and conditions that affect an individual. The physical environment and family, cultural, social, and community systems all have an impact.
- Health is dynamic and viewed as a continuum.
- There are numerous definitions of health.
- Nurses view health holistically, including its effect on an individual's physical, emotional, social, and spiritual functioning, as well as its effect on the family.
- Health is affected by health beliefs and health behaviors.
- As an open system, nursing integrates person, environment, and health into a meaningful whole.
- Nursing assists people to achieve health at the highest possible level, given their environmental and genetic constraints.

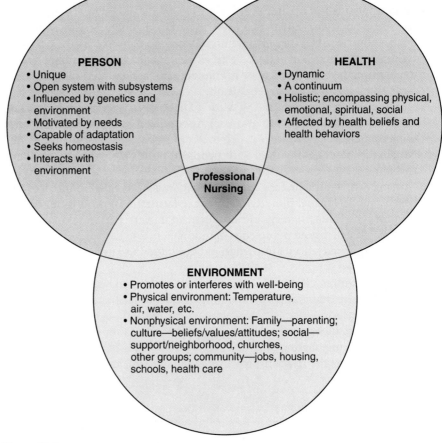

PERSON
- Unique
- Open system with subsystems
- Influenced by genetics and environment
- Motivated by needs
- Capable of adaptation
- Seeks homeostasis
- Interacts with environment

HEALTH
- Dynamic
- A continuum
- Holistic; encompassing physical, emotional, spiritual, social
- Affected by health beliefs and health behaviors

Professional Nursing

ENVIRONMENT
- Promotes or interferes with well-being
- Physical environment: Temperature, air, water, etc.
- Nonphysical environment: Family—parenting; culture—beliefs/values/attitudes; social—support/neighborhood, churches, other groups; community—jobs, housing, schools, health care

Figure **10-5**
Concepts and subconcepts basic to professional nursing.

CRITICAL THINKING QUESTIONS

1. Discuss systems in relation to your family. What are the family equivalents of inputs, throughputs, subsystems, suprasystems, outputs, evaluation, and feedback? Does your family tend to be an open or closed system?
2. Describe Maslow's hierarchy of needs and place yourself on the hierarchy today, 1 week ago, and when you were a senior in high school. Were you at a different level each time? Consider what factors—internal and external—may have been involved in your placement at each of these times. If possible, compare and discuss your findings with at least one other person.
3. Write your own personal definition of health and share it with one other person. Evaluate your definition in terms of holism.
4. What are factors that influence an individual's personal health behaviors? Make a list of your health behaviors, including those that promote health and those that

diminish health. Analyze why you continue both the healthy and the nonhealthy behaviors. Identify population-based initiatives that could influence you to make more health-generating choices.

5. Using a search engine, assess the array of support groups online. Enter the discussion group of one group that interests you, and simply observe. How would you evaluate the quality of the support and information being shared?

6. Look through your local Yellow Pages under "Social Services" and "Organizations." What types of social support do you find that might be useful to patients? Compare these with the online choices. Which type of support—face-to-face or online—is more appealing to you? Why?

7. Conduct an assessment of your community in terms of one of the following: availability of jobs, quality of public education, availability of health services, environmental hazards, and quality of air and water. What is the impact of the factor you selected on the health of the community's citizens? What can you do to strengthen the environmental health of your community?

8. Find out what your state and community are doing to link their health objectives to those of the *Healthy People 2010* initiatives. Discuss these in class. Design a project to assist your school of nursing to support the national effort.

REFERENCES

Ahmann E: Supporting families' savvy use of the Internet for health research, *Pediatr Nurs* 26(4):419-423, 2000.

Bandura A: A social cognitive approach to the exercise of control over AIDS infection. In DiClemente RJ, editor: *Adolescents and AIDS: a generation in jeopardy,* Newbury Park, CA, 1992, Sage Publications.

Bandura A: *Self-efficacy: exercise of control,* New York, 1997, WH Freeman.

Beyea SC: Evaluating evidence found on the Internet, *AORN J* 72(5):906-910, 2000.

Chase M: Health journal: a guide for patients who turn to the Web for solace and support, *Wall Street Journal* September 17, 1999, B1.

Dunn HL: High-level wellness for man and society, *Am J Pub Health* 49(6):786-792, 1959.

Dunn HL: *High-level wellness,* Thorofare, NJ, 1961, Slack.

Grossman D: Enhancing your cultural competence, *Am J Nurs* 94(7):58-62, 1994.

Half of single moms get support, *Citizen-News* (Dalton, GA), October 14, 1991, 4A.

Holmes TH, Rahe RH: The social readjustment rating scale, *J Psychosomat Res* 11(2):213-218, 1967.

Maslow AH: *Motivation and personality,* New York, 1954, Harper & Row.

McGinnis JM, Lee PR: Healthy People 2000 at mid-decade, *JAMA* 273(14):1123-1129, 1995.

Miller MA, Rahe RH: Life changes scaling for the 1990s, *J Psychosomat Res* 43(3):279-292, 1997.

Parsons T: Definitions of health and illness in light of American values and social structure. In Jaco EG, editor: *Patients, physicians and illness,* New York, 1959, Free Press, pp 165-187.

Pratt JP, Overfield T, Gill-Hilton H: Health behaviors of nurses and general population women, *Health Values* 18(3):41-46, 1994.

Rogers C: *On becoming a person,* Boston, 1961, Houghton Mifflin.

Rosenstock IM: Why people use health services, part II, *Milbank Mem Fund Quart* 44(3):94-124, 1966.

Rosenstock IM: The health belief model: explaining health behavior through expectancies. In Glans K, Lewis FM, Rimer BK, editors: *Health behavior and health education: theory, research, and practice,* San Francisco, 1990, Jossey Bass, pp 39-62.

Smith K, Bazini-Barakat N: A public health nursing practice model: melding public health principles with the nursing process, *Pub Health Nurs* 20(1):42-48, 2003.

Smuts JC: *Holism and evolution,* New York, 1926, Macmillan.

Steptoe A, Wardle J: Locus of control and health behaviour revisited: a multivariate analysis of young adults from 18 countries, *Br J Psychol* 92(4):659-673, 2001.

U.S. Census Bureau: Growth in single fathers outpaces growth in single mothers, Census Bureau reports, Online, 1998 *(www.census.gov/Press-Release/cb98-228.html).*

U.S. Census Bureau: *Households and families for the United States, regions, and states, and for Puerto Rico: 1990 and 2000,* Washington, DC, 2000a, Government Printing Office.

U.S. Census Bureau: More custodial parents receive full amount of child support, Census Bureau reports, Online, 2000b *(www.census.gov/Press-Release/www/2000/cb00-170.html).*

U.S. Census Bureau: *Profile of the foreign-born population in the United States: 2000,* Washington, DC, 2001, Government Printing Office.

U.S. Census Bureau: Poverty, income see slight changes: child poverty rate unchanged, Census Bureau reports, Online, 2003 *(www.census.gov/Press-Release/www/2003/cb03-153.html).*

U.S. Department of Health and Human Services: *Healthy people 2000: fact sheet,* Washington, DC, 1990, Government Printing Office.

U.S. Department of Health and Human Services: *Healthy people 2000: review 1998-1999,* Washington, DC, 1999a, Government Printing Office.

U.S. Department of Health and Human Services: *Healthy people 2010: fact sheet,* Washington, DC, 1999b, Government Printing Office.

U.S. Department of Health and Human Services: Healthy people 2010: implementation, Online, 2003 *(www.healthypeople.gov/Implementation/default.htm#partners).*

von Bertalanffy L: *General systems theory: foundations, development, applications,* New York, 1968, George Braziller.

World Health Organization: *Constitution,* Geneva, 1947, World Health Organization.

Nursing Theory: The Basis for Professional Nursing

Martha Raile Alligood

Key Terms

Abstract
Adaptation
Patricia Benner
Concept
Conceptual Model
Criteria
Framework
Virginia Henderson
Dorothy Johnson
Imogene King

Knowledge
Madeleine Leininger
Metaparadigm
Middle-Range Theory
Myra Levine
Florence Nightingale
Betty Neuman
Margaret Newman
Dorothea Orem
Ida Orlando

Rosemarie Parse
Phenomena
Philosophy
Martha Rogers
Callista Roy
Structure of Knowledge
Systems
Theory
Jean Watson

Learning Outcomes

After studying this chapter, students will be able to:

- Explore elements of selected nursing philosophies, nursing conceptual models, and theories of nursing.
- Consider how selected nursing theoretical works guide the practice of nursing.
- Delineate the role of nursing theory for different levels of nursing education.
- Describe the function of nursing theory in research and theory-based practice.
- Relate the role of nursing theory in education, research, and practice to the development of the profession.

WHAT IS THEORY?

The purpose of this chapter is to introduce you to the major theoretical works of nursing. Some of you may be asking, "What is theory, and why is it important for us to study nursing theory?" The term **theory** has many definitions, but generally it refers to a group of related concepts, definitions, and statements that propose a view of nursing **phenomena** from which to describe, explain, or predict outcomes (Chinn and Kramer, 1998; Powers and Knapp, 1995). More simply, theory is "a group of related concepts that propose actions to guide practice" (Alligood and Tomey, 1997, p. 225). Furthermore, "these systematic organized perspectives serve as guides for nursing action in administration, education, research, and practice" (Alligood and Tomey, 2002, p. 487). Theories represent **abstract** ideas rather than concrete facts. As such, theories are tentative and when new knowledge becomes available, theories that are no longer useful are modified or discarded. Therefore theories are considered propositions that suggest new understandings, and although some may be used for centuries, new theories are always being generated.

Professional nurses are conscious of the need for nursing theory development and theory-based practice to be complementary activities. As nursing has developed as a professional practice and a scholarly discipline, interest in the theoretical basis of nursing has increased. Scholars understand that continued theory development and theory-based nursing practice are among the most crucial challenges facing professional nursing today (Alligood, 2002a; Chinn and Kramer, 1998; Fawcett, 2002; Holder and Chitty, 1997; Meleis, 1997).

Theory is important for many reasons; we will discuss three of those reasons here. First, as seen in Chapter 6, one criterion for a profession is a distinct body of **knowledge** as the basis for practice. Nursing's interest in developing a body of substantive nursing knowledge has been a major driving force within the profession throughout the twentieth century (Alligood, 2002a). Theory testing and the development of new theory in theory-based research is a means of building that knowledge and strengthening nursing as a profession.

Second, commitment to theory-based nursing practice using sound, reliable knowledge is intrinsically valuable to nursing; that is to say, by its very nature, knowledge is desirable (Alligood, 2002b). The evolving development of knowledge in and of itself is an important activity for nurse scholars to pursue. Progress and development of the profession depend on continued recognition and respect for nursing as a scholarly discipline that contributes to society.

Third, theory is a useful nursing practice tool for reasoning, critical thinking, and decision making (Alligood, 2002c; Alligood and Tomey, 2002; Tomey and Alligood, 2002). Nursing practice settings are complex, and the amount of data (information) confronting nurses is virtually endless. Nurses must analyze a vast amount of information about each patient and decide what to do. A theoretical approach helps practicing nurses not to be overwhelmed by the mass of information confronting them and to progress through the nursing process in an orderly manner. Theory enables nurses to organize and understand what happens in practice, to analyze patient situations critically and recognize pertinent evidence for clinical decision making; to plan care and propose appropriate nursing interventions; and to predict patient outcomes from that care and evaluate its effectiveness. Box 11-1 summarizes the ways theory guides practicing nurses.

Because theory is abstract, it is useful to consider theoretical works in the context of a **structure of knowledge.** Figure 11-1 illustrates the structure of nursing knowledge as conceptualized by Fawcett (2000). This structure is useful in that it specifies a metaparadigm consisting of the major concepts of the discipline: person, environment,

Box **11-1** Nursing Theory and the Practicing Nurse

Theory assists the practicing nurse to:
- Organize patient data
- Analyze patient data
- Recognize pertinent evidence in the data
- Understand patient data
- Make decisions based on evidence and understanding
- Plan patient care
- Predict outcomes of care
- Evaluate patient outcomes

health, and nursing. It also differentiates types of theoretical works based on the nature of the works themselves (philosophies, models, and theories) and their levels of abstraction. Although nursing theory has been traced back to **Florence Nightingale,** most nursing theory was developed in the latter half of the twentieth century (Alligood, 2002a; Tomey and Alligood, 2002).

A number of nursing theory textbooks are available that provide an overview and critique of developments in nursing theory (see Alligood and Tomey, 2002; Fawcett, 2000; Fitzpatrick and Whall, 1996; George, 2002; McEwen and Wills, 2002; Parker 2001; Tomey and Alligood, 2002). Although these texts may differ in their approach, each addresses person, environment, health, and nursing as the major nursing concepts. Together, these concepts compose the most abstract aspect of the

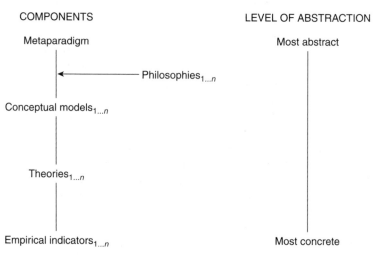

COMPONENTS   LEVEL OF ABSTRACTION

Metaparadigm   Most abstract

Philosophies$_{1...n}$

Conceptual models$_{1...n}$

Theories$_{1...n}$

Empirical indicators$_{1...n}$ Most concrete

Figure **11-1**
A structure of nursing knowledge. (Adapted from Fawcett J: *Analysis and evaluation of contemporary nursing knowledge: models and theories,* Philadelphia, 2000, FA Davis.)

structure of nursing knowledge, which is known as a metaparadigm for a discipline (Fawcett, 2000; Powers and Knapp, 1995). A **metaparadigm** is defined as "the most global perspective that subsumes the more specific views and approaches to the central concepts with which a discipline is concerned" (Alligood and Tomey, 2002, p. 485).

Whereas the best source for in-depth understanding of each of the theoretical works is the primary source (actual writing) of the theorist, explanatory texts are also very helpful but in a different way. They introduce students to the theoretical basis of the discipline of nursing from a comprehensive, metatheoretical, nursing science perspective that is much broader than any one of the individual works. That is, these explanatory texts trace the historical development of the philosophy, model, or theory and specify **criteria** to analyze, critique, and evaluate them. The explanatory texts began to be published in the early 1980s with a completely different purpose than the theorists' original writings. They contribute to the general understanding of nursing theory and theoretical developments in nursing in a unique but complementary way. These books have served and continue to serve this purpose for undergraduate and graduate students, for faculty, and for practicing nurses who have found that these comprehensive theory texts make a significant contribution to their knowledge and understanding of nursing science in their own right.

In this chapter, three general types of nursing theoretical works will be considered: nursing philosophies, nursing models, and theories of nursing (Tomey and Alligood, 2002). Selected works from each of the three types provide a broad overview of theory within the discipline of nursing. This introduction is designed to help you develop a beginning understanding of nursing theory on which to build as you pursue your nursing education and career in the profession of nursing.

Nursing Philosophies

Chapter 9 introduced nursing philosophy and discussed its function in nursing practice and educational institutions. A **philosophy** provides a broad, general view of nursing that clarifies values and answers broad disciplinary questions such as "What is nursing?" "What is the profession of nursing?" "What do nurses do?" "What is the nature of human caring?" and "What is the nature of nursing practice and the development of practice expertise?" For our discussion here, four philosophies have been selected because they represent different positions in the development of nursing theory.

Nightingale's Philosophy

Florence Nightingale's work represents the beginning of professional nursing, as noted in Chapter 1. In her most frequently cited work, *Notes on Nursing: What It Is and What It Is Not* (1969, originally published in 1859), Nightingale answered the philosophical question "What is nursing?" She envisioned nursing as different from the work of household servants, which were common in her day. She also developed a logical distinction between medicine and nursing by clarifying the major concern of nursing as health rather than illness.

Though we draw many ideas from the writings of Nightingale, her unique perspective for nursing practice focused on the relationship of patients to their surroundings. She set forth principles that were foundational to nursing and remain relevant to nursing practice today. For example, her description of the importance of observing the patient and accurately recording information and her principles of cleanliness, which clarified clean areas from dirty ones, can be seen in hospital-based nursing practice today.

Using Nightingale's philosophy in practice

Nightingale believed that the health of patients was related to their surroundings. She discussed the need for pure air and water, efficient drainage, cleanliness, and light. She emphasized the necessity of ventilation and sunlight and encouraged moving patients' beds to change their view and give them access to direct sunlight. Her discussion of diet spoke not only to the necessity of a balanced diet but also to the nurse's responsibility to observe and record what was eaten. She emphasized cleanliness of the patient, the bed linens, and the room itself. Her discussion of noise was especially interesting in light of attention to noise pollution in recent years. She recognized the problem of noise in the room or in the hall for patients confined to bed. She emphasized the importance of rest and discouraged sudden disruption of sleep.

Nightingale gave nurses the responsibility for protecting patients from possible harm by visitors who mean well but may provide false hope, discuss upsetting news, or idly chatter, thereby tiring the patient. Furthermore, she focused on the nurse's responsibility for patients even when the nurse was off duty. Finally, she suggested that patients might benefit from visits by small pets, yet another idea that speaks to the timeless relevance of her work.

The nurse whose practice is guided by Nightingale's philosophy is keenly aware of the importance of surroundings to health or recovery from illness. Her work presented an implicit theory that proposed changing patients' surroundings (environment) to bring about changes in their health. She held nurses responsible for patients and their surroundings.

Henderson's Philosophy

Virginia Henderson was another early philosopher of nursing. Henderson's work appeared at a time when efforts to clarify nursing as a profession emphasized defining nursing. As mentioned in Chapter 7, she provided a comprehensive definition: the "unique function of the nurse … is to assist the individual, sick or well, in the performance of those activities contributing to health or its recovery (or a peaceful death) that he would perform unaided if he had the necessary strength, will or knowledge" (Henderson, 1966, p. 15). Although Henderson was recognized for many contributions to nursing throughout her career, this early work, which defined nursing and specified the role of the nurse in relation to the patient, remains particularly noteworthy and relevant.

Henderson's philosophy of nursing linked her definition of nursing, which emphasized the functions of the nurse and the assisting aspects of nursing, with a list of basic patient needs that are the focus of nursing care. Her work proposed an answer to the questions "What is the nursing profession?" and "What do nurses do?" She described the nurse's role as that of a substitute for the patient, a helper to the patient, or a partner with the patient.

Box 11-2 **Henderson's 14 Basic Needs of the Patient**

1. Breathe normally.
2. Eat and drink adequately.
3. Eliminate body wastes.
4. Move and maintain desirable position.
5. Sleep and rest.
6. Select suitable clothes—dress and undress.
7. Maintain body temperature within normal range by adjusting clothing and modifying the environment.
8. Keep the body clean and well groomed and protect the integument (skin).
9. Avoid dangers in the environment and avoid injuring others.
10. Communicate with others in expressing emotions, needs, fears, or opinions.
11. Worship according to one's faith.
12. Work in such a way that there is a sense of accomplishment.
13. Play or participate in various forms of recreation.
14. Learn, discover, or satisfy the curiosity that leads to normal development and health and use the available health facilities.

Reprinted with permission of Henderson V: *The nature of nursing: a definition and its implications for practice, research, and education,* New York, 1996, Macmillan.

Henderson's 14 basic needs provided a general focus for patient care. She proposed that these needs clarified the elements of nursing care. The function of nurses was to assist patients if they were unable to perform these 14 functions themselves. Box 11-2 lists Henderson's 14 basic needs of the patient.

Henderson's work has been used by nurses all over the world for direction in nursing education and practice. The needs she included might at first be viewed as physical, psychological, emotional, sociological, spiritual, and developmental areas. However, a more careful analysis reveals a holistic view of human development and health.

The first nine needs on Henderson's list stress the importance of breathing, eating and drinking, elimination, movement and positioning, sleep and rest, suitable clothing, maintenance of suitable environment for the body temperature, cleanliness, and avoidance of danger or harm. Next, she included the psychological or sociological need to communicate and the spiritual need for worship and faith. She concluded with three needs that might be viewed as developmental: the need for work and the sense of accomplishment, the need for play and recreation, and the need to learn, discover, and satisfy curiosity.

Using Henderson's philosophy in practice

Nursing practice based on Henderson's work focuses on nursing care that is consistent with her definition of nursing. The nurse approaches patients from the perspective of the 14 basic needs. Henderson's clarity about the role and function of the nurse is a strength of her work. She used her definition of nursing and the basic needs approach in her well-known case study of a young patient who had undergone a leg amputation. Using this case, Henderson demonstrated how the nurse's role changes on a day-to-day, week-to-week, and month-to-month basis in relation to the patient's changing needs and the contributions of other members of the health care delivery team (Henderson, 1966).

Watson's Philosophy

Jean Watson published her initial philosophical work, *The Philosophy and Science of Caring*, in 1979. In this work, she issued a call for a return to the earlier values of nursing and emphasized the caring aspects of nursing. Watson's work is recognized as human science. Themes of caring can also be noted in her other professional accomplishments. For example, she established the Center for Human Caring at the University of Colorado in Denver, where nurses can incorporate knowledge of human caring as the basis of nursing practice and scholarship. Watson proposed 10 factors, which she labeled *carative* factors, a term she contrasted with *curative* to differentiate nursing from medicine. Watson's 10 carative factors are listed in Box 11-3.

Watson's work (1979, 1988, 1999) addressed the philosophical question of the nature of nursing when viewed as a human-to-human relationship. She focused on the relationship of the nurse and the patient, drawing on philosophical sources for a new approach that emphasized how the nurse and patient change together through transpersonal caring. She proposed that nursing be concerned with spiritual matters and the inner knowledge of nurse and patient as they participate together in the transpersonal caring process. She equated health with harmony, resulting from unity of body, mind, and soul, for which the patient is primarily responsible. Illness or disease was equated with lack of harmony within the mind, body, and soul experienced in internal or external environments (Watson, 1979). According to Watson, nursing, based on human values and interest in the welfare of others, is concerned with health promotion, health restoration, and illness prevention. Her most recent work (1999) interprets her earlier works in light of postmodern thought for the twenty-first century.

Box **11-3** **Watson's Ten Carative Factors**

1. The formation of a humanistic-altruistic system of values.
2. The instillation of faith-hope.
3. The cultivation of sensitivity to one's self and others.
4. The development of a helping-trust relationship.
5. The promotion and acceptance of the expression of positive and negative feelings.
6. The systematic use of the scientific problem-solving method for decision making.
7. The promotion of interpersonal teaching-learning.
8. The provision for a supportive, protective, and/or corrective mental, physical, sociocultural, and spiritual environment.
9. Assistance with the gratification of human needs.
10. The allowance for existential-phenomenological forces.

Reprinted with permission of Tomey AM, Alligood MR: *Nursing theorists and their work,* ed 5, St. Louis, 2002, Mosby.

Using Watson's philosophy in practice

Watson's carative factors guide nurses who use transpersonal caring in practice. Carative factors specify the meaning of the relationship of nurse and patient as human beings. Nurses are encouraged to share their genuine selves with patients. Patients' spiritual strength is recognized, supported, and encouraged for its contribution to health. In the process of transpersonal relationships, nurses develop and encourage openness to understanding of self and others. This leads to the development of trusting, accepting relationships in which feelings are shared freely and confidence is inspired.

Watson recognized the scientific method as a tool for systematic solutions to problems and a guide for making decisions. She suggested that teaching and learning of patients, vital aspects of nursing practice, be carried out in an interpersonal manner true to the philosophy and nature of the caring relationship.

The nurse guided by Watson's work has responsibility for creating and maintaining an environment supporting human caring while recognizing and providing for patients' primary human requirements. In the end, this human-to-human caring approach leads the nurse to respect the overall meaning of life from the perspective of the patient. Watson's 1988 work formalized the theory of human caring from this philosophy.

Benner's Philosophy

The work of **Patricia Benner** (1984) centers on the nature of nurses' personal knowledge of nursing practice. It emerged from research studies aimed toward understanding nurses' knowledge more completely. She sought personal and practical knowledge from nurses about how they acquired nursing expertise. As a result, the focus of Benner's work is nursing practice.

Using Benner's philosophy in practice

Benner proposed seven domains of nursing practice that identify the role of the nurse in relation to the patient: helping, teaching-coaching, diagnosing and monitoring, managing changes, administering and monitoring therapeutic interventions, monitoring for quality care, and organizing to enact the work role. From her study of nurses within these domains she proposed five stages in the development of expertise. These stages—novice, advanced beginner, competent practitioner, proficient practitioner, and expert practitioner—were summarized in Chapter 8 (Table 8-3).

Benner's more recent work is extremely useful to practicing nurses (Benner, Hooper-Kyriakidis, and Stannard, 1999). Detailed interpretations of the practice of nurses at various levels of proficiency have contributed to in-depth understanding of the complexities of nursing practice and the unique value they have for patients. Benner's work has also been helpful to the profession of nursing for differentiating levels of nursing practice. Whereas earlier in nursing history levels were mainly differentiated by educational preparation or longevity of service, Benner's work described specific behaviors for different levels of expertness in nursing practice documenting empirical competency indicators.

NURSING CONCEPTUAL MODELS

Conceptual models (or conceptual frameworks) are the second type of theoretical work in the structure of nursing knowledge (Fawcett, 2000). They are broad conceptual structures providing comprehensive, holistic perspectives of nursing through the interrelationship of delineated concepts. They provide organizational frameworks for critical thinking about the processes of nursing (Alligood, 2002c; Fawcett, 2000). As seen in Figure 11-1, models are less abstract and more formalized than the philosophies just discussed in this chapter; models are more abstract, however, than theories of nursing, which will be discussed later. It is important to note that nursing conceptual models are structures from which nursing theory may be derived. To illustrate, Box 11-4 lists seven nursing conceptual models, along with an example of a theory that has been derived from each of them. The name of a nursing conceptual model usually includes the name of the theorist who developed the model, for example, Rogers' Science of Unitary Human Beings (Alligood, 2002c). Each of the nursing conceptual models addresses the four major nursing concepts—person, environment, health, and nursing—and defines those concepts in its own way.

The conceptual models to be reviewed in the following sections were developed by Johnson, King, Levine, Neuman, Orem, Rogers, and Roy. The focus and perspective of each model is discussed, followed by a brief overview of how that model guides nursing practice.

Johnson's Behavioral System Model

The work of **Dorothy Johnson** (1968, 1980) focuses on human behavior. She proposed a system of nursing based on the observation of patient behavior. The behavioral phenomena of persons are presented as a single system with seven subsystems: achievement behavior, affiliative behavior, aggressive/protective behavior, dependency behavior, eliminative behavior, ingestive behavior, and sexual behavior. An eighth subsystem, restorative behavior, was later added (Holaday, 1997). Johnson distinguished the phenomena of concern with her framework from others by contrasting her behavioral system approach for nursing with the physiological system approach of medicine or the social system approach of sociology.

Box **11-4** Conceptual Models of Nursing With a Theory Example for Each	
Conceptual Models of Nursing	**Theory Example**
Johnson's Behavioral System	Theory of the person as a behavioral system
King's Interacting Systems	Theory of goal attainment
Levine's Conservation Model	Theory of therapeutic intention
Neuman Systems Model	Theory of optimal client stability
Orem's Conceptual Model	Orem's self-care deficit theory
Rogers' Science of Unitary Human Beings	Theory of accelerating change
Roy's Adaptation Model	Theory of the person as an adaptive system

From Alligood MR: Philosophies, models and theories: critical thinking structures. In Alligood MR, Tomey AM, editors: *Nursing theory: utilization and application*, ed 2, St. Louis, 2002c, Mosby, pp 41-61.

Using Johnson's model in practice

When using Johnson's work as a guide for nursing practice, nurses view patients' behaviors in a systematic way according to the subsystems outlined above. Observation of patient behavior is paramount in this model. Each subsystem has its own structure, which assists nurses in considering what may be contributing to a patient's actual behaviors. Subsystem structures include a goal, which is based on universal drive, a set, a choice, and an action. An example of a "universal drive" is to maintain health; "set" is the usual behaviors of the patient that might help maintain health; "choice" is the range of behaviors the person considers to maintain health; and "action" is the observable healthy behavior (Holaday, 2002).

The nurse identifies the subsystem involved by observing a patient's behavior, then assesses the patient's set (usual behavior) in relation to the goal of the system. If the goal of the subsystem is not being met, the behavioral choices are reviewed in relation to action or the patient's actual behavior. An environmental assessment (internal and external) is also carried out to understand the impact of environment on a patient's behavior and to discover behavioral alternatives. A diagnostic analysis determines whether the behavior of the subsystem is dominant, incompatible, discrepant, or insufficient. Based on the diagnosis within the subsystem, nurse and patient select mutual goals and develop a plan for intervention.

If you wish to read more about the use of Johnson's model in practice, Holaday (2002) and Alligood (2002b) are suggested resources.

King's Interacting Systems Framework and Theory of Goal Attainment

The work of **Imogene King** (1981) focused on persons, their interpersonal relationships, and social contexts with three interacting **systems:** *personal, interpersonal,* and *social.* Within each of these three systems King identified concepts that provide a conceptual structure describing the processes in each system. The three systems and their concepts are presented in Box 11-5.

King's interacting systems form a framework to view whole persons in their family and social contexts: the *personal system* identifies concepts that provide an understanding of individuals, personally and intrapersonally; the *interpersonal system* deals with interactions and transactions between two or more persons; and the *social system* presents concepts that consider social contacts, such as those at school,

---

Box 11-5 **King's Three Systems and Their Concepts**

Personal System	Interpersonal System	Social System
Perception	Role	Organization
Self	Interaction	Power
Body image	Communication	Authority
Growth and development	Transaction	Status
Time	Stress	Decision making
Space		

From King IM: *A theory for nursing: systems, concepts, process,* New York, 1981, John Wiley & Sons.

at work, or in social settings. King's work is unique because it provides a view of persons from the perspective of their interactions (or communications, both verbal and nonverbal) with other people at three interacting systems levels.

Using King's model in practice

When using King's work, nurses are guided by the framework as well as the theory of goal attainment. First, the traditional steps of the nursing process—assessment, planning, goal setting, intervention, and evaluation—are augmented in several ways. It is less clear to describe the process as a linear progression, because when understood as a process, it becomes clear that more than one of the steps is occurring simultaneously. The steps of the process describe the type of action the nurse is taking, and they each help the nurse gather and use information to provide care.

Second, the focus of the process is guided by concepts at each of the system levels. For example, the personal system leads the nurse to pay close attention to the patient's perceptions, the interpersonal system steers the nurse to notice patients' roles and their stresses in each role, and the social system cues the nurse to consider what seems to influence the patient's decision making.

A third aspect of the process focuses on interactions with the patient. Nurses are aware of their communication with patients, identifying steps from the first encounter through to the attainment of the specified goal. King describes these steps as a progression from perception, judgment, action, reaction and interaction, to transaction (King, 1981).

King emphasized the importance of joint goal setting by nurse and patient, reminding nurses that this relationship involves mutuality. King's process provided a structure for the nurse to monitor the relationship's progress. King clearly specified the goal of nursing to be health.

Examples of applications of King's work in nursing practice are available in the nursing literature (see Alligood, 1995; Alligood and May, 2000; Norris and Frey, 2002; Frey and Sieloff, 1995; Sieloff, 2002).

Levine's Conservation Model

Myra Levine (1973, 1991) developed a model based on three major concepts: wholeness, adaptation, and conservation. The framework, which was first used to organize nursing school curricula, set forth a set of conservation principles as a comprehensive guide for nursing. Simply stated, Levine viewed human life as a process of maintaining wholeness through **adaptation,** which is facilitated by conservation. She believed that wholeness, defined as "keeping together," continues throughout life. According to Levine, the integrity of wholeness is sustained by adaptation or change, as humans interact with their environments. Wholeness is defined as health or well-being of persons, that is, the outcome of properly functioning adaptive change. Illness and disease interrupt the normal process of adaptation and produce the need for nursing.

Levine asserted that nursing is a human interaction designed to promote human adaptation until wholeness is regained or the person can adapt without assistance. Nurses promote adaptation through conservation, which is guided by four principles: conservation of energy, structure, personal integrity, and social integrity. She proposed two theories from her model, the theory of redundancy and the theory of therapeutic intention. Both are testable in nursing practice and research (Schaefer, 2002).

Using Levine's model in practice

When using Levine's model to guide nursing practice, nurses use the four conservation principles in assessing patients. With information from this assessment, they make nursing judgments and propose hypotheses for interventions that promote adaptation. The hypotheses are then tested for their use as guides in selecting nursing interventions and evaluating patients' responses. Interventions are designed with Levine's theory of redundancy in mind. This means that nurses involve patients in choosing interventions to avoid conflicts with the patient's own conservation efforts (Schaefer, 2002). Schaefer and Pond (1991), Schaefer (2002), and Alligood (2002b) are resources for more information about the use of Levine's model in nursing practice.

Neuman Systems Model

Betty Neuman (1995) designed a systems model in response to student requests for an organizing **framework** for the mass of information they encountered in nursing practice. The Neuman Systems Model, now in its fourth revision, views persons from the perspective of actual and potential stressors and associated health risk factors. Strengths and weaknesses are identified in relation to those stressors, and stress reduction goals are set as nursing outcomes. According to Neuman, the client (referred to as the core and source of basic energy) possesses unique survival capabilities in five areas: physiological, psychological, sociological, developmental, and spiritual. The client system includes the core as well as its system of resistance and defenses. The client is continuously exposed to internal and external factors, which are met by the lines of defense and/resistance.

Nursing interventions build on client strengths to shore up defenses and strengthen weaknesses. To this end, nursing interventions are based on the strengths and weaknesses in three possible levels of prevention. Primary prevention is for the promotion of health or wellness retention; secondary prevention is for treatment of symptoms, as well as for conserving energy and strengthening the lines of resistance; and tertiary prevention is similar to what we sometimes call "recuperation," wherein strengths are supported while the client returns to health or wellness. This comprehensive model may be applied in all practice areas and is especially useful when working with families and communities.

Using Neuman's model in practice

Nurses practicing with the Neuman Systems Model interact with clients to identify actual and potential stressors in five client variables: physiological, psychological, sociocultural, developmental, and spiritual. Next, the nurse and client identify strengths and weaknesses in relation to the stressors. The approach is holistic and systematic. Based on the client's level of stress and health goals, a plan is developed. Nursing care provides primary, secondary, and tertiary prevention in relation to the identified strengths and weaknesses. Throughout the process the client is supported and assessed according to the many facets of the model. The emphasis is on maintaining client system balance, or stability, which Neuman specifies as the goal of nursing.

Applications of Neuman's work in nursing practice are available in secondary sources (Alligood, 2002b; Sohier, 2002), as well as in her own text, *The Neuman Systems Model* (1995). Betty Neuman remains active in writing and speaking about the model. The Neuman Systems Model Trustee Group is active internationally and meets biannually to continue refining and developing the model as a community of scholars.

Orem's Self-Care Model

As an early nurse theorist, **Dorothea Orem** published *Concepts of Nursing* in 1971. This work is now in its sixth edition (2001). Over the years Orem formalized three interrelated theories: theory of self-care, theory of self-care deficit, and theory of nursing system. The model focuses on the patient's self-care capacities and the process of designing nursing actions to meet the patient's self-care needs. In this model, the nurse prescribes and regulates the nursing system for self-care.

Orem's (2001) work is widely used in nursing education and practice. It sets forth a comprehensive system for nursing practice in a variety of clinical settings.

Orem and nursing practice

When using Orem's work as a guide, the nurse carries out a systematic series of four operations: diagnosis, prescription, regulation, and control. Each of these specifies activities for the patient and the nurse.

Diagnostic operations begin with the establishment of the nurse-patient relationship and include contracting with the patient to explore current and potential self-care demands. Diagnosis is accomplished by examining basic conditioning factors in relation to the universal, developmental, and health care deviation requisites and related self-care actions of the patient. For example, recognizing a patient's inability to carry out self-care (called deficits) is a diagnostic operation. Prescriptive operations occur when therapeutic self-care requisites (based on deficits) are determined and the nurse reviews various methods, actions, and priorities with the patient. In regulatory operations the nurse designs, plans, and produces a system for care (Berbiglia, 2002).

This model has wide practical application. There is a biannual Orem Conference, an Orem Newsletter, and Orem websites. Numerous examples of nursing care using Orem's model are available in the nursing literature (Alligood, 2002b; Berbiglia, 2002; Renpenning and Taylor, 2003).

Rogers' Science of Unitary Human Beings

Another early theorist, **Martha Rogers,** first published her model in 1970. Rogers believed that if nurses needed only knowledge from other disciplines to practice nursing, there was no need for higher education in nursing. To prove that this was not the case, she set about identifying and developing a body of unique nursing knowledge.

Rogers clarified *nursing* as a noun and defined it as "a body of knowledge necessary for practice." She called this organized body of abstract knowledge nursing science and specified nursing art as the imaginative and creative application of knowledge in practice. Thus she believed that nursing was both science and art and described nursing as a learned profession that focuses on the nature and direction of human development and human betterment.

Rogers' work focused on the process of humans and their environments. Her model has four main concepts: energy fields, openness, pattern, and pan-dimensionality, which Rogers used to describe the human developmental process in life.

Many theories have been derived from Rogers' conceptual system, a number by Rogers herself and many others by Rogerian scholars. Two theories derived from Rogers' work will be addressed in the later theory section of this chapter.

The Society of Rogerian Scholars, formed in the 1980s, is an organization for nurses who use Rogerian science in their practice, education, administration, or research and who wish to promote its development in the future. The organization sponsors annual meetings, biennial conferences, a newsletter, and a journal titled *Visions: The Journal of Rogerian Science,* which celebrated 10 years of publication in 2003 and is devoted to the development and dissemination of Rogerian science.

Using Rogers' model in practice

Rogers' model (1970, 1992) provides a very different view of nursing practice compared with other nursing models. Not only is hers an abstract model, but it is also *acausal,* which means life events are viewed as emerging from the simultaneous actions of persons and the environment rather than from actions and reactions, or causes and effects, which are traditional views. This perspective allows nurses and patients to join in their life processes, participating in one another's patterns, while the nurse provides care and information. Nurses participate knowingly with patients toward increased understanding of patterns. Nursing care must be pertinent to the patient's life process.

Rogers' framework leads the nurse to respect the patient's preferences in all matters. The nurse and patient progress toward an outcome of well-being specified by the patient. Box 11-6 provides observations of a nurse who is a Rogerian practitioner. There are many examples of the use of Rogers' work in the nursing literature. For case applications see Bultemeier (2002), Alligood (2002b), Barrett (1990), and Madrid (1994); for a theory of the art of nursing practice, see Alligood (2002e).

Roy's Adaptation Model

Sister **Callista Roy** first presented her adaptation model as a conceptual framework for a nursing curriculum in 1970 and updated all of her writing in a comprehensive text in 1999 (Roy and Andrews, 1999). Her model is widely used for education, research, and nursing practice today. She focused on the individual as a biopsychosocial adaptive system and described nursing as a humanistic discipline that emphasizes the person's adaptive or coping abilities. Roy's work is based on adaptation and adaptive behavior, which is produced by altering the environment.

According to Roy, the individual and the environment are sources of stimuli that require modification to promote adaptation in the patient. Roy viewed the person

Box **11-6** Using Nursing Science in Practice: Observations of a Rogerian Practitioner

Practice within the Rogerian model (framework) is ever dynamic and centers on continual pattern appraisal. The Rogerian framework is an abstract guide to nursing practice as it encompasses the simultaneous process of the human-environmental field. This dynamic emergent conceptual framework provides guidance for my practice toward systematic, innovative, and individualized care.

My practice is conceptually centered on the Rogerian concepts of resonancy, helicy, and integrality. These concepts guide my practice in selection of tools, which facilitate pattern appraisal, mutual patterning, and evaluation of the human-environmental field. Pattern appraisal tools are based on mutual participation (of the patient and the nurse) and observation of emergent patterns. These patterns are often evident through perceived colors, smells, descriptive words, physical symptoms, and overt physical manifestations. The emergent pattern guides the patterning process always remembering the pandimensionality of the human-environment process. Patterning modalities frequently used in my practice include meditation, contemplation, reflection, journaling, therapeutic touch, massage, humor, music, metaphors, color, light, sleep, vitamins, and exercise. Evaluation is ongoing, integral, and centers on perceptions emerging via the mutual patterning of the patient and the nurse.

My professional practice is working with women at Women's Health Associates in Oak Ridge, Tennessee. I am an adjunct faculty member at the University of Tennessee, College of Nursing, in Knoxville and precept graduate students in my practice. In addition, I provide massage therapy to individuals in their homes. Nursing practice within the Rogerian model is ever evolving and rewarding. …

Courtesy Kaye Bultemeier, PhD, RNCS, Oak Ridge, Tennessee, 1999.

as an adaptive system with physiological, self-concept, role function, and interdependent modes. According to Roy, these modes are manifestations of cognator and regulator coping responses to stimuli.

Roy's model provides a comprehensive understanding of nursing from the perspective of adaptation. When the demands of environmental stimuli are too high or the person's adaptive mechanisms are too low, the person's behavioral responses are ineffective for coping. Effective adaptive responses promote the integrity of the individual by conserving energy and promoting the survival, growth, reproduction, and mastery of the human system. Nursing promotes the patients' adaptation and coping, with progress toward integration as the goal (Phillips, 2002).

Using Roy's model in practice

The nurse using Roy's model focuses on the adaptation of the patient and on the environment. Adaptation, specifically patients' adaptation behavior and stimuli in the internal and external environments, is assessed and facilitated. Based on these assessments, the nurse develops nursing diagnoses to guide goal setting and interventions aimed at promoting adaptation. Simply stated, the nurse modifies the environment to facilitate patient adaptation.

Observable behavior is recognized and understood in the context of Roy's physiological, self-concept, role function, and interdependent modes. Descriptions of the behaviors included in each mode provide the nurse with a means of making evaluative judgments about the patient's progress toward the goal of adaptation (Phillips, 2002). Case applications are presented in Phillips (2002). Roy's model is very widely used in nursing practice and comprehensively described in the literature (Alligood, 2002b; Phillips, 2002; Roy, 1999).

THEORIES OF NURSING

Nursing theories are the third type of theoretical work in the structure of nursing knowledge to be reviewed in this chapter. Theories are composed of sets of **concepts** that are related in statements or propositions. Theories are less abstract than nursing conceptual models, and they are more prescriptive; that is, they propose an explicit outcome that is testable in practice and research (Alligood, 2002c). Fawcett (2000) classified theories according to their breadth and depth. For example, a grand theory is very broad, a theory is less broad, and a **middle-range theory** is the most specific. Theories are usually named for the outcome they propose or for specific characteristics of their content—for example, Parse's theory of human becoming or Newman's theory of health as expanding consciousness (Alligood, 2002c).

Orlando's Nursing Process Theory

Ida Orlando first proposed her theory of effective nursing practice in 1961. She later revised it as a nursing process theory (1990). Her work actually proposed both: it is a theory about how nurses process their observations of patient behavior and also about how they react to the patients based on inferences from their behavior, including what they say. Her early research revealed that processing observations as specified in the theory led to effective nursing practice and good outcomes.

Orlando's theory is specific to nurse-patient interactions. The goal of the nurse is to determine and meet patients' immediate needs and to improve their situation by relieving distress or discomfort. Orlando emphasized deliberate action (rather than automatic action) based on observation of the patients' verbal and nonverbal behavior, which leads to inferences. Inferences are confirmed or disconfirmed by the patient, leading the nurse to identify the patients' needs and provide effective nursing care.

Using Orlando's theory in practice

As a nursing practice theory, Orlando's theory specified how patients are involved in nurses' decision making. When used in practice, Orlando's theory guides interactions to predictable outcomes, which are different from outcomes that occur when the theory is not used. Nurses individualize care for each patient by attending to behavior, confirming with the patient ideas and inferences the nurse draws from interactions, and identifying pressing needs.

Use of Orlando's theory improves the effectiveness of the nurse. It might be said that the nurse gets to the bottom line more quickly when observing, listening to, and confirming with patients. Therefore, use of this theory saves time and energy for both the patient and the nurse. An excellent example of the use of Orlando's theory in nursing practice may be found in Schmieding (2002).

Leininger's Theory of Culture Care Diversity and Universality

The work of **Madeleine Leininger** (1978, 1991) in cultural care grew out of her early nursing experiences. She observed that children of different cultures had widely varying behaviors and needs. After discussing the parallels between nursing and anthropology with the famed anthropologist Margaret Mead, Leininger pursued doctoral study in cultural anthropology. Through her doctoral work she became more convinced about the relationship of cultural differences and health practices. This led her to begin developing a theory of cultural care for nursing.

Leininger's work is formalized as a theory rather than as a conceptual model. It has stimulated the formation of the Transcultural Nursing Society, transcultural nursing conferences, newsletters, the *Journal of Transpersonal Caring,* and the awarding of master's degrees in the specialty area known as transcultural nursing.

Transcultural nursing's goal involves more than simply being aware of different cultures. It involves planning nursing care based on knowledge that is culturally defined, classified, and tested—and then used to provide care that is culturally congruent (Leininger, 1978).

Leininger described theory as a creative and systematic way of discovering new knowledge or accounting for phenomena in a more complete way (Leininger, 1991). She encouraged nurses to use creativity to discover cultural aspects of human needs and use these findings to make culturally congruent therapeutic decisions. Her theory is broad, since it considers the impact of culture on all aspects of human life, with particular attention to health and caring practices.

As global migration continues and all societies become more diverse, Leininger's theory is more relevant than ever before.

Using Leininger's theory in practice

Leininger specified caring as the essence of nursing, and nurses who use Leininger's theory of cultural care in their practices view patients in the context of their cultures. Practice from a cultural perspective begins by respecting the culture of the patient and recognizing the importance of its relationship to nursing care. Use of the "sunrise model" (Figure 11-2) guides the assessment of cultural data for an understanding of its influence in the patient's life (Leininger, 1991). The nurse plans nursing care, recognizing the health beliefs and folk practices of the patient's culture as well as the culture of traditional health services. To this end, nursing care is then focused on culture care preservation, accommodations, or repatterning, depending on the patient's need. The nursing outcome of culturally congruent nursing care is health and well-being for the patient. Case applications of Leininger's theory in nursing practice may be found in Morgan (2002).

Newman's Theory of Health as Expanding Consciousness

Margaret Newman (1986, 1994) developed a theory of health derived from Rogers' Science of Unitary Human Beings. She focused on pattern and the life process to come to a new understanding of health and illness. Newman proposed a redefinition of health based on the original concept of wholeness. She saw health not as something apart from the person, as in "How is your health?" or as something to be gotten over, as with an illness, but as a manifestation of the person's pattern of wholeness. As such, she proposed health as a manifestation of each person's wholeness: something to be understood progressively over time. She sought to design a means

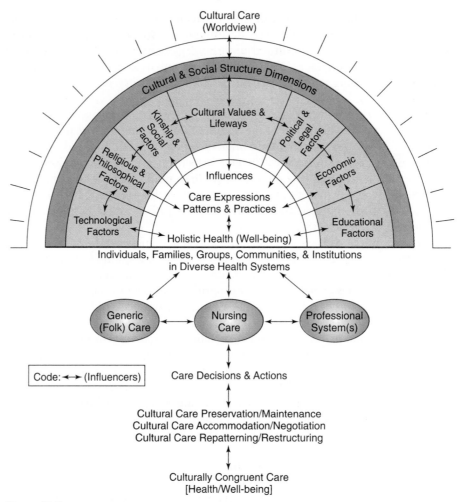

Figure 11-2
Leininger's sunrise model, created to facilitate the application in practice of the Theory of
Culture Care Diversity and Universality. (Courtesy Dr. Madeleine Leininger.)

of recognizing the pattern of whole persons and their expanding consciousness
throughout the process of life.

Using Newman's theory in practice

When using Newman's theory in nursing practice, the nurse's goal is to form meaningful relationships with patients and participate in their use of inner strengths as they
move through higher and higher levels of consciousness (Fawcett, 2000; Newman,
1986, 1994). Newman (1994) emphasized viewing patients in the context of their
holistic patterns, or "pattern of the whole." Patients' perceptions of time are assessed
in relation to their movement in space and time.

Newman's inclusive view incorporates all aspects of the person's process of living. Illness and disease are understood as they are revealed in the patient's pattern. The nurse participates with patients toward this goal: to establish relationships to facilitate the discovery of their inner strength as consciousness of their pattern unfolds. Health emerges from the patient's improved consciousness of life processes. See Witucki (2002) for excellent examples of the application of Newman's theory in nursing practice.

Parse's Theory of Human Becoming

The work of **Rosemarie Parse** was first published as "theory of man-living-health" (1981) and later renamed "theory of human becoming" (1992). Parse derived her theory from two main sources: Martha Rogers' Science of Unitary Human Beings and existential phenomenology. Therefore, like Rogers, Parse viewed nursing as participation with the patient. Her work focused on the importance of health throughout life. She emphasized the nursing profession's history of focusing on health and contrasted that with the medical profession's history of treating illness and disease.

According to Parse, health is a cocreation with the universe as patients experience the being and becoming of life. Parse described this process (which, like Rogers' model, is acausal) in three existential phenomenological principles: The first principle proposed human meaning as a developing structure of valuing and imaging from which reality emerges through languaging; the second principle proposed a patterned unity of person and universe in rhythm of human behavioral patterns of revealing-concealing, enabling-limiting, and connecting-separating; the third principle proposed cotranscendence as the human capacity to grow (become) in process with the universe. She described transcendence as a rhythmical process originating from the intents and purposes of one's activity as the possibilities become realities (Parse, 1981).

Using Parse's theory in practice

Nursing practice with Parse's theory involves participation with the patient. Within the relationship the nurse gains a perspective of the patient in the universe, being and becoming. This theory does not view nursing practice as an adjunct to medicine. Rather, nursing is seen as a profession in its own right focused on human becoming and health. The three principles help the nurse to recognize patient patterns and participate with patients in their becoming. Mitchell (2002) presents a most engaging description and application of Parse's theory in nursing practice.

THEORETICAL CHALLENGES FOR NURSING EDUCATION, PRACTICE, AND RESEARCH

These examples of nursing theoretical works illustrate the vital role theory plays in nursing education, practice, and research. To continue the forward movement of nursing and to improve the quality of nursing care, theory-based practice, theory testing, and theory-generating research are required. Sound curricula based on nursing knowledge are essential.

Theory-Based Education

The nursing profession has grown exponentially throughout the theory development era. Schools of nursing have proliferated, preparing nurses from the associate degree level to the PhD level. Nurses prepared at each level of nursing are involved with nursing theory, as noted in Box 11-7.

The nursing profession has evolved from an applied vocation dependent on knowledge from other disciplines to its current stage of development, with its own knowledge base. This period of growth has stimulated—and been stimulated by—the development of the nursing PhD, a research degree that requires the generation of new, discipline-specific knowledge.

At the doctoral level nurses are concerned with the philosophy of science—that is, the nature of knowledge and how it is known; philosophy of nursing science and the generation of nursing knowledge; theory testing; and the development of new theory through research. The master's level nurse may be a primary provider in advanced practice, going beyond the generic nursing process. Master's-level nurses use theoretical perspectives focused on the patient for specific nursing outcomes. Many nurses conduct their first research studies as master's students, and they are focused on nursing practice and the testing of nursing interventions with specific patient groups.

The baccalaureate nurse is introduced to the research process and the use of theory to guide it. The research emphasis for baccalaureate-level students is on learning to critique nursing research, to become informed consumers of research relevant to nursing practice. Many curricula of bachelor's of science in nursing programs are based on a selected nursing theoretical perspective; others introduce students to a variety of nursing theoretical perspectives. Whether the curriculum is built around one or many nursing theoretical works, the focus for the baccalaureate level is utilization and application of nursing theory as a guide for nursing practice.

Box 11-7 Levels of Education and Use of Nursing Theory

Level of Nursing Education	Use of Nursing Theory
PhD in nursing	Conducts theory testing and theory development research for nursing science development; frames practice, administration, or research in nursing works
Master of science in nursing	Frames advanced practice with a nursing model or theory; uses theory to guide research with practice questions
Bachelor of science in nursing	Learns the nursing perspective in a nursing model or theory-based curriculum or courses; uses models, theories, and middle-range theories to guide nursing practice
Associate degree in nursing	May have a nursing model or theory-guided curriculum or courses; may be introduced to middle-range theories for nursing practice

The associate degree level of nursing education may also use nursing theoretical works to teach the unique perspectives of nursing. Nurses with associate degrees often find middle-range theories, which are specific to patient care, useful in their practice.

Basing nursing education on nursing theory not only benefits nursing students but also contributes to the growth of schools and colleges of nursing. Holding scholarly discussions about the application of nursing theory in education, research, and practice establishes an environment of critical thinking, imagining, questioning, and learning. Hosting theorists as guest lecturers helps students and faculty see the theorists in a realistic light, as persons with seminal knowledge of nursing. Programs featuring endowed distinguished lecturers draw audiences from campus and the surrounding nursing community for the opportunity to hear nursing theorists discuss their work in person. Figure 11-3 shows Dr. Madeleine Leininger, the 1999 Mary T. Boynton Distinguished Lecturer at the University of Tennessee, College of Nursing in Knoxville, pictured with Mary T. Boynton, the retired faculty member for whom the lecture series is named.

Theory-Based Practice

How is theory translated into practice? The answer to that question lies with theory-based practice. Theory-based practice occurs when nurses intentionally structure their practice around a particular nursing theory and use it to guide them as they

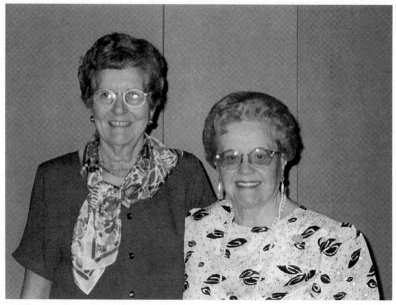

Figure **11-3**
Madeleine Leininger, RN, PhD, FAAN *(right)* and Mary T. Boynton at the 1999 nursing theorist lecture at the College of Nursing, The University of Tennessee, Knoxville. (Photo by Sally Helton, Courtesy the College of Nursing, University of Tennessee, Knoxville.)

assess, plan, diagnose, intervene, and evaluate nursing care. Theory provides a systematic way of thinking about nursing that is consistent and guides the decision making process as data are collected, analyzed, and used in the planning and administration of nursing practice. Theory empowers nurses to challenge the conventional views of patients, illness, the health care delivery system, and traditional nursing interventions.

As this chapter on nursing theory comes to a conclusion, we hope that these introductions to various nursing theoretical works will lead you to identify works that resonate with your values and that you will select one or two for in-depth study. With increased understanding you will develop the use of nursing theory in your practice. Many benefits are gained from theory-based practice. First, you will be able to explain your practice to other members of the health care team. That is, nursing theory provides language for you to explain what you do, how you do it, and why you do it. Second, this language of practice facilitates the transmission of nursing knowledge to you as students who are new to the profession, as well as to other health professionals. Third, theory contributes to professional autonomy by providing a nursing-based guide for practice, education, and research. Finally, nursing theory develops your analytical skills, challenges your thinking, and clarifies your values and assumptions (Holder and Chitty, 1997).

Many nurses have developed their own ideas about nursing and continue to develop nursing assumptions based on education, experience, observation, and reading. Most nurses do not formally develop their own personal theories, even though their ideas certainly influence the way they practice nursing. According to Wardle and Mandle (1989), who studied nurses who think that their own ideas of practice are "their theories," nurses' personal theories tend to be incomplete and inconsistent as a basis for nursing practice. When you rely on your personal ideas as a basis for practice or when faculty members use their own ideas as a "framework for curricula," the outcome is ineffective. Wardle and Mandle recommended using a theory that has been tested or developed through nursing research and critiqued, analyzed, and evaluated for usefulness in nursing practice. Each of the philosophies, models, and theories presented in this chapter meets their recommendation. Application of these works in your practice with specific patient groups is an opportunity to test middle-range theories. In addition, many practice areas and patient populations may be addressed in formalized middle-range theories (Alligood, 2002d).

As you engage in theory-based practice, remember to provide feedback to nurse researchers and theorists concerning your experiences. You can do this through the Internet, where you will find groups of nurses using, discussing, and refining the theoretical works that have been discussed in this chapter. You can also assist these scholars and the discipline of nursing by developing manuscripts and submitting your experiences for publication, joining the many nurses who have discovered the benefits of theory-based practice.

Theory-Based Research

Great strides have been made in the last 25 years in nursing research. The expansion of graduate nursing education at the master's level and the proliferation of nursing doctoral programs played a major role, as more nurses than ever before were equipped with the knowledge and skills to conduct research. Nursing research tests and refines the knowledge base of nursing. Ultimately, research findings enable nurses to improve the quality of care and understand how nursing actions influence patient outcomes.

Research is vital to the future of nursing, and theory is integral to research. Historically, an emphasis on method has overshadowed the subject of our research and the theory for developing nursing knowledge. In addition, many nurses have continued to use theories that address the phenomena of other disciplines—theories that do not view persons holistically or provide a nursing perspective. Therefore, the outcome of their research is often valued by adjunct disciplines as much as by the discipline of nursing. However, more and more nurse researchers have come to understand the vital role of nursing theory in their research for knowledge development in their own discipline. These nurses are meeting the challenge of using nursing theory to structure nursing research that tests theory or that interprets the findings of qualitative research for theory development.

Chapter 12 is devoted to understanding the research process. It is important for nurses to recognize that theory, nursing practice, and research are interrelated. Each of these components stimulates, improves, and advances the others. An example of how nurses used theory as a framework for research that contributed knowledge to nursing practice is presented in the Research Note on p. 294.

Summary of Key Points

- Theory development is not a mysterious activity restricted to a few nursing scholars. It is an activity that combines education, knowledge, and skill in a sustained effort.
- Nursing philosophies, models, and theories offer many perspectives on nursing, varying in their levels of abstraction and their definitions of four major concepts: person, environment, health, and nursing.
- As nurses devise theories of nursing, present them for review by their colleagues in a peer review process, publish them in the nursing literature, and test their efficacy in nursing practice, the discipline moves forward in the development of its unique knowledge base.
- Scholarly contributions may be made by nurses at every level of educational preparation. To the extent that nurses question, read, study, network, and write about nursing practice, they contribute to the development of nursing knowledge.
- Nurses in practice settings have invaluable insights and observations, thereby contributing to the knowledge base for nursing. Nursing theorists rely on practicing nurses to test clinical interventions and explore the usefulness of their theories.
- Clinical research requires the support of practicing nurses who recognize the importance of theory-based practice and research. Nurses contribute to the development of the profession by participating in research studies when possible and supporting research in practice settings.
- Nurse theorists whose works were reviewed in this chapter, as well as others too numerous to include, have made significant contributions to the development of the unique body of nursing knowledge.

RESEARCH note

A Study Illustrating the Interrelationship of Theory, Research, and Practice

Even though breast cancer is the leading cause of cancer mortality in African-American women, fewer than half of these women who are older than 50 years report ever having had a mammogram and breast examination. Two thirds report not practicing regular breast self-examination. Puzzled by these findings, Brown and Williams used Leininger's Culture Care Theory and the Health Belief Model to explore factors that prevented these women from using screening services.

According to Leininger's work, African-Americans value extended family networks, religious values, interdependence with other African-Americans, daily survival, folk foods, and folk-healing modes. The five variables of the Health Belief Model are susceptibility, seriousness, benefits, barriers, and health motivation.

After an extensive literature review, the researchers determined that some barriers to breast screening programs experienced by older African-American women were unique to their culture, whereas others were shared with all older women. Some barriers they identified that were unique to the African-American culture included heightened fear of cancer, underestimating its incidence, pessimism about cure, lack of awareness of screening tests, and use of a lay referral system that may delay treatment. In common with other older women, they attributed breast changes to age, were embarrassed, lacked knowledge about mammogram and breast self-examination, and believed that screening programs were too much trouble, inconvenient, or unnecessary. In addition, African-American individuals thought that health care providers were insensitive to their cultural and social needs.

Several guidelines for practice were identified as a result of this literature review. Nurses may:

- Encourage the use of screening methods daily in their interactions with older African-American women.
- Reduce expenses by planning reduced-cost services.
- Increase the availability and accessibility of screening programs by using mobile units and community sites during evening and weekend hours.
- Plan and implement breast health educational programs using culturally sensitive materials.
- Work with African-American community leaders to promote breast cancer screening.

Adapted with permission of Brown LW, Williams RD: Culturally sensitive breast cancer screening programs for older black women, *Nurse Pract* 19(3):21, 25-26, 31, 35, 1994. ©Springhouse Corporation *(www.springnet.com).*

- Nurse scholars continue to develop and refine the works of the nursing theorists. Each theoretical work has a community of scholars (Kuhn, 1970) who use the work in their research and practice and continue to expand, clarify, and refine these original works (Alligood and Tomey, 2002; Fawcett, 2000; Tomey and Alligood, 2002).

CRITICAL THINKING QUESTIONS

1. Recognizing that your understanding of the theoretical works of nursing is only beginning, which works introduced in this chapter appeal to you the most? Which ones describe nursing in the way you think about it? What is it about these works that intrigues you?
2. Which of the theoretical works seem the most useful to help you organize your thoughts for critical thinking and decision making in nursing practice?
3. Interview two practicing nurses and ask them which nursing philosophies, models, or theories have influenced their thinking and practice of nursing.
4. Describe the use of nursing theory for nurses at your current level of nursing education.
5. Explain why theory development is important to the profession of nursing.

REFERENCES

Alligood MR: Theory of goal attainment: application to adult orthopedic nursing. In Frey MA, Sieloff C, editors: *Advancing King's systems framework and theory,* Thousand Oaks, CA, 1995, Sage Publications, pp 209-222.

Alligood MR: The nature of knowledge needed for nursing practice. In Alligood MR, Tomey AM, editors: *Nursing theory: utilization and application,* ed 2, St. Louis, 2002a, Mosby, pp 3-14.

Alligood MR: Nursing models: normal science for nursing practice. In Alligood MR, Tomey AM, editors: *Nursing theory: utilization and application,* ed 2, St. Louis, 2002b, Mosby, pp 15-39.

Alligood MR: Philosophies, models and theories: critical thinking structures. In Alligood MR, Tomey AM, editors: *Nursing theory: utilization and application,* ed 2, St. Louis, 2002c, Mosby, pp 41-61.

Alligood MR: Areas for further development of theory-based nursing practice. In Alligood MR, Tomey AM, editors: *Nursing theory: utilization and application,* ed 2, St. Louis, 2002d, Mosby, pp 453-463.

Alligood MR: A Theory of the art of nursing discovered in Rogers' Science of Unitary Human Beings, *Int J Hum Caring* 6(2):55-60, 2002e.

Alligood MR, Choi EC: Evolution of nursing theory development. In Tomey AM, Alligood MR, editors: *Nursing theorists and their work,* ed 3, St. Louis, 1998, Mosby, pp 55-66.

Alligood MR, May BA: A nursing theory of personal system empathy: interpreting a conceptualization of empathy in King's Interacting Systems, *Nurs Sci Q* 13(3):243-247, 2000.

Alligood MR, Tomey AM: *Nursing theory: utilization and application,* ed 2, St. Louis, 2002, Mosby.

Alligood MR, Tomey AM: *Nursing theory: utilization and application,* St. Louis, 1997, Mosby.

Barrett E: *Visions of Rogers' science-based nursing,* New York, 1990, National League for Nursing.

Benner PM, Hooper-Kyriakidis P, Stannard D: *Clinical wisdom and interventions in critical care: a thinking-in-action approach,* Philadelphia, 1999, WB Saunders.

Benner P: *From novice to expert: excellence and power in clinical nursing practice,* Menlo Park, CA, 1984, Addison-Wesley.

Berbiglia V: Orem's self-care deficit theory in nursing practice. In Alligood MR, Tomey AM, editors: *Nursing theory: utilization and application,* ed 2, St. Louis, 2002, Mosby, pp 239-266.

Brown LW, Williams RD: Culturally sensitive breast cancer screening programs for older black women, *Nurse Pract* 19(3):21, 25-26, 31, 35, 1994.

Bultemeier K: Rogers' science of unitary human beings in nursing practice. In Alligood MR, Tomey AM, editors: *Nursing theory: utilization and application,* ed 2, St. Louis, 2002, Mosby, pp 267-288.

Chinn P, Kramer M: *Theory and nursing: a systematic approach,* ed 5, St. Louis, 1998, Mosby.

Fawcett J: *Analysis and evaluation of contemporary nursing knowledge: models and theories,* Philadelphia, 2000, FA Davis.

Fawcett J: Conceptual models of nursing, nursing theories, and nursing practice: future directions. In Alligood MR, Tomey AM, editors: *Nursing theory: utilization and application,* ed 2, St. Louis, 2002, Mosby, pp 465-481.

Fitzpatrick J, Whall A: *Conceptual models of nursing: analysis and application,* ed 3, Norwalk, CT, 1996, Appleton & Lange.

Norris D, Frey MA: King's systems framework and theory in nursing practice. In Alligood MR, Tomey AM, editors: *Nursing theory: utilization and application,* ed 2, St. Louis, 2002, Mosby, pp 173-196.

Frey MA, Sieloff CL: *Advancing King's systems framework and theory for nursing,* Thousand Oaks, CA, 1995, Sage Publications.

George JB: editor: *Nursing theories: the base for professional nursing practice,* ed 5, Norwalk, CT, 2002, Appleton & Lange.

Henderson V: *The nature of nursing: a definition and its implications for practice, research, and education,* New York, 1996, Macmillan.

Holaday B: Johnson's behavioral system model in nursing practice. In Alligood MR, Tomey AM, editors: *Nursing theory: utilization and application,* ed 2, St. Louis, 2002, Mosby, pp 149-171.

Holder PJ, Chitty KK: Theory as a basis for professional nursing. In Chitty KK, editor: *Professional nursing: concepts and challenges,* ed 2, Philadelphia, 1997, WB Saunders.

Johnson D: *One conceptual model for nursing,* Paper presented in Nashville, TN, 1968, Vanderbilt University.

Johnson D: The behavioral systems model for nursing. In Riehl J, Roy C, editors: *Conceptual models for nursing practice,* ed 2, New York, 1980, Appleton-Century-Croft, pp 207-216.

King IM: *A theory for nursing: systems, concepts, process,* New York, 1981, John Wiley & Sons.

Kuhn TS: *The structure of scientific revolutions,* ed 2, Chicago, 1970, University of Chicago Press.

Leininger M: *Transcultural nursing: concepts, theories, and practices,* New York, 1978, John Wiley & Sons.

Leininger M, *Culture care diversity and universality: a theory of nursing,* New York, 1991, National League for Nursing.

Levine M: *Introduction to clinical nursing,* ed 2, Philadelphia, 1973, FA Davis.

Levine M: The conservation model: a model for health. In Schaefer KM, Pond JB, editors: *The conservation model: a framework for nursing practice,* Philadelphia, 1991, FA Davis, pp 1-11.

Madrid M, Barrett EAM: *Rogers' scientific art of nursing practice,* New York, 1994, National League for Nursing.

McEwin M, Wills EM: *Theoretical basis for nursing,* Philadelphia, 2002, Lippincott Williams & Wilkins.

Meleis A: *Theoretical nursing: development and progress,* ed 3, Philadelphia, 1997, JB Lippincott.

Mitchell GJ: Parse's theory of human becoming in nursing practice. In Alligood MR, Tomey AM, editors: *Nursing theory: utilization and application,* ed 2, St. Louis, 2002, Mosby, pp 403-428.

Morgan MG: Leininger's theory of culture care diversity and universality in nursing practice. In Alligood MR, Tomey AM, editors: *Nursing theory: utilization and application,* ed 2, St. Louis, 2002, Mosby, pp 385-402.

Neuman B, Fawcett J: *The Neuman Systems Model,* ed 4, Upper Saddle River, NJ, 2001, Prentice Hall.

Newman M: *Health as expanding consciousness,* St. Louis, 1986, Mosby.

Newman M: *Health as expanding consciousness,* ed 2, New York, 1994, National League for Nursing.

Nightingale F: Notes on nursing: what it is and what it is not, New York, 1969, Dover Publications (originally published in 1859).

Orem D: *Nursing: concepts of practice,* ed 6, St. Louis, 2001, Mosby.

Orlando I: *The dynamic nurse-patient relationship: function, process and principles,* New York, 1990, National League for Nursing (originally published in 1961).

Parker M: *Nursing theories and nursing practice,* Philadelphia, 2001, FA Davis.

Parse RR: *Man-living-health: a theory for nursing,* New York, 1981, John Wiley & Sons.

Parse RR: Human becoming: Parse's theory of nursing, *Nurs Sci Q* 5(1):35-42, 1992.

Phillips KD: Roy's adaptation model in nursing practice. In Alligood MR, Tomey AM, editors: *Nursing theory: utilization and application,* ed 2, St. Louis, 2002, Mosby, pp 289-314.

Powers BA, Knapp TR: *A dictionary of nursing theory and research,* ed 2, Thousand Oaks, CA, 1995, Sage.

Renpenning KM, Taylor SG: *Self-care theory in nursing,* New York, 2003, Springer.

Rogers M: *An introduction to the theoretical basis of nursing,* Philadelphia, 1970, FA Davis.

Rogers M: Nursing science and the space age, *Nurs Sci Q* 5(1):27-34, 1992.

Roy C Sr: Adaptation: a conceptual framework for nursing, *Nurs Outlook* 18(3):42-45, 1970.

Roy C Sr, Andrews HA: *The Roy adaptation model: the definitive statement,* Norwalk, CT, 1991, Appleton & Lange.

Roy C Sr, Andrews HA: *The Roy adaptation model,* ed 2, Norwalk, CT, 1999, Appleton & Lange.

Schaefer KM: Levine's conservation model in nursing practice. In Alligood MR, Tomey AM, editors: *Nursing theory: utilization and application,* ed 2, St. Louis, 2002, Mosby, pp 197-217.

Schaefer KM, Pond JB: *The conservation model: a framework for practice,* Philadelphia, 1991, FA Davis.

Schmeiding NJ: Orlando's nursing process theory in nursing practice. In Alligood MR, Tomey AM, editors: *Nursing theory: utilization and application,* ed 2, St. Louis, 2002, Mosby, pp 325-337.

Sohier R: Neuman's systems model in nursing practice. In Alligood MR, Tomey AM, editors: *Nursing theory: utilization and application,* ed 2, St. Louis, 2002, Mosby, pp 219-238.

Tomey AM, Alligood MR: *Nursing theorists and their work,* ed 5, St. Louis, 2002, Mosby.

Wardle MG, Mandle CL: Conceptual models used in clinical practice, *West J Nurs Res* 11(1):108-114, 1989.

Watson J: *Postmodern nursing and beyond,* Edinburgh, 1999, Churchill Livingstone/WB Saunders/Harcourt Health Sciences.

Watson J: *Nursing: human science and human care,* New York, 1988, National League for Nursing.

Watson J: *Nursing: the philosophy and science of caring,* Boston, 1979, Little, Brown.

Witucki J: Newman's theory of health as expanding consciousness in nursing practice. In Alligood MR, Tomey AM, editors: *Nursing theory: utilization and application,* ed 2, St. Louis, 2002, Mosby, pp 429-449.

12

The Scientific Method, Nursing Research, and Evidence-Based Practice

Carol T. Bush

Key Terms

Applied Science
Conceptual Framework
Confidentiality
Data
Deductive Reasoning
Disseminate
Ethnographic Research
Evidence-Based Practice
Experimental Design
Generalizable
Holistic Nursing
Hypothesis

Inductive Reasoning
Informed Consent
Institutional Review Board
Nonexperimental
  Design
Nursing Research
Peer Review
Phenomena
Phenomenological Research
Population
Problem Solving
Protocol

Pure Science
Qualitative Research
Quantitative Research
Reliable
Replicate
Research Process
Research Question
Sample
Scientific Method
Subjects
Valid

Learning Outcomes

After studying this chapter, students will be able to:

- Differentiate between pure and applied science.
- Describe the historical development of the scientific method.
- Give examples of inductive and deductive reasoning.
- Discuss the limitations of the scientific method when applied to nursing.
- Differentiate between problem solving and research.
- List the steps in the research process.
- Describe the phases in the design of a qualitative study.
- Discuss contributions nursing research has made to nursing practice and to health care.
- Describe the relationship of nursing research to nursing theory and practice.

- Identify sources of support for nursing research.
- Discuss the roles of nurses in research.
- Define evidence-based practice.
- Differentiate between research and evidence-based practice.
- Discuss the pros and cons of evidence-based practice in nursing.

In the 1960s, the nursing profession was poised on the threshold of a higher level of development. It was recognized that mature professions had strong scientific bases, which were lacking in nursing. Nursing scholars realized that nursing could achieve its potential and desired professional status only to the extent that the discipline was based on a scientifically derived body of knowledge unique to nursing. As a result of that recognition, nursing researchers set about developing knowledge, and nursing theorists began developing theories and testing them.

About the same time, nurses realized that a similar professionalization of patient care practices was needed. Using traditional methods to deal with familiar patient problems and relying on trial and error or intuition to deal with unfamiliar ones were no longer seen as acceptable ways to care for patients and move the profession toward evidence-based practice. Practitioners of nursing, therefore, also developed a more scientific approach to patient care that is an adaptation of the classic scientific method. This problem-solving approach is called the nursing process and is presented in more depth in Chapter 15. An understanding of the scientific method is helpful in appreciating both nursing research and the nursing process.

SCIENCE AND THE SCIENTIFIC METHOD

The study of any subject by using the **scientific method** or other methods of reasoning can be considered science. The scientific method is an orderly, systematic way of thinking about and solving problems. It has been used by scientists for centuries to discover and test facts and principles. When used under carefully planned and controlled conditions, the scientific method becomes research. The scientific method is the same, regardless of the discipline using it.

Pure and Applied Science and Research

Scientists divide scientific knowledge into two categories: pure and applied. **Pure science** or pure research, sometimes called basic science or basic research, summarizes and explains the universe without regard for whether the information is immediately useful. When Joseph Priestly discovered oxygen in 1774, he did not have an immediate use for that information. Therefore, that discovery could be classified as pure science—that is, information gathered solely for the sake of obtaining new knowledge. **Applied science** or applied research seeks to *use* scientific theory and laws in some practical way. The use of oxygen in caring for premature infants is an example of applied science. The testing of this method to refine treatment guidelines is applied research. From this example, it can be seen that today's pure science can become tomorrow's applied science. Nursing makes use of applied scientific principles and is most effective in conducting applied research to improve patient outcomes through nursing care.

History of the Scientific Method

In Western cultures, until the time of Hippocrates (ca. 460-377 B.C.), illness was believed to be caused by evil spirits. Gradually, over the years and through the efforts of many scientists, humankind has learned a great deal about the human body, health, and illness. Most of this knowledge was developed after the scientific method came into widespread use.

A period of great intellectual activity, known as the Age of Reason, began in the 1600s and lasted until the late 1700s. During that time, scientists, by using reason and experimentation, made unparalleled advances in understanding the laws by which nature operates. Galileo (1564-1642), the Italian physicist and astronomer, and Sir Isaac Newton (1642-1727), the English philosopher and mathematician, are usually credited with developing and refining the scientific method. A scientific revolution and technological explosion resulted from the use of the scientific method. In the area of health care alone, profound and far-reaching scientific discoveries have changed human life dramatically. Selected important scientific discoveries related to health are listed in Box 12-1.

Each era has been characterized by scientific advances. For example, the 1990s became known as the "Decade of the Brain," with impressive findings such as brain scans illustrating differences between the brains of persons with mental illness and substance abuse addictions and those of so-called normal persons. The future looks bright for continuation of brain-related research, which may someday unlock the secrets of human behavior. The National Institute of Nursing Research (NINR) is a member of the Council of Federal Liaisons. This group has endorsed the initiative "Decade of Behavior: 2000-2010," which highlights contributions already made by the behavioral and social sciences in addressing national challenges in health, education, and safety and potential future advances. You can learn more about the NINR's activities in this important area of research online *(www.decadeof-behavior.org/people.html)*.

Inductive and Deductive Reasoning

The scientific method requires the use of two types of logic: inductive and deductive reasoning. In **inductive reasoning,** the process begins with a particular experience and proceeds to generalizations. Repeated observations of an experiment or event enable the observer to draw general conclusions. For example, the statement "All the St. Bernard dogs I have encountered are gentle; therefore, St. Bernards are gentle" is an example of inductive reasoning. It is obvious from this example that this type of logic leads to probabilities—not certainties—unless the world's entire population of St. Bernard dogs is observed.

Scientists also use **deductive reasoning,** a process through which conclusions are drawn by logical inference from given premises. Deductive reasoning proceeds from the general case to the specific. For example, if the premises "All schoolchildren like chocolate" and "Missie is a schoolchild" are accepted, the conclusion

Box 12-1	Important Health-Related Events in the Evolution of Science
ca. 400 B.C.	Hippocrates taught that diseases have natural, not supernatural, causes.
100 A.D.	Galen laid the foundation for the study of anatomy and physiology.
ca. 1500	Leonardo da Vinci recognized the importance of observation and experimentation in learning.
1543	Andreas Vesalius published a book on human anatomy, based on observation.
1628	William Harvey published his theory on the circulation of blood.
1774	Joseph Priestly discovered oxygen.
ca. 1796	Edward Jenner discovered a method of smallpox vaccination.
1839	Matthias Schleiden and Theodor Schwann developed the theory that all living things are composed of cells.
1866	Gregor Mendel demonstrated the laws of heredity.
ca. 1876	Louis Pasteur demonstrated that microorganisms cause fermentation and disease.
1882	Robert Koch isolated the bacterium that causes tuberculosis.
1895	Wilhelm K. Roentgen discovered x-rays.
1898	Marie and Pierre Curie isolated the element radium.
ca. 1900	Paul Ehrlich originated chemotherapy, the treatment of diseases with chemicals (drugs).
1928	Alexander Fleming discovered penicillin.
1953	Jonas Salk developed the first effective polio vaccine.
1957	Arthur Karnberg grew deoxyribonucleic acid (DNA), the basic component of genes, in a test tube.
1978	The world's first test tube baby was delivered.
1982	William DeVries implanted the world's first artificial heart.
1989	The first authorized use of genetic engineering, injecting genetically altered cells into patients with malignant melanoma, was undertaken.
1998	A team of Scottish scientists, led by Dr. Ian Wilmut, reported the first successful cloning of an adult mammal, resulting in Dolly, the world's most famous sheep.
2003	The Human Genome Project ended with the successful completion of the human genetic sequence.

From Kuhn TS: The structure of scientific revolutions. In Nurath O, editor: *International encyclopedia of unified science*, ed 2, vol 2, Chicago, 1970, University of Chicago Press; Ware CF, Panikkar KM, Romein JM: *The twentieth century: history of mankind, cultural and scientific development*, vol 6, New York, 1966, Harper & Row; and *Time Magazine*, Online (*www.time.com/time/newsfiles/cloning/*).

"Missie likes chocolate" can be drawn. It may be entirely possible, however, that Missie, although a schoolchild, does not like chocolate at all. In deductive reasoning, the premises used must be correct or the conclusions will not be. Conclusions drawn through deductive processes are called valid rather than true. **Valid** is a term meaning "soundly founded," whereas true means "in accordance with the fact or reality" (Flexner, Stein, and Su, 1980). It is possible for a conclusion to be solidly founded without being true. There is a subtle but real difference in the two terms.

As seen by these examples, neither inductive nor deductive processes alone are adequate. If scientists used only deductive logic, experience would be ignored. If they used only inductive logic, relationships between facts and principles would be ignored. A combination of both types of reasoning processes in science unifies the theoretical and the practical, which is the basis for the scientific method and research.

Limitations of the Scientific Method in Nursing

Polit and Beck (2004, p. 16) asserted that the "traditional scientific approach used by quantitative researchers has enjoyed considerable stature as a method of inquiry and it has been used productively by nurse researchers studying a wide range of nursing problems. This is not to say, however, that this approach can solve all nursing problems." Many authorities believe that the use of any other method should be avoided. There are at least four reasons, however, why the scientific method has limitations when applied to nursing.

The first and most obvious drawback is that health care settings are not comparable to laboratories. There are realities and priorities operating in health care settings that must take precedence over laboratory protocols. The safety and security of human patients are of the utmost importance and cannot be jeopardized.

Second, human beings are far more than collections of parts that can be dissected and subjected to examination or experimentation. A strength of nursing is its ability to view patients holistically, whereas the basis of the scientific method is to divide a problem into manageable problem statements, each of which can be tested. Because humans are complex organisms with interrelated parts and systems, the classic scientific method loses much of its usefulness.

A third limitation of the scientific method as the only approach to solving patient problems is its objectivity; it fails to consider the meaning of patients' own experiences, that is, their subjective view of reality. Nurses are keenly aware that patients' perceptions of their experiences, or subjective data, are just as important as objective data.

Finally, there are definite ethical implications involved in experimenting with humans that make reliance on the scientific method impractical. The rights of human subjects in research are paramount, as discussed elsewhere in this chapter. Research on the influence of prayer in health care of patients and their families is an example of research that cannot be done with a strictly scientific method. Research Note 1 provides examples of nursing research on the role of prayer in healing and health care.

NURSING RESEARCH BASED ON THE SCIENTIFIC METHOD

For many undergraduates their only exposure to research is in introductory psychology or sociology courses, in which they may be subjects in a professor's research project. In these cases, all they see of research are the boring forms they fill out or the nonsense syllables they memorize. This kind of orientation leads them to wonder what research has to do with their ability to care for patients.

Before students of nursing write off research altogether, they should consider the value of a different kind of research—patient care research. The National Institute of Nursing Research (NINR) "seeks to understand and ease the symptoms of acute and chronic illness, to prevent or delay the onset of disease or disability or slow its progression, to find effective approaches to achieving and sustaining good health, and

---

RESEARCH note 1

Nursing Research on the Role of Prayer in Healing and Health Care

Nurses are recognizing the importance of spirituality, including prayer, in the way patients respond to their illnesses and to the illnesses of loved ones. Some examples include:

- The role of prayer for nurses who practice **holistic nursing.** Addressing the spirituality needs of the patient is important. Prayer may also enrich the holistic nurse-client interaction (Lewis, 1996).
- A review of research articles and personal clinical experience were reported by Brown-Saltzman (1997). The conclusion was that prayer is a valuable component of care for patients who have cancer and for their families.
- Hawley and Irurita (1998) studied patients who had been discharged following coronary artery bypass graft surgery. They used a type of qualitative research known as **ethnographic research** using interviews. Seeking comfort through prayer had three stages: maintaining or reestablishing a relationship with God; making peace with God; and asking God to be with them during the hospitalization.
- A critical analysis of the literature was done by Meraviglia (1999). The finding was that prayer and meaning in life can be used as indicators of spirituality.
- Intercessory prayer was found to have positive effects on persons with rheumatoid arthritis. It is interesting to note, however, that distant prayer had no measurable effect. Williams (2002) concluded that nurses should be educated on the potential benefits of prayer.
- Another study with patients with cancer was conducted by Taylor and Outlaw (2002). They used phenomenological methods of qualitative research to observe a range of approaches to prayer and topics for prayer. Suggestions were made for clinical practice and future research.

---

to improve the clinical settings in which care is provided. Nursing research involves clinical care in a variety of settings including the community and home in addition to more traditional health care sites" *(www.nih.gov/ninr/research/themes.doc)*.

For example, nurses are often the key to life or death for low-birth-weight infants. What do nurses need to know to tip the balance in favor of life for those babies? A group of researchers at the University of Pennsylvania, led by nurse Barbara Medoff-Cooper (Gibson, Medoff-Cooper, Nuama, et al., 1998; Medoff-Cooper, 2000; Medoff-Cooper, McGrath, and Bilker, 2000; Medoff-Cooper and Ray, 1995), has considered this question in studying neonatal sucking behaviors. According to these researchers, "Effective sucking behaviors or feeding is not only a prerequisite for survival, but also implies that an infant has achieved the neurologic, behavioral, and physiologic maturity required for safe, effective oral feeding" (Medoff-Cooper and Ray, 1995, p. 195). Their finding that for premature or sick infants breast-feeding is easier and requires less energy expenditure than bottle-feeding is important in infant care.

Then there is the question of pacifiers—are they useful or harmful? Known in the research literature as "nonnutritive sucking," pacifier usage for 5 minutes before feeding has been demonstrated to increase the time infants are awake. This knowledge provided the basis for nurses to experiment with giving pacifiers to infants who were being tube-fed. The use of the pacifier was found to help the tube-fed infants move more rapidly to normal oral feedings (Medoff-Cooper and Ray, 1995). Another group studied neonates given sucrose-dipped pacifiers to determine whether the pain from certain procedures (such as heel sticks to obtain blood samples) would be somewhat ameliorated (Gibbins, Stevens, Hodnett, et al., 2002; Gibbins, Stevens, Asztalos, et al., 2003; Stevens, Johnson, Franch, et al., 1999).

Another nurse researcher, Dr. Patricia Becker of the University of Wisconsin, has also studied low-birth-weight infants and the stress they experience during routine feeding, bathing, and intrusive procedures in neonatal intensive care units (NICUs). Her findings are expected to change NICU care-giving routines, thereby reducing complications and improving weight gain (Becker, Grunwald, Moorman, et al., 1993; Becker and Grunwald, 2000). The sooner the infants gain weight, the sooner they can be discharged to their homes and families. From these examples, it is easily seen that studying newborn behavior yields a great deal of useful information that can improve nursing care and ultimately improve the health of infants. This is only one area in which evidence-based nursing practice benefits patients.

Another example of nursing research that makes a difference in health care is the study of falls in geriatric patients. Some older persons lose strength in their lower extremities or lose their balance from time to time, leading to hip fractures and other injuries suffered during falls. Fractures can be set and hips surgically replaced, but it would be better if older people did not fall.

Elizabeth McNeely, a nurse who specializes in working with older persons, collaborated with researchers from other disciplines to study falls in elderly individuals. A group of older persons were taught tai chi, a form of martial arts, to see whether they would fall less often than those who did not practice tai chi (Kutner, Barhart, Wolf, et al., 1997; Wolf, Barnhart, Kutner, et al., 1996). The moves performed in tai chi exercises promote balance and strengthen muscles. When elderly people have better balance and greater strength, they are not as likely to fall, and they may avoid breaking bones. This study is expected to have an impact on the health of elderly persons in the future.

Another example is provided by nurses who work with children. These nurse researchers use imagery to decrease the nausea and vomiting of children receiving cancer treatment. Imagery, sometimes used in stress reduction exercises, involves creating positive mental images that counteract unpleasant experiences. The nurse researchers design individual imagery programs for the children with whom they work. They make a tape with the child's favorite music in the background and talk the patient into relaxing while listening to the music. For children who have a favorite recording artist, the nurses play that artist's recordings and talk the child through a sequence of pleasant mental images. Children who have cancer respond in a positive way to music and images to which they can relate and thereby tolerate their treatments better (Hockenberry, 1989, 2003).

The rest of this chapter describes some basic concepts of **nursing research.** The purpose is to introduce nursing research, demonstrate its merit, and provide a basic vocabulary. The ultimate goal is for nurses to participate in the research process and apply research findings to clinical practice. This is what is known as **evidence-based practice.**

WHAT IS NURSING RESEARCH?

Nursing research is the systematic investigation of **phenomena** (events or circumstances) related to improving nursing care. When nurses have a question that they believe must be answered to provide better care for patients, and they have the time, money, skill, and energy to study that question, they should do nursing research. Although the chosen research topic may be in a new area of investigation, much can be gained from choosing research problems that are connected to work already done. This builds nursing knowledge in an orderly way.

Research problems should be pursued if they meet all three of the following tests:
1. A conceptual framework exists; that is, the researcher's ideas about the problem fit logically and dovetail with what is already known about the topic.
2. The proposed research project is based on related research findings published in professional journals or is networked with similar ongoing research in other settings, thereby building nursing knowledge.
3. The proposed research is carefully designed so that the results will be applicable in similar situations.

In addition to building nursing knowledge, studies that build on previous work are more likely to receive financial support. Research is expensive and often requires funding beyond what one nurse, hospital, or university can supply. Nurses who want to do research usually find it necessary to obtain outside funding or compete with other aspiring researchers for limited internal (from within the agency) funding. Therefore, to receive funding, nurses must do research that interests others and that a funding agency is willing to support.

The agencies that fund nursing research look for ideas that build on and advance nursing knowledge. Thus, although nursing research may be broadly defined as anything that interests nurses and helps them provide better care, controversy exists over what can legitimately be included. When choosing a research question, the wise nurse researcher considers the practical issues of background and financial support.

Research is different from **problem solving.** Problem solving is specific to a given situation and is designed for immediate action, whereas research is **generalizable** (transferable) to other situations and deals with long-term solutions rather than immediate ones. For example, Mrs. Abney is an elderly patient who frequently is found wandering in the halls of the nursing home, unable to find her way back to her room. This is quite distressing to her and time-consuming for the nursing staff who help her find her way "home." A nurse notices that Mrs. Abney has no difficulty recognizing her daughter, so she tapes a photograph of the daughter to Mrs. Abney's door. Now Mrs. Abney can find her room easily. She is less agitated, and the nursing staff time can be spent on other priorities.

Table 12-1　Comparison of Problem Solving and Research

Characteristic	Research	Problem Solving
Type of problems addressed	Widely experienced	Situation-specific
Conceptual basis	Theoretical framework	Often none; trial and error
Knowledge base needed	Extensive review of literature to determine latest thinking and research	Practical knowledge, common sense, and experience
Scope of application	Generalizable to similar situations	Useful in immediate situation; transferability must be determined

Mrs. Abney's case is an example of problem solving. It is effective in one set of circumstances and has immediate application. But the solution that worked for Mrs. Abney may not work for all confused patients. In fact, it may not continue to work for Mrs. Abney if her cognitive abilities decline further. Table 12-1 compares problem solving and research.

Research Process

The nursing **research process** is the same as any other research process; it simply addresses a nursing-related problem. Research starts with a problem or stimulus. The stimulus for a research project may be the feeling that something needs to be addressed, that something is not right. It may be that there are insufficient data for resolving a problem, or the literature is unclear, or the data presented in the literature are conflicting. When there is a need for more information and no adequate information exists, research is in order.

There are two major categories of research: quantitative and qualitative. **Quantitative research** is generally considered objective and uses data-gathering techniques that can be repeated by others and verified. Data collected are quantifiable; that is, they can be counted, measured with standardized instruments, or observed with a high degree of agreement among observers.

Qualitative research is more subjective. Finding may be presented from more than one perspective (multiple realities) and the report may be a rich narrative (Streubert and Carpenter, 1999). Questions that cannot be answered by quantitative designs must be addressed by qualitative methods. Answering "why" questions requires the use of qualitative approaches. Why do persons with diabetes choose not to follow the diet prescribed for them? Why do chronically mentally ill individuals choose not to take the medications that would reduce psychotic symptoms? Qualitative research is useful in understanding the perceptions, feelings, and motivations of the research subjects.

Whether quantitative or qualitative, all research must be rigorously planned, carefully implemented, and scrupulously analyzed. Therefore, most research follows a formal process known as the research process. Students in baccalaureate nursing programs often take a semester-long course in nursing research in which both qualitative and quantitative methods are described, so this chapter will serve as a brief introduction to the research process. First, the several steps (listed below) in the quantitative research process are presented; then the importance of research for nursing theory and practice and general considerations in doing research are discussed.

1. Identification of a research problem
2. Review of literature
3. Formulation of the research question or hypothesis
4. Design of the study
5. Implementation
6. Drawing conclusions based on findings
7. Discussion of implications
8. Dissemination of findings

Identification of a research problem

Problems generally come from three sources: clinical situations, the literature, or theories. Clinical situations are rich sources for research problems. Nurses want to prevent elderly clients from wandering off the unit and getting lost. How can they do it? Asking this question can lead to a research problem. Or perhaps a nurse wonders if a time-honored method of providing care is, in fact, the best way. A research problem may result from her curiosity.

Sometimes researchers become interested in a problem because it has been written about in the literature. They may decide to **replicate** (repeat) the study or may design a similar one to test part of the original study in a new way.

The third source of research problems, theory, relates to testing theoretical models. Chapter 11 discussed several models of nursing theory that have been developed. If a theoretical model is designed to predict patients' responses to nursing actions, whether or not it actually does predict patients' responses can be tested through research. The researcher can create certain conditions and determine whether, in fact, the events happen as the theoretical model predicted. Most ideas for nursing research projects come from one of these three sources.

Review of literature

Once a problem is identified, the professional literature must be reviewed. A review of the literature is comprehensive and covers all relevant research and supporting documents in print. Doing a thorough review of the literature requires a great deal of library time or computer search efforts and detective work. Computer-generated searches of the literature can assist tremendously with this step but cannot totally replace the efforts of a dedicated researcher.

The literature review is essential to locate similar or related studies that have already been completed and upon which a new study can build. The review is helpful in creating a **conceptual framework,** or organization of supporting ideas, on which to base the study. The review of literature answers the question, "What have other researchers and theorists written about this problem?"

Formulation of the research question or hypothesis

Once researchers have identified a research problem, are intimately acquainted with the relevant literature, and have chosen a conceptual framework that helps to focus the topic, they need to formulate the **research question.** The question may be stated in one of three forms: a statement, a question, or a hypothesis. If researchers are going to describe something, they may make a statement, such as, "The purpose of this study is to identify the five most frequently expressed needs of family members in intensive care unit waiting rooms." They could also ask a question, such as, "What are the characteristics of mothers who have difficulty bonding to their newborn babies?" If comparing the relationship of two variables, a different type of question might be asked, such as, "What is the relationship of time spent studying and grade point averages?" If conducting an experiment, researchers must have a **hypothesis** (educated guess) as to what the outcome will be so that hypothesis-testing statistics may later be applied. For example, "First-time mothers who attend childbirth classes will demonstrate earlier bonding with their newborn babies than mothers who do not attend the classes" is a testable hypothesis. Whatever the form used, the research question must be expressed succinctly and clearly and it should answer the question, "Exactly what am I trying to determine with this study?"

Design of the study

Once the research question is identified, the study must be designed. There are two broad categories of research designs: experimental and nonexperimental. If the researcher influences the subjects in any way, the research is experimental. If not, the research is nonexperimental. There are numerous types of research under each of these two categories, but the main difference between experimental and non-experimental research is whether or not the researcher manipulates, or influences, the subjects.

True **experimental designs** provide evidence of a cause-and-effect relationship between actions. For example, testing the hypothesis "Patients who receive preoperative teaching need less pain medication in the first 72 hours postoperatively than those who do not" would provide evidence of a cause-and-effect relationship between teaching and pain. Sometimes it is impossible to conduct a true experimental study with human beings, because to do so might endanger them in some way. In those instances, modified experimental studies are used.

Nonexperimental designs are frequently referred to as "descriptive designs" because the researcher describes what the situation is or was at some point in the past. There are many types of nonexperimental designs: surveys, descriptive comparisons, evaluation studies, exploratory studies, and historical-documentary research.

Whether the researcher chooses an experimental or nonexperimental design influences the data collection process. The data collection process includes selection of data collection instruments, design of the data collection protocol, the data analysis plan, subject selection, and informed consent and institutional review plans. The data collection process answers the question, "How will we conduct the study?"

Data collection instruments. When designing a study, researchers must consider how the data will be collected. Data collection instruments, sometimes called data collection tools, range from simple survey forms to complex radiographic scanning devices. The instrument used must be **reliable,** or accurate. A reliable instrument is one that yields the same values dependably each time the instrument is used to measure the same thing. The tool must also be valid, which, when applied to a research instrument, means that it must measure what it is supposed to be measuring.

If body temperature is being measured, a thermometer is an obvious data collection tool. When measuring an abstract factor, such as anxiety or depression, the best data collection tool is not as clear. The selection of a data collection instrument answers the question, "What tool(s) will we use to collect the data?" To minimize measurement errors, beginning researchers should choose published instruments with established reliability and validity, rather than designing their own.

Data collection protocol. Another aspect of designing the study is deciding on the data collection **protocol** (procedure). The quality of the data depends on strict adherence to the plan. If, for example, the plan calls for administering a questionnaire to renal dialysis patients after dialysis, the data collectors must be sure to give the questionnaire to all subjects—and only after their treatments. The data collection protocol answers the question, "How will we go about gathering our data?"

Data analysis plan. It may seem premature to decide how the data will be analyzed before it is even collected, but careful planning for the analysis is important. The research design is developed with data analysis in mind. The analysis must be part of the planning process, because the data and the protocols for collecting them depend on how the data will be analyzed. Unless the nurse researcher is an expert in statistics or there is already a statistician on the research team, consultation with a statistician well versed in human subject research is recommended in designing the data analysis plan, which answers the question, "What will we do with the data once we gather it?"

Subject selection. Once the researcher knows what is to be done, the specifics of who will be included are decided. The individual people or laboratory animals being studied are known as research **subjects.** If the researchers plan to study pain control in postoperative patients, for example, they have to decide the specific type of surgery and the age, sex, ethnicity, and geographic location of the patients, as well as a variety of other factors in planning the subject selection (Figure 12-1). Subject selection answers the question, "Who qualifies to be a participant in this study?"

In the past, women have not been well represented as research subjects. Today there is recognition that women must be included as study subjects if the research findings are to be applicable to women. This is considered such a high priority that the National Institutes of Health, a major funding source for health-related research, has established a policy regarding inclusion of women as study subjects. The policy is available online (*www4.od.nih.gov/orwh/inclusion.html*). Box 12-2 provides further information about including women in research. Sometimes nurses themselves are the subjects of research. Research Note 2 gives a brief description of the Nurses' Health Study.

Rarely, all subjects in a particular group are studied. The term **population** refers to all subjects who meet the selection criteria. Usually, researchers have to use a **sample** (subgroup) of the entire population, however, and valid results can be obtained if the sample is properly selected.

Variations in design: qualitative methods of inquiry. The planning and design of the second type of research process, qualitative research, is more fluid and dynamic than the process of quantitative research. Polit and Beck (2004) emphasized the

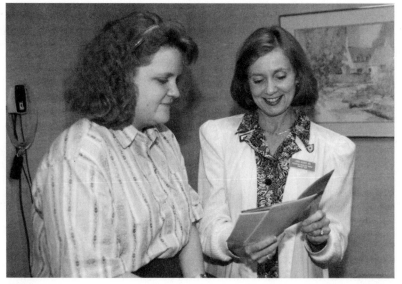

Figure **12-1**
Research subjects are selected based on factors such as age, gender, condition, and location. They must then be informed about certain aspects of the proposed research in order to make a decision about participating. That decision, which is written and signed, is known as "informed consent." (Courtesy Memorial Hospital, Chattanooga, Tennessee.)

need for advanced planning, although the researcher must be flexible. The researcher typically does not seek to control research conditions but tries to observe natural environments. Some of the strategies used to collect information are focus groups, interviews, and field notes (Streubert and Carpenter, 1999).

Phenomenological research is a frequently used qualitative approach. The focus of this method is what people experience in regard to a particular phenomenon and how they interpret those experiences. The main source of data is extensive interviews with the subjects. The researcher poses planned and follow-up questions depending on the subjects' responses, modifying the investigation according to the responses of the subjects. A major difference between quantitative and qualitative methods is that with qualitative methods the subject is generally more aware of the aims of the research. Although researchers do not attempt to influence subjects, they are coparticipants in the experience (Polit and Beck, 2004).

Informed consent and institutional review. Next, researchers who use human subjects must plan to protect the rights of those subjects by asking them to sign an **informed consent** form that describes the details of the study and what participation means. Any risks involved in participating must be explained. No one should be pressured in any way to participate, and the **confidentiality** (privacy) of participants must be ensured.

A related step when using human subjects is submitting the proposal to the institution, such as a hospital or clinic, where the research will take place. It must be

Box 12-2 Including Women in Research

Nurses have a responsibility to apply appropriate ethical standards as they incorporate research findings into practice. Additionally, qualified nurses conducting research must do so in an ethical manner. Although these two statements may seem obvious, the practice is not as obvious or as easy as one might think.

For example, women have traditionally been excluded as subjects from research for seemingly appropriate reasons: (a) the drugs being tested in some experiments could be harmful to fetuses if women in the study were pregnant or became pregnant during the study; and (b) the recognition that women might react differently to some experiments due to hormonal changes was a deterrent in some studies.

There have been more serious problems with the misuse of women as subjects in research. An example was the use of gynecological patients in a pilot study to test antibody reaction to transplanted cancer cells without obtaining written permission from the subjects (although signed permission was obtained from male prison volunteers who were the healthy subjects). Another example was a study to determine the side effects of hormone contraceptives. Most of the women subjects were poor and from an ethnic/minority population who were seeking effective contraceptive measures after having had several pregnancies. More pregnancies resulted in the placebo group. It was determined that the women were not adequately informed about the risk of pregnancy before participating in the study.

Such examples provided the stimulus for the National Institutes of Health to publish guidelines for including women and minorities in research. The guidelines mandate:
- The inclusion of women and members of minorities in all human research.
- The inclusion of women and minorities in clinical trials to the degree that differences in intervention effect can be accomplished in the statistical analysis.
- The exclusion of cost as an acceptable reason to exclude groups.
- The initiation of programs and support for outreach efforts to recruit these groups into clinical studies.

The nurse's increased awareness of these potential dilemmas and subsequent action to prevent biased and discriminatory treatment can result in decreased vulnerability and oppression for women.

Pinch SJ: Women in research, *ANA Center for Ethics and Human Rights Communique* 3(3):4-5, 1994. Used by permission.

approved by the **institutional review board.** Usually composed of individuals from different disciplines, these boards exist to ensure that research is well designed and ethical and does not violate the policies and procedures of the institution or the rights of the subjects. Only after the institutional review board approves the proposal can the study begin.

Implementation

Up until this point, only planning has taken place. Careful planning is, however, the key to a successful study. In the implementation phase, the actual study is conducted. The two main tasks during this phase are data collection and data analysis.

Data collection. **Data** (research-generated information) should be collected only by those who are thoroughly familiar with the study. All research assistants should understand the purpose of the data and the importance of accuracy and careful record keeping. No matter who is collecting the data, the integrity of the project is ultimately the responsibility of the primary researcher.

RESEARCH note 2

Nurses as Research Subjects

In 1976, with funding from the National Institutes of Health (NIH), Dr. Frank Speizer established the Nurses' Health Study. The purpose of the study was to evaluate the long-term effects of oral contraceptives. Nurses were chosen as the subjects, because they were able to respond with a high degree of accuracy to technical questionnaires. Of the 170,000 original questionnaires mailed, 122,000 nurses responded. Subjects were married nurses who were 30 to 55 years old in 1976. In 1980 questions about food intake were added to the questionnaire. Mailings were repeated in 1984, 1986, and every 4 years since then. Additionally, toenail samples were obtained to determine mineral content, and blood samples were obtained to identify hormone levels and genetic markers. Response rates to the questionnaires have been 90 percent.

In 1989 Dr. Walter Willett and colleagues established the Nurses' Health Study II, also funded by NIH. The purpose of this study was to examine the effects of oral contraceptives, diet, and lifestyle risk factors in a group of women younger (25 to 42 years old) than those in the previous study. (Note that the youngest subjects in the earlier study were approximately 42 years old at the time of initiation of the second study.) A total of 116,686 women were involved in the Nurses' Health Study II.

Every 2 years the subjects in the Nurses' Health Study II have received follow-up questionnaires with inquiries about diseases they have had and other health-related topics, including tobacco use, hormone use, pregnancy history, and menopausal status. A food frequency questionnaire was added in 1991 and is administered every 4 years. A quality of life assessment was included in 1993 and repeated in 1997. Blood and urine samples were collected in the late 1990s.

The response rate to the questionnaires administered at 2-year intervals has also been 90 percent.

From Nurses' Health Study, Online *(www.channing.harvard.edu/nhs/hist.html)*.

Data analysis. If all goes well, the data are analyzed exactly as proposed. In analyzing the data, most researchers use the same statistical consultants who assisted in planning the study. The researcher is well advised to work closely with the statistician in interpreting as well as analyzing the data. The nurse researcher is in charge, however, and he or she has the final word on what interpretations are made.

Analyzing the findings of qualitative research presents formidable challenges for several reasons. First, the data are voluminous, often consisting of lengthy dialogues between researchers and subjects. Next, dialogues must be transcribed verbatim, yielding hefty stacks of pages. Then comes the task of organizing the transcripts, identifying themes, and arranging the themes into meaningful patterns. Fortunately, computer programs are now available to assist in this process.

Drawing conclusions based on findings

In writing the research report, the findings directly related to the research question are presented first. Findings are presented factually—without value judgments. The facts must speak for themselves. Simple presentation of the facts is the only requirement. After findings related to the research question are reported, unexpected findings can be reported. Conclusions are then drawn. Conclusions answer the question, "What do these findings mean?" Here researchers can be more subjective and inject some of their own thinking but should stay within the boundaries of the study.

Discussion of implications

Researchers are always alert to the implications of their studies. Implications are suggestions of things that should be done in the future. Every good study raises more questions than it answers. In nursing studies, there may be indications for modifications in nursing education or nursing practice. Nearly every study has implications for further research, and if the findings turn out as expected, almost all studies should be carefully replicated. Replication can answer these and other questions: "What needs to be known to develop more confidence in the findings? Will the research instrument produce similar results in a similar population in a different geographic location? Will the procedure be effective with patients having a slightly different diagnosis, condition, or type of surgery? Will age make a difference? Will cultural beliefs make a difference? What else do we need to know to improve the care of patients?"

Dissemination of findings

A research study is not useful unless the results are communicated to others who may use them. Most funding agencies want to know in advance how the researcher plans to **disseminate** the findings. The two major vehicles for dissemination of knowledge are articles published in professional journals and presentations given at conferences. Examples of nursing research journals include *Clinical Nursing Research, Journal of Nursing Scholarship, Nursing Research, Research in Nursing and Health Care,* and the *Western Journal of Nursing Research.* Because there are relatively few research journals in nursing, the competition for publishing may seem fierce; however, editors say they have great difficulty acquiring well-written manuscripts on topics of interest to readers. A review process, called **peer review,** is the method most journals use to determine whether or not to publish a research report. During peer review, a manuscript is circulated to a review panel consisting of one or more experts in the area of study. They evaluate its appropriateness and accuracy and recommend that it be published, resubmitted with changes, or rejected. Most research that is carefully conceived, conducted, and presented can get published, although the researcher must be persistent and resilient in taking criticism and reworking manuscripts.

A somewhat easier, yet still discriminating, route to dissemination is presentation at one or more of the numerous nursing research conferences. Many research conferences also use the peer review process. In general, however, the proportion of abstracts (summaries of research) selected for presentation at conferences is higher than the proportion of manuscripts chosen for publication.

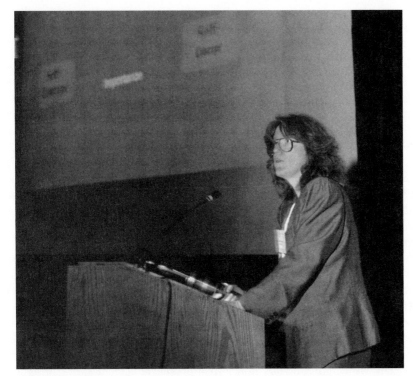

Figure **12-2**
Dissemination of findings is an essential aspect of the research process. Here nurse researcher Maureen Killeen presents her findings at a psychiatric nursing conference. (Courtesy Maureen Killeen.)

Whether research is published or presented, it is important to disseminate research results to other nurses, who may choose to use them either to improve patient care practices or to replicate the study (Figure 12-2).

INTERVIEWS WITH NURSE RESEARCHERS

The field of nursing research is growing, with many nurses actively involved in the process. In Interviews 1 and 2, two nurse researchers talk about their work.

These interviews demonstrate how these nurse researchers feel about the work they do. Nationwide there are hundreds of nurses who, like Killeen and McNeely, are excited about nursing research and the contributions it makes to improving nursing through evidence-based practice.

RELATIONSHIP OF NURSING RESEARCH TO NURSING THEORY AND PRACTICE

Relationships among nursing research, practice, and theory are circular. As mentioned earlier, research ideas are generated from three sources: (1) clinical practice, (2) literature, and (3) theory.

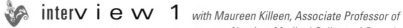

interv i e w 1 *with Maureen Killeen, Associate Professor of Nursing, Medical College of Georgia*

Interviewer: Maureen, your research is with children and self-esteem; exactly what do you do?

Killeen: I go into people's homes and ask children about themselves, and I ask the parents about the children. I ask the children, "What kinds of things are you good at?" And I ask them how important certain words are to them.

Interviewer: What are some examples of the important words?

Killeen: Pretty, smart, honest, messy, lazy, active, careful, happy—things like that. In another study, I am interested in the relationship between obesity and self-esteem. I go into a fifth-grade classroom and give everyone a self-concept scale and measure height and weight. I ask if they are heavier or thinner than others their age.

Interviewer: How do you happen to be doing this kind of work?

Killeen: I read about research on self-esteem in a "Social Psychology and the Self" course I took in graduate school. I read a lot of studies, and every study indicated that if you think of yourself in a certain way, this leads to certain behaviors. But there was nothing about how people come to think of themselves in certain ways. What are the characteristics or traits that get people thinking that way? I wanted to know the answer to that question.

Interviewer: What impact do you hope your research will have on the care of children?

Killeen: If we can figure out how other people affect children's ideas about themselves, how talk about children and talk to children affects them, then we can teach parents how to talk more effectively with their children. We can increase the relevance of treatment and therapy. We will know how to change how people feel about themselves. That is the treatment implication of this research.

Interviewer: What has been most helpful to you in the process of becoming a nurse researcher?

Killeen: Mentoring by more experienced researchers. I have benefited from the kindness of senior researchers who shared ideas. Experience is the best teacher, and I have been fortunate to have had good mentoring. Also, getting a funded grant to pay the bills while I do research has helped a lot!

Interviewer: With regard to your professional life, what is the most enjoyable for you?

Killeen: Some aspects of research are enjoyable, but teaching is close behind. If I can use my research in teaching—that's a lot of fun!

Interviewer: What do you least enjoy in your work as a researcher?

Killeen: Writing. Writing is hard because there are constant revisions. Sometimes it seems it will never be finished.

Interviewer: What are some of your recent research activities?

Killeen: Recently I have been collecting preliminary data for a study of perinatal depression. As a result of my work on self-esteem, I became interested in examining maternal perceptions of their children.

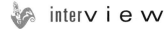

interv i e w 1 *with Maureen Killeen, Associate Professor of Nursing, Medical College of Georgia—cont'd*

I am conducting the study at a nurse-midwifery clinic. We collect data during pregnancy and at six to ten weeks postpartum. Through questionnaires, interviews, histories, and videotaping, we are trying to answer the question of whether depression in mothers and their ability to recognize infant facial expressions influences their interactions with their babies. There is some evidence that depressed women have difficulty identifying facial emotional expressions and in parenting.

If difficulty in recognizing facial expressions is linked to depressed mothers' parenting difficulties, then we may be able to develop interventions targeted at helping mothers recognize infants' nonverbal cues and respond appropriately to them.

Interviewer: What would you like to say to nursing students about research?

Killeen: Research can be a lot of fun. Find a mentor who believes it's fun and who asks interesting research questions. Nursing research is a very exciting field!

Questions about how best to deal with patient problems regularly arise in clinical situations. As shown in the earlier example of Mrs. Abney, the elderly lady who could not find her room, problems often can be "solved" for the present. However, when the same questions recur, long-term answers may be needed. Research develops solutions that can be used with confidence in different situations.

Published articles about nursing research often generate interest in further studies. If there is published research on a particular nursing care problem, other researchers may be stimulated to investigate the subject further and refine the solutions. This is how nursing knowledge builds.

Nursing theorists also generate research ideas. They piece together postulates or premises that "explain" what has been discovered. The explanation is "tested" to determine whether it is robust or strong enough to be useful. If so, there may be more implications for applications in clinical practice.

Nursing research journals are filled with clinical studies that have made a difference in patient care. A few examples of changes in nursing practice stimulated by research include the following:

1. Improved care of patients with skin breakdown from pressure ulcers
2. Decreasing light and noise in critical care units to prevent sleep deprivation
3. Using caps on newborns to decrease heat loss and stabilize body temperature
4. Positioning patients following chest surgery to facilitate respiration
5. Scheduling pain medication more frequently following surgery
6. Preoperative teaching to facilitate postoperative recovery

Nursing research findings not only improve patient care but also affect the health care system itself. For example, research studies have demonstrated the cost-effectiveness of nurses as health care providers. This is discussed further in Chapter 16.

interv i e w 2 *with Elizabeth McNeely, Gerontological Nurse Practitioner*

The second nurse researcher interviewed was Elizabeth McNeely, who did the tai chi research with older people mentioned earlier in this chapter. McNeely was an assistant professor in Emory University's Nell Hodgson Woodruff School of Nursing and is currently a gerontological nurse practitioner in private practice. Her research collaborators were in the Emory School of Medicine and the Atlanta Veterans Administration Medical Center.

Interviewer: How did you happen to become a nurse researcher?

McNeely: Accidentally. It was the last thing I envisioned. I happened to have a specialization in a field [gerontology] where research was growing. I became recognized as an expert in that field. One day my supervisor told me to go to a meeting where my expertise was needed. The meeting turned out to be a planning meeting for the multidisciplinary research I do now.

Interviewer: How do you believe your research has contributed to better patient care?

McNeely: There are so many things health care professionals do because they "know" they work. But this knowledge doesn't get communicated beyond the walls of the institution. With hard data that comes from research, the information can be published so others can know how to do it. This improves patient care.

Interviewer: What are some examples?

McNeely: This tai chi grant. They have been doing tai chi in China for hundreds of years. But thousands of testimonials to the benefits won't lead to its being recommended by medical professionals in this country. We have to study the effects systematically before it will be supported by the medical profession.

Interviewer: How do you like your work as a nurse researcher?

McNeely: It's intriguing. Everyone needs to realize the importance of getting hard data to support practice.

Interviewer: What do you like best about your work?

McNeely: The air of excitement and discovery that comes when we see that some of our ideas are working. Also, my association with other researchers and the opportunities for thinking.

Interviewer: What do you like the least?

McNeely: There is a lot of tedium. It's hard to realize how long it takes to get from idea to publication. You have to be "long-term" oriented.

Interviewer: What would you like to say to nursing students?

McNeely: I would tell them that nurses have a unique contribution to make to the multidisciplinary research team. The problems are complex and require complex approaches, including the nursing perspective. As a clinician in a multidisciplinary practice, I have seen the concept of interdisciplinary clinical practice become more and more acceptable, especially in the present managed care environment. As a result, the number of interdisciplinary research studies conducted and published has increased. The combination of the knowledge and skills from several disciplines has enhanced health care toward a more holistic approach. The health care consumer has benefited from this trend.

Box **12-3** Relating Nursing Research to Practice and Theory

Behavior theory suggests that behavior can be modified with reinforcement (reward or punishment). Incontinence is behavior characterized by involuntary urination before the patient can get to the bathroom or get positioned on a bedpan or with a urinal. Some researchers wondered, "Can incontinence be modified with positive reinforcements such as a special treat or additional time in the television room?" Specifically, they believed that patients could be "taught" to control urination if effective reinforcers were applied. Several subsequent studies suggest that patients can learn to control incontinence in specific situations. In this case, a theory—behavior theory—was useful in planning research, the results of which enable nurses to improve the clinical nursing care of incontinent patients.

Another contribution of nursing research to practice is in the area of power. A person who possesses knowledge that is useful to others has power. Nurses gain much knowledge through clinical practice. Yet practical knowledge, as important as it is, lacks the power of research-validated knowledge. Research can be used to demonstrate, for example, that one nursing action is more effective than another. When knowledge from practice is validated through research, that knowledge is more powerful. Thus, it could be said that research empowers practice.

A final point about the influence of research on practice has to do with professionalism. In Chapter 6, the characteristics of professions were presented. One of the criteria commonly mentioned is a scientific body of knowledge that is expanded through research. Nursing research enhances the status of nursing as a profession by expanding nursing's scientific knowledge base. A brief example that may clarify the interplay between nursing research, practice, and theory is provided in Box 12-3.

COLLABORATION IN NURSING RESEARCH

The history of nursing research spans 40 years. Since the 1960s, with awareness of the need for a nursing body of knowledge based on research, nursing research today has matured to the level of collaboration with other disciplines to generate knowledge that would be limited if done only by members of one discipline. The Open Letter to Nursing Students from nurse researcher Larry Scahill (Box 12-4) illustrates the effectiveness and excitement of collaborative research relationships.

Another example of collaborative research relationships is found in the research partnerships of Judith Noble Halle (Goldsmith, 1995). Halle, a doctoral student at the University of California at Los Angeles School of Nursing, worked with women who were experiencing difficult pregnancies. Halle's concern was for the health of the infant, and she did physiological research to develop methods for preventing brain damage due to a lack of oxygen at birth. Her research was based on a major finding of a physician with whom she collaborated. Other researchers who collaborated with Halle include another nurse, Christine Kasper, who administered a nursing cell physiology laboratory, and the director of a pediatric neurosurgery research laboratory.

| Box **12-4** | **Open Letter to Nursing Students Regarding Research in Child Psychiatry** |

Child psychiatry is in the midst of tremendous change. Recent findings from several related fields, including neuroanatomy, developmental neuroscience, pharmacology, genetics, molecular biology, and epidemiology have propelled this change. Because no one discipline can embrace all of these fields, research in child psychiatry is increasingly multidisciplinary. Although nursing education does not prepare students for careers in basic biological research, nurses can and do collaborate in clinical research. What is clinical research in child psychiatry, and what part do nurses play in clinical research?

Clinical research refers to research endeavors that are closely connected to the care of patients. In child psychiatry, this might include a medication trial in children with autism, an evaluation of a cognitive-behavioral intervention program in attention-deficit hyperactivity disorder, a neuroimaging study of brain function in Tourette's syndrome, or a family genetic study in obsessive-compulsive disorder. Each of these research studies requires comprehensive assessment of subjects, careful management of the data collected, and analysis of results.

As with other fields of research, clinical research usually involves a question about the relationship between two things. The research question may emerge from theory or from clinical practice. For example, the question of whether the vulnerability for obsessive-compulsive disorder is inherited emerged because clinicians noticed that it recurred in families at a higher-than-expected rate compared with the rate in the general population. To investigate the relationship between childhood obsessive-compulsive disorder and family history, researchers interview family members to ascertain the frequency of obsessive-compulsive disorder in the family and the pattern of inheritance. By contrast, the neuroimaging study of Tourette syndrome evolved from a theory that dysregulation of specific brain circuits underlies this disorder.

Another area of increasing importance in child psychiatry is psychopharmacology. The proliferation of pharmacologic agents for the treatment of psychiatric disorders of childhood offers hope for children afflicted with mental illness. Despite the promise of this growing list of medications, however, the scientific support for their use is limited. Indeed, only a few of the drugs commonly used in child psychiatry have demonstrated efficacy in rigorous studies. The method for showing that a medication is effective for a given problem is the randomized controlled trial. For some, studies of this sort are questionable, because a child may receive a placebo rather than the active treatment. On the other hand, in the absence of clear evidence that a given medication is effective in children, there may be ethical concerns about exposing children to an untested psychotropic medication. Thus, the value of placebo-controlled trials is that they provide information about the efficacy and safety of a medication from which the risks and benefits can be evaluated.

Research involves the systematic investigation of the relationship between two or more phenomena. Research in child psychiatry is expanding and embraces a wide range of disciplines from basic scientists to clinicians. Especially relevant for nurses is clinical research, such as placebo-controlled medication trials. These studies require careful assessment, close monitoring during the trial, and accurate assessment of outcome. The future of child psychiatry will increasingly rely on neuroscience, psychopharmacology, and clinical measurement. Nurses interested in these fields can consider a career in clinical research in child psychiatry.

Larry Scahill, M.S.N., M.P.H.
Yale University

According to Kasper, "Many of the unique questions that nurses ask when they begin to address new areas of research are supported by existing fields of science, such as cell physiology, or the behavioral sciences. Rather than reinventing the wheel, collaborating with scientists outside of nursing contributes to nursing science, and nursing contributes to others" (Goldsmith, 1995, p. 7). As the experiences of these nurses illustrate, interdisciplinary collaboration can be a rewarding aspect of nursing research.

SUPPORT FOR NURSING RESEARCH

Nursing research is expensive, and support takes many forms. It can include encouragement, consultation, computer and library resources, money, and release time from researchers' regular work responsibilities. Each of these forms of support is important, but none alone is adequate. Early in the development of nursing research, encouragement was often the only support available, and not all nurse researchers had that. Gradually over the years, funding sources have developed, but financial support is still difficult to obtain, particularly for new researchers.

The National Institute of Nursing Research (NINR) was created in 1992 from what had been the National Center for Nursing Research (NCNR), part of the National Institutes of Health. NINR supports clinical and basic research to establish a scientific basis for the care of individuals across the life span—from management of patients during illness and recovery to the reduction of risks for disease and disability, the promotion of healthy lifestyles, the promotion of quality of life in those with chronic illness, and the care for individuals at the end of life. In the years of NCNR/NINR's existence, its budget has quadrupled; however, it is still able to fund only a small portion of the proposals it receives. To establish priorities for funding, the National Nursing Research Agenda (NNRA) was launched in 1987. Themes were developed in a series of meetings, discussed at the National Advisory Council for Nursing Research and the National Nursing Research Roundtable and presented at the American Association of Colleges of Nursing meeting. The five research themes of the future are the following:

1. Changing Lifestyle Behaviors for Better Health—The need for this research is strong, as illustrated by a recent Department of Health and Human Services (HHS) report. This report found that 40 percent of premature deaths can be attributable to individual unhealthy behaviors. Conversely, of the 30-year gain in life expectancy, HHS states that 25 of these years came from advances in public health, principally from prevention.
2. Managing the Effects of Chronic Illness to Improve Quality of Life—As the population ages, chronic illnesses are also increasing, with implications for patients, families communities, and the health care system. Chronic disease conditions are the leading cause of illness, disability, and death, and affect at least 100 million people.
3. Identifying Effective Strategies to Reduce Health Disparities—National health surveys identify substantial disparities among different segments of the population, including certain members of ethnic groups, in access to health care, incidence of disease, length of life, and mortality rates.
4. Harnessing Advanced Technologies to Serve Human Needs—With advances in genetics increasingly applied to disease screening and therapies, sometimes with

complex ethical implications, researchers have new issues to address. Technologies should be integrated into practice and training to promote their optimal application for the physical and emotional health of individuals.

5. Enhancing the End-of-Life Experience for Patients and their Families—A significant number of Americans continue to be dissatisfied with the way the health care system provides care for the dying. In fact, according to the National Institutes of Health (NIH), 93 percent of Americans believe that improving end-of-life care is important. You can read more about all of these research themes for the future from a September 29, 2003, online posting *(www.nih.gov/ninr/research/themes.doc).*

Several other federal agencies accept proposals that meet their funding guidelines when submitted by qualified nurse researchers. These include the National Institute on Aging, the National Cancer Institute, the National Institute of Mental Health, the National Institute of Alcohol Abuse and Addiction, the National Institute on Drug Addiction, and the Centers for Disease Control and Prevention. Competition with researchers from other disciplines is keen, however, and generally only experienced nurse researchers are successful in obtaining funding from these sources.

Nursing associations also fund nursing research. The American Nurses Foundation, Sigma Theta Tau, and many clinical specialty organizations provide research awards, even for novice researchers. State and local nursing associations sometimes have seed money for pilot projects. Universities, schools of nursing, and large hospitals also may provide small amounts of research funds. Generally, however, finding adequate funding for large-scale studies continues to be a problem faced by researchers.

ROLES OF NURSES IN RESEARCH

The *Code of Ethics for Nurses* states: "The nurse participates in the advancement of the profession through contributions to practice, education, administration, and knowledge development." (American Nurses Association, 2001). Ideally, every nurse should be involved in research, but practically, all nurses should, as a minimum, use research results to improve their practices. Evidence-based nursing practice requires staying informed about current literature, especially studies done in one's own specific area of clinical practice.

As seen in Table 12-2, in addition to using research to improve practice, all professional nurses can contribute to one or more aspects of the research process. Baccalaureate nurses can read, interpret, and evaluate research for applicability to nursing practice. Through clinical practice, they can identify nursing problems that need to be investigated. They can also participate in the implementation of scientific studies by helping principal researchers collect data in clinical settings or elsewhere. These beginning researchers must know enough about the purpose of the research to follow the research protocols explicitly or know when it is necessary to deviate from the protocol for a patient's well-being. Baccalaureate nurses also can help disseminate research-based knowledge by sharing useful research findings with colleagues.

The master's-prepared nurse may be ready to replicate studies that have been previously conducted. Researchers cannot be sure that their findings are true until studies are repeated with similar results. Nurse researchers have learned that it is not necessary (or even desirable) always to generate a totally new and disconnected idea

Table 12-2 LEVELS OF EDUCATIONAL PREPARATION AND LEVELS
OF PARTICIPATION IN NURSING RESEARCH

Level of Preparation	Level of Research Participation
Student nurse	Consumer
BSN nurse	Problem identifier
	Data collector
MSN nurse	Replicator
	Concept tester
Doctoral nurse	Theory generator
Postdoctoral nurse	Funded program director

BSN, Bachelor of science in nursing; *MSN,* master of science in nursing.

to do research. As mentioned earlier, to be most useful, research must be based on a conceptual framework and related to previous research.

Depending on education, clinical and research experiences, and interests, some nurses at the master's level are better prepared to conduct research than others. In addition to education and experience, a crucial factor is the support system the nurse has available. To do research, nurses need time, money, consultation, and subjects. With rich resources in a research environment, master's-prepared nurses can and do make vital research contributions.

Usually, to be a nationally recognized researcher and obtain federal funding for a research program, nurses need doctoral and even postdoctoral preparation. Researchers across the United States in all professions compete for a limited pool of research dollars available each year. Only those nurses with strong academic and experiential backgrounds and the best proposals succeed in obtaining federal funding.

Nurses who aspire to careers as competitive nurse researchers should plan a specific program of research. This means limiting one's research to a defined set of phenomena. For example, May Wykle, who is at Case Western Reserve, has a research program producing stimulating studies about persons who care for their elderly dependent relatives (Son, Wykle, and Zauszniewski, 2003; Wykle, 1995; Wykle, 1986; Dunkle and Wykle, 1988; Fitzpatrick, Wykle, and Morris, 1990). Sandra Dunbar of Emory University is focusing her research program on ways to help patients who are experiencing heart failure to participate in the management of their care (Clark, Deaton, and Dunbar, 2003; Dunbar, Jacobson, and Deaton, 1998). These researchers realize that only by becoming specialists in a particular area of research can they receive the kind of funding they need to support their research and the national recognition it takes to get the results of their studies published so that they can have the desired impact—better nursing care for patients through evidence-based practice.

EVIDENCE-BASED PRACTICE: BRIDGING THE GAP BETWEEN RESEARCH AND PRACTICE

The best efforts of nurse researchers are fruitless unless nurses make use of their research findings to improve patient care in their day-to-day practices. Patients have become more knowledgeable consumers of health care and nurses must ensure that they provide the latest and best available care. One way to ensure positive patient outcomes is through evidence-based practice.

Evidence-based practice (EBP) means using the best available research findings "to make clinical decisions that are most effective and beneficial for patients" (Cope, 2003, p. 97). EBP was originally created in the 1980s by a Canadian university as an approach to clinical learning. The Centre for Evidence-Based Medicine (EBM) at Oxford University in England defines EBM as "the conscientious, explicit, and judicious use of current best evidence in making decisions about the care of individual patients. The practice of evidence-based medicine means integrating individual clinical expertise with the best available external clinical evidence from systematic research" (Sackett, Rosenberg, Gray, et al., 1996, p. 71). The motivation behind EBP was the belief that most of medical practice was based on intuition, experience, clinical skills, and guesswork, rather than science. The value of EBP in clinical practice, as well as in learning situations, was recognized, and its study and use spread rapidly to the nursing profession.

Questions regarding best practices are raised daily by nurses in direct patient care roles. It is not always feasible to conduct a study to answer those questions. In fact, answers may already be available in the nursing literature. Nurses have traditionally used various research methods to answer questions arising from clinical practice. EBP represents a new way of using the now-substantial body of nursing research that has been compiled during the past several decades.

According to Cope, EBP is a multistep process. An advanced practice oncology nurse in Florida, Cope outlined seven steps in the evidence-based practice process (2003, p. 97). They are:
1. Precise definition of a patient problem
2. Identification of information necessary to solve the problem
3. Efficient and thorough search of the literature
4. Critical appraisal of the evidence
5. Extraction of the clinical answer as it applies to the patient problem
6. Clinical guideline or protocol development and implementation
7. Evaluation

Not surprisingly, EBP in nursing has aroused some controversy (Salazar, 2003). There are differences of opinion among nurses about what types of studies constitute the strongest evidence and what weight to give to each. They disagree, for example, about the relative merits of randomized controlled trials, long considered the "gold standard" in research, versus descriptive and qualitative studies. Where do clinical expertise, intuition, and patient preference come into the hierarchy of importance? These issues are being debated in numerous evidence-based practice conferences and symposia.

Sigma Theta Tau International, Honor Society of Nursing, has long supported nursing research and dissemination of research findings through its publications. This association has adopted a position statement on evidence-based nursing that demonstrates its importance to the members of that organization (Box 12-5).

Today's students can be assured that they will be hearing much more about EBP and participating in evidence-based nursing practice initiatives in the future.

Box **12-5** **Sigma Theta Tau International's Position Statement on Evidence-Based Nursing**

As a leader in the development and dissemination of knowledge to improve nursing practice, the Honor Society of Nursing, Sigma Theta Tau International, supports the development and implementation of evidence-based nursing (EBN). The society defines EBN as an integration of the best evidence available, nursing expertise, and the values and preferences of the individuals, families, and communities who are served. This assumes that optimal nursing care is provided when nurses and health care decision makers have access to a synthesis of the latest research, a consensus of expert opinion, and are thus able to exercise their judgment as they plan and provide care that takes into account cultural and personal values and preferences. This approach to nursing care bridges the gap between the best evidence available and the most appropriate nursing care of individuals, groups, and populations with varied needs. The society, working closely with key partners who provide information to support nursing research and EBN around the world, will be a leading source of information on EBN with an integrated cluster of resources, products, and services that will foster optimal nursing care globally. The society, along with its strategic partners, will provide nurses with the most current and comprehensive resources to translate the best evidence into the best nursing research, education, administration, policy, and practice.

Sigma Theta Tau International, Position statement on evidence-based nursing, Online, 2003 (*www.nursingsociety.org/research/main.html#ebp*).

Visit Evolve for WebLinks related to the content of this chapter: **http://evolve.elsevier. com/Chitty/professional/.**

Summary of Key Points

- The scientific method is the name given to a systematic, orderly process of solving problems. It has been used for centuries and is applicable in many different situations.
- Knowledge can be categorized as either pure knowledge (that is, knowledge that is not immediately useful) or applied knowledge (that is, knowledge that can be used in a practical way).
- Much of the scientific knowledge we take for granted today was discovered through use of the scientific method.
- The scientific method has been particularly useful in the fields of medicine and health care, and human existence has been profoundly affected by discoveries made through its use.
- The scientific method uses two types of logic: inductive and deductive reasoning.
- Both inductive and deductive reasoning are necessary to combine the theoretical and the practical aspects of the scientific method.
- For safety and ethical reasons, there are limitations on the use of the scientific method with human beings.

- Nursing research is defined as the systematic investigation of phenomena related to improving nursing care.
- The major steps in the research process are identification of a research problem, review of the literature, formulation of the research question, design of the study, implementation, drawing conclusions based on findings, discussion of implications, and dissemination of findings.
- Nurse researchers have made significant contributions to improvements in nursing care practices.
- Nursing research is related to and informed by nursing theory and nursing practice and in turn influences them.
- Nurses of all educational backgrounds have a role in research.
- Evidence-based nursing practice is the goal of nursing research.

CRITICAL THINKING QUESTIONS

1. Why is nursing called an applied science? Explain why you agree or disagree with this description.
2. Name and describe the two types of reasoning used in the scientific method. Explain why neither alone is adequate to advance knowledge.
3. List and discuss each step of the research process.
4. Explain why a purely experimental model is an inadequate one for nursing.
5. Discuss the reasons for using nurses as research subjects. Do you think this is a good plan? Why or why not?
6. Go to your college library and see which nursing research journals are in the collection. Thumb through some recent issues and notice the types of studies reported. Compare them with studies done 20 years ago. What similarities and differences do you note?
7. Read a research article that interests you. See whether you can identify each of the steps in the research process. If not, what is missing? Discuss with your teacher and classmates what the significance of the missing steps might be.
8. Find out what research is being done in your school or hospital. If possible, talk with those involved, including data collectors, data analysts, research directors, subjects, families of subjects, and nurses who work on units where research is being conducted. What do they know about the research? What are their concerns? What do they hope will be learned from the research?
9. Obtain job descriptions for nurses at varying experience levels at different agencies. Are research functions included in the job descriptions? If not, what research functions do you think might be appropriate to include?
10. Of the following studies, identify which are nursing research and which are not, giving your rationale for each:
    a. The investigation of optimum staffing patterns in a long-term care facility.
    b. A study of effective methods of clinical supervision of nursing students.
    c. A comparison of two behavioral techniques for managing incontinence in spinal cord–injured patients.
11. As a class, explore the EBP websites and debate the pros and cons of evidence-based practice.

REFERENCES

American Nurses Association: *Code of ethics for nurses with interpretive statements,* Washington, DC, 2001, American Nurses Publishing.

Becker PT, Grunwald PC: Contextual dynamics of ethical decision making in the NICU, *J Perinat Neonatal Nurs* 14(2):58-72, 2000.

Becker PT, Grunwald PC, Moorman J, et al: Effects of developmental care on behavioral organization in very-low-birth-weight infants, *Nurs Res* 42(4):214-220, 1993.

Brown-Saltzman K: Replenishing the spirit by meditative prayer and guided imagery, *Semin Oncol Nurs* 13(4), 255-259, 1997.

Clark PC, Deaton C, Dunbar SB: Identifying possible depression in clinical research: ethical and outcome considerations for the investigator/clinician, *Appl Nurs Res* 16(1), 53-59, 2003.

Cope D: Evidence-based practice: making it happen in your clinical setting, *Clin J Oncol Nurs* 7(1):97-98, 2003.

Dunbar SB, Jacobson LE, Deaton C: Heart failure: strategies to enhance patient self-management, *AACN Clin Iss* 9(2):244-256, 1998.

Dunkle RE, Wykle ML: *Decision making in long-term care: factors in planning,* New York, 1998, Springer.

Fitzpatrick JJ, Wykle ML, Morris DL: Collaboration in care and research, *Arch Psychiatr Nurs* 4(1):53-61, 1990.

Flexner SB, Stein J, Su PY, editors: *The Random House dictionary,* New York, 1980, Random House.

Friends of the National Institute of Nursing Research: *Nursing research: advancing science for health,* Washington, DC, 1995, Friends of the National Institute of Nursing Research.

Gibbins S, Stevens B, Asztalos E: Assessment and management of acute pain in high-risk neonates, *Expert Opin Pharmacother* 4(4):475-483, 2003.

Gibbins S, Stevens B, Hodnett E, et al: Efficacy and safety of sucrose for procedural pain relief in preterm and term neonates, *Nurs Res* 51(6):375-382, 2002.

Gibson E, Medoff-Cooper B, Nuama IF, et al: Accelerated discharge of low birth weight infants from neonatal intensive care: a randomized, controlled trial, The Early Discharge Study Group, *J Perinatol* 18(6):17-23, 1998.

Goldsmith J: Newborn research depends on partnerships, *Sigma Theta Tau Int Reflections* 21(3):6-8, 1995.

Hawley G, Irurita V: Seeking comfort through prayer, *Int J Nurs Pract* 4(1):9-18, 1998.

Hockenberry MH: Guided imagery as a coping measure for children with cancer, *J Assoc Pediatr Oncol Nurses* 6(2):29, 1989.

Hockenberry MH: Pediatric oncology nursing, *J Pediatr Nurs* 18(2):85-86, 2003.

Kuhn TS: The structure of scientific revolutions. In Nurath O, editor: *International encyclopedia of unified science,* ed 2, vol 2, Chicago, 1970, University of Chicago Press.

Kutner NG, Barhart H, Wolf SI, et al: Self-report benefits of tai chi practice by older adults, *J Gerontol B Psychol Sci Soc Sci* 52(5):242-246, 1997.

Lewis PJ: A review of prayer within the role of the holistic nurse, *J Holist Nurs* 14(4):308-315, 1996.

Medoff-Cooper B: Multisystem approach to the assessment of successful feeding, *Acta Paediatr* 89(4):393-394, 2000.

Medoff-Cooper B, McGrath JM, Bilker W: Nutritive sucking and neurobehavioral development in preterm infants from 34 weeks PCA to term, *MCN Am J Matern Child Nurs* 25(2):64-70, 2000.

Medoff-Cooper B, Ray W: Neonatal sucking behaviors, *Image J Nurs Schol* 27(3):195-200, 1995.

Meraviglia MG: Critical analysis of spirituality and its empirical indicators, *J Holist Nurs* 17(1):18-33, 1999.

Pinch SJ: Women in research, *ANA Center for Ethics and Human Rights Communique* 3(3):4-5, 1994.

Polit DF, Beck CT: *Nursing research: principles and methods,* ed 7, Baltimore, 2004, Lippincott Williams and Williams.

Sackett DL, Rosenberg WM, Gray JA, et al: Evidence-based medicine: what it is and what it isn't, *Br Med J* 312:71-72, 1996.

Salazar MK: Evidence-based practice: relevance to occupational health nurses, *AAOHN J* 51(3):109-112, 2003.

Sigma Theta Tau International: Position statement on evidence-based nursing. Online, 2003 *(www.nursingsociety.org/research/main.html#ebp).*

Son GR, Wykle ML, Zauszniewski JA: Korean adult child caregivers of older adults with dementia: predictors of burden and satisfaction, *J Gerontol Nurs* 29(1):19-28, 2003.

Stevens B, Johnson C, Franch L, et al: The efficacy of developmentally sensitive interventions and sucrose for relieving procedural pain in very low birth weight neonates, *Nurs Res* 48(1):35-41, 1999.

Streubert HJ, Carpenter DR: *Qualitative research in nursing: advancing the humanistic imperative,* ed 2, Philadelphia, 1999, JB Lippincott.

Taylor EJ, Outlaw FH: Use of prayer among persons with cancer, *Holist Nurs Pract* 16(3): 46-60, 2002.

Ware CF, Panikkar KM, Romein JM: *The twentieth century: history of mankind, cultural and scientific development,* vol 6, New York, 1966, Harper & Row.

Williams T: Intercessory prayer and its effect on patients with rheumatoid arthritis, *Ky Nurse* 50(1):16, 2002.

Wolf SL, Barnhart HX, Kutner NG, et al: Reducing frailty and falls in older persons: an investigation of tai chi and computerized balance training, *J Am Geriatr Soc* 44(5):489-497, 1996.

Wykle ML: Mental health nursing: research in nursing homes. In Harper MS, Lebowitz B, editors: *Mental illness in nursing homes: a research agenda,* Rockville, MD, 1986, U.S. Department of Health and Human Services, pp 221-234.

Wykle ML: Geriatric mental health interventions in the home, *J Gerontol Nurs* 21(3):47-48, 1995.

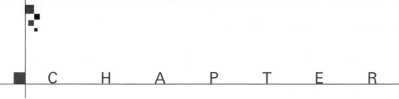

CHAPTER 13

The Health Care Delivery System

*Jennifer E. Jenkins**

Key Terms

Capitation
Chief Executive Officer (CEO)
Chief Nurse Executive
Chief of Staff
Continuous Quality
    Improvement (CQI)
Cross-Functional Team
Decentralization
Dietitian
Disease Management
For-Profit Agency
Gatekeeper
Governmental (Public) Agency
Health Maintenance
    Organization (HMO)

Health Promotion
Home Health Agency
Illness Prevention
Institutional Structure
Interdisciplinary Team
Long-Term Care
Managed Care
Managed Care Organization (MCO)
Multiskilled Worker
Not-for-Profit Agency
Organizational Structure
Paramedical Staff
Patient-Focused Care
Performance
    Improvement (PI)

Physician Hospital
    Organization (PHO)
Point-of-Service (POS)
    Organization
Preferred Provider
    Organization (PPO)
Primary Care
Reengineering
Rehabilitation Services
Secondary Care
Social Services
Subacute Care
Tertiary Care
Therapists
Voluntary (Private) Agency

Learning Outcomes

After studying this chapter, students will be able to:

- Describe the four basic types of services provided by the health care delivery system.
- Identify the three main classifications of health care agencies.
- Explain the traditional internal structures of health care agencies.
- Identify the key members of the interdisciplinary health care team and explain what each contributes.
- Describe how managed care has changed the health care delivery system.
- Explain the impact of changes in consumers' expectations on the health care delivery system.
- Describe how health care organizations have changed through reengineering.
- Relate two major mechanisms used to maintain quality in health care agencies.

*The author wishes to acknowledge the contributions of Karen J. Wisdom in the preparation of this chapter.

The health care delivery system in the United States is a misnomer. Far from providing *health* care, our system has traditionally provided care for *illness*. Its complexity, with multiple types of financing and many different settings where patients can receive services, has resulted in a fragmented system that is difficult to understand and navigate. Although this country has the best technology, the most sophisticated procedures, and the best educated health care providers in the world, many people do not have access to even the most basic care, much less prevention. During the last two decades, the system, for financial and health reasons, has undergone major reform.

This chapter describes the present health care delivery system and makes some predictions about its future. Most planners believe that one of the essential parts of an improved health care system will be an emphasis on prevention, early detection of disease, and wellness. Active participation of patients in their own health choices will be encouraged as health care services increasingly emphasize the importance of holism and treatment of the whole person, not just the diseased part.

The delivery system of the future will be more efficient than the current one. Life-threatening illnesses and injuries will continue to be treated in centers where technology and intensive care services are available. Primary care, or basic health services, however, will be provided in a variety of settings—workplaces, schools, homes, and community-based facilities such as neighborhood clinics. Health care workers will be educated to provide holistic, efficient, and cost-effective care.

A system that answers the following questions will ensure that these objectives are met:

1. What services does the patient need and want?
2. Who can best provide these services (patient, health care worker, family, others)?
3. Where is the most effective and efficient place to provide these services?
4. How will these services affect the quality and cost of care, as well as patient and health care worker satisfaction?

The U.S. government has not yet devised a definitive national health policy. An important first step, however, has been taken. As discussed in Chapter 10, a consortium of nearly 300 national health organizations, the U.S. Public Health Service, and state health departments met in 1980 to establish goals and objectives for improving the health of U.S. citizens by the year 2000. The resulting report, *Healthy People 2000: National Health Promotion and Disease Prevention Objectives*, established three broad goals (U.S. Department of Health and Human Services, 2003):

1. Increase the span of healthy life for Americans.
2. Reduce health disparities among Americans.
3. Achieve access to preventive services for all Americans.

Many specific objectives and priorities were accomplished toward these goals, but health practices and technology changed dramatically during the 1990s. Policymakers agreed that these changes necessitated updating the *Healthy People 2000* objectives to reflect the impact of managed care on the system and of the changing demographics of the United States, which created an older and more culturally diverse population. The new plan, *Healthy People 2010: Healthy People in Healthy Communities*, emphasized community involvement and focused on the responsibility of consumers, individuals, and families (U.S. Department of Health and Human Services, 2003). With this brief look at the future in mind, let us now take a look at today's health care delivery system and build a framework for understanding tomorrow's system.

MAJOR CATEGORIES OF HEALTH CARE SERVICES

Regardless of the setting in which services are provided—clinics, hospitals, homes, primary care provider's offices—there are basically only four major categories of health services: health promotion, illness prevention, diagnosis and treatment, and rehabilitation and long-term care. Each of these categories is briefly explained below.

Health Promotion

Health promotion services assist patients to remain healthy, prevent diseases and injuries, detect diseases early, and promote healthier lifestyles. These services require patients' active participation and cannot be performed solely by a health care provider. Health promotion services are based on the assumption that patients who participate in lifestyle changes are likely to avoid heart attacks, lung cancers, certain infections, and other lifestyle-related diseases.

An example of health promotion services is prenatal classes. By learning good nutritional habits, an expectant mother can take care of herself and her baby during pregnancy and after delivery. This increases the chances of a normal pregnancy and the birth of a healthy baby. Other examples include aerobic exercise and smoking-cessation classes aimed at increasing the health of an individual's cardiovascular and respiratory systems.

Health promotion also includes the detection of warning signs indicating the presence of a disease in early stages. Early detection often allows the treatment to be minimal and less costly and results in a good outcome.

Illness Prevention

With the identification of risk factors such as a family history of heart disease, **illness prevention** services assist patients in reducing the impact of those risk factors on their health and well-being. These services also require the patient's active participation.

Prevention services differ from health promotion services in that they address health problems after risk factors are identified, whereas health promotion services seek to prevent development of risk factors. For example, a health promotion program might teach the detrimental effects of alcohol and drugs on a person's health to prevent the person from using alcohol and drugs. Illness prevention services are used when the patient has been using alcohol or drugs and is at risk for developing health problems as a result. The boundary between health promotion, early detection, and illness prevention is often blurred. Box 13-1 gives examples of activities in these three areas.

Diagnosis and Treatment

Traditionally, in the U.S. health care system, heavy emphasis has been put on diagnosis and treatment. Modern technology has enabled the medical profession to refine methods of diagnosing illnesses and disorders and to treat them more effectively than

Box **13-1** Examples of Illness Prevention, Early Detection, and Health Promotion Activities

Illness Prevention

- Community health programs
- Promotion of healthy lifestyles to counteract risk factors
- Occupational safety programs (use of eye guards for work that endangers the eyes)
- Environmental safety programs (proper disposal of hazardous waste)
- Legislation that prevents injury or disease (seat belt/child restraint laws)

Early Detection

- Mammograms
- Vision and hearing screening
- Cholesterol screening
- Periodic histories and physical examinations
- Blood glucose screening
- Osteoporosis screening

Health Promotion/Maintenance

- Health education programs (prenatal classes)
- Exercise programs
- Health fairs
- Wellness programs (worksite/school)
- Nutrition education

in the past. Scientific advances permit many noninvasive tests and treatments to be performed. Widely available technologies that were unheard of only a few years ago include the use of ultrafast CT scans to detect calcification in coronary arteries and live three-dimensional ultrasonography that creates 3-D images of structures such as the fetal face, hand, or spine. The future promises more "high-tech" noninvasive technologies.

Laparoscopic instruments have transformed surgery techniques, allowing incisions of 1 inch or less. This technology has reduced postoperative pain, reduced hospital stays from days to hours, and enabled individuals to return to normal function much more rapidly.

Unfortunately, high-tech services can lead patients to feel dehumanized. This occurs when caregivers focus on machines rather than on patients. Nurses must remember that patients benefit most when they understand their diagnoses and treatments and can be active participants in the development and implementation of their own treatment plans. Partnering with patients is a recurring theme in the philosophies, models, and theories discussed in Chapter 11.

Rehabilitation, Disease Management, and Long-Term Care

Rehabilitation services help restore the patient to the fullest possible level of function and independence following injury or illness. Rehabilitation programs deal with conditions that leave patients with less than full functioning, such as strokes, broken bones, or severe burns. Both patients and their families must be active participants in this care if it is to be successful. Rehabilitation services should begin as soon as the patient's condition has stabilized after an injury or stroke. These services may be provided in institutional settings such as hospitals, in special rehabilitation facilities, in long-term care facilities such as nursing homes, or in the home and the community. The objectives are to assist patients to achieve their full potential and return to a level of functioning that permits them to be contributing members of society.

Disease management services grew exponentially at the turn of the twenty-first century. This has a direct correlation with the aging of the baby boomer population. Diseases such as congestive heart failure, diabetes, coronary artery disease, chronic obstructive pulmonary disease, and conditions such as low back pain, hypertension, and hyperlipidemia all contribute to higher health care costs and a reduced quality of life. Disease management companies use nurses and other health professionals to help participants understand and manage their chronic conditions more effectively through phone calls, coaching and education, symptom prevention and management, and collaboration with the participant's provider. Proactive disease management companies send providers information collected from participants between office visits—information such as trended biometric measurements, alerts outside national clinical guidelines for specific diseases, medication lists (prescription, over-the-counter, and herbal), and subjective data gleaned in the outbound calls to participants. This gives providers information between office visits, not normally available to them, so that they can proactively manage the participant's condition before emergency or hospital services are required—thus reducing health care costs and improving the quality of life for their patients.

Long-term care is provided in residential facilities such as assisted-living homes, skilled and intermediate nursing homes, and personal care homes. Each facility is tailored to provide services that the patient or family cannot provide but at a level that maintains the individual's independence as long as possible. With the aging of the population, and with more patients surviving severe trauma and disease with impairments in physical or mental functioning or both, these long-term care facilities are expected to experience rapid growth.

CLASSIFICATIONS OF HEALTH CARE AGENCIES

There are many agencies involved in the total health care delivery system. Organizations that deliver care can be classified in three major ways: as governmental or voluntary agencies; as not-for-profit or for-profit agencies; or by the level of health care services they provide.

Governmental (Public) Agencies

Many **governmental (public) agencies** contribute to the health and well-being of U.S. citizens. All of these public agencies are primarily supported by taxes, administered by elected or appointed officials, and tailored to the needs of the communities served.

Federal agencies

Federal agencies focus on the health of all U.S. citizens. They promote and conduct health and illness research, provide funding to train health care workers, and assist communities in planning health care services. They also develop health programs and services and provide financial and personnel support to staff them. Federal agencies establish standards of practice and safety for health care workers and conduct national health education programs on subjects such as the benefits of not smoking, prevention of acquired immunodeficiency syndrome (AIDS), and the need for prenatal care. Examples of federal agencies are the U.S. Public Health Service (PHS), the National Institutes of Health (NIH), the U.S. Department of Health and Human Services (DHHS), the Occupational Safety and Health Administration (OSHA), the Centers for Medicare and Medicaid Services, and the Centers for Disease Control and Prevention (CDCP).

As a result of the changing health care delivery system, complementary and alternative medicine are now recognized by the federal government. In 1998 under provisions of the Omnibus Appropriations Bill, the NIH established the National Center for Complementary and Alternative Medicine. The center serves as a public information clearinghouse and a research center (National Institutes of Health, 1999).

State Agencies

State health agencies oversee programs that affect the health of citizens within an individual state. Examples of state governmental health agencies include state departments of health and environment, departments that regulate and license health professionals such as state boards of nursing, and those that administer Medicaid insurance programs for the poor. These agencies are not typically involved in providing direct patient care but support local agencies that do provide direct care.

Under increasing influence from managed care organizations, the federal government has transferred responsibility for managing governmental health care funds to some states, at the request of the states. The rationale used to justify this move was that states would be able to exercise more flexibility in designing and administering health care programs tailored to the needs of citizens. However, many believed the danger existed that traditional "safety nets" of federal mandates for services for the poor, elderly, or disadvantaged would be lost. Some feared the long-term outcome would be patients who put off seeking care until they were so sick that their diseases were even more expensive to treat, thus defeating the purpose of state control. In fact, these fears were realized during the early days of state control of Medicaid funds and some problem still continue.

Local agencies

Local agencies serve one community, one county, or a few nearby counties. They provide services to both paying and nonpaying citizens. Public health departments are examples of local governmental agencies found in almost every county in the United States. All citizens, whether or not they can pay, are eligible for health care through local public health departments. These services usually include immunizations, prenatal care and counseling, well-baby and well-child clinics, sexually transmitted disease clinics, tuberculosis clinics, and others. Public health nurses sometimes make home visits as well.

Voluntary (Private) Agencies

Citizens often voluntarily support agencies working to promote or restore health. When private volunteers support an agency providing health care, it is called a **voluntary (private) agency.** Support is generally through private donations, although many of these agencies apply for governmental grants to support some of their activities.

Voluntary agencies often begin when a group of individuals band together to address a health problem. Volunteers may initially perform all their services. Later, they may obtain enough donations to hire personnel, staff an office, and expand services. They may be able to secure ongoing funding through grants or organizations such as the United Way. Examples of voluntary health agencies are the Visiting Nurses Association, the American Heart Association (Figure 13-1), Hospice, the American Cancer Society, and the Mental Health Association.

Not-for-Profit or For-Profit Agencies

The second major way to classify health service delivery agencies is by what is done with the income earned by the agency. A **not-for-profit agency** is one that uses profits to pay personnel, improve services, advertise services, provide educational programs, or otherwise contribute to the mission of the agency. A common misconception is that not-for-profit agencies do not ever make a profit. Actually, they may make profits,

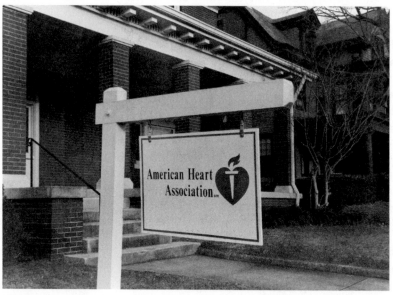

Figure 13-1
Private, not-for-profit agencies, such as the American Heart Association, provide a variety of health-related services to the citizens of their communities. (Photo by Kelly Whalen.)

but the profits must be used for the improvement of the agency. Most voluntary agencies, such as the ones listed previously, are not-for-profit agencies, as are many private hospitals.

Proprietary agencies, or **for-profit agencies,** may distribute profits to partners or shareholders. The growth in for-profit health care agencies has mushroomed over the past two decades. Health care is big business and has the potential to be very profitable.

For-profit agencies include numerous home health care companies that send nurses and other health personnel to care for patients at home. Several large national chains of for-profit health care providers also exist and have demonstrated that it is possible to provide quality patient care and make a profit while doing so. Examples include national nursing home networks, specialty outpatient centers for ambulatory surgery, heart hospitals, and rehabilitation centers. An issue hotly debated is that for-profit health care organizations do not typically treat nonpaying patients. These people must go to publicly funded facilities that are rapidly becoming overburdened with patients who are unable to pay their bills.

Level of Health Care Services Provided

The third major way health care services are classified is by the level of health care services they provide. These levels have traditionally been primary care, secondary care, and tertiary care. A new level, subacute care, has recently emerged. These four levels are discussed below.

Primary care services

Care rendered at the point at which a patient first enters the health care system is considered **primary care.** This care may be provided in a student health clinic, health centers in the community, an emergency department, physicians' offices, nurse practitioners' clinics, or health clinics at work sites. The major goals of the primary health care system are providing the following:

1. Entry into the system
2. Emergency care
3. Health maintenance
4. Long-term and chronic care
5. Treatment of temporary health problems that do not require hospitalization

In addition to treating common health problems, primary care centers are, for many citizens, where much of prevention and health promotion takes place. Unfortunately, these centers are plagued by many problems, such as lack of adequate financing, staffing, space, and community support. However, this pattern is changing, in large part because of the increasing influence of managed care. Access to primary care in the least costly setting is now mandated by managed care organizations.

Secondary care services

Secondary care involves assisting in the prevention of complications from disease, treating temporary dysfunction requiring medical intervention such as hospitalization, evaluating long-term care or chronic patients who may need treatment changes, and providing counseling and therapy that are not available in primary care settings.

Although hospitals have traditionally been associated with this level of care, agencies that increasingly provide secondary health services are **home health agencies,** ambulatory care agencies, skilled nursing agencies, and surgical centers. These agencies offer skilled personnel, easy access, convenient parking, compact equipment and monitoring systems, medications and anesthesia services, and a financial reimbursement program that rewards shorter lengths of stay and home or community care.

A new addition to secondary care is the disease management industry. Health services are provided through outbound/inbound calls with nurses and health professionals, patients interactive voice response (using touchtone phone to respond to questions that are entered into an electronic health record), educational videos/ books sent to the patient, and Internet-based tools. To use these services, patients do not have to leave their homes; they have access to health education, coaching, and tools 24 hours a day, 7 days a week. Another advantage is that patients develop a longitudinal relationship with their disease management nurse/health professional.

It is expected that the trend toward providing community-based secondary care will continue. However, reimbursement has decreased as the terms of the Balanced Budget Act of 1997 have been implemented, eliminating many home health services and skilled nursing care previously covered. The full effect of that Act on this segment of the health care industry has yet to be evaluated.

Tertiary care services

Tertiary care services are those provided to acutely ill patients, to those requiring long-term care, to those needing rehabilitation services, and to terminally ill patients. Tertiary care usually involves many health professionals working together on interdisciplinary teams to design treatment plans.

Examples of tertiary agencies are specialized hospitals such as trauma centers and specialized pediatric centers; long-term care facilities offering skilled nursing, intermediate care, and supportive care; rehabilitation centers; and hospices, where care is provided to the terminally ill and their families in the hospital, in the home, or in special hospice "houses."

Subacute care services

A growing segment of health care, **subacute care** services emerged in the 1990s. According to the Joint Commission on Accreditation of Healthcare Organizations (JCAHO), subacute care is defined as:

> goal-oriented, comprehensive, inpatient care designed for an individual who has had an acute illness, injury, or exacerbation of a disease process. It is rendered immediately after, or instead of, acute hospitalization to treat one or more specific, active, complex medical conditions or to administer one or more technically complex treatments in the context of a person's underlying long-term conditions and overall situation. Generally, the condition of an individual receiving subacute care is such that the care does not depend heavily on high-technology monitoring or complex diagnostic procedures.

Subacute care requires the coordinated services of an interdisciplinary team, including physicians, nurses, and members of other relevant professional disciplines who are knowledgeable and trained to assess and manage these specific conditions and perform the necessary procedures. It is given as part of a specifically defined program, regardless of the site.

Subacute care is generally more intensive than traditional nursing facility care and less intensive than acute inpatient care. It requires frequent (daily to weekly) patient assessment and review of the clinical course and treatment plan for a limited time period (several days to several months), until a condition is stabilized or a predetermined treatment course is completed (Joint Commission on Accreditation of Healthcare Organizations, 1995, p. 3).

The realm of subacute care lies between hospital care and long-term care. By the mid-1990s, this was one of the fastest-growing segments of the health care delivery system and provided employment opportunities for nurses and other health care team members who lost jobs when hospitals downsized. The goal was to provide lower-cost health care and create a seamless transition for patients moving through the health care system. By the end of the decade, growth in the subacute care sector had slowed, owing to two major factors: increasing government regulation had driven the costs up, and lower third-party reimbursement for services rendered in subacute settings made them less profitable.

TRADITIONAL INTERNAL STRUCTURES OF HEALTH CARE AGENCIES

The health care delivery system consists of agencies such as hospitals, clinics, associations, long-term care facilities, and home health services that provide any of the four major types of health services.

Institutional Structure

Institutional structure refers to how an agency is organized to accomplish its mission. The institutional structure of most agencies includes a governing body, a board of trustees, which may also be called a board of directors.

Board of trustees

In the past, board members were often chosen from two groups: community philanthropists, who were expected to donate generously to the facility, and physicians who practiced in the institution. Boards were large, met infrequently, and had mainly ceremonial functions.

But as the health care environment became more complex, board members were chosen to represent various business and political interests of the community. They were expected to bring knowledge and expertise from the business world, as well as to have an appreciation and understanding of health care agencies and how they operate.

Boards now tend to be smaller and carry significant responsibility for the mission of the organization, the quality of services provided, and the financial status of the organization. Boards are not involved in the day-to-day running of the agency, but they are legally responsible for establishing policies governing operations and for ensuring that the policies are executed. They delegate responsibility for running the agency to the chief executive officer (CEO). Box 13-2 outlines a typical hospital board's primary responsibilities.

Box **13-2** **Board of Directors' Responsibilities**

- Mission development and long-range planning
- Ensuring high-quality care
- Oversight of medical staff credentialing
- Financial oversight
- Selection and evaluation of the hospital chief executive officer
- Board self-evaluation and education

From American Hospital Association: *Welcome to the board: an orientation for the new health care trustee*, Chicago, 1999, AHA Press.

Chief executive officer

The **chief executive officer (CEO)** is the individual responsible for the overall operation on a daily basis. He or she usually has a minimum of a master's degree in business or hospital administration. Responsibilities include making sure that the institution runs efficiently and is cost-effective and carrying out policies established by the board. The CEO also has an important external role addressing health care issues in the community and usually sits on the board of trustees and reports to the board. A chief operating officer (COO) often assists the CEO in larger organizations.

Nurses with advanced degrees and experience in administration, business, and health care policy increasingly occupy both of these positions. Boards, who are responsible for hiring CEOs, have found that the broad holistic education and clinical experience of nurses prepares them unusually well for these positions.

Medical staff

A medical staff consists of physicians, who may be either employees or independent practitioners. In either case they must be granted privileges by the board of trustees to see patients at that particular institution. They cannot simply decide to admit patients to an institution. A credentials committee, composed of members of the medical staff, performs the credentialing process. This committee is charged with the responsibility of assuring the board of trustees that every physician admitted to the medical staff of that facility is a qualified and competent practitioner and that, over time, each one keeps his or her skills and knowledge updated.

The medical staff, through its credentials committee, is often charged with the responsibility for credentialing nonphysician providers who admit or consult with patients. These include advanced practice nurses, psychologists, optometrists, podiatrists, and others.

In large organizations, medical staffs are usually organized by service (e.g., department of surgery, department of medicine, and department of obstetrics). The entire medical staff usually elects a **chief of staff.** The chief of staff and the chiefs of the various services work together with the chief executive officer and other administrative representatives through the medical executive committee to make important decisions about medical policy for the institution. The rules and regulations that govern these activities are called bylaws. The board of trustees, to whom the physicians are responsible, must approve the actions of the medical staff.

Service on committees and leadership positions of the medical staff are time-consuming activities; therefore, some institutions pay members of the medical staff a fee for special services in recognition that time away from seeing patients reduces their income.

Nursing staff

The senior administrative nurse in an organization is known as the **chief nurse executive** or chief nursing officer, vice president for nursing, or director of nursing. Once excluded from broad institutional decision making, nurse executives today are often members of the board of trustees. Many organizations now consider the nurse executive and the chief of the medical staff of equal importance.

The educational preparation of nurse executives usually includes a minimum of a master's degree in nursing administration or business administration or a joint master's of science in nursing and master's of business administration (MSN/MBA). Nurse executives are responsible for overseeing all the nursing care provided in the institution and serve as clinical leaders and administrators. Because of the need to coordinate patient care and outcomes among all disciplines, the role has been expanding during recent years to include administrative responsibilities with departments other than nursing, such as pharmacy, respiratory therapy, and social services.

The nursing staff consists of all the registered nurses, licensed practical nurses/licensed vocational nurses, nursing assistants, and clerical assistants employed by the department of nursing. These staff members are usually organized according to the units on which they work.

Each patient care unit has its own budget and staff, for which the manager is responsible. The manager, who is usually a nurse, is also a communication link between the staff and the next level of management.

In large or networked organizations, there may be an additional level of management between the nurse executive and the manager of a unit. These are middle managers, known as clinical directors or supervisors. In most cases, they are also nurses, but they may come from other clinical disciplines or from a business background. These directors are responsible for multiple units or for specific projects or programs. They ensure that nursing and all other services they manage are integrated with other hospital services. They also serve as the communication link between the unit managers and the executive staff.

Other nurses combine direct patient care responsibilities with research, education, and management responsibilities, such as nurse educators, nurse researchers, clinical nurse specialists, and infection control nurses. Nurses in these roles support direct care nurses and serve as expert resources to them in their areas of specialization.

Others

Physicians, nurses, and all the other individuals who work with patients are called the health care team, or **interdisciplinary team.** They are supported in their work by a number of other departments, such as nutrition services, environmental services, and laundry services.

Health care organizations are complex facilities. The way they are organized may vary, but each has an organizational chart that shows its unique structure and explains lines of authority. When considering employment in a health care organization, you can learn a great deal by examining its organizational chart to see how nursing is governed and how it relates to senior management and the board of directors.

THE HEALTH CARE TEAM

Within the almost dizzying array of health care settings discussed in this chapter are the people who provide care to patients—the health care team. At one time, physicians and nurses were the only members of the health care team, but as health care became complex and technology expanded, a number of other health disciplines developed. Today, there are many different health care team members who come from a variety of backgrounds. The decision about which of these various personnel should be involved in the care of a patient depends on the desired patient outcomes.

In the past, physicians were the only coordinators of patient care. In contemporary practice, the coordination of services is likely to be led by a case manager. Case managers, who may be nurses, recognize the contribution of each discipline in achieving the desired outcomes and bring a team together to plan, deliver, and evaluate such care in the most cost-effective manner. Case managers are used in many health care settings other than in managed care organizations, as previously described. The case management model is discussed more fully in Chapter 14.

Key Members of the Health Care Team

In addition to nurses, there are dozens of health care workers who serve from time to time on interdisciplinary health care teams. Several of the key members who are most likely to be involved in the care of patients are discussed below.

Physicians

Physicians have completed college and three or four years of medical school and are licensed by a state board of medical examiners. Although a hospital residency is not required to practice medicine in all states, most physicians have completed one, and many do postgraduate work in a specialty area and then take examinations to become board-certified in the specialty area.

Physicians are responsible for the medical diagnosis and therapies designed to restore health. Although physicians have traditionally been involved mainly in restorative care, many are beginning to recognize the value of illness and injury prevention and health promotion. Most insurance companies have not reimbursed these activities, and until recently there has been little financial incentive to do so. But now managed care plans have dramatically increased reimbursement for preventive care. Some physicians are also integrating nontraditional or alternative treatment choices such as chiropractic medicine, acupuncture, herbal treatments, and massage therapy into their practices.

Dietitians

Many patients require management of their nutritional intake as part of the healing process. Others need to know how to prepare and eat a healthy diet (Figure 13-2). **Dietitians** have baccalaureate degrees and may have completed internships.

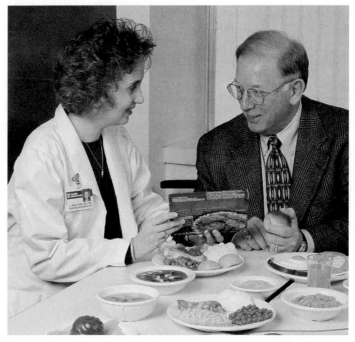

Figure 13-2
Dietitians assist patients to facilitate their own healing and health maintenance through therapeutic diets and healthful nutritional practices. (Photo courtesy Hamilton Medical Center, Dalton, Georgia.)

They understand how the diet (oral or intravenous) can affect a patient's recovery and promote and maintain health. Dietitians focus on the therapeutic value of foods and on teaching people about therapeutic diets and healthful nutrition.

Pharmacists

Pharmacists prepare and dispense medications, instruct patients and other health workers about medications, monitor the use of controlled substances such as narcotics, and work to reduce medication errors. The number and complexity of drugs available today necessitates special education and training in their preparation and dispensing and in monitoring the effects on patients. Clinical pharmacists spend time on hospital units working closely with physicians and nursing case managers to coordinate complex chemotherapy drug administration. They assist in monitoring the drug interactions resulting from a patient taking many different medications because some medications can be rendered ineffective when given with another drug (Figure 13-3).

Pharmacists may pursue either a bachelor's degree in pharmacy, which takes 5 years, or a doctor of pharmacy, which takes 6 years. Depending on state licensing requirements, they may also be required to complete an internship. Pharmacy technicians assist them.

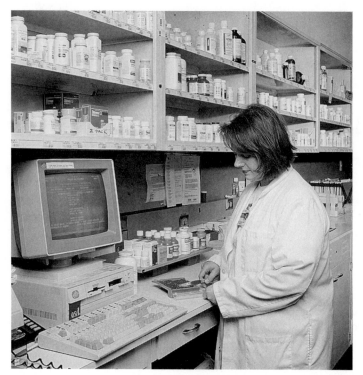

Figure **13-3**
Pharmacists are responsible for preparing and dispensing drugs and monitoring their effects on patients, in addition to numerous other duties. (Photo courtesy Hamilton Medical Center, Dalton, Georgia.)

Paramedical personnel

A number of personnel are educated to assist physicians in the diagnosis of patient problems. This connection with medicine identifies them as **paramedical staff.**

Laboratory technologists handle patient specimens, such as blood, sputum, feces, urine, and body tissues to be examined for cancer or other abnormalities (Figure 13-4). Laboratory technologists carefully subject these body substances to various tests to determine whether or not the patient needs treatment. Technologists have at least a bachelor's degree and are often assisted by laboratory technicians, who have 2-year degrees. They must pass a licensing examination to practice.

Radiology technologists perform x-ray procedures. Although patients still need routine x-ray studies, technology in this field has become much more sophisticated. Subspecialties such as computed tomography (CT), magnetic resonance imaging (MRI), and positron-emission-tomography (PET) have developed (Figure 13-5). All of these techniques are ways of "seeing" what is going on inside the body without surgery. All require specially educated technicians who operate multimillion-dollar equipment. Although some radiology technicians are still trained "on the job,"

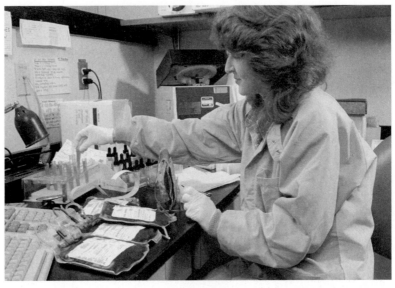

Figure **13-4**
This laboratory technologist works in a critically important setting—a blood bank. Here she prepares several units of blood for administration. (Photo courtesy Hamilton Medical Center, Dalton, Georgia.)

most are educated in formal programs lasting from 1 to 4 years. Radiology technologists have a bachelor's degree. They must be registered with the state in which they practice.

Respiratory technologists

Acutely ill or injured patients often require assistance in breathing. Respiratory technologists operate equipment such as ventilators, oxygen therapy devices, and intermittent positive-pressure breathing machines. They also perform some diagnostic procedures, such as pulmonary function tests and, in some facilities, blood gas analysis. With the increase in respiratory care in the home and community, these health care team members are working closely with home health agencies and community health centers. They must complete either a 2-year (technician) or 4-year (technologist) educational program; in some states they must complete an internship.

Social workers

The **social services** worker is specifically educated and trained to assist patients and their families as they face the impact of illness and injury. They help patients and their families deal with financial problems caused by interruption of work or inadequate insurance benefits; they also direct them to the appropriate community support systems or facilities for home health care or long-term care.

Social workers hold either a bachelor's or master's degree. They serve as liaisons between hospitalized patients and the resources and services available in the community. In addition, social workers frequently are called on to assist other health

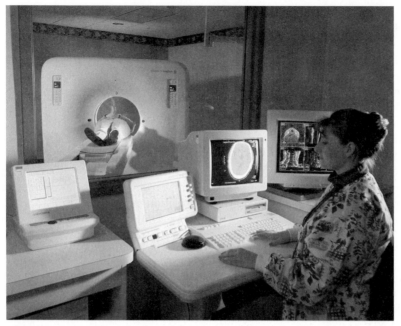

Figure **13-5**
Advances in radiology include a new generation of magnetic resonance imaging (MRI), seen here. Radiological technologists are prepared to operate multimillion-dollar equipment such as this in addition to assisting patients during procedures. (Photo courtesy Hamilton Medical Center, Dalton, Georgia.)

care personnel to cope more effectively with the stresses associated with caring for patients in crisis.

Therapists

Several types of **therapists** help patients with special challenges. Physical therapists, or physiotherapists, assist patients to regain maximum possible physical activity and strength. They focus on assessing preillness or preinjury function, current damage, and potential for recovery. They then develop a long-term plan for gradual return to function through exercise, rest, heat, and hydrotherapy. Physical therapists, who have a minimum of a bachelor's degree, also supervise physical therapy assistants, who hold associate degrees.

Occupational therapists work with physical therapists to develop plans to assist patients in resuming the activities of daily living after illness or injury. They may help patients learn to cook, carry out their personal hygiene, or drive a specially equipped car. In addition, they assist patients to learn skills to return to their previous jobs or retrain patients for new employment options. Occupational therapists have bachelor's degrees. Other types of therapists include recreational therapists, art and music therapists, speech therapists, and massage therapists.

Administrative support personnel

In all organizations, administrative support staff members are needed for clerical jobs such as answering phones, directing visitors, scheduling patient tests, filing insurance claims, filing forms, paying bills, facilitating payroll, and other support functions. These activities require considerable time. Hiring administrative staff members frees the clinical staff to concentrate on direct patient care.

Keeping complete and accurate medical records is an extremely important administrative function that ensures proper insurance billing, eligibility for accreditation, and legal protection of the hospital and its staff. Registered records administrators are vital members of the administrative staff. These professionals staff the medical records department (Figure 13-6). Many organizations today now refer to the medical records departments as "health information services."

The administrative staff ensures that the operations of the facility run smoothly and that clinicians have the resources necessary to meet patient needs. These staff members also educate the clinical staff on financial constraints and work with the staff to find ways to provide quality care at the lowest possible cost.

FORCES CHANGING THE HEALTH CARE DELIVERY SYSTEM

The last decade of the twentieth century was described as the most turbulent time of transition and reform that the United States health care system ever experienced.

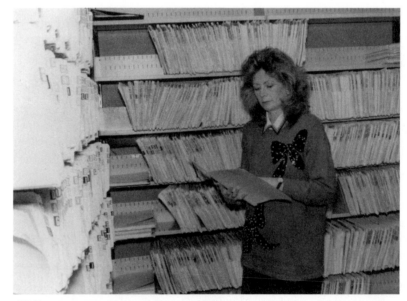

Figure 13-6
This registered records administrator is a highly trained professional whose work is vital to the health care agency by which she is employed. (Photo by Kelly Whalen.)

Total expenditures on health care in the United States exceeded $1 trillion for the first time in 1996 and by 2001 had grown to $1.424 trillion, according to a report by the Centers for Medicare and Medicaid Services (2003). Hospital spending and prescription drug expenditures fueled this increase. As escalating costs of delivery of services hit record levels, a major change in reimbursement for services took place. During that same period, the explosion of information technology contributed to a revolution in consumer knowledge and changing expectations for information and treatment options.

Managed Care

The term **managed care** is used to describe a wide variety of organizations and activities that attempt to control health care costs. Issues of access and quality are key factors in determining the success of various managed care strategies. It is interesting to note that managed care has health promotion, not illness treatment, as one of its primary goals. As the 1990s progressed, several factors led to the development of a variety of managed care models (Figure 13-7), which included the rising cost of providing health care benefits, growing taxpayer unrest about the expense of tax-funded health care programs, unequal access to services, and concerns about quality.

Types of Managed Care Organizations

Managed care organizations (MCOs) can be categorized into four basic models: health maintenance organizations (HMOs), preferred provider organizations (PPOs), point-of-service (POS) plans, and physician hospital organizations (PHOs).

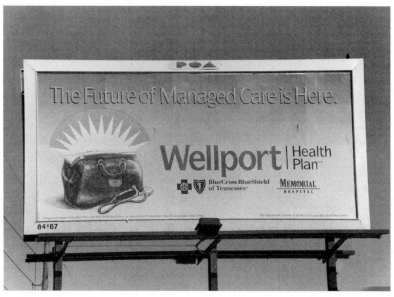

Figure **13-7**
Managed care has created a highly competitive health care market, as this billboard illustrates. (Photo by Kelly Whalen.)

Health maintenance organizations

In contrast to the traditional fee-for-service system, the **health maintenance organization (HMO)** is a system in which a defined group of people receives health care services for a predetermined fixed fee. This method of financing is called **capitation,** and it is paid on a per-member per-month basis. The same amount is paid to the provider each month regardless of whether services were provided or how much the services cost. The fee is usually negotiated for a period of 1 to 3 years. The patient's access to services is coordinated and managed by a primary care provider. The primary care provider, sometimes called a **gatekeeper,** is responsible for all referrals for tests and to specialists. Keeping patients healthy means that the primary care provider gets to keep more of the fee. Some people worry that this will discourage gatekeepers from ordering diagnostic tests and referring patients to specialists, even when indicated.

Preferred provider organizations

The **preferred provider organization (PPO)** contracts with independent providers such as physicians and hospitals for a negotiated discount for the services provided to its members.

Point-of-service organizations

The **point-of-service (POS) organization** is a form of MCO with more options. Members may choose to receive services within the defined network, or they may go outside the network and pay a higher deductible or copayment.

Physician hospital organizations

As managed care organizations penetrated the market and threatened the financial viability of hospitals and many physicians' practices, the providers of health services created another type of organization, **physician hospital organizations (PHOs).** The PHO is a separate corporation formed by a hospital and a group of its medical staff for the purpose of joint contracting with managed care organizations. This structure allows hospitals and physicians to work together to negotiate fees for services directly with self-insured employers and managed care organizations.

In spite of this collaboration, both hospitals and physicians continued to face cutbacks in reimbursement. Physicians began to fight against the high profits of managed care organizations. In June 1999, the physicians of the American Medical Association voted to develop a national labor union. Their claim was that such action was necessary to help them more effectively treat patients. Committed to remaining faithful to the ethical traditions of professionalism in the practice of medicine, physicians assured their patients there would be no strikes (Smoak, 1999).

Hospitals had similar concerns. They saw reimbursement shrink both from managed care and as a result of the Balanced Budget Act of 1997. The Balanced Budget Act outlined progressive cuts in services and reimbursement rates over a 5-year period. In preparation for the declining revenues, mergers and acquisitions between hospitals took place at a staggering rate during the 1990s. These strategies were intended to consolidate services and cut costs.

Registered nurses are used extensively throughout managed care systems. Many HMOs utilize advanced practice nurses in the primary care role in ambulatory and community settings. Another key role for the registered nurse is that of case manager. The case manager coordinates care for a patient throughout the health care system to decrease fragmentation, contain costs, and enhance the quality of life. Nurses also serve in a triage role, deciding the most appropriate course of intervention. Nurses are often employed as utilization reviewers to determine the most appropriate and cost-efficient level of care. This role often facilitates moving a patient out of the hospital and into a rehabilitation center, a nursing home, or home, with home health services.

The consumers' perspective toward managed care and their experiences with it vary. Some consumers have good access, a full range of services, providers they trust, and lower costs. Others have experienced access problems, denial of treatment, and limited coverage. As consumers became more educated, they began to fight for their rights to health care through political reform and the legal system. The collective power of consumers created changes in the health care system, mainly in terms of safeguards to prevent such abuses as "drive-through deliveries," discussed in the following section.

Changes in Consumers' Expectations

The computer age has afforded access to global information at explosive rates. Society has embraced the information technology age and has become increasingly dependent on instant global news, information, and service. By the end of the twentieth century consumers had instant service touching every area of life, such as drive-through banking, fast food service, and car maintenance and 1-hour eyeglass prescriptions and photography services. The proliferation of Internet websites has also affected the knowledge and expectation of health care consumers.

In 1998 more than 22 million U.S. adults reported using the Internet to obtain health information. Experts predicted that in 2000 more than 33 million would have researched health issues online. That prediction was dwarfed by the actual numbers. According to a comprehensive report by the Pew Internet & American Life Project, about 52 million American adults relied on the Internet in making health decisions in 2000. By 2002, that number had risen to 73 million (Fox and Rainie, 2002, p. 4). "We're seeing a remarkable transition in health care," says Mitchell Morris, a surgeon and vice president at the University of Texas M. D. Anderson Cancer Center in Houston. "The Internet is going to irrevocably affect how patients and doctors interact. This is not going to go away" (*USA Today*, July 14, 1999, p. 1A). The News Note on p. 350 provides more on this topic.

Health-related websites offer a wide range of topics, such as wellness, nutrition, general health information, live surgery and births, women's health, medication reference books, government health agencies, professional associations, referrals and information about hospitals, physicians, managed care, patient rights, and libraries filled with medical textbooks and journals. Live interactive websites even offer diagnosis, treatment, and medication prescription services without a hands-on assessment and examination. Long-term outcomes of electronic care have not been researched and documented at this time.

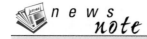

Net Empowering Patients: Millions Scour the Web to Find Medical Information

In ever-growing numbers, patients clutching Internet printouts and a list of smart questions are marching into doctor's offices nationwide, sometimes knowing more about their disease and ways to treat it than their physicians.

This explosion of medical knowledge—and misinformation—among lay people is causing a dramatic shift in the balance of power between doctor and patient, changing how medicine is practiced more profoundly than anything since the advent of managed care.

"That is going to change the whole paradigm we've been used to in medicine," says former surgeon general C. Everett Koop, whose site was once the most popular medical area on the Web. "Patients are getting more and more control because of the knowledge they have ... which enables them to make decisions with their doctor about diagnosis, procedures, and treatment."

From Davis R, Miller L: Net empowering patients: Millions scour the Web to find medical information, *USA Today,* July 14, 1A, 1999. Reprinted with permission.

Physicians today are not surprised when patients come to their offices with complete research, a potential diagnosis, and treatment options from the Internet. This has led some health care leaders to be concerned about consumers' ability to discern the quality of information from such a vast array of choices. The Federal Trade Commission (FTC) cracked down on companies and individuals posting misleading health information on the Internet in 1998 after investigators found 800 websites making fraudulent claims. In June 1999 the FTC launched Operation Cure All, a campaign to stop false health information on the Internet. The FTC now monitors health sites on the Internet on an ongoing basis (Flaherty, 1999).

HEALTH CARE'S RESPONSE TO MANAGED CARE AND CONSUMER EXPECTATIONS

The impact of managed care and advanced information technology has forced the health care system to undergo massive transformation to meet the demands of new reimbursement structures and consumer expectations. The reengineering of health care organizations has included the redesign not only of patient care delivery but also of the **organizational structures** necessary to support the changes.

Reengineering

During the 1990s, health care organizations recognized the full impact of managed care and changes in consumer expectations. Hospitals were so complex, bureaucratic, and convoluted that many were failing to deliver high-quality products and services consistently. In health care, for example, it was not unusual for a patient staying 5 to 7 days in a typical hospital to travel by wheelchair or stretcher 8 or 9 miles during that stay. A simple laboratory test might require 40 to 60 separate activities or steps before results could be reported. Excessive and duplicative paperwork and trivial tasks burdened care providers and left patients dissatisfied and angry. The patient was no longer the center of the system. At times, it seemed patients and families were nuisances that got in the way of bureaucratic activities.

Health care organizations recognized that becoming more efficient was imperative for survival. The challenge to provide high-quality care at the right cost with the expected outcome has become the focus of the last decade of the twentieth century. A dramatic new paradigm was needed. The continuous quality improvement movement had laid the groundwork and provided the tools necessary to transform patient care from being designed around various specialized departments to an integrated process-driven system. **Reengineering** is the "fundamental rethinking and radical redesign of business processes to bring about dramatic improvement in performance" (Hammer and Stanton, 1995). **Patient-focused care,** also known as patient-centered care, means placing the patient at the center of activity and designing processes that efficiently and effectively attain desired patient outcomes.

Management experts believe that reducing layers of management is an essential component of any reengineering initiative. One key to the new organization and structure is decentralization. **Decentralization** empowers staff, allowing them to exercise their own good judgment rather than waiting to be told what to do. Decision-making authority is given to those most affected by the decision, rather than being limited to a few executives or managers. This means fewer layers in an organizational chart and is in agreement with the philosophy that all professionals should be encouraged to use their talents fully.

For empowerment to be effective, the board of trustees and top executives must clearly articulate their vision, goals, and expectations so that all employees understand the direction of the organization and their roles in it. Decentralization and empowerment involve the development and use of many skills, including consensus, decision making, positive discipline, worker independence and interdependence, negotiation, collaboration, and critical thinking.

Reengineering and patient-focused care are accomplished by cross-functional teams, who are involved with all aspects of achieving a specific patient-focused outcome. **Cross-functional teams** are composed of people from all areas of the organization who contribute to a particular process and outcome. They redesign, from scratch, how the work will be done and who will do it and in what time frame and location. In some new models staff members are cross-trained to be able to complete several different tasks, each of which was formerly performed by a different worker. Workers who are cross-trained to perform different tasks are also known as **multiskilled workers.** For example, a single worker may be trained to collect admission demographic information, draw blood for tests ordered, and perform an electrocardiogram. With these changes, patient satisfaction is typically higher than with the older fragmented bureaucratic methods.

When done well, reengineering addresses the purpose of the business; the organizational culture needed for success, processes, and performance; and the people, knowledge, and skills needed to accomplish the redesigned work. When done poorly, reengineering is often a euphemism for downsizing or staff reductions or layoffs. Although it is true that as the work is redesigned, fewer people may be needed, staff reduction is not the main goal of reengineering.

Downsizing without proper work redesign simply leaves fewer people to accomplish already inefficient and ineffective work. Unfortunately, many companies, both in and outside health care, take this shortsighted approach to reengineering. The result is poor morale, loss of competent staff, lower-quality outcomes, patient dissatisfaction, and loss of market share. Studies continue to show that empowerment, job satisfaction and organizational commitment remain closely linked (Kuokkanen, Leino-Kilpi, and Katajisto, 2003). Box 13-3 lists key components for successful reengineering. The accompanying Research Note discusses the specific outcomes resulting from restructuring at a Pennsylvania health care facility.

Tomorrow's health care workers are facing a different work environment. They will probably have seven to ten different jobs during an average work career rather than the three jobs or fewer held by previous generations. Even when employed in the same position, they should expect that position to undergo major evolution and change. You may ask yourself, "How can I thrive in this constantly changing environment?" The following suggestions should help you keep your options open, even as the health care system changes:

- Take every opportunity to learn new skills.
- Read widely both inside and outside your field.
- Identify emerging trends and new opportunities.
- Find new ways to apply your knowledge and skills.
- Volunteer for community activities that will stretch your skills, help you learn new ones, and allow you to meet people who can be helpful to you.
- Keep your resume current, but do not change jobs too often because this implies instability.
- Develop flexibility, including openness to new challenges.

Hospitals Respond With New Organizational Models

After 15 years of restructuring efforts in hospitals, there are several basic organizational models in use, each with numerous variations. Five representative structures

---

Box 13-3 Keys to Successful Reengineering

- Strong leadership
- Support from the top (financial, cultural, time, resources)
- Team members who love ambiguity, creativity, risk taking, and holism
- An irreverence for the past
- Optimism, persistence
- Ability to answer these questions: What is our business? What culture do we want? How do we need to do our work? What people do we want to work with?

RESEARCH note

Nursing administrators are interested in evaluating how redesigning patient care delivery and organizational restructuring affect the quality of patient care. Eighteen months after Lehigh Valley Hospital in Allentown, Pennsylvania, completed restructuring, a study of how the redesign affected patient and nurse satisfaction, cost of care, and clinical quality was conducted on four medical-surgical units. The redesign efforts had included the following: facility changes to improve the convenience of the location of supplies, nurses' stations, and patient records; enhanced telecommunication and information systems; and redesign of all work processes and many staff roles.

Using the Press-Ganey Patient Satisfaction Survey, seven dimensions of nursing care were measured in the evaluation of patient satisfaction: friendliness, promptness, taking problems seriously, attention to special needs, being inform-ative about tests, technical skill, and consideration of patients as individuals.

The clinical quality outcomes measured were patient falls, medication errors, hospital-acquired infections, and intravenous-related complications. Hospital mortality data, length of stay, and the costs of care were also evaluated.

Results of the study revealed that patient satisfaction scores declined during implementation of changes, but after 18 months, scores increased significantly on three of the four units. Nurses also experienced improved collaboration with physicians following the restructuring. All of the clinical quality outcomes were either improved or maintained at the time of the 18-month follow-up. Hospital mortality data could not be completely linked to redesign initiatives, but the data indicated that the restructuring had not adversely affected patient outcomes. There were varied results in the degree to which costs and length of stay declined. Overall results on the four pilot units were positive enough that nursing leaders decided to expand the redesign initiative to other parts of the hospital.

The researchers pointed out a lack of comprehensive research analyzing long-term effects of hospital restructuring. They also observed that nursing journals have published numerous articles about organizational redesign and concluded that according to many reports, results of organizational redesign have been disappointing. They stress the importance of establishing goals and outcomes for restructuring before implementation and the need to evaluate changes systematically over a period of time to obtain scientific evidence about the impact on patient care.

From Bryan YE, Hitchings KS, Fuss MA, et al: Measuring and evaluating hospital restructuring efforts, *J Nurs Admin* 28(9):21-27, 1998.

are described below. Readers should recognize that the models overlap and few "pure" models are in use.

Functional model

The traditional functional model clearly defines each major function of the organization and establishes clear lines of managerial authority. Examples of the major functions are inpatient care, outpatient care, surgery, professional services, facility operations, marketing and planning, and human resources.

Service line model

The service line model establishes management responsibilities around specific types of services wherever they occur in the hospital or in its associated clinics and offices. Examples of major service lines include cardiology, orthopedics, oncology, obstetrics, ambulatory services, and behavioral health.

Matrix model

The matrix model is a complex model with multiple authority and support systems. Consider this model as a blend of the functional and service line models. In the matrix model there is one overall manager who directs dual lines of authority. It is a team concept with one manager overseeing the specialized functional areas and another manager providing the expertise to the particular service. In this model some employees report to two managers. For example, the housekeeping supervisor in the surgical department would report to both the head of housekeeping and the director of the surgical services.

Process model

The process model is a newer approach that organizes management of care around phases in the process of health care delivery. These phases include access, treatment, transition, and evaluation. Responsibilities of managers in the process model span all departments.

Regional model

The regional model is another new approach addressing more complex health care systems that have emerged through the expansion of services and organizations beyond the single hospital. It is organized according to the individual service providers. Examples include hospital functions, home health, nursing homes, managed care organizations, rehabilitation centers, and smaller hospitals that have been acquired as part of a larger system.

MAINTAINING QUALITY IN HEALTH CARE AGENCIES

Maintaining high-quality services should be the goal of every health care agency. As pressure increases to control costs, it becomes even more important to ensure that quality is not sacrificed simply to save dollars. This can be accomplished in a variety of ways, chiefly through accreditation and quality care initiatives.

Accreditation of Health Care Agencies

As you learned in Chapter 2, schools of nursing may choose to participate in a process called accreditation. Health care organizations such as hospitals, home health agencies, and long-term care facilities are also accredited. Their accrediting body is the Joint Commission on the Accreditation of Health Care Organizations (JCAHO). Accreditation by JCAHO is important and requires that a number of standards be met in every department. The goal of accreditation is to improve patient outcomes. Considerable agency resources of time and money are spent making sure accreditation criteria are met. Another strategy through which most organizations choose to work toward improvement in patient outcomes is continuous quality improvement.

Continuous Quality Improvement/Total Quality Management

The concept of **continuous quality improvement (CQI)** was first developed by management expert W. Edwards Deming in the 1940s when he suggested that managers in industry should rely on groups of employees, which he called quality circles, as they made decisions about how work was to be done. His work was not widely accepted in this country, but when the Japanese government asked him to help them rebuild their workplaces after the devastation of World War II, Deming went to Japan. His ideas revolutionized Japanese industry, which became superior to American industry in many ways by the 1970s, leading to a belated acceptance of Deming's ideas in this country.

In today's health care systems, one of the most important management concepts borrowed from industry is CQI, also called total quality management (TQM). Rather than trying to identify mistakes after they have occurred, these systems focus on establishing procedures for ensuring high-quality patient care. Using quality improvement concepts, groups of employees from different departments decide how care will be provided (Figure 13-8). They decide what outcomes are desired and design systems and assign roles and activities to create those outcomes. Every effort is made to anticipate potential problems and prevent their occurrence. Management delegates authority to the providers of services to plan and carry out quality improvement programs. Programs in CQI/TQM reinforce the belief that quality is everyone's responsibility.

Recently **performance improvement (PI)** has been used to describe organizational efforts to improve corporate performance. Incorporating aspects of quality management, PI focuses efforts on increasing individual and group competence and productivity. When done well, the company and its employees and customers gain many advantages. Employees who are more efficient may find job enrichment opportunities. When done poorly, however, quality can be compromised in the process of increasing productivity. Reduction in labor force is often a result of these efforts and can lead to lowered employee morale.

Nurses are actively involved in quality and performance improvement and in accreditation processes, but these activities are not the responsibility of nursing alone. They are institution-wide initiatives, and everyone, at all levels, gets involved. Working together to improve patient care builds cooperation among departments and clinical

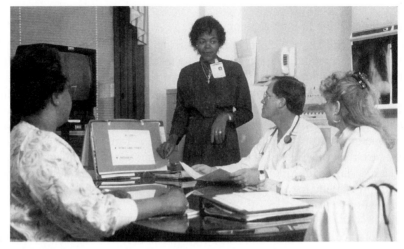

Figure 13-8
This group of professionals works together to implement continuous quality improvement processes in an acute care hospital with the goal of improving efficiency and patient care while reducing costs. (Photo by Wilson Baker.)

disciplines and boosts morale. In the accompanying Interview, a nurse describes her role in performance improvement.

Summary of Key Points
- The health care delivery system in the United States is a complex system that provides health promotion, illness prevention, diagnosis and treatment, and rehabilitation and long-term care.
- Health care agencies may be classified as governmental or voluntary, as for-profit or not-for-profit, or according to level of care provided. A single agency may fit into all three categories.
- Health care agencies have traditionally been structured with boards of trustees, chief executive officers, medical and nursing staffs, and members of a variety of other disciplines.
- An interdisciplinary health care team consists of an array of professionals, including physicians, nurses, dietitians, pharmacists, paramedical personnel, respiratory technologists, social workers, various therapists, and administrative support personnel. Each member has an important part to play in ensuring the best patient outcomes.
- Managed care has forced major changes in the health care delivery system.
- Information technology, leading to increased consumer expectations, has contributed to revolutionary change that will continue in the future and will affect professional nursing in many ways, most of which are yet unknown.
- As a result of managed care and changes in consumer expectations, organizations have gone through reengineering, reducing layers of management, and empowering the workforce to take part in decision making.

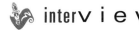 inter v i e w *with Pamela G. Stelmack, RN, BSHA, CPHQ, Director,*
Performance Improvement/Utilization Management,
Hamilton Medical Center, Dalton, Georgia

Interviewer: What does a utilization management nurse do?

Stelmack: My primary duties in utilization management are to provide clinical information concerning the patient's admission to third-party payers to obtain reimbursement for services. We review all inpatient and observation admissions for both appropriateness and quality of care provided. We review both commercially insured patient records and Medicare, Medicaid, and other payer categories. We are responsible for obtaining the precertification authorization for all emergency, inpatient Medicaid admissions, which is required for both the hospital and physician to get reimbursed.

Interviewer: How has managed care changed your role as a nurse?

Stelmack: I have seen the role of nursing expanding as a result of managed care. We used to focus only on the clinical issues surrounding patient care, not the reimbursement aspects. With today's emphasis on cutting costs in health care while maintaining quality, nurses need to understand the financial impact of providing care for their patients. Patients may not have access to or be able to afford the care they need to maintain optimal health or prevent readmission to the hospital. In our role as patient advocates, nurses try to minimize the financial impact of the condition or disease process.

Interviewer: How can nurses serve as patient advocates in minimizing the financial impact of a patient's illness? Is nursing documentation on the patient's record used in receiving approval for a hospitalization or continued stay?

Stelmack: Yes, definitely. In doing these reviews, we are looking at what is documented in the record to support severity of illness, intensity of service, and discharge criteria. Admission assessments, which include vital signs, symptoms, onset of those symptoms, previous medical history, and discharge, help to support the severity of illness. Intensity of service refers to the treatments/medications ordered for the patients. Nursing documentation should focus on the patient's response to treatment and what additional needs they have. When we review the record, the nursing documentation is a key component in supporting the need for the admission and determining when it is appropriate to consider an alternate level of care. If the documentation does not support the need for services, then either the organization does not get reimbursed or the patient will be responsible for a larger portion of the bill than they might expect. This can have a significant impact on the patient/family's ability to cope with the situation. So you see, nursing documentation is very important.

Continued

interv i e w *with Pamela G. Stelmack, RN, BSHA, CPHQ, Director, Performance Improvement/Utilization Management, Hamilton Medical Center, Dalton, Georgia—cont'd*

Interviewer: Managed care organizations have received a lot of negative press. Are they really interested in quality of care? If so, what are some examples of quality indicators they monitor?

Stelmack: Managed care organizations are definitely interested in quality of care. They have a national organization, the National Committee for Quality Assurance (NCQA), that assesses health care plans and managed care organizations in a manner similar to JCAHO surveys. They serve as a watchdog for the organizations to help ensure quality patient care. Managed care organizations monitor patient outcomes by tracking physician practice patterns and various organizational indicators such as mortality rates, nosocomial [hospital-acquired] infections, and c-section rates. Managed care organizations also are judged by their coverage for preventive or early detection health services such as cervical cancer screening, diabetic eye exams, and prenatal care.

- New organizational structures for hospitals include functional, service line, matrix, process, and regional models.
- Accreditation and continuous quality improvement are efforts to ensure public safety and institutional effectiveness and accountability.

CRITICAL THINKING QUESTIONS

1. Using the yellow pages of your telephone directory or a directory of social services, identify local health services in the following areas: health promotion, illness prevention, diagnosis and treatment, rehabilitation, and long-term care. Judging from the number of agencies for each service, where does the health care emphasis seem to be? What implications does this have for citizens of your community?

2. Obtain the organizational chart of a health care facility. Determine how it compares with one of the organizational structures described. Examine it to see how nursing fits into the overall structure. Who reports to the nurse executive, and to whom does the nurse executive report? What other administrative staff members are on the same level with the nurse executive?

3. Hold a panel discussion on reimbursement. Invite representatives from government, a managed care organization, a hospital, a major employer, and a nonprofit charity to discuss how managed care has affected their organizations.

4. Interview nurses in the hospital, home health, disease management and case management settings. Look for the similarities and the differences in their work and interactions with patients. How do they work together to provide seamless care for the patient?

5. Interview a nurse and one or more nonnurse health professionals. Ask them to share some of their experiences as members of interdisciplinary health care teams

during reengineering or restructuring of their institutions. What impact have these initiatives had on the way they care for patients?

6. Go to the Internet and search for websites that provide information on menopause and hormone replacement therapy. Include sites on prevention, wellness, and alternative medicine. Search for a virtual hospital, referrals to physicians, and patient rights. Analyze the information to determine how many different options for diagnosis and treatment were found. How might patients use this information as they interact with health care professionals?

REFERENCES

American Hospital Association: *Welcome to the board: an orientation for the new health care trustee,* Chicago, 1999, AHA Press.

Bell CT, editor: *Modern Healthcare's by the Numbers,* July 19(29):17-24, 1999.

Bryan YE, Hitchings KS, Fuss MA., et al: Measuring and evaluating hospital restructuring efforts, *J Nurs Admin* 28(9):21-27, 1998.

Centers for Medicare and Medicaid Services: Report details national health care spending increases in 2001, Baltimore, MD, 2003, Centers for Medicare and Medicaid Services.

Davis R, Miller L: Net empowering patients: Millions scour the Web to find medical information, *USA Today,* July 14, 1A, 1999.

Deming WE: *Quality, productivity, and competitive position,* Cambridge, MA, 1982, Massachusetts Institute of Technology, Center for Advanced Engineering Study.

Deming WE: Out of the crisis, Cambridge, MA, 1986, Massachusetts Institute of Technology, Center for Advanced Engineering Study.

Flaherty M: FTC targets Internet health fraud, *Nurse Week/Health Week,* July 5, 1999, Online *(www.nurseweek.com/new/00-7/36d.html).*

Fox S, Rainie L: Vital decisions: How Internet users decide what information to trust when they or their loved ones are sick, Washington, DC, Released May 22, 2002, Pew Internet & American Life Project, Online *(www.pewinternet.org/reports/toc.asp?Report=59).*

Hammer M, Stanton S: *The reengineering revolution,* New York, 1995, Harper Business.

Joint Commission on Accreditation of Health Care Organizations: Survey protocol for subacute programs, Oakbrook Terrace, IL, 1995, Joint Commission on Accreditation of Healthcare Organizations.

Kuokkanen L, Leino-Kilpi H, Katajisto J: Nurse empowerment, job-related satisfaction, and organizational commitment, *J Nurs Care Qual* 18(3):184-192, 2003.

National Institutes of Health: National center for complementary and alternative medicine: General information, Online, 1999 *(www.nccam.nih.gov).*

Smoak RD: *American Medical Association news release,* Online, 1999 *(www.ama-assn.org/advocacy/statemnt/990623s.htm).*

U.S. Department of Health and Human Services: *Healthy people 2000: national health promotion and disease prevention objectives,* Washington, DC, 1990, Government Printing Office.

U.S. Department of Health and Human Services: *Healthy people 2010,* fact sheet, Washington, DC, 2003, Government Printing Office.

14

Nursing Roles in the Health Care Delivery System

*Jennifer E. Jenkins**

Accountability
Autonomy
Case Management Nursing
Change Agent
Collaboration

Delegate
Differentiated Practice
Entrepreneur
Functional Nursing
Patient Advocate

Primary Nursing
Professional
  Accountabilities
Shared Governance
Team Nursing

■ **L e a r n i n g O u t c o m e s**

After studying this chapter, students will be able to:
- Differentiate among four nursing care delivery systems.
- Discuss a variety of roles for the nurse in the health care delivery system.
- Discuss the purpose of differentiated levels of practice.
- Describe the shared governance council model in nursing organizational structure.
- Describe five professional accountabilities within the shared governance model.
- Identify skills the nurse needs when working with interdisciplinary teams.

C hapter 13 covered aspects of our changing health care delivery system, discussed the organizational structure of health agencies, and explained the impact of managed care and how health care organizations are redesigning their work processes. It also reviewed the classifications of health care agencies and responsibilities of the various members of the health care delivery team. This chapter takes a closer look at nursing from a historical perspective and examines how nursing is integral to the interdisciplinary health care delivery team of today and into the future.

*The author wishes to acknowledge the contributions of Karen J. Wisdom to the preparation of this chapter.

TYPES OF NURSING CARE DELIVERY SYSTEMS HISTORICALLY USED IN ACUTE CARE SETTINGS

Before World War I, nurses visited the sick in their homes to care for them. As hospital care improved and nursing education evolved, more sick people were treated in hospitals. Providing care to groups of patients rather than to individuals required nurses to be efficient and use their time effectively. An organizing structure was needed, and various types of care delivery systems were designed to meet the goals of efficient and effective nursing care. Several types of patient care delivery systems have been used in acute care settings. Four systems—functional nursing, team nursing, primary nursing, and case management nursing—are reviewed in this chapter.

Functional Nursing

By the 1930s, advances in medical technology had evolved to a point at which hospital treatment surpassed that which could be provided at home. As more patients were admitted to hospitals, more nurses were employed to care for them.

The functional approach to nursing care grew out of a need to provide care to large numbers of patients. It focused on organizing and distributing the tasks, or functions, of care. Trained nurses provided care that required high skill levels, and untrained workers with little skill or education performed many less complex tasks.

In **functional nursing,** personnel worked side by side, each performing the assigned task. The goal of functional nursing was efficient management of time, tasks, and energy. Although this practice saved hospitals money, patient care was fragmented, and patients had to relate to many different people. There was no one person they could call, "my nurse."

Today, functional nursing is still used in some settings. It is particularly useful when there are few staff members available, such as at night, on weekends, and on holidays. It often is combined with another method, however, and is rarely used as

---

case study

Functional Nursing

A registered nurse (RN) on the evening shift at a local nursing home has been assigned to administer special skin care treatments to bed-bound patients, change dressings, and give all medications. A licensed practical nurse (LPN) monitors all patient temperatures and blood pressures, weighs patients, records the amount they eat and drink, and monitors the blood sugar of diabetic patients. The nursing assistants have each been assigned a different group of patients for whom they are responsible during the shift. They help these patients with personal hygiene, see that they receive their meals and snacks, and assist them with eating, toileting, and other tasks. Because it is evening, the head nurse is not there. In her place is a charge nurse, who signs all charts, indicating that care was administered; talks with physicians and family members; and orders supplies and medications. As nursing assistants go about their work, there is infrequent interaction. Often they can be heard telling a patient who asks for something, "I'm not assigned to do that tonight. I'll tell the other nursing assistant that you need something."

Box **14-1** Advantages and Disadvantages of Functional Nursing

Advantages

- Efficient—can complete many tasks in a reasonable time frame.
- Workers do only tasks they are educated to do and become very efficient.
- Promotes organizational skills—each worker must organize his or her own work.
- Promotes worker autonomy.

Disadvantages

- Lack of holistic view of patient—emphasis on task, not person.
- Lacks continuity—patients often do not know who their nurse is.
- Registered nurses have little time to talk with patients or render personal care.

---

the sole care delivery method (Bernhard and Walsh, 1990). Box 14-1 lists advantages and disadvantages of functional nursing.

Team Nursing

In response to the frustration some nurses felt when using the functional approach to patient care, Lambertson (1953) designed **team nursing.** She envisioned nursing teams as democratic work groups with different skill levels represented by different team members. They were assigned as a team to a group of patients.

Team nursing has been widely used in hospitals and long-term care facilities. The team usually consists of a registered nurse, who serves as team leader, a licensed practical nurse, and one or more certified nursing assistants (Figure 14-1).

The team leader, although ultimately responsible for all the care provided, **delegates** (assigns responsibility for) certain patients to each team member. Each member of the team provides the level of care for which he or she is best prepared. The least skilled and experienced members care for the patients who require the least complex care, and the most skilled and experienced members care for the most seriously ill patients who require the most complex care.

Team nursing allows the team leader to shift, match, and redistribute patient assignments to team members according to their level of education and expertise. For example, because of the acuity level (extent of illness) of a group of patients, a team leader may make a "trade" with another team leader, for instance, trading a nursing assistant for an additional registered nurse. The nursing assistant would work on the team with less acutely ill patients, and the team with the more seriously ill patients would have an extra registered nurse.

Team nursing enables the team leader to supervise, coordinate, and manage the care given to all the team's patients for the assigned shift. Often the team approach is closer to functional nursing because the team leader delegates without overseeing the care given by team members or patient outcomes. The team leader reports to the head nurse.

Today, team nursing is still used, but the model is usually modified. Many of the patient-focused care models implemented during patient care redesign use registered

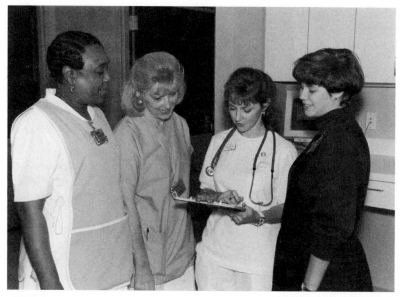

Figure 14-1
Communication and coordination are keys to effective use of team nursing as a model of nursing care delivery. Here team members brief the team leader on their patients. (Photo by Kelly Whalen.)

nurses as team leaders coordinating care for a group of patients and supervising multiskilled workers who have been trained to perform a variety of comfort measures, such as positioning, and technical procedures, such as taking vital signs or drawing blood.

case study

Team Nursing

The team leader for 12 patients on a medical-surgical unit during the night shift has one licensed practical nurse and one certified nursing assistant (CNA) on his team. First, the registered nurse team leader makes visits to all patients' rooms to assess their conditions. Based on those assessments, he assigns the licensed practical nurse to five patients. Three of those patients had surgery within the past 3 or 4 days and are recovering without complication. The other two have routine conditions.

The nursing assistant is assigned to two patients who are ready for discharge tomorrow, two more who are within 2 days of discharge, and one newly admitted patient who will have surgery tomorrow.

One patient has had surgery today. He is receiving intravenous fluids and has a lot of pain. There is a family member spending the night with him. The team leader takes this patient assignment but does not take an overload of patients because he needs the flexibility to assist where needed and to supervise the other team members. During the night, the team leader also develops and updates nursing care plans on all the team's patients.

Box **14-2** Advantages and Disadvantages of Team Nursing

Advantages
- Potential for building team spirit.
- Provides comprehensive care.
- Each worker's abilities are used to the fullest.
- Promotes job satisfaction.
- Decreases nonprofessional duties of registered nurses.

Disadvantages
- Constant need to communicate among team members is time-consuming.
- All must promote teamwork, or team nursing is unsuccessful.
- Team composition varies from day to day, which can be confusing and disruptive and decreases continuity of care.
- May result in blurred role boundaries and resulting confusion and resentment.

In team nursing, the RN team leader oversees all care for a particular shift, makes assessments, and documents responses to care. The licensed practical nurse team member provides direct care by performing treatments and procedures and reports patient responses to the team leader. The certified nursing assistant provides routine direct, personal care. If multiskilled, nonlicensed workers are used, the role of the licensed practical nurse or certified nursing assistant is often eliminated.

As with functional nursing, team nursing has both advantages and disadvantages; these are presented in Box 14-2.

Primary Nursing

Developed by Manthey (1980), **primary nursing** was designed to promote the concept of an identified nurse for every patient during the patient's stay on a particular

---

case study

Primary Nursing

A primary nurse in a rehabilitation hospital is assigned a new patient. He is a 25-year-old man who sustained a spinal cord injury in a diving accident. This patient has been in a trauma intensive care unit, and now that his condition has stabilized, he has been transferred. He is paralyzed from the shoulders down.

In addition to providing direct care and writing the care plan, the primary nurse assesses the emotional status of the patient's wife of 2 months and discovers she has few sources of emotional support and is growing anxious about the future. In addition, the wife feels guilty about her anger and frustration over this dramatic change in their life plans.

The primary nurse acknowledges and discusses these feelings. She explains that patients and family members often have angry feelings under similar circumstances. She refers the couple to a rehabilitation psychologist, who works with them in replanning and reprioritizing their life goals.

unit. The goal of primary nursing is to deliver consistent, comprehensive care by identifying one nurse who is responsible, has authority, and is accountable for the patient's nursing care outcomes for the period during which the patient is in a unit.

In primary nursing, each newly admitted patient is assigned to a primary nurse. Primary nurses assess their patients, plan their care, and write the plan of care. While on duty, they care for their patients and delegate responsibility to associate nurses when they are off duty. Associate nurses may be other registered nurses or licensed practical nurses.

Patients are divided among primary nurses in such a manner that each nurse is responsible for the care of a group of patients 24 hours a day. Unless there is a compelling reason to transfer a patient, the primary nurse cares for the patient in the unit from the time of admission to the time of discharge. These nurses know their patients well and can enjoy a feeling of accomplishment and completion when the patients leave the hospital.

Primary nursing is similar to practice in other professions because there is a continuing relationship between the professional nurse and the patient. It promotes both **autonomy** and **accountability** because one nurse is responsible for all the nursing care for the patient. The primary nurse may be assisted by other care providers (such as other nurses, aides, and technicians) but retains accountability for care outcomes 24 hours a day while the patient is in the unit. Some organizations have implemented the primary care model with registered nurses assuming total care for the patient, thereby eliminating the need for other care providers. The primary nurse communicates effectively with associate nurses caring for the patient on other shifts and with primary nurses in other units when the patient is transferred (e.g., to the operating room and intensive care unit).

Today, primary nursing is used in a variety of settings. As the restructuring of patient care delivery occurred, primary nursing also evolved and was modified. Many of the hospitals using only registered nurses as primary nurses found the cost too great as managed care and lowered reimbursement rates forced organizations to reduce the costs of providing care. Adding nonlicensed personnel to assist the registered nurse in a variety of tasks was widely adopted. Instead of bringing back the nursing assistant role, the newer role of the multiskilled worker was adapted to fit the organizational redesign. The registered nurse still functioned as the primary nurse but no longer did everything for the patient.

Primary nursing has several advantages. Because of the amount of time they spend with patients, primary nurses are in a position to care for the entire person— physically, emotionally, socially, and spiritually. Other advantages and disadvantages of primary nursing are listed in Box 14-3.

Case Management Nursing

The most recent evolution in nursing care delivery systems is **case management nursing.** In many ways, it is a return to the type of nursing practiced before patients were cared for primarily in hospitals. Begun in the late 1980s as another attempt to improve the cost-effectiveness of patient care, case management ensures that patients receive the services they need from the entire health care team in an efficient manner while holding costs down (Fagin, 1990). In many case management

Box **14-3** Advantages and Disadvantages of Primary Nursing

Advantages
- High patient and family satisfaction.
- Promotes registered nurse responsibility, authority, and accountability.
- Patient knows nurse well, and nurse knows patient well.
- Promotes patient-centered decision making.
- Increases coordination and continuity of care.
- Promotes professionalism.
- Promotes job satisfaction and sense of accomplishment for nurses.

Disadvantages
- Difficult to hire all registered nurse staff.
- Expensive to pay all registered nurse staff.
- Nurses do not know other patients—difficult to "cover" for each other.
- May create conflicts between primary and associate nurses.
- Stress of round-the-clock responsibility.
- Heavy responsibility, especially for new nurses.

systems, nurses serve in the role of case manager. In the accompanying Interview, two health care providers discuss the implementation of case management at their hospital.

In 2003 the Case Management Society of America (CMSA) revised its 1995 standards of practice for case management, which have become nationally recognized in defining case management, its functions, settings for services, relationships with patients, and the standards of care and performance. The CMSA has approved the definition of case management as:

> a collaborative process which assesses, plans, implements, coordinates, monitors and evaluates options and services to meet an individual's health needs through communication and available resources to promote quality and cost-effective outcomes (Case Management Society of America, 2003).

Two models of case management nursing have evolved over time. These are characterized by either an "internal" focus, in which the case manager works within a treatment facility, or an "external" approach, in which the case manager oversees patients and the delivery of services over the continuum of an illness or long-term disease. Although different in scope, these two models share the same principles.

Key functions of the case manager role include assessor, planner, facilitator, and advocate (Box 14-4). Key skills for nurses in these roles include critical thinking, communication, advocacy, negotiation, holistic planning and evaluation, and the ability to set both long-term and short-term goals.

The New England Medical Center and the Center for Case Management in Boston, Massachusetts, developed the internal approach using the nursing case manager to coordinate care for select patients—about 20 percent of the hospital

inter v i e w *with Hiroko Pellom, RN, Director Case Management, and Carlton D. Lancaster, Jr., MD, Medical Consultant, Hamilton Medical Center, Dalton, Georgia*

Interviewer: Why was case management implemented at your hospital?

Pellom: The goal was to improve coordination of the discharge planning and to reduce fragmentation in patient care.

Interviewer: How was the program started?

Pellom: First, the selection of the case managers for this new role was very important. The nurses selected had demonstrated expertise in their clinical knowledge, experience, clinical judgment, and their coordination and communication skills. Second, time was invested to enhance relationships with our physicians, since collaboration as a team was critical to success. Third, clinical data collection was a priority, so we provided each case manager with a laptop computer. Then we formed multidisciplinary teams, which included physicians. Over the next one and one-half years we developed and implemented 22 clinical pathways. We also developed patient versions of the pathway to educate patients and their families and to encourage their active participation.

Interviewer: What would you say have been the benefits of clinical pathways in your facility?

Lancaster: Clinical pathways have reduced variation in care, and this was our main goal. In many cases there have been other benefits, including decrease in length of stay and resource utilization, and decrease in time required for the physician to complete orders. Case management is also helping with our disease management programs.

Interviewer: What are your next steps with case management?

Pellom: After we were comfortable with clinical pathways, it was time for us to begin coordinating the care of the high-risk, high-cost patients. We have integrated social workers and the chaplain into the case management department to provide a stronger multidisciplinary team approach. We have also expanded case management into focused areas of disease management, such as asthma, that reaches patients in the community and physician's offices.

Interviewer: How will case management benefit patient care in the future?

Lancaster: As we transition from inpatient clinical pathways to disease management, involving management of care across the continuum, case management will be the clinical core which coordinates this process. We expect to see progressive involvement in quality of care even as we strive to hold down the cost of delivering that care. We feel that combining a patient focused approach with ongoing refinement of our clinical processes will offer improved patient outcomes.

population—whose care is complex or requires the use of many health care resources (Bower, 1992). These nursing case managers are primary nurses on various units, usually medical-surgical units. They not only care for these patients while on their assigned units but also manage the plans of care from admission to

Box **14-4**	Case Manager Functions

Assessor

- Gathers all relevant data and obtains information by interviewing patient/ family and performing careful evaluation of the entire situation.
- Evaluates all information related to the current treatment plan objectively and critically to identify barriers, clarify or determine realistic goals and objectives, and seek potential alternatives.

Planner

- Works with patient/family to develop a treatment plan that enhances the outcomes and reduces the payer's liability.
- Includes the patient/family as the primary decision maker and goal setter.
- Incorporates contingency plans for each step in the process to anticipate treatment and service complications.
- Initiates and implements plan modifications as necessary through monitoring and reevaluation to accommodate changes in treatment or progress.

Facilitator

- Actively promotes communication among team members, patient, family, provider, and all parties involved.
- Collaborates between the patient and the health care team to maximize outcomes.
- Coordinates the health delivery process by eliminating unnecessary steps and by promoting timely provision of care.

Advocate

- Incorporates the patient's individualized needs and goals throughout the case management process. Supports and educates the patient to become empowered and self-reliant in self-advocacy.
- Obtains consensus of all parties to achieve optimal outcomes.
- Promotes early referral to provide optimum care and cost containment.
- Represents the patient's best interest through advocacy for necessary funding, treatment alternatives, coordination of health services, and frequent reevaluation of progress and goals.

discharge, crossing interdepartmental lines. Although nursing case managers do not physically provide care in all units, they actively collaborate with primary nurses assigned to the patients in those units. This model is similar to the one used by a family practice physician who coordinates medical care for a hospitalized patient but defers to the expertise of a specialist physician if the patient is in the intensive care unit.

In this nursing model, critical paths are used for all patients. A critical path, such as the congestive heart failure CareTrac, which can be found on the Evolve website (**www.evolve.elsevier.com/Chitty/professional/**), is an interdisciplinary agreement showing who will provide care in a given timeframe to achieve agreed-upon out-comes. The use of critical paths is intended to standardize patient care and allow hospitals to plan staffing levels, lengths of stay, and other factors that heretofore could not be anticipated. Variances in the path are identified. Using continuous quality improvement methodology, health care team members review data period-ically to determine whether variations are patient-induced, staff-induced, or system-induced. Once the causes are identified, team members attempt to plan solutions to reduce variances.

The external model of case management nursing began at Carondelet St. Mary's Hospital and Health Center in Tucson, Arizona (Bower, 1992). The nurse case managers spend about 30 percent of their work time in the hospital and 70 percent outside the hospital. Similar to their counterparts in New England, the St. Mary's team members are partners with their patients. Other similarities include a profes-sional practice model of nursing that uses principles of shared governance, acuity-based billing for nursing care, and salaried, rather than hourly, pay status for the case managers. The nurse case manager in this "multisetting case management model" is part of a large network (i.e., hospital, clinic, home health agency, long-term care) and may provide services anywhere in the system (Figure 14-2).

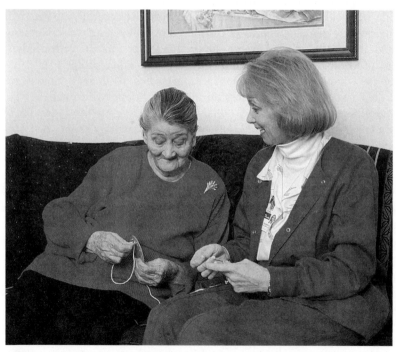

Figure **14-2**
The case management nurse's responsibilities continue following the patient's discharge. This case manager follows up with one of her patients at home. (Photo courtesy Hamilton Medical Center, Dalton, Georgia.)

case study

Case Management Nursing

A registered nurse case manager is working with a patient scheduled for a modified mastectomy the following day. He explains the sequence of events to the patient and family and tells them what to expect. He gives the patient and family a tour of the hospital, including the surgical suite and postanesthesia care unit.

As the patient's case manager, he follows the patient after surgery and may or may not provide direct nursing care. He makes sure a "Reach to Recovery" volunteer from the American Cancer Society is called to visit his patient before she leaves the hospital and that she has a follow-up home visit planned with the volunteer. He talks with the patient's family members, especially her spouse, to help them understand their own feelings and anticipate those of the patient.

Before his patient is discharged, he provides any discharge planning or teaching she may need. He makes sure she has a follow-up appointment scheduled with the surgeon and that she has transportation to the appointment. After she is discharged, he makes a home visit to check on her progress and reports back to the physician. If indicated, he refers her to an ongoing support group, such as Y-ME.

Other case management models may be found in health maintenance organizations (HMOs), managed care organizations (MCOs), third-party payers (e.g., insurance companies), public health departments, physicians' offices, home health agencies, and long-term care facilities. As can be seen from the type of activities in which they engage, case managers perform complex and challenging work. Nurses generally need about 5 years of clinical experience to fill this role effectively. Social workers, psychologists, rehabilitation counselors, or other professionals may also serve as case managers. All case managers, regardless of their discipline, work to reduce the cost of providing services through coordination of providers across the continuum of care.

Advantages and disadvantages of case management nursing are shown in Box 14-5.

Box 14-5 Advantages and Disadvantages of Case Management Nursing

Advantages
- Promotes interdisciplinary collaboration.
- Increases quality of care.
- Is cost-effective.
- Eases patient's transition from hospital to community services.

Disadvantages
- Nurse has increased responsibility.
- Requires additional training.
- Requires nurses to be off the unit for periods of time.
- Is time-consuming.
- Is most useful only with high-risk/high-cost/high-volume patients.

HOW PATIENTS DEFINE EXCELLENT NURSING CARE

It is important for nurses to understand how patients describe quality nursing care. Although patients probably could not name any model of patient care delivery, the levels of practice, the various roles of registered nurses, or nurses' professional accountabilities, they have a clear idea about what they expect from nursing care. While these models and roles provide a framework for practice, it is critical to stay focused on patients' perceptions of what makes a good nurse. The accompanying Research Note describes a study that quantified eight qualities of good nursing as defined by patients.

DIFFERENTIATING LEVELS OF PRACTICE: AN ONGOING DEBATE

A continuing issue in the delivery of nursing care is differentiating among the levels of nursing practice. Historically, nurses with different levels of education

RESEARCH note

Researcher Laurel Radwin, PhD, RN, an assistant nursing professor at the University of Massachusetts, Lowell, believes that most professionals have a good idea of what constitutes good quality nursing care but that they do not stop to ask patients what they think often enough. Radwin's study quantified eight qualities of good nursing as defined by patients. She interviewed 22 oncology patients, asking them what characteristics make a good nurse. They responded with these eight qualities:

- Attentiveness (promptness)
- Care coordination (communication with other providers)
- Caring
- Continuity (same nurse as often as possible)
- Individualized care (humanized approach)
- Partnership (shared decision making)
- Professional knowledge (including technical competence)
- Rapport (human connection)

Radwin reported that the effect of quality care was profound. Patients who felt they received excellent care were more optimistic about the future and felt a greater sense of fortitude to fight their illness. The study also found that good nurses inspired a sense of "authenticity," helping the patient feel comfortable about being honest and open.

The study also demonstrated a change in the type of personal attachment nurses have with their patients. Nurses are no longer trained to maintain a purely clinical relationship with their patients, a change from the days when divulging any personal information was considered unprofessional. Patients in this study appreciated it when nurses had experiences that could be related to them.

From Schreiber C: A closer look: patients explain what they think makes excellent nursing, *Nurse Week/Health Week,* Online, 6/10/99 *(www. nurseweek.com/features/99/ptswant.html).*

were used interchangeably in hospitals. Nursing graduates qualify for the same license, and in many settings, diploma, associate degree, and baccalaureate nurses all function under the same job description. This sometimes creates a discrepancy between the competencies nurse managers expect of new graduates and their actual competencies.

The goal of **differentiated practice** is to define two levels of practice, implying two levels of education and possibly leading ultimately to two levels of licensure.

Clearly differentiating two levels of practice would promote understanding of nursing practice in terms of technical skills needed to provide care, interpersonal skills needed to facilitate care, and leadership skills needed to manage care. In the mid-1980s, a group of donors, including the Kellogg Foundation, funded the South Dakota Statewide Project for Nursing and Nursing Education, which lasted 2 years. The project participants differentiated the competencies for the associate degree in nursing (ADN) and the bachelor of science in nursing (BSN) as follows:

> The BSN cares for focal clients who are identified as individuals, families, aggregate, and community groups. The level of responsibility of the BSN is from admission to post-discharge. The unstructured setting is a geographical and/or situational environment that may not have established policies, procedures, and protocols and has the potential for variation requiring independent nursing decisions. The ADN cares for focal clients who are identified as individuals and members of a family. The level of responsibility of the ADN is for a specified work period and is consistent with the identified goals of care. The ADN is prepared to function in a structured health care setting. The structured setting is a geographical and/or situational environment where the policies, procedures, and protocols for the provision of health care are established and there is recourse to assistance and support from the full scope of nursing expertise (Primm, 1988, p. 2).

Box 14-6 compares selected competencies of nurses with associate degrees in nursing versus those with a bachelor of science in nursing.

Box 14-6 Comparison of Differentiated ADN and BSN Competencies

Clients
- ADN: Individuals and family members
- BSN: Individuals, families, aggregates, and community groups

Level of Responsibility
- ADN: For a specified work period
- BSN: From admission to after discharge

Type of Setting
- ADN: Structured; other personnel available
- BSN: Unstructured; other personnel may not be available

ADN, Associate degree in nursing; *BSN,* bachelor of science in nursing.
From Primm P: Differentiated practice for ADN and BSN prepared nurses, *J Prof Nurs* 3(4):218-225, 1987.

During the 1990s an issue that affected differentiated levels of practice moved to center stage: mutual recognition for licensure. This means that nursing licensure would move from the single-state model to a system similar to the one used for a driver's license: multistate regulation (MSR). Reasons to change the current system were identified in 1995 through the Pew Task Force on Health Care Work Force Regulation. Since then, the National Council of State Boards of Nursing (NCSBN) has evaluated the work of the Pew Task Force and added additional supportive arguments for reform. In 1997 the NCSBN endorsed the mutual recognition model, approved a 10-step implementation model, agreed that no interstate model would be implemented until after January 1, 2000, and stipulated that implementation would be contingent on an electronic database and the supporting technology required to support the system. Some nurse leaders objected, believing that if the mutual recognition model was implemented, it would further complicate support for differentiated levels of licensure (Chaffee, 1998).

In October 2002, the American Organization of Nurse Executives endorsed the Nurse Licensure Compact (NLC), as this effort has become known, citing the threat of bioterrorism and the need for competent nurses to be mobilized quickly from various parts of the country. As of 2004, 20 states have enacted the NLC. You can read more about the issue of multistate regulation at the National Council of State Boards of Nursing website *(www.ncsbn.org/n/c/index.asp)*.

THE NURSE'S ROLE ON THE HEALTH CARE TEAM

Whatever the setting, nurses fulfill a number of roles on the health care team. As the health care delivery system changes, the evolving role of the registered nurse requires new competencies and skills in each of the roles described below.

Provider of Care

Nurses provide direct, hands-on care to patients in all health care agencies and settings. As providers, they take an active role in illness prevention and health promotion and maintenance. They offer health screenings, home health services, and an array of health care services in schools, workplaces, churches, clinics, physicians' offices, and other settings. They are instrumental in the high survival rates in trauma centers and newborn intensive care units, among others. Nurses with advanced nursing degrees are increasingly providing care at all levels of the health care system. Managed care has created opportunities for nurses to provide direct care as gatekeepers in primary care settings. Their breadth and depth of knowledge, their ability to care holistically for patients, and their natural partnership with physicians are making them some of the most sought-after care providers.

Educator

Nurse educators teach patients and families, the community, other health care team members, students, and businesses. In hospital settings as patient and family educators, nurses provide information about illnesses and teach about medications, treatments, and rehabilitation needs. They also help patients understand how to deal

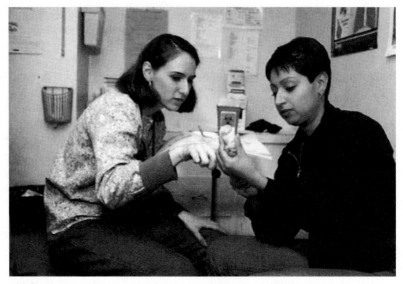

Figure 14-3
In the role of educator, this nurse teaches a newly diagnosed diabetic patient about insulin self-administration. (From Lindeman CA, McAuthie M: *Fundamentals of nursing practice,* Philadelphia, 1999, WB Saunders, p 229.)

with the life changes necessitated by chronic illnesses (Figure 14-3) and teach how to adapt care to the home setting when that is required.

In community settings, nurses offer classes in injury and illness prevention and health promotion. Often, these classes are jointly taught with other health care team members. For example, a nutritionist and a nurse may teach a group of expectant parents how to prepare formula and feed their infants. School settings offer opportunities for nurses to fulfill aspects of several roles inherent in professional practice, as illustrated in the accompanying News Note. Nurses also have a responsibility to understand and teach how a healthful or unhealthful environment may affect both the short-term and long-term health of the community.

In a recent developing trend, nurses serve as patient educators in disease management companies. By educating patients about their chronic diseases and coaching them in effective self-care behaviors, nurses proactively work with the patient and the primary care provider to keep the patient healthier and thus reduce the cost of providing health care. Additional outcomes from this are reduced health care utilization and cost.

Another community setting for nurse educators is parish nursing. Discussed in Chapter 5, parish nursing has grown to become a discipline that offers educational opportunities with a holistic emphasis in a setting that is ideal for ongoing education.

Nurses are often the key educators on the health care team. They teach other team members about the patient and family and why different interventions may have varying degrees of success. Nurses help other team members find cost-effective,

news
note

"Nurse Honored, Helps Pregnant Students"

Keeping pregnant teenagers in school is Ann Richey's goal, but it isn't achieved by following a pat formula. Mrs. Richey is a Hamilton County school nurse who serves the system's three Teen Learning Centers and three other schools that have parent support groups.

Richey was named Nurse of the Year by the Tennessee Association of School Nurses in recognition of her excellence in school nursing practice and leadership in school health. Her specific jobs include talking to classes about issues related to adolescent pregnancy and health issues, doing health assessments and home visits, and participating in WIC (Women, Infants and Children program) and immunization clinics for teen mothers and their infants.

Not all Mrs. Richey's work is directed at teenage parents or parents-to-be. She sees other students if the need arises. "Sometimes I see 20 or 30 people in a day, and I have to make judgments," she said. And she finds herself juggling a variety of things all at once.

Reprinted with permission of McDonald E: *Chattanooga Times/Free Press*, June 8, 1999, B1.

quality interventions that are desired and needed by the patient rather than wasting resources on ineffective, inefficient, undesired, or unneeded services.

Nurses also serve as teachers of the next generation of nurses. Nursing students need educators who set high standards and ideals and who help students understand the ethical choices that all health care providers must make.

As discussed in Chapter 13, the Internet is transforming the access and dissemination of information. Nurses can play an important role in assisting patients to use the Internet as an enhancement to traditional education. "Nursing is about information and the transmission of that information from professional to healthcare consumer. There's an increasing number of information resources on the Internet that provide far more current information than we're seeing in the literature," said Carol Bickford, RN, MS, a certified informatics nurse with the American Nurses Association. "To become Internet-savvy, nurses don't need to be informatics specialists. They just need to learn to surf the Net," Bickford said during a recent interview. Tips from the experts for referring patients to the Internet are found in Box 14-7.

Counselor

People who experience illness or injury often have strong emotional responses. It is clear that the relationships among the emotions, the mind, and the body are critical to promotion of and restoration to health. As counselors, nurses provide basic counseling and support to patients and their families.

Box **14-7** Referring Patients to the Internet: Advice From the Experts
■ Familiarize yourself with Internet resources in your field.
■ Refer patients to sites you know have reputable information.
■ Caution patients to consider the source before believing online information.
■ Encourage patients to print out what they find and bring it to their next appointment.
■ Answer patients' questions about information they have gleaned from the Internet.
■ Advise patients not to make decisions based solely on what they have read in cyberspace.

Federwisch A: Plugged in: point your patients to the Web for health information, *NurseWeek/HealthWeek,* 5/27/99, Online *(www.nurseweek.com/features/99-5/webuse.html).*

Using therapeutic communication techniques, nurses encourage people to discuss their feelings, to explore possible options and solutions to their unique problems, and to choose for themselves the best alternatives for action. They also serve as bereavement counselors to terminally ill patients and their families. Nurses may, with advanced education and certification, provide psychotherapy services that extend beyond the basic counseling role.

The nurse's role as counselor often overlaps with the roles of social workers, psychiatrists, spiritual advisers, and mental health specialists. Because nurses spend more time with patients than these other professionals, they have opportunities to respond to the emotional needs of patients as they occur.

Manager

The effective management of nursing resources is essential. With budgets ranging from hundreds of thousands to many million dollars, nurse managers of patient care units in hospitals manage "businesses" larger than many small companies. Nurse managers must have strong leadership, financial, marketing, system design, outcome research, and organizational behavior skills.

Chief nurse executives may manage more than 1,000 employees and multimillion-dollar budgets. They interact with other top executives and community leaders, often sitting on the health care organization's board of directors. Nurse executives must ensure the quality of nursing care within financial, regulatory, and legislative constraints. As noted in Chapter 13, nurses may serve as patient care executives, chief operating officers, and chief executive officers.

In their daily work, all nurses are managers. The bedside staff nurse must manage the care of a group of patients and decide priorities, which staff members to assign to patients, and how to accomplish all the activities during an 8- or 12-hour period. Nurses are also involved in case management or managed care. In this role, nurses review patient cases and coordinate services so that quality care can be achieved at the lowest cost.

Researcher

As discussed in Chapter 12, whether or not research is a nurse's primary responsibility, all nurses should be involved in nursing research. Nurse researchers investigate whether current or potential nursing actions achieve their expected outcomes, what options for care may be available, and how best to provide care. Nursing research looks at patient outcomes, the nursing process, and the systems that support nursing services.

Outcomes research has become an integral part of the health care delivery system. Managed care organizations and regulatory agencies require outcome data related to quality of care, which requires research by nurses. Participation by all nurses in research is essential to the growth and development of the nursing profession.

Collaborator

With so many health care workers involved in providing patient care, collaboration among the professions is increasingly important. The collaborator role is a vital one for nurses to ensure that everyone agrees on the same patient outcomes. Multidisciplinary teams require collaborative practice, and nurses play key roles as both team members and team leaders. **Collaboration** requires that nurses understand and appreciate what other health professionals have to offer. They must also be able to interpret to others the nursing needs of patients. More information about collaboration with professional colleagues is in Chapter 18.

An often-overlooked collaborative function of nurses is collaboration with patients and families. Involving patients and their families in the plan of care from the beginning is the best way to ensure their cooperation, enthusiasm, and willingness to work toward the best patient outcomes.

Change Agent (Intrapreneur)

When changes are needed in the nursing system, nurses themselves can serve as agents of change. Most professional nursing education programs include change theory as part of their management courses, and graduates are prepared to become change agents in their work settings. The role of **change agent** is one that requires a combination of tact, energy, creativity, and interpersonal skills. Change is often resisted, particularly if people are comfortable with the "old way" and believe it works. The role of change agent within a health care organization has been dubbed *intrapreneurship* (Manion, 1990) in the belief that it requires the same kind of initiative and risk taking that entrepreneurship requires (Box 14-8).

Entrepreneur

Nurse **entrepreneurs** are becoming more common. As you learned in Chapter 5, nurses now have businesses of their own that provide direct patient services in hospitals, community settings, businesses, schools, homes, and many other settings. Nurse entrepreneurs provide consultation and educational services to nurses and other health team members. They provide services to businesses by conducting work site wellness programs and by advising human resource staff on how to provide high-quality health benefits to employees while reducing costs.

Box **14-8** **Self-Assessment: How Intrapreneurial Are You?**

- Do you like to spend time thinking of ways to make things work better?
- Are you willing to take risks that you view as reasonable?
- Do you enjoy ambiguity because it stimulates your creativity?
- Do you think of new ideas while driving to work, taking a shower, or exercising?
- When you have a new idea, can you visualize the steps to take to get it done?
- Do you have more energy than most people you know?
- Do you like the challenge of new tasks and projects?
- Are you willing to work extremely hard at problems or tasks when you believe you can make a difference in how they turn out?
- Are you good at influencing others to accept new ways of doing things?
- Do you have a good sense of humor? Can you laugh at yourself?
- Do you like to consider the possibilities rather than the limitations in a situation?
- Can you mobilize the necessary resources (time, energy, people, and materials) when a job needs to be done?
- Can you work collaboratively with others on your ideas?
- Do you learn from your failures?
- Have you found ways to give yourself positive feedback so you are less reliant on the feedback of others?

If you answer "yes" to more of these questions than you answer "no," you have the personality characteristics to become an intrapreneur.

Adapted from Manion J: Nurse intrapreneurs: the heroes of health care's future, *Nurs Outlook* 39(1):18-21, 1991. Used with permission.

Patient Advocate

Rules and regulations designed to help a complex hospital run efficiently can often get in the way of a patient's treatment, and an impersonal health care system frequently infringes on the patient's rights.

Therefore health care institutions often employ **patient advocates.** Nurses who occupy patient advocate positions know how to cut through the levels of bureaucracy and red tape and will stand up for the patient's rights, advocating his or her best interests at all times. They must value patient self-determination, that is, patient independence and decision making. In this role, nurses sometimes help patients bend the rules when it is in the patient's best interests and doing so will harm no one else. Patient advocates are nurses who realize that policies are important and govern most situations well but occasionally can, and should, be broken. For example, special care units often have strict visiting hours. Family members may be allowed in to see the patient for only 10 minutes each hour. If a patient's recovery will be faster if the family is present, the nurse, serving as a patient advocate, will allow the family members more generous visitation than the policy provides. Whether or not a nurse is employed as a patient advocate, every nurse should advocate for patients daily.

Box 14-9 Five Professional Accountabilities in the Shared Governance Model

Practice

- Define standards of care (patient outcomes).
- Define standards of practice (interventions).
- Define standards of performance (job/position descriptions and expectations).
- Manage interdisciplinary collaborative relationships.
- Define career advancement criteria.
- Select and manage the conceptual framework and/or care delivery system.

Quality Improvement

- Develop measurement tools and methods for applying to standards of care, standards of performance, standards of practice, and career advancement.
- Develop and administer the nursing plan for continuous quality improvement, referring to the appropriate group or individual for resolution of variances.
- Integrate unit-based quality improvement activities.

Research

- Review the literature for nursing research pertinent to current work environment.
- Identify opportunities for nursing research.
- Develop mechanisms and forums for validating current practice.
- Develop mechanisms for studying ways to improve care through new nursing interventions and/or new ways of applying existing interventions.
- Disseminate information on nursing research to the nursing staff.
- Review requests for nursing research and approve as appropriate, ensuring safety of clients and staff, full disclosure, and minimized risk.

Education (Competency)

- Foster a positive environment for learning and teaching.
- Evaluate need for and develop competency-based educational programs (orientation, inservice, continuing education).
- Measure the outcomes of nursing education programs.
- Manage the relationship between schools of nursing and the care facility.
- Monitor effectiveness of nursing's communication and develop interventions for improvement as needed.
- Recognize that both the individual and the organization have responsibility for ensuring competency.

Management

- Coordinate, allocate, and manage human, fiscal, material, support, information, and system resources needed to deliver care to patients and to foster healthy, productive relationships.

Adapted from Porter O'Grady T: *Shared governance implementation manual,* St. Louis, 1992, Mosby; Jenkins J: Professional governance: the missing link, *Nurs Manage* 22(8):26-28, 30, 1991. Used with permission.

NURSING ORGANIZATION GOVERNANCE

In most health care agencies, nurses have a nursing staff organization. In some settings it serves mainly as a communication vehicle. In other more enlightened settings, nurses are expected to govern themselves through the organization, much as the medical staff is expected to govern itself through the medical staff organization. The concept of **shared governance** is founded on the philosophy that employees have both a right and a responsibility to govern their own work and time within a financially secure, patient-centered system. Nursing has led the way in implementing the shared governance model. It is presented here as an example of how self-governance can be structured.

Shared Governance Model

This governance model consists of councils that are patterned after five professional accountabilities.

In this model, the five **professional accountabilities** for which professional nurses are responsible are practice, quality improvement, research, education, and management. Each accountability takes on more or less importance depending on the role a nurse assumes in a particular setting. For example, staff nurses' accountabilities are primarily in the areas of clinical practice and quality improvement. They also may have secondary accountabilities in other areas if, for example, they advise managers about management of resources, precept new nurses, or join a research discussion group to learn about research being done by other nurses.

Nurse managers have primary accountability to manage resources so that the clinical staff has what they need to provide care. They also advise the clinical staff in areas of practice and quality improvement. They collaborate with nurse educators on staff orientation and continuing education programs. They may also work with nurse researchers to identify needs for research to define new and better nursing practices.

Novice nurses usually concentrate on the accountabilities central to their jobs. Later, as they gain confidence and competence, they gradually expand their scope to include all five professional accountabilities. There is a management council made up of the chief nurse executive and the chairpersons of four subcouncils (clinical practice council, education council, research council, and quality council). The management council establishes management practices, sets broad goals and objectives, oversees resources, and facilitates communication about nursing's vision. This group also ensures that successes are shared and that learning rather than punishment is the result of risk taking.

The other councils have the responsibility, authority, and accountability within their designated areas—clinical, research, education, and quality of practice—for setting the standards, policies, procedures, and behaviors necessary for nurses to carry on their work. Each council works closely with the others to ensure that decisions are well thought out. At the patient care unit level, a unit committee (or council) is elected by the staff to represent all jobs and shifts on that unit. This group is authorized to translate the organizational council decisions at the unit level.

Shared governance promotes decentralization and participation at all levels in nursing. This form of organizational structure in nursing has been successful in improving patient outcomes and enhancing job satisfaction among nurses.

NURSES AND INTERDISCIPLINARY TEAMS

For years nurses have tried to implement care teams that included all disciplines providing care to a particular patient and that would discuss, agree on, and deliver complex care. Too often, nurses were frustrated in their attempts by a variety of problems: a lack of skill in developing and managing teams, a lack of incentive for other health care team members to participate, and a failure of the system to sanction, support, create, and encourage opportunities for this type of team work.

Because of the emphasis on continuous quality improvement, reengineering, restructuring, and changing reimbursement patterns, nurses now find themselves at the center of interdisciplinary teams (Newhouse and Mills, 2002). Interdisciplinary teams "are characterized by shared leadership, frequent communication among members, and coordination of care leading to optimal client outcomes" (Sandor, Copeland, and Robinson, 1998, p. 290).

Nurses managing interdisciplinary teams must know how to manage people as equals and not as subordinates because other team members are frequently experts in their fields (e.g., radiology technicians, physicians, social workers, physical therapists, or laboratory technicians). Nurses must be prepared to participate both as leaders and as members of these teams and to assume and relinquish the leadership role to best meet the needs of patients and the team.

Managing this diverse group requires tact, diplomacy, a genuine respect for the contribution of each team member, flexibility, and the ability to "think outside the box." The last-mentioned quality is demonstrated when a person's mind is open to solutions that are nontraditional and that challenge current thinking and practice. For many nurses who have fought hard for their "turf," sharing it with others is intimidating. For others, it is a freeing experience that permits them to experience truly collaborative relationships on equal footing with other professionals (Figure 14-4).

Leaders in health care organizations have recognized that special leadership training is necessary for employees to assume both leadership and team member roles on multidisciplinary teams. Training is often provided in several sessions to equip participants with the understanding of what it takes to develop a successful team. Training includes how to structure meetings, rules of conduct, use of the tools available in data gathering and decision making, and conflict resolution. Box 14-10 identifies the characteristics that are necessary for a highly effective team.

A complete discussion of team-building skills goes beyond the scope of this book. For further exploration of this topic, an excellent continuing education resource, complete with a case study and discussion of team-building skills, can be found online at the University of Chicago Hospitals nursing career fitness website (*www.nsweb.nursingspectrum.com/ce/ce90.htm*).

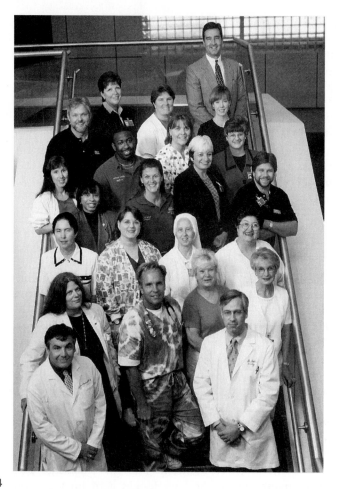

Figure 14-4
This multidisciplinary team is trained to stop the progression of strokes and rehabilitate stroke patients. The team includes paramedics, nurses, care managers, imaging technologists, laboratory technologists, physical therapists, chaplains, neurologists, emergency physicians, and volunteers. The nurse is required to use all his or her team-building skills to work successfully with the group. (Courtesy Memorial Hospital, Chattanooga, Tennessee.)

Summary of Key Points
- Historically, there have been a number of systems of nursing care delivery, each of which has advantages and disadvantages.
- Functional nursing is task-oriented and can be impersonal, but it is efficient.
- Team nursing makes use of the skills of team members, who are assigned as a team to care for a group of patients.
- Primary nursing promotes the concept of having an identified nurse for every patient.

Box 14-10 Key Components in Highly Effective Teams

- Team goals are as important as individual goals; members are able to recognize when a personal agenda is interfering with the team's direction.
- The team understands the goals and is committed to achieving them; everyone is willing to shift responsibilities.
- The team climate is comfortable and informal; people feel empowered; individual competitiveness is inappropriate.
- Communication is spontaneous and shared among all members; diversity of opinions and ideas are encouraged.
- Respect, open-mindedness, and collaboration are high; members seek win/win solutions and build on one another's ideas.
- Trust replaces fear, and people feel comfortable taking risks; direct eye contact and spontaneous expression are present.
- Conflicts and differences of opinion are considered opportunities to explore new ideas; the emphasis is on finding common ground.
- The team works on improving itself constantly by examining its procedures, processes, and practices and experimenting with change.
- Leadership is rotated; no one person dominates.
- Decisions are made by consensus and have the acceptance and support of members.

From Harrington-Macklin D: *The team building tool kit*, New York, 1994, American Management Association, p 21.

- Case management nursing involves collaboration between nurse and patient and coordination of services to meet health needs in a cost-effective manner.
- Many variations and combinations of the major nursing care delivery systems are in use today.
- Satisfaction or frustration can result from the match between nurses' expectations and the system of care in use in the employing agency.
- When interviewing for a position, nurses must assess the delivery system carefully to make sure it is congruent with their values about nursing practice.
- Nurses use a variety of roles, such as provider of care, teacher, counselor, manager, researcher, collaborator, change agent, and patient advocate in meeting patients' needs.
- As members of interdisciplinary care teams, nurses are often in leadership roles.
- An understanding of team-building skills is critical to working effectively with interdisciplinary teams.

CRITICAL THINKING QUESTIONS

1. Compare and contrast the four types of nursing care delivery systems from the viewpoint of the patient. If you were a consumer of nursing care, which system would you prefer? Why?

2. Look at the same question from the standpoint of the nurse. Which system would you find most satisfying in terms of your practice? Which would you like least?
3. Talk to a practicing nurse and find out which systems he or she has used to deliver care. What were the strong and weak points?
4. Interview nurses in practice in an acute care setting in your community to determine what type of governance structure is used by the nursing staff. What do they see as the positive and negative aspects of the type identified?
5. From your own experiences as a consumer of nursing care, identify all the nursing roles you have encountered. Share these with at least one classmate.
6. If possible, interview nurses from different countries. How does their approach to providing nursing care differ from nursing in the United States? In what ways is it similar?

REFERENCES

Bernhard LA, Walsh M: *Leadership: the key to the professionalism of nursing*, ed 2, St Louis, 1990, Mosby.

Bower FA: *Case management by nurses*, Washington, DC, 1992, American Nurses Publishing.

Case Management Society of America: *Standards of practice for case management*, Little Rock, AR, 2003, Case Management Society of America, pp 8-12.

Chachas M: Maureen Keefe speaks from experience: nursing, a profession with potential, *Health Sciences Report* (University of Utah) 26(2), 2002.

Chaffee M: Changes proposed for RN licenses, *Pediatr Nurs* 24(1/2):75-77, 1998.

Fagin CM: Nursing's value proves itself, *Am J Nurs* 90(10):17-30, 1990.

Federwisch A: Plugged in: point your patients to the Web for health information, *NurseWeek/ HealthWeek*, 5/27/99, Online *(www.nurseweek.com/features/99-5/ webuse.html)*.

Friese CG, Flevrant S, Sanders S, et al: Nursing council coordination within decentralization, *Nurs Manage* 29(3):40-41, 1998.

Harrington-Mackin D: *The team building tool kit*, New York, 1994, American Management Association.

Lambertson E: *Nursing team organization and functioning*, New York, 1953, Columbia University.

Manion J: *Change from within: nurse intrapreneurs as health care innovators*, Kansas City, MO, 1990, American Nurses Association.

Manthey M: *The practice of primary nursing*, Boston, 1980, Blackwell Scientific Publications.

McDonald E: Nurse honored; helps pregnant students, *Chattanooga Times/Free Press*, June 8, 1999, B1.

Newhouse RP, Mills ME: *Nursing leadership in the organized delivery system for the acute care setting*, Washington, DC, 2002, American Nurses Publishing.

Porter O'Grady T: *Shared governance implementation manual*, St. Louis, 1992, Mosby.

Primm PL: Differentiated practice for ADN and BSN prepared nurses, *J Prof Nurs* 3(4):218-225, 1987.

Primm PL: *Differentiated nursing care management/patient care delivery system*, Kansas Nurse, April 1988, 2.

Sandor MK, Copeland D, Robinson S: Team-building interventions for interdisciplinary teams: a case study of a pediatric client, *Rehab Nurs* 23(6):290-294, 1998.

Schreiber C: A closer look: patients explain what they think makes excellent nursing, *Nurse Week/Health Week*, Online, 6/10/99 *(www. nurseweek.com/features/99/ptswant.html)*.

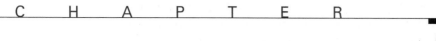

C H A P T E R

15

Critical Thinking, the Nursing Process, and Clinical Judgment

Kay Kittrell Chitty

Key Terms

Affective Goal
Analysis
Assessment
Clinical Judgment
Cognitive Goal
Consultation
Critical Path
Defining Characteristics
Dependent Intervention
Evaluation
Human Responses
Implementation
Independent Intervention

Interdependent
  Intervention
Long-Term Goal
NANDA International
Nursing Diagnosis
Nursing Interventions
  Classification (NIC)
Nursing Order
Nursing Outcomes
  Classification (NOC)
Nursing Process
Objective Data
Outcome Criteria

Patient Interview
Planning
Primary Source
Protocol
Psychomotor Goal
Reflective Thinking
Secondary Source
Short-Term Goal
Signs
Subjective Data
Symptoms
Taxonomy
Tertiary Source

Learning Outcomes

After studying this chapter, students will be able to:

- Define critical thinking in nursing.
- Contrast the characteristics of "novice thinking" with those of "expert thinking."
- Explain the purpose and phases of the nursing process.
- Differentiate between nursing orders and medical orders.
- Explain the differences between independent, interdependent, and dependent nursing actions.
- Describe evaluation and its importance in the nursing process.
- Define clinical judgment in nursing practice.
- Discuss the benefits of a unified, standardized nursing language to the profession.
- Develop a personal plan to use in developing sound clinical judgment.

A lmost every nurse-patient encounter is an opportunity for the nurse to assist the patient in moving to a higher level of wellness. Whether or not this actually happens depends in large measure on the nurse's ability to think critically about the patient's particular needs and how best to meet them. It also depends on the nurse's ability to use a reliable problem-solving approach that leads to sound clinical decisions about the patient's priority nursing needs. Underlying this admittedly simplistic description is the assumption that patients are not passive recipients of nursing care but active participants in care to the extent of their ability.

This chapter explores several important and interdependent aspects of thinking and decision making in nursing: critical thinking, the nursing process, and clinical judgment.

CRITICAL THINKING IN NURSING

The ability to think critically can be learned. It involves paying attention to how one thinks and making thinking itself a focus of concern. A nurse who is exercising critical thinking asks, "What assumptions have I made about this patient?" "How do I know my assumptions are accurate?" "Do I need any additional information?" and "How might I look at this situation differently?" Nurses just beginning to pay attention to their thinking processes may ask these questions *after* nurse-patient interactions have ended. This is known as **reflective thinking.** Reflective thinking is an active process valuable in learning, changing behaviors, perspectives, or practices. Nurses can also learn to examine their thinking processes *during* an interaction as they learn to "think on their feet." This is a characteristic of expert nurses.

Critical thinking in nursing involves more than good problem-solving strategies. It is a complex process that has specific characteristics that make it different from run-of-the-mill problem solving. Critical thinking in nursing involves a purposeful, disciplined process, consciously developed, to improve patient outcomes. It is motivated by the needs of the patient and family, and determined in part by elements of the scientific method. Critical thinking in nursing is undergirded by the standards and ethics of the profession. Nurses who think critically seek to build on patients' strengths while honoring patients' values and beliefs (Alfaro-LeFevre, 1999). They are engaged in a process of constant evaluation, redirection, improvement, and increased efficiency. Box 15-1 summarizes these characteristics and offers an opportunity for you to evaluate your progress as a critical thinker.

In earlier chapters you read about Dr. Patricia Benner (1984, 1996), who studied the differences in expertise of nurses at different stages in their careers, from novice to expert. So it is with critical thinking; novices think differently than experts. Novices tend to act as soon as they recognize a pattern, while experts may spend time gathering more information before acting, recognizing that other patterns may emerge. For example, when confronted with a patient who has not voided postoperatively, the novice might quickly decide to intervene by catheterizing. The expert, before intervening, may palpate the patient's suprapubic area for distention, check the chart to see how much intravenous fluid the patient has received, assess the amount of discomfort and vomiting, if any, and determine how

Box **15-1** Self-Assessment: Critical Thinking

Directions: Listed below are 15 characteristics of critical thinkers. Mark a plus (+) next to those you now possess; mark IP (in progress) next to those you partly have mastered; and mark a zero (0) next to those you have not yet mastered. When you are finished, make a plan for developing the areas that need improvement. Share it with at least one person and report on progress weekly.

Characteristics of Critical Thinkers: How Do *You* Measure Up?

___+___ Inquisitive/curious/seeks truth
___+___ Self-informed/finds own answers
___IP___ Analytical/confident in own reasoning skills
___IP___ Open-minded
___+___ Flexible
___+___ Fair-minded
___+___ Honest about personal biases/self-aware
___+___ Prudent/exercises sound judgment
___+___ Willing to revise judgment when new evidence warrants
___IP___ Clear about issues
___+___ Orderly in complex matters/organized approach to problems
___IP___ Diligent in seeking information
___IP___ Persistent
___IP___ Reasonable
___IP___ Focused on inquiry

Adapted from American Philosophical Association: Critical thinking: a statement of expert consensus for purposes of educational assessment and instruction, *The Delphi Report: Research Findings and Recommendations Prepared for the Committee on Pre-College Philosophy,* ERIC Document Reproduction Services, 315-423, 1990.

long the patient was kept on an NPO (nothing by mouth) order prior to surgery before considering catheterization. Box 15-2 summarizes the differences in novice and expert thinking.

As mentioned earlier, critical thinking skills can be learned. The learning process requires both an understanding of what constitutes critical thinking and insight into how you and others think. Critical thinking involves far more than stating your opinion. You must be able to describe how you came to a conclusion and support your conclusions with explicit rationales. This is a different way of thinking for most people and requires practice.

Dimensions of critical thinking include both cognitive skills and "habits of the mind" (Scheffer and Rubenfeld, 2000). The habits or characteristics of critical thinkers were listed in Box 15-1. The necessary cognitive skills and a definition of each are found in Table 15-1.

An excellent continuing education self-study module designed to improve your ability to think critically can be found online *(www.nsweb.nursingspectrum.com/ce/ce168.htm)*. You can also begin to learn about the many facets of critical thinking by participating with classmates in the Critical Thinking Exercise on p. 391.

Box **15-2** **Novice Thinking Compared With Expert Thinking**

Novice Nurses

- Tend to organize knowledge as separate facts. Must rely heavily on resources (texts, notes, preceptors). Lack knowledge gained from actually doing (e.g., listening to breath sounds).
- Focus so much on actions that they tend to forget to assess before acting.
- Need clear-cut rules.
- Are often hampered by unawareness of resources.
- Are often hindered by anxiety and lack of self-confidence.
- Must be able to rely on step-by-step procedures. Tend to focus more on procedures than on the patient response to the procedure.
- Become uncomfortable if patient needs preclude performing procedures exactly as they were learned.
- Have limited knowledge of suspected problems; therefore, they question and collect data more superficially.
- Tend to follow standards and policies by rote.
- Learn more readily when matched with a supportive, knowledgeable preceptor or mentor.

Expert Nurses

- Tend to store knowledge in a highly organized and structured manner, making recall of information easier. Have a large storehouse of experiential knowledge (e.g., what abnormal breath sounds sound like, what subtle changes look like).
- Assess and think things through before acting.
- Know when to bend the rules.
- Are aware of resources and how to use them.
- Are usually more self-confident, less anxious, and therefore more focused.
- Know when it's safe to skip steps or do two steps together. Are able to focus on both the parts (the procedures) and the whole (the patient response).
- Comfortable with rethinking procedure if patient needs require modification of the procedure.
- Have a better idea of suspected problems, allowing them to question more deeply and collect more relevant and in-depth data.
- Analyze standards and policies, looking for ways to improve them.
- Are challenged by novices' questions, clarifying their own thinking when teaching novices.

From Alfaro-LeFevre R: *Critical thinking in nursing: a practical approach,* ed 2, Philadelphia, 1999, WB Saunders. Reprinted with permission.

Table 15-1   Cognitive Skills Needed by Critical Thinkers

Skill	Definitions
Analyzing	Separating or breaking a whole into parts to discover the nature, function, and relationships.
Applying standards	Judging according to established personal, professional, or social rules or criteria.
Discriminating	Recognizing differences and similarities among things or situations and distinguishing carefully as to category or rank.
Information seeking	Searching for evidence, facts, or knowledge by identifying relevant sources and gathering objective, subjective, historical, and current data from those sources.
Logical reasoning	Drawing inferences or conclusions that are supported or justified by evidence.
Predicting	Envisioning a plan and its consequences.
Transforming knowledge	Changing or converting the condition, nature, form, or function of concepts among contexts.

Scheffer BK, Rubenfeld MG: A consensus statement on critical thinking, *J Nurs Ed* 39:352-359, 2000.

THE NURSING PROCESS IN HISTORICAL PERSPECTIVE

The **nursing process** is a method of thinking critically about how to solve patient problems in professional practice. It is an outgrowth of the scientific method and can be used as a framework for approaching almost any problem. Yura and Walsh (1983) defined the nursing process as "a designated series of actions intended to fulfill the purposes of nursing—to maintain the patient's wellness—and, if this state changes, to provide the amount and quality of nursing care the situation demands to direct the patient back to wellness." They continued to state that "if wellness cannot be achieved, then [the purpose of the nursing process is] to contribute to the patient's quality of life, maximizing his resources as long as life is a reality" (p. 71).

A simple example of using a process approach to problem solving is illustrated by examining a daily decision that you and most other people face: how to dress for the day. Before putting on your clothes, there are several factors you need to consider. What is the expected temperature? Will it be clear, raining, or snowing? How much time will be spent outdoors? Are there any activities planned that require special dress? Next, you probably look at the possible clothing choices. Some clothes may be out of season, and others need repairs, are too dressy or casual, or don't fit quite right. After considering the environmental factors, the day's activities, and your mood, you select the day's clothing. After dressing, you may look in a mirror to evaluate how you look. You may then modify your outfit based on your image in the mirror. At this point, you have solved the problem of clothing yourself. You have identified a problem, considered various factors related to the problem, identified possible actions, selected the best alternative, evaluated the success of the alternative selected, and made adjustments to the solution based on the evaluation. This is the same general process nurses use in solving patient problems through the nursing process.

CRITICAL THINKING *Exercise*

Six Caps

This is an hour-long group activity designed to clarify the various types of thinking that constitute critical thinking. For every six participants, you will need six pieces of colored paper (1 white; 1 red; 1 black; 1 yellow; 1 green; and 1 blue). You will also need six straight pins. Divide the group into smaller groups of six and give each group member a pin and piece of colored paper. Each person draws a cap on the paper and pins it to his or her shirt in plain view. These represent the six "thinking caps"—that is, the various types of thinking to be explored:

- White cap = Information. Asks the questions, "What information do we have, what is needed, and how can we get it?"
- Red cap = Feelings, intuition, and emotion. Asks the questions, "What are we, the patient, and the family feeling, and how do we know?"
- Black cap = Policies, codes, standards, protocols, laws. Asks the questions, "What are the standards we should consider, and what are the risks?"
- Yellow cap = Optimism. Asks the questions, "What are the benefits, who benefits, and what are the values being expressed?"
- Green cap = Growth. Asks the questions, "Why don't we try it this way?" and "What are some different alternatives?"
- Blue cap = Focuses on thinking. Asks the questions, "How are we going to proceed in thinking through this situation?" and "What have we achieved and what do we want to achieve?"

Read the case study below (or one prepared by your teacher) and discuss it from the viewpoint of each "cap." Identify issues for reflection. Then switch "thinking caps." Discuss the case study again. How easy or difficult was it to change your type of thinking? Do some types of thinking come more naturally to you than others? Which ones will you have to work to develop? Do you see value in each type of thinking? When the group reconvenes, summarize what you have learned on a flip chart.

Case Study

Marianne is a 79-year-old woman who was admitted to the emergency department yesterday with a severe headache. Shortly after admission, she became unresponsive; a brain scan revealed she had suffered a hemorrhagic stroke. Marianne's pupils are dilated and do not respond to light; she is breathing with the assistance of a respirator. Her elderly husband and three adult children are all assembled. The physician has recommended surgery to remove the blood clot but cannot offer much assurance that she will recover function. She has no advanced directives, but her husband wants to "try everything." The children believe that she would not want to undergo this surgery only to be kept alive with poor quality of life, which they agree is the likely outcome. The ethics committee is assembled to assist the family in making the decision. Before meeting with the family, the committee meets to discuss the situation.

Modified from De Bono E: *Edward de Bono's mind pack,* London, 1995, Dorling-Kindersley; Kenney LJ: Using Edward de Bono's six hats game to aid critical thinking and reflection in palliative care, *Int J Palliat Nurs* 9(3):105-112, 2003.

For individuals outside the profession, nursing is commonly and simplistically defined in terms of tasks nurses perform (i.e., give injections). Even within the profession, the intellectual basis of nursing practice was not articulated until the 1960s, when nursing educators and leaders began to identify and name the components of nursing's intellectual processes. This marked the beginning of the nursing process.

During the 1970s and 1980s, debate about the use of the term *diagnosis* began. Up until that time, diagnosing was considered to be within the scope of practice of physicians only. Nurses were not supposed to diagnose patients. All this began to change in 1973 when the National Group for the Classification of Nursing Diagnosis, now called **NANDA International,** published its first list of nursing diagnoses. The purpose of this group was (and is) to identify terminology and definitions that may be used and tested as nursing diagnoses.

The nursing process as a method of clinical problem solving is taught in nursing curricula across the United States, and many states refer to it in their nurse practice acts. The operations of the nursing process are described in detail in the American Nurses Association's *Nursing: Scope and Standards of Practice* (2003), which serves as the profession's guide to a national standard of care.

In recent years some nursing leaders have questioned the use of the nursing process, describing it as linear, rigid, and mechanistic. They believe that the tabular format of the nursing process contributes to linear thinking and stymies critical thinking. They are concerned that this format, and rigid faculty adherence to it, encourages students to copy from published sources when writing care plans, thus inhibiting the development of a holistic, creative approach to patient care (Mueller, Johnson, and Bligh, 2002). Certainly the nursing process *can* be taught, learned, and used in that manner. It can also be used as a creative approach to thinking and decision making in nursing. Since the nursing process is an integral aspect of nursing education, practice, and law nationwide, learning to use it as a dynamic approach to patient care and a tool for critical thinking is a worthwhile endeavor.

Whether you are a beginning student or a registered nurse, you may be wondering about the value of the nursing process in your own practice. The letter in Box 15-3 from a student nearing graduation describes her thoughts about the nursing process and how they have changed since she first began using it.

Further support for the nursing process can be found in the 2003 revision of *Nursing: Scope and Standards of Practice,* which includes steps of the nursing process as an organizing framework for standards of professional nursing practice (ANA, 2003, pp. 21-32). The nursing process remains a cornerstone of nursing standards, legal definitions, and practice and, as such, should be well understood by every nurse.

PHASES OF THE NURSING PROCESS

As in the scientific method, presented in Chapter 12, a series of steps make up the nursing process. Identifying specific steps makes the process clear and concrete but can cause nurses to use them rigidly. Keep in mind that this is a process, that

Box **15-3** **Letter From a Senior Nursing Student**

Dear Fellow Students:

I recall sitting in my first nursing class wondering how long my professor would lecture about the "nursing process." I didn't want to learn about problem-solving techniques. I didn't want to get bogged down in all the time-consuming paperwork. I wanted to save lives. You know what I mean—I was only interested in learning about the diseases, traumas, and surgeries I was sure I would be dealing with on a daily basis. What was all this assess, diagnose, plan, etc., stuff? I was impatient to be finished with this material and thought that once I got through the exam covering the nursing process, I would be home free. I was so naive!

I can also remember the day I realized that the nursing process had become as natural to me as walking and talking. It was during my acute care rotation when I walked into a patient's room to find him experiencing respiratory difficulty. I immediately assessed the patient and began to take steps to alleviate his distress. I admit I felt a little anxious, yet I was able to take the necessary steps to bring the situation under control. If not for my knowledge of the nursing process, I am positive that I would have been unable to organize my thoughts and actions in an efficient manner while under pressure.

So my message to you is this: Relax and don't resist learning the nursing process. I guarantee this tool will help you feel more self-confident and better able to organize your time and thoughts.

Good Luck!

At the time this was written, Elizabeth Baird was a senior nursing student at The University of Tennessee, Chattanooga. (Courtesy Elizabeth Baird.)

progression through the process may not be linear, and that it is a tool to use, not a road map to slavishly follow. For example, if a newly hospitalized patient is experiencing a great deal of pain, a novice nurse might proceed with the admission interview, focusing on the task at hand. An expert nurse would realize that performing an initial assessment under those circumstances would not contribute to the patient's well-being and would instead reposition, massage, or administer medication first, deferring the interview for a time.

Phase 1: Assessment

Assessment is the initial phase in the nursing process. During this phase, information or data about the individual patient, family, or community are gathered. Data may include physiological, psychological, sociocultural, developmental, spiritual, and environmental information. The patient's available financial or material resources also need to be assessed and recorded in a standard format; each institution usually has a slightly different method of recording assessment data.

Types of data

There are two types of data that nurses obtain about patients: subjective and objective. **Subjective data** are obtained from patients as they describe their needs, feelings, strengths, and perceptions of the problem. Subjective data are frequently referred to as **symptoms.** Examples of subjective data are statements such as, "I am in pain" and "I don't have much energy." The *only* source for these data is the patient. Subjective data should include physical, psychosocial, and spiritual information. Subjective data can be very private. Nurses must be sensitive to the patient's need for confidence in the nurse's trustworthiness.

The second type of patient data is **objective data.** These are data that the nurse obtains through observation, examination, or consultation with other health care providers. These data are factual, not colored by patients' perceptions, and include patient behaviors as observed by the nurse. Objective data are frequently called **signs.** An example of objective data that a nurse might gather includes the observation that the patient, who is lying in bed, is diaphoretic, pale, and tachypneic and holding his hand to his chest.

Objective data and subjective data usually are congruent; that is, they usually are in agreement. In the situation just mentioned, if the patient told the nurse, "I feel like a rock is sitting on my chest," the subjective data would substantiate the nurse's observations (objective data) that the patient is having chest pain. There are times, however, when subjective and objective data are in conflict. An example of incongruent subjective and objective data would be an emaciated teenager stating, "I'm too fat." In this example, the conflict reveals a perceptual error by the patient.

Sources of patient data

Patient data can be obtained from many sources (Figure 15-1). The patient is considered the only **primary source.** Sources of data such as the nurse's own observations or reports of family and friends of the patient are considered **secondary sources.** **Tertiary sources** of data include medical records and information gathered from other health care providers such as physical therapists, physicians, or dietitians.

Methods of collecting patient data

A number of methods are used when collecting patient data. An important one is the **patient interview.** This usually involves a face-to-face interaction with the patient and requires the nurse to use the skills of interviewing, observation, and listening. The environment in which the interaction occurs or other internal and external factors can influence the amount and the type of data obtained. For example, when interviewing a patient who is having difficulty breathing, the verbal data obtained by the interview may be limited, but observation and listening can reveal much about the patient's condition. Likewise, if an interview takes place in a cold, noisy, or public place, the type of data obtained may be affected by environmental distractions.

A second method of obtaining data is through **consultation.** Consultation is discussing patient needs with health care workers and others who are directly

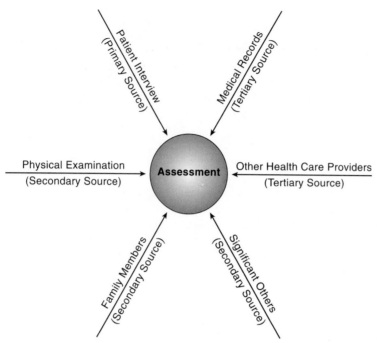

Figure 15-1
Patient data come from primary, secondary, and tertiary sources.

involved in the care of the patient. Nurses also consult with patients' families to obtain background information and their perceptions about the patients' needs. Physical examination is the third method for obtaining data. Nurses use physical assessment techniques of inspection, auscultation, percussion, and palpation to obtain these data (Figure 15-2).

Organizing patient data

Once patient data have been collected, they must be sorted or organized. A number of methods have been developed to assist nurses in organizing patient data. These methods include Abdellah's 21 nursing problems, Henderson's 14 nursing problems, Yura and Walsh's human needs approach, and Gordon's 11 functional health patterns. Contemporary nursing theorists continue to develop other organizing frameworks, including those of Madeleine Leininger, Sister Callista Roy, Dorothy Orem, and others you read about in Chapter 11. Nurses choose different methods of organizing patient data depending on personal preference and the method used in the agencies where they are employed.

Confidentiality of patient data

A word of caution is needed in regard to patient data. Earlier, it was mentioned that patients confide personal information to nurses only if they believe the nurse is trustworthy. Patients need to know and trust that nurses share such information

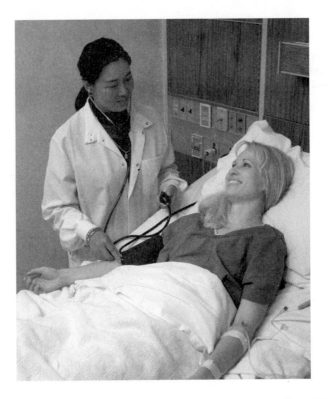

Figure **15-2**
Physical examination is a secondary source of objective assessment data. (Photo courtesy Hamilton Medical Center, Dalton, Georgia.)

only with the other treatment team members. Nurses must respect patients' privacy rights and should never discuss patient information with anyone who does not have a work-related need to know.

A complicating factor in ensuring patients' privacy in this age of information technology is that vast amounts of patient data may be stored and retrieved relatively easily. Although the issues of confidentiality and access to electronically stored data have yet to be fully resolved, each nurse should commit himself or herself never to violate a patient's privacy by revealing patient information except to other members of that patient's treatment team.

Phase 2: Analysis and Diagnosis

As mentioned, during the data-gathering phase of the nursing process, nurses obtain a great deal of information about their patients. These data must be validated, then compared with norms to sort out data that might indicate a problem or identify a pattern. Next, the data must be clustered or grouped so that problems can be identified and their cause discerned. This process is known as data **analysis** and results in the identification of one or more nursing diagnoses. Knowledge from the biological sciences, social sciences, and nursing enables nurses to analyze relationships among various pieces of patient data.

Nursing diagnosis

Nursing diagnosis was defined by Gordon (1976) as "actual or potential health problems which nurses, by virtue of their education and experience, are capable and licensed to treat" (p. 1299). In 1990, NANDA defined nursing diagnosis as "a clinical judgment about individual, family, or community responses to actual or potential health problems/life processes … (which) provide the basis for selection of nursing interventions to achieve outcomes for which the nurse is accountable" (North American Nursing Diagnosis Association, 1990).

NANDA diagnoses

For three decades the NANDA has worked to develop a comprehensive list of nursing diagnoses. The composition of the NANDA originally included nursing educators, theorists, and practitioners from the United States and Canada who first met in 1973 at the National Conference Group to develop standard terminology, content, and format for nursing diagnoses. The group became NANDA in 1982 and has continued to meet every 2 years to revise the original list of approved diagnoses. After each revision, new diagnoses are tested by nurses in practice settings to evaluate their appropriateness and usefulness. This is a continuing process. Membership in the NANDA is now open worldwide to nurses and nursing groups interested in advancing nursing diagnosis. A list of the 2003-2004 NANDA-approved nursing diagnoses can be found on the Evolve website (**www.evolve. elsevier.com/Chitty/professional/**).

NANDA-approved nursing diagnoses consist of five components (NANDA, 2003, pp. 263-264):

- Label—Concise term or phrase that names the diagnosis.
- Definition—Clearly delineates meaning and helps differentiate from similar diagnoses.
- Defining characteristics—Clusters of observable cues or inferences.
- Risk factors—Factors that increase vulnerability to an unhealthful event.
- Related factors—Factors that precede, are associated with, or relate to the diagnosis.

All nursing diagnoses must be supported by data, which NANDA refers to as **defining characteristics,** also known as signs and symptoms. Remember that a sign is observable, whereas a symptom is reported by the patient.

Writing NANDA nursing diagnoses

Accurate diagnosis of human responses is very important. All nursing actions flow from the diagnosis, and inaccurate diagnoses can lead to lost time and wasted resources and may endanger the patient. Accuracy of diagnosis is a professional behavior, one of nursing's accountabilities (Lunney, 2001).

A format used to write the diagnostic statement, called the PES format (Box 15-4), was developed by Gordon (1987). In this format, the P stands for the concise description of the *problem,* using the NANDA diagnostic label—for example, *ineffective breathing pattern.*

The E part of the statement stands for *etiology,* or cause, and begins with the words *related to.* These related factors are conditions or circumstances that can cause or

Box 15-4	Writing Nursing Diagnoses

P = Problem (NANDA diagnostic label)
E = Etiology (causal factors)
S = Signs and symptoms (defining characteristics)

contribute to the development of the problem. To extend the previous example, *ineffective breathing pattern related to anxiety,* explains the cause of the ineffective breathing pattern as the patient's high anxiety level. The etiology part of the statement is important, because if the cause were decreased energy or fatigue rather than anxiety, the nurse would need to select different nursing actions to solve the problem.

The last part of the diagnostic statement is S, which stands for *signs and symptoms,* or as the NANDA calls them, defining characteristics. Thus, the complete diagnostic statement for our sample diagnosis might be *ineffective breathing patterns related to anxiety as manifested by dyspnea, nasal flaring, use of accessory muscles to breathe, and respiratory rate >24/minute.*

Prioritizing nursing diagnoses

After diagnoses are identified, the nurse must put them in order of priority. There are two common frameworks used to establish priorities. One of these considers the relative danger to the patient. Using this framework, diagnoses that are life-threatening are the nurse's first priority. Next come those that have the potential to cause harm or injury. Last in priority are those that are related to the overall general health of the patient. Thus, a diagnosis of "ineffective airway clearance" would be dealt with before "sleep pattern disturbance," and "sleep pattern disturbance" would have priority over "knowledge deficit."

Another framework that may be used to prioritize diagnoses is Maslow's (1970) hierarchy of needs (refer to Chapter 10, Figure 10-2). When this framework is used, there is an inverse relationship between high-priority nursing diagnoses and high-level needs. In other words, highest priority is given to diagnoses related to basic physiological needs. Diagnoses related to higher-level needs such as love and belonging or self-esteem, although important, have priority only after basic physiological needs are met.

Except in life-threatening situations, nurses should take care to involve patients in identifying priority diagnoses. Because varied sociocultural factors have a great impact on the manner in which patients prioritize problems, nurses must be aware of these factors and take them into consideration when planning patient care.

Medical diagnosis and nursing diagnosis

Nursing diagnosis is different from medical diagnosis and was never intended to be a substitute for it. Rather than focusing on what is wrong with the patient in terms of a disease process, a nursing diagnosis identifies the problems the patient is experiencing as a *result* of the disease process, that is, the **human responses** to the illness, injury, or threat.

Another important difference between nursing diagnosis and medical diagnosis is that nursing diagnoses cover patient problems that nurses can legally treat. It would do little good for nursing diagnoses to include "appendicitis" because appendicitis is a medical diagnosis requiring surgery, and it is not legal for nurses to perform surgery. An appropriate nursing diagnosis for a patient after an appendectomy might be "ineffective airway clearance related to incisional pain." Because it is legal in all states for nurses to provide comfort measures and to assist patients to cough and deep breathe, this would be both an appropriate and a legal nursing diagnosis.

Phase 3: Planning

Planning is the third phase in the nursing process. **Planning** begins with the identification of patient goals. These are goals that are used by the patient and the nurse to guide the selection of interventions and to evaluate patient progress.

Just as nursing diagnoses are written in collaboration with the patient, goals should also be agreed on by both nurse and patient unless collaboration is impossible, such as when the patient is unconscious. In that event, family members or significant others can collaborate with the nurse. Goals give the patient, family, significant others, and nurse direction and make them active partners.

Writing patient goals and outcomes

The terms *goal* and *objective* are frequently used interchangeably. These terms are statements of what is to be accomplished and are derived from the diagnoses. Because the problem or diagnosis is written as a patient problem, the goal should also be stated in terms of what the *patient* will do rather than what the nurse will do. The goal begins with the words "the patient will" or "the patient will be able to." The goal sets a general direction, includes an action verb, and should be both attainable and realistic for the patient.

Outcome criteria are specific and make the goal measurable. Outcome criteria define the terms under which the goal is said to be met, partially met, or unmet.

Each diagnosis has at least one patient goal, and each patient goal may have several outcome criteria. Effective outcome criteria state under what conditions, to what extent, and in what time frame the patient is to act. A sample patient goal with outcome criteria might be "The patient will demonstrate effective bowel elimination as evidenced by having one soft, formed stool every other day without the use of laxatives or enemas within 2 weeks." It is easy to see that this goal is written in terms of what the patient will do (have a bowel movement at least every other day), is measurable (one soft, formed stool), gives conditions (without the use of laxatives or enemas), and has a specified time frame for accomplishment (2 weeks).

Types of patient goals. There are three types of patient goals: psychomotor, cognitive, and affective goals. A goal that requires motor skills or actions by the patient is a **psychomotor goal;** for example, "The patient will walk 10 feet in the hallway with a walker three times per day within 1 day after surgery." **Cognitive goals** deal with a desired change in a patient's knowledge level. An example of a cognitive goal might be: "The patient will list three effects of a high cholesterol level on the heart prior to discharge from the hospital." **Affective goals** involve a change in mood,

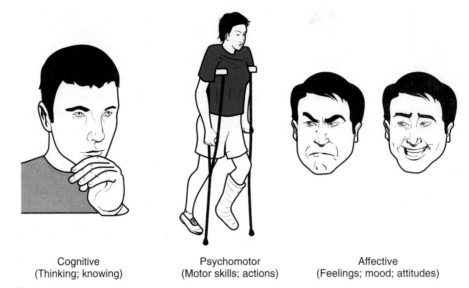

| Cognitive | Psychomotor | Affective |
| (Thinking; knowing) | (Motor skills; actions) | (Feelings; mood; attitudes) |

Figure **15-3**
Patient goals may be in one or more of three domains: cognitive, psychomotor, or affective.

values, attitudes, or belief systems. An example of an affective goal is: "The patient will express an increased sense of well-being after participating in an exercise program for 1 month." A single patient may have a combination of psychomotor, cognitive, and affective goals (Figure 15-3).

Establishing time frames for patient goals. One aspect of goal setting not yet discussed is the estimated length of time needed to accomplish the goal. **Short-term goals** may be attainable within hours or days. They are usually specific and are small steps leading to the achievement of broader, long-term goals. For example, "The patient will lose 2 pounds" is a short-term goal, and the time limit for accomplishment can be brief, perhaps a week or 10 days.

Long-term goals usually represent major changes. A goal such as "The patient will lose 75 pounds" may take months or perhaps even years to accomplish, and the time frame should be set accordingly.

It is extremely important to assist patients to set realistic goals for themselves. Setting their sights too high causes frustration and discouragement in patients, families, and nurses.

Nursing Outcomes Classification (NOC). A standardized system of classification of patient outcomes sensitive to nursing interventions has been developed by a group of researchers at the University of Iowa. The purpose of this effort was to evaluate the effects of nursing care, believing that this was essential if nursing was to become "a full participant in clinical evaluation science along with other health disciplines" (Center for Nursing Classification, 2003). The work began in 1991 with a team of 43 nurses from all aspects of nursing—service, education, and research. As the work progressed, they were funded by a grant from the National Institute of Nursing Research (NINR). From 1993 through 1997, these researchers identified, labeled, validated, and classified nursing outcomes and tested them in the field. Their work is ongoing. **Nursing Outcomes Classification (NOC)** is the result.

There are 260 standard NOC outcomes, each with a label, definition, and a set of indicators and measures to determine achievement of the outcome. Examples of outcomes include *ambulation, mobility level,* and *cognitive orientation.* You can learn more about NOC online *(www.nursing.uiowa.edu/centers/cncce/index.htm).*

Selecting interventions and writing nursing orders

After short-term and long-term goals are identified through collaboration between nurse and patient, the nurse writes nursing orders. **Nursing orders** are actions designed to assist the patient in achieving a stated goal. Every goal has specific nursing orders, which may be carried out by a registered nurse (RN) or delegated to other members of the nursing staff.

Nursing orders and medical orders differ. Nursing orders refer to interventions that are designed to treat the patient's response to an illness or medical treatment, whereas medical orders are designed to treat the actual illness or disease. An example of a nursing order is "Teach turning, coughing, and deep-breathing exercises prior to surgery." These activities are designed to prevent postoperative respiratory problems due to immobility. They are appropriate nursing orders because prevention of complications due to immobility is a nursing responsibility. Nursing orders may include instructions about consultation with other health care providers, such as the dietitian, physical therapist, or pharmacist.

Types of nursing interventions. Nursing interventions are of three basic types: independent, dependent, or interdependent. **Independent interventions** are those for which the nurse's intervention requires no supervision or direction by others. Nurses are expected to possess the knowledge and skills to carry out independent actions safely. An example of an independent nursing intervention is teaching a patient how to examine her breasts for lumps. The nursing practice act of each state usually specifies general types of independent nursing actions.

Dependent interventions do require instructions, written orders, or supervision of another health professional, usually a physician. These actions require knowledge and skills on the part of the nurse but may not be done without explicit directions. An example of a dependent nursing intervention is the administration of medications. Although a physician or advanced practice nurse must order most medications, it is the responsibility of the nurse to know how to administer them safely and to monitor their effectiveness.

The third type, **interdependent interventions,** includes actions in which the nurse must collaborate or consult with another health professional before carrying out the action. One example of this type of action is the nurse implementing orders that have been written by a physician in a protocol. **Protocols** define under what conditions and circumstances a nurse is allowed to treat the patient, as well as what treatments are permissible. They are used in situations in which nurses need to take immediate action without consulting with a physician, such as in an emergency department, a critical care unit, or a home setting.

Nursing Interventions Classification (NIC). Classification research conducted at the University of Iowa College of Nursing resulted in the development of the

Nursing Interventions Classification (NIC). This classification describes the treatments that nurses perform in all specialties and in all settings. NIC provides a list of 486 interventions. Each is defined and includes a set of activities that a nurse performs to carry out the intervention. Interventions are coded and organized for ease of computerization. Examples of interventions include acid-base management, anxiety reduction, shock management, fall prevention, exercise promotion, and emergency cart checking. Note that the last is an indirect care intervention. You can learn more about NIC online *(www.nursing.uiowa.edu/centers/cncce/index.htm)*.

Writing the plan of care

Once interventions are selected, a written plan of care is devised. Some health care agencies use individually developed plans of care for their patients. The nurse creates and develops a plan for each patient. Others use standardized plans of care that are based on common and recurring problems. The nurse then individualizes these standard plans of care. One of the advantages of using standardized plans is that they can decrease the time spent in generating a completely new plan each time a patient is seen. These plans are easily computer-generated, with the nurse making selections from menus to individualize the plan to the particular patient. The amount of time needed to update and document these plans is thereby vastly decreased. Computer use also facilitates data collection for research.

Because of the decreasing average length of stay for patients in health care facilities, the increasing focus on achieving timely patient outcomes in the specific time frame permitted by reimbursement systems, and the JCAHO's emphasis on multidisciplinary care, many agencies have adopted the use of multidisciplinary plans of care known as **critical paths,** care tracks, or care maps. A critical path for congestive heart failure can be found on the Evolve website (**www.evolve.elsevier.com/Chitty/professional**). Multidisciplinary care plans such as critical paths are written in collaboration with physicians and other health care providers and establish a sequence of short-term daily outcomes that are easily measured. This type of care planning facilitates communication and collaboration among all members of the health care team. It also permits comparisons of outcomes between treatment plans as well as among health care facilities. As with the nursing process, slavish adherence to the critical path without taking individuality into consideration can negatively affect patient outcomes and is a detriment to holistic nursing care.

The development of appropriate plans of care depends on the nurse's ability to think critically. Nurses must be able to analyze information and arguments, make reasoned decisions, recognize many viewpoints, and question and seek answers continuously. At the same time, nurses must be logical, flexible, and creative and take initiative while considering the holistic nature of each patient.

Phase 4: Implementation of Planned Interventions

When nursing orders are actually carried out, the fourth phase of the nursing process, **implementation,** begins. Most people think of nursing as "doing something" for or to a patient. Notice, however, that in using the nursing process, nurses must do a great deal of thinking, analyzing, and planning before the first actual nursing action takes place.

Nurses who skip the essential first three phases of the nursing process and jump immediately into action are not behaving in a responsible, professional manner. Patients feel a greater sense of trust in a nursing staff if both physicians' and nurses' orders are carried out in an orderly, planned, and competent manner.

It is difficult to make general statements about this phase of the nursing process because interventions vary widely, depending on the nursing diagnosis and patient goals. Typical nursing interventions include such actions as monitoring patients' responses to medications, teaching patients, and performing certain procedures, such as changing dressings on a wound. As the nurse carries out planned interventions, he or she is continually assessing the patient, noting responses to nursing interventions and modifying the care plan or adding nursing diagnoses as needed. Integral to the implementation phase of the nursing process is the documentation of nursing actions.

Very sick patients require intense nursing care. As patients improve, however, they are gradually able to assume responsibility for their own care. It is important for nurses to allow patients to do as much for themselves as their illnesses allow. Patient independence is an important step in recovery.

To implement the plan of care, nurses must possess a triad of skills: thinking, or cognitive skills; doing, or psychomotor skills; and communicating or interpersonal skills. If any one set of skills is lacking, the nurse's ability to implement the nursing process is significantly decreased. Implementation involves performing actions, delegating, teaching, counseling, consulting, reporting, and documenting, all while continuously assessing.

Phase 5: Evaluation

The next phase in the nursing process is **evaluation.** In this phase, the nurse examines the patient's progress in relation to the goals and stated outcome criteria to determine whether a problem is resolved, is in the process of being resolved, or is unresolved. In other words, the outcome criteria are the basis for evaluation of the goal. Evaluation may reveal that data, diagnosis, goals, and nursing interventions were all on target and that the problem is resolved.

Evaluation may also indicate a need for a change in the plan of care. Perhaps inadequate patient data were the basis for the plan, and further assessment has uncovered additional needs. The nursing diagnoses may have been incorrect or placed in the wrong order of priority. Patient goals may have been inappropriate or unattainable within the designated time frame. It is possible that nursing actions were incorrectly implemented.

Evaluation is a critical phase in the nursing process and one that is often slighted. It is not enough to continue to do the "right things" if the patient is not improving in the expected manner. If, on evaluation, the problem has not been resolved, the nursing care plan must be revised to reflect the necessary changes, and the process must begin again.

In addition to evaluating the individual plan of care, nurses are responsible for evaluating the quality of care that all patients receive. As discussed in Chapter 13, many terms are currently used for this process, including *total quality management* (TQM), *continuous quality improvement* (CQI), and *quality improvement* (QI).

Regardless of the terminology, the goal is the same: to improve health care and the way in which it is delivered.

DYNAMIC NATURE OF THE NURSING PROCESS

Although the phases in the nursing process are discussed separately here, in practice they are not so clearly delineated, nor do they always proceed from one to another in a linear fashion. As seen in Figure 15-4, the nursing process is dynamic, meaning that nurses are continuously moving from one phase to another and then beginning the process again. Often a nurse performs two or more phases at the same time, for instance, observing a wound for signs of infection (assessment) while changing the dressing on the wound (intervention) and asking the patient whether pain has been relieved by the pain medication (evaluation).

Now that you have reviewed the phases of the nursing process, let us look back at the opening scenario. The problem that was identified was the necessity to don appropriate clothing. Data, both objective (the temperature outdoors) and subjective (the mood one is in), were gathered. Selection was made and implemented, and an evaluation of the implementation was carried out by looking in the mirror. This comparison reveals that problem solving is something each person does every day. The use of the nursing process simply provides professional nurses with a patient-oriented framework with which to solve clinical problems.

An example of using the nursing process in a clinical situation is found in Box 15-5. This case study demonstrates how using the nursing process becomes so natural that experienced nurses go through the phases fluidly and automatically.

UNIFIED NURSING LANGUAGE SYSTEMS

In the preceding pages you read about three different classification systems being developed: NANDA (nursing diagnosis), NIC (nursing intervention) and NOC (nursing outcomes). These classification systems were formulated by groups working independently. The result was three separate structures and languages (Dochterman and Jones, 2003). This fragmentation is now being addressed. Work is under way to develop a standardized system of nursing terminology incorporating all three systems.

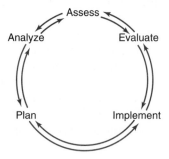

Figure 15-4
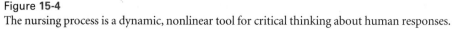
The nursing process is a dynamic, nonlinear tool for critical thinking about human responses.

Box 15-5 **Nursing Process Case Study**

You have just received a report from the day shift about Mr. Burkes. You were told that he had been admitted with a diagnosis of cancer of the tongue and that he had had a radical neck dissection. He has a tracheostomy and requires frequent suctioning. He is alert and responds by nodding his head or writing short notes.

When you enter his room, you note that he is apprehensive and tachypneic, and is gesturing for you to come into the room. You auscultate his lungs and note coarse crackles and expiratory wheezes. You can see thick secretions bubbling out of his tracheostomy. He has poor cough effort.

Based on these data, you realize that a priority nursing diagnosis is ineffective airway clearance. You immediately prepare to perform tracheal suctioning. As you are suctioning, you watch the patient's nonverbal responses and note that he is less apprehensive when the suctioning is completed. You also auscultate the lungs and note that decreased crackles and the expiratory wheezes are no longer present. Mr. Burkes writes "I can get my breath now" on his note pad.

I. Assessment
   A. Subjective data
      1. None due to inability to speak
   B. Objective data
      1. Tracheostomy with copious, thick secretions
      2. Tachypnea
      3. Gesturing for help
      4. Coarse crackles and expiratory wheezes
      5. Poor cough effort
II. Analysis
   A. Ineffective airway clearance related to copious, thick secretions
III. Plan
   A. Short-term goal: Patient will maintain patent airway as evidenced by absence of expiratory wheezes and crackles.
   B. Long-term goal: Patient will have patent airway as evidenced by his ability to clear the airway without the use of suctioning by the time of discharge.
IV. Implementation
   A. Assess lung sounds every hour for crackles and wheezes
   B. Suction airway as needed
   C. Elevate head of bed to 45 degrees
   D. Teach patient abdominal breathing techniques
   E. Encourage patient to cough out secretions
V. Evaluation
   A. Short-term goal: Achieved as evidenced by decreased crackles and absent wheezes when auscultating the lungs.
   B. Long-term goal: To be evaluated prior to discharge.

Known as the NNN Alliance, the working group is composed of leaders from NANDA International, NIC, and NOC. They are moving toward the development of a unified nursing classification that will enable nurses "to consistently communicate nursing practice to others" (p. 7). An August 2001 NNN Conference Group (NNNCG) stated the purpose of their efforts: "Nurses worldwide need to be able to use and expand the language they use so that nursing practice can be articulated, evaluated, and included in discussions of cost-effective, quality patient care" (p. 7). Specific examples of the purposes of a standardized language system include:

- The consistent description, communication, and evaluation of nursing care.
- Easier documentation and retrieval of information in computerized systems.
- The improved quality of information available for care decisions.
- Enhanced communication across providers and settings.
- The potential for wide-scale studies of nursing effectiveness (Keenan, Killeen, and Clingerman, 2003, p. 162).

As a first step in the integration of the three systems, the NNN Conference Group developed a proposed *Taxonomy of Nursing Practice* (Table 15-2) to assist in organizing or indexing nursing content (Dochterman and Jones, 2003). A **taxonomy** is simply a framework for classifying and organizing information. The taxonomy proposed by NNNCG consists of 4 domains and 28 classes into which all diagnoses, outcomes, and interventions can be organized. Although it may appear daunting at first, profession-wide use of this or other taxonomy will ultimately simplify research, teaching, and quality patient care.

The three systems discussed here are not the only nursing classification systems being developed and used. A great deal of effort has gone into the development of other nursing nomenclatures. Among the first to be developed was the Omaha System, developed by the Omaha Visiting Nurses Association. This system classifies the problems that nurses identify in home health settings, including nursing interventions and expected and actual patient outcomes. The Home Health Care Classification (HHCC), developed at Georgetown University, and the Patient Care Data Set (PCDS), developed at the University of Virginia, are among other notable efforts.

You will be hearing much more in the future about the development of a common nursing language system to support evidence-based practice.

DEVELOPING CLINICAL JUDGMENT IN NURSING

Becoming an effective nurse involves more than critical thinking and the ability to use the nursing process. It depends heavily on developing what is known as **clinical judgment.** Clinical judgment consists of informed opinions and decisions based on theoretical knowledge and experience. Nurses develop clinical judgment gradually as they gain a broader, deeper knowledge base and clinical experience. There is no substitute for extensive direct patient contact in developing clinical judgment.

Critical thinking and clinical reasoning used in the nursing process are both important aspects of clinical judgment. A nurse who has developed sound clinical judgment knows what to look for (elevation of temperature in a surgical patient), draws valid conclusions about what the signs mean (possible postoperative infection), and knows what to do about it (listen to breath sounds, assess for dehydration,

Table 15-2 TAXONOMY OF NURSING PRACTICE

DOMAINS

I. Functional Domain	II. Physiological Domain	III. Psychosocial Domain	IV. Environmental Domain
Includes diagnoses, outcomes, and interventions to promote basic needs.	Includes diagnoses, outcomes, and interventions to promote optimal biophysical health.	Includes diagnoses, outcomes, and interventions to promote optimal mental and emotional health and social functioning.	Includes diagnoses, outcomes, and interventions to promote and protect the environmental health and safety of individuals, systems, and communities.

CLASSES

Include diagnoses, class outcomes, and interventions that pertain to:

Activity/Exercise—Physical activity, including energy conservation and expenditure.	**Cardiac Function**—Cardiac mechanisms used to maintain tissue profusion.	**Behavior**—Actions that promote, maintain, or restore health.	**Health Care System**—Social, political, and economic structures and processes for the delivery of health care services.
Comfort—A sense of emotional, physical, and spiritual well-being and relative freedom from distress.	**Elimination**—Processes related to secretion and excretion of body wastes.	**Communication**—Receiving, interpreting, and expressing spoken, written, and nonverbal messages.	**Population**—Aggregates of individuals or communities having characteristics in common.
Growth and Development—Physical, emotional, and social growth and development milestones.	**Fluid and Electrolyte**—Regulation of fluid-electrolytes and acid-base balance.	**Coping**—Adjusting or adapting to stressful events.	**Risk Management**—Avoidance or control of identifiable health threats.
Nutrition—Processes related to taking in, assimilating, and using nutrients.	**Neurocognition**—Mechanisms related to the nervous system and neurocognitive functioning, including memory, thinking, and judgment.	**Emotional**—A mental state or feeling that may influence perceptions of the world.	**Roles/Relationships**—Maintenance and/or modification of expected social behaviors and emotional connectedness with others.
Self-Care—Ability to accomplish basic and instrumental activities of daily living.	**Pharmacological Function**—Effects (therapeutic and adverse) of medications or drugs and other pharmacologically active products.	**Knowledge**—Understanding and skill in applying information to promote, maintain, and restore health.	**Self-Perception**—Awareness of one's body and personal identity.

Continued

Table 15-2 TAXONOMY OF NURSING PRACTICE—CONT'D

DOMAINS, *cont'd*

I. Functional   **II. Physiological**
Domain, *cont'd*   **Domain,** *cont'd*

CLASSES

Sexuality—   **Physical Regulation**—
  Maintenance or   Body temperature,
  modification of   endocrine, and
  sexual identity   immune system
  and patterns.   responses to regulate
Sleep/Rest—The   cellular processes.
  quantity and quality   **Reproduction**—
  of sleep, rest, and   Process related to
  relaxation patterns.   human procreation
Values/Beliefs—   and birth.
  Ideas, goals,   **Respiratory**
  perceptions,   **Function**—
  spiritual, and other   Ventilation adequate
  beliefs that   to maintain arterial
  influence choices   blood gases within
  or decisions.   normal limits.
                          Sensation
                            Perception—Intake
                            and interpretation
                            of information
                            through the senses,
                            including seeing,
                            hearing, touching,
                            tasting, and smelling.
                          Tissue Integrity—
                            Skin and mucous
                            membrane protection
                            to support secretion,
                            excretion, and healing.

Source: NANDA International: *Nursing diagnoses: definitions and classification, 2003-2004,* Philadelphia, 2003, NANDA International.

check incision for redness and drainage, seek another opinion, notify the physician, and so forth). Developing sound clinical judgment requires recalling facts, recognizing patterns in patient behaviors, putting facts and observations together to form a meaningful whole, and acting on the resulting information in an appropriate way.

An important aspect of clinical judgment is knowing the limitations of your expertise. Most nurses have an instinctive awareness of when they are approaching their limits and should seek consultation with another professional. Your state's nurse practice act, health agency policies, school policies, and the professions' standards of practice all provide guidance in making the decision about nursing actions within your scope of practice. Nursing students, whether new to nursing or registered nurses in baccalaureate programs, must consider policies and standards in determining their scope of practice in any given nursing situation.

Rosalinda Alfaro-LeFevre (1999) developed a list of nine key questions to consider when seeking to improve clinical judgment. These are found in Box 15-6.

Nurses are responsible for developing sound clinical judgment and are accountable for their decisions. Whatever your current level of clinical judgment may be, it can always be improved. You may want to devise a personal plan for improving your own clinical decision making. Thoughtfully completing the self-assessment in Box 15-7 will help you begin.

Summary of Key Points

- Critical thinking in nursing is a purposeful, disciplined, active process that improves clinical judgment and thereby improves patient care.
- Thinking by novice nurses is different from that of expert nurses in identifiable ways.
- The nursing process is a systematic problem-solving strategy that is based on the scientific method. It is used by nurses when delivering patient care.
- The phases of the nursing process are assessment, analysis and diagnosis, planning, implementation, and evaluation.
- Properly used, the nursing process is cyclic and dynamic rather than rigid and linear.
- Nurses may initially find that using the nursing process feels awkward or slow. After practice, however, most find it becomes a natural, yet organized way to approach patient care.
- When all nurses use the nursing process effectively, patient care is consistent, comprehensive, and coordinated.
- Through the use of the nursing process, nurses are able to work toward resolving patient problems in a systematic manner, thus advancing both the scientific basis of nursing and professionalism.
- Developing a unified nursing language will advance the nursing profession.
- Critical thinking; creative use of the nursing process; current knowledge about health, illness, and scope of practice; and abundant clinical experience combine to create sound clinical judgment.

CRITICAL THINKING QUESTIONS

1. Explain the "habits of mind" that are characteristic of critical thinkers.
2. List at least four ways in which novice thinking and expert thinking differ and give an example that illustrates each.
3. Describe the phases in the nursing process and the activities of each phase.
4. List a short-term personal goal and a long-term personal goal using all the essential elements of effective goals. Evaluate your progress toward these goals.
5. Compare the nursing process with the scientific method (Chapter 12) and state how they are similar and how they differ.
6. Explain the difference between independent, dependent, and interdependent nursing interventions and give an example of each.
7. Describe and critique the PES format for writing a nursing diagnosis.
8. Explain the difference between medical and nursing diagnoses.

Box **15-6** Clinical Judgment: Nine Key Questions

1. What major outcomes (observable beneficial results) do we expect to see in this particular person, family, or group when the plan of care is terminated? Example: The person will be discharged infection free, able to care for himself, 3 days after surgery. Outcomes may be addressed on a standard plan, or you may have to develop these outcomes yourself. Be sure that you check to make sure any predetermined outcomes in standard plans are appropriate to your patient's specific situation.

2. What problems or issues must be addressed to achieve the major outcomes? Answering this question will help you set priorities. You might be faced with a long list of actual or potential health problems. You need to narrow down your list to those that must be addressed.

3. What are the circumstances? Who is involved (e.g., child, adult, group)? How urgent are the problems (e.g., life-threatening, chronic)? What are the factors influencing their presentation (e.g., when, where, and how did the problems develop)? What are the patient's values, beliefs, and cultural influences?

4. What knowledge is required? Knowledge required includes problem-specific facts (e.g., how health problems usually present, how they're diagnosed, what their common causes and risk factors are, what common complications occur, and how these complications are prevented and managed); nursing process and related knowledge and skills (ethics, research, health assessment, communication, priority setting); related sciences (anatomy, physiology, pathophysiology, pharmacology, chemistry, physics, psychology, sociology). You must also be clearly aware of the circumstances, as addressed in question 3 above.

5. How much room is there for error? In the clinical setting, there is usually minimal room for error. However, it depends on the health of the individual and the risks of interventions. Example: In which of the following cases do you think you have more room for error? (1) You're trying to decide whether to give a healthy child a one-time dose of acetaminophen for heat rash without checking with the doctor. (2) You have a child who's been sick for 3 days with a fever, and the mother wants to know whether she should continue giving acetaminophen without checking with the doctor.
If you chose the first example, you're right. In the second case, the symptoms have continued for 3 days without a diagnosis. If you continue to give acetaminophen without checking with a physician, you might be masking symptoms of a problem requiring medical management.

6. How much time do I have? Time frame for decision making depends on (1) the urgency of the problems (e.g., there's little time in life-threatening situations, such as cardiac arrest) and (2) the planned length of contact (e.g., if your patient will be hospitalized only for 2 days, you have to be realistic about what can be accomplished, and key decisions need to be made early).

7. What resources can help me? Human resources include clinical nurse educators, nursing faculty, preceptors, more experienced nurses, advance practice nurses, peers, librarians, and other health care professionals (pharmacists, nutritionists, physical therapists, physicians). The patient and family are also valuable resources (usually they know their own problems best). Other resources include texts, articles, other references, computer databases, decision-making support, national practice guidelines, and facility documents (e.g., guidelines, policies, procedures, assessment forms).

8. Whose perspectives must be considered? The most significant perspective to consider is the patient's point of view. Other important perspectives include those of the family and significant others, caregivers, and relevant third parties (e.g., insurers).

9. What's influencing my thinking? Be sure you identify personal biases and any other factors influencing your critical thinking.

From Alfaro-LeFevre R: *Critical thinking in nursing: a practical approach,* ed 2, Philadelphia, 1999, WB Saunders. Reprinted with permission.

Box **15-7** Self-Assessment: Developing Sound Clinical Judgment

Answer the following questions honestly. When finished, make a list of the items you need to work on in your quest to develop sound clinical judgment. Keep the list with you and review it frequently. Seek opportunities to practice needed activities.

1. Use References
   - Do I look up new terms when I encounter them to make them part of my vocabulary?
   - Do I familiarize myself with normal findings so that I can recognize those outside the norm?
   - Do I bother to find out why abnormal findings occur?
   - Do I learn the signs and symptoms of various conditions, what causes them, and how they're managed?
2. Use the Nursing Process
   - Do I always assess before acting, stay focused on outcomes, and make changes as needed?
   - Do I always base my judgments on fact, not emotion or hearsay?
3. Assess Systematically
   - Do I have a systematic approach to assessing patients to decrease the likelihood that I will overlook important data?
4. Set Priorities Systematically
   - Do I evaluate both the problem and the probable cause before acting?
   - Am I willing to obtain assistance from a more knowledgeable source when indicated?
5. Refuse to Act Without Knowledge
   - Do I refuse to perform an action when I don't know the indication, why it works, and what risks there are for harm to this particular patient?
6. Use Resources Wisely
   - Do I look for opportunities to learn from others—teachers, other experts, even my peers?
   - Do I seek help when needed, being mindful of patient privacy issues?
7. Know Standards of Care
   - Do I read facility policies, professional standards, school policies, and state board of nursing rules and regulations to determine my scope of practice?
   - Do I know the clinical agency's policies and procedures affecting my particular patients?
   - Do I attempt to understand the rationales behind policies and procedures?
   - Do I follow policies and procedures carefully, recognizing that they are designed to help me use good judgment?
8. Know Technology and Equipment
   - Do I routinely learn how to use patient technology such as IV pumps, patient monitors, computers?
   - Do I learn how to check equipment for proper functioning and safety?
9. Give Patient-Centered Care
   - Do I always remember the needs and feelings of the patient, family, and significant others?
   - Do I value knowing my patients' health beliefs and values within their own cultural contexts?
   - Do I "go the extra mile" for patients?
   - Do I demonstrate the belief that every patient deserves my very best efforts?

Adapted from Alfaro-LeFevre R: *Critical thinking in nursing: a practical approach,* ed 2, Philadelphia, 1999, WB Saunders, pp 88-92. Used with permission.

9. Describe what is meant by the statement, "The nursing process is a cyclic process."
10. Explain what is meant by "a unified nursing language" and discuss how this could benefit nursing.
11. Using what you learned about yourself from the Self-Assessment: Developing Sound Clinical Judgment (Box 15-7), set short-term goals for improvement in each of the nine areas. Make a checklist to take to your next clinical laboratory experience and consciously work on improving your clinical judgment.

REFERENCES

Alfaro-LeFevre R: *Critical thinking in nursing: a practical approach,* ed 2, Philadelphia, 1999, WB Saunders.

American Nurses Association: *Nursing's social policy statement,* ed 2, Washington, DC, 2003, nursesbooks.org.

American Nurses Association: *Nursing: scope and standards of practice,* Washington, DC, 2003, nursesbooks.org.

American Philosophical Association: Critical thinking: a statement of expert consensus for purposes of educational assessment and instruction, *The Delphi Report: Research Findings and Recommendations Prepared for the Committee on Pre-College Philosophy,* ERIC Document Reproduction Services, 315-423, 1990.

Benner P: *From novice to expert,* Menlo Park, CA, 1984, Addison-Wesley.

Benner P, Tanner CA, Chesla CA: *Expertise in nursing practice: caring, clinical judgment, and ethics,* New York, 1996, Springer.

Center for Nursing Classification: Nursing outcomes classification, Online, 2003 *(www.nursing.uiowa.edu/centers/cncce/index.htm).*

De Bono E: *Edward de Bono's mind pack,* London, 1995, Dorling-Kindersley.

Dochterman JM, Jones DA: Unifying nursing languages: the harmonization of NANDA, NIC, and NOC, Washington, DC, 2003, nursesbooks.org.

Gordon M: *Nursing diagnosis: process and application,* ed 2, New York, 1987, McGraw-Hill.

Gordon M: Nursing diagnosis and the diagnostic process, *Am J Nurs* 76(5):1298-1300, 1976.

Keenan GM, Killeen MB, Clingerman E: NANDA, NOC, and NIC: Progress toward a nursing information infrastructure, *Nurs Ed Perspect* 23(4):162-163, 2003.

Kenney LJ: Using Edward de Bono's six hats game to aid critical thinking and reflection in palliative care, *Int J Palliat Nurs* 9(3):105-112, 2003.

Lunney M: *Critical thinking and nursing diagnosis: case studies and analyses,* Philadelphia, 2001, North American Nursing Diagnosis Association.

Maslow AH: *Motivation and personality,* New York, 1970, Harper & Row.

Mueller A, Johnston M, Bligh D: Joining mind mapping and care planning to enhance student critical thinking and achieve holistic nursing care, *Nurs Diagn* 13(1):24-27, 2002.

NANDA International: *Nursing diagnoses: definitions and classification, 2003-2004,* Philadelphia, 2003, NANDA International.

Scheffer BK, Rubenfeld MG: A consensus statement on critical thinking, *J Nurs Ed* 39:352-359, 2002.

Yura H, Walsh MB: The nursing process: assessing, planning, implementing, evaluation, ed 4, Norwalk, CT, 1983, Appleton-Century-Crofts.

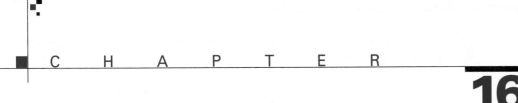

CHAPTER 16

Financing Health Care

Frances A. Maurer

Key Terms

Acuity
Capitation
Centers for Medicare and
  Medicaid Services (CMS)
Certificate of Need (CON)
Copayment
Cost Containment
Deductible
Diagnosis-Related Groups
  (DRGs)
Gatekeeper
Health Care Network
Health Insurance Portability and
  Accountability Act (HIPAA)

Health Maintenance
  Organization (HMO)
Hill-Burton Act
Managed Care Organization
  (MCO)
Medicaid
Medicare
Out-of-Pocket Payment
Patient Classification System
  (PCS)
Personal Payment
Point-of-Service (POS)
Preferred Provider Organization
  (PPO)

Premium
Private Insurance
Professional Review
  Organization (PRO)
Prospective Payment
  System (PPS)
Quality Management
Retrospective
  Reimbursement
Self-Insurance
Skill Mix
Third-Party Payment
Universal Care
Workers' Compensation

Learning Outcomes

After studying this chapter, students will be able to:

- Explain the economic principle of supply and demand and its relevance to health care costs.
- Cite examples of causes of health care cost escalation.
- Describe the major methods of payment for health care.
- Explain cost-containment efforts since 1975 and their impact on nursing practice.
- Describe the impact of managed care on cost containment and health care consumers.
- Describe the relationship between cost containment and quality management initiatives.
- Identify current and proposed strategies aimed at changing segments of the health care delivery system.
- Identify general guidelines for evaluating national health insurance proposals.

arly in the twenty-first century there is renewed vigor to the public debate over financing health care in the United States. Health care costs continue to climb, as does the number of uninsured citizens. Legislative reforms and managed care efforts have had mixed success at cutting health care costs and increasing access to health care. The nation's dilemma remains: how to provide high-quality health care services to all citizens while keeping costs down.

In 2001, the nation's health care expenditures reached $1.4 trillion and consumed 14.1 percent of the gross domestic product (GDP). This percentage has increased 3500% since 1960, making health care the nation's largest single budget item (Levit, Smith, Cowan, et al., 2003). Estimates for the year 2011 indicate that health care costs are expected to reach $2.8 trillion (Centers for Medicare and Medicaid Services, [CMS], 2003). If this trend is allowed to continue until the year 2010, 40% of all national resources will be spent on health care. Yet the health of American citizens is not as good as it should be. As a result, almost everyone agrees that there is a crisis in health care and that reform is needed.

Americans are concerned about rising health care costs. Today the public's concern is about the ability of our health care system to maintain the Medicare program, provide for the growing number of uninsured, and ensure the quality of managed care. It seems that at a time when health care breakthroughs are at an all-time high, public support for the system that created those breakthroughs is eroding.

The March 2, 2002, issue of *Time* magazine contained an article that illustrated numerous examples of public health care worries (Tumulty, 2002). For example, TennCare, the Tennessee health plan designed to cover the working poor, is costing the state $6 billion/year, far more than anticipated. As a result, TennCare is contemplating dropping one-half million enrollees to reduce costs. Another example involved the high cost of insurance premiums. The article described the dilemma of a 25-year-old single mother of two who works for an employer who does not offer health insurance. The best individual policy she found cost $400/month ($4800/year) in premiums with a $2300 deductible. She could not afford to purchase this insurance. These are but two examples of the multitude of health care problems faced by individuals, businesses, and governments today.

Most Americans believe that health care is a right, not a privilege. In 1993, former President Bill Clinton attempted national health care reform, addressing rising health care costs and restricted access for many Americans. His plan was heavily attacked by various special interest groups and failed to pass Congress. Enthusiasm for health care reform faded. Recently, however, there has been a resurgence of interest in universal coverage because the number of uninsured people climbs ever higher, low-income individuals have difficulty accessing health care services, and prescription drugs costs place a substantial burden on the elderly.

Despite governmental inaction on health care reform in the 1990s, business interests forced major changes in health care access and delivery. Corporations and other large employers were in the vanguard of efforts to reduce health care costs, primarily because health care benefits represent a significant cost to employers. For example, General Motors, Chrysler, and Ford spend $9,000 or more each year in health care benefits for each employee. The same companies spend about $15,000 annually to cover each retiree and retiree family (Hakin, 2003). Employers generally pay more health care costs for retirees than for active workers. Ford, for example, paid a startling $2.8 billion in retiree health care during 2002.

The cost-reduction strategies implemented by businesses placed limits on employees' treatment options and altered the payment structure of health care for many employed Americans. Even without planned, organized, comprehensive change in the structure of the health care system, significant change nevertheless continued. Finding a solution to the health care finance dilemma while maintaining quality and improving access to services remains a challenge that will not easily be achieved.

Financial issues profoundly affect nurses and nursing practice. Therefore, students of professional nursing need to understand the overall economic context in which nursing care is provided. The financial component of health care affects nurses professionally, in their nursing practice, and personally, in the type of insurance and health services they and their families are able to afford. This chapter explores several major concepts necessary to understanding health care finance: basic economic theory, a brief historical review of the causes of health care cost escalation, current methods of payment, cost-containment efforts, the economics of nursing care, and the impact of cost containment on nursing care. Criteria to evaluate health reform proposals are summarized.

BASIC ECONOMIC THEORY

Nursing school curricula do not typically require undergraduates to take courses in economics; yet there is an urgent need for nurses to understand the economic context in which they practice. Economics influences the type and quality of health services provided, as well as employment opportunities for nurses.

Supply and Demand

A basic economic theory is the *law of supply and demand*. According to this theory, a normal economic system consists of two parts: suppliers, who provide goods and services, and consumers, who demand and use goods and services. In a monetary environment, that is, one in which money is used as a unit of exchange, consumers exchange money for desired goods and services.

In an efficient marketplace, the market price of goods and services serves to create an equilibrium in which supply roughly equals demand, and demand roughly equals supply. When demand exceeds supply, prices rise. When supply exceeds demand, prices fall. The relationship between price and equilibrium can be seen at the clothing store. During an unusually mild winter for example, the demand for heavy coats is likely to be low. Because demand is low, manufacturers cut back on production, and retailers stop ordering coats and place their current stock of coats on sale. If the sale price is low enough, however, people will continue to buy coats. Through fluctuations in supply and demand, created by price, equilibrium is approached. This example illustrates the principle of price sensitivity, that is, a change in demand for goods or services is a function of the change in the price of those goods or services (Feldstein, 1998). Figure 16-1 illustrates the relationships among price, supply, and demand.

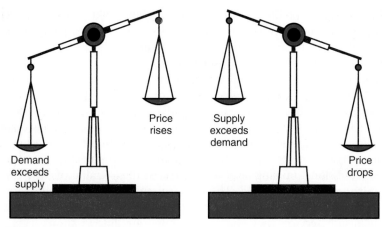

Figure **16-1**
Price sensitivity in a normal economic environment.

IS BASIC ECONOMIC THEORY APPLICABLE TO HEALTH CARE?

There are problems associated with applying basic economic theory to the health care market. This chapter highlights a few of those problems.

Health Care as a Right or Privilege

In a free-market economy, consumption of any good or service is determined by an individual's ability to pay. In a pure free market, a portion of the population would be denied health care if they were unable to pay. People who support this position consider health care a privilege. Others believe that everyone should have access to basic health care and consider health care a right.

Despite the United States' leanings toward a free-market economy in general, health care is largely considered a right, not a privilege. Rather than allowing economically disadvantaged citizens to do without health services, the federal government has taken steps to ensure certain groups access to health care services through publicly funded programs such as **Medicare** and **Medicaid.** Although this is generally considered an ethical policy, it is nevertheless a policy decision that interferes with the functioning of free-market principles.

Price Sensitivity in Health Care

In the days before health insurance existed, people paid their own medical bills, and providers set their fees with some sensitivity to what patients could pay. When costs were high, patients complained. Health insurance created an indirect payment structure, **third-party payment,** that removed price sensitivity from the concern of most health care consumers because they pay only a small portion of the actual costs. A third party (the employer, insurance company, or government) pays the rest. If someone other than the consumer pays, demand can increase because the consumer is insensitive to cost. This is an important point to keep in mind when reviewing the history of health care finance. History has demonstrated that when there is little or no out-of-pocket expense to the consumer, economic equilibrium is upset because consumers use more health care services (Jacob and Rapoport, 2002).

Additional Influences on the Health Care Market

Economists have identified a number of other factors that affect the health care market in ways that violate the assumptions surrounding an effective free-market system. For example, consumers cannot always control demand for health care services. With ordinary products, a consumer can delay a purchase until there is a sale or forego the purchase altogether. Health care is different because often health care needs are immediate. The consumer might suffer serious harm or even death by a delay in seeking services.

From this brief discussion, readers can see that the health care market differs from the free market system in several key ways. Box 16-1 summarizes some of the

---

Box 16-1 Barriers to a Free Market Economy in Health Care

Poor Consumer Information

Individual consumers are not accustomed to "shopping" for the best available prices for medical services, supplies, and equipment. Even when the consumer is motivated to compare costs, getting that information from the suppliers of health care is difficult and time-consuming. Most consumers require services quickly and cannot afford long delays to seek information, even if they have the expertise to search out the needed information.

Ineffective Pricing System

When the price of services is based on "reasonable and customary costs of similar services" in an area, health care providers have an incentive to continue to increase their prices rather than compete by lowering prices. Eventually the new, higher price becomes the "reasonable and customary" price. Reform efforts have had some success at reducing the impact of this phenomenon by establishing prospective funding and capping reimbursement for the cost of selected services.

Health Care Providers' Interests May Conflict With Consumers'

Health care providers have economic interests that can be in opposition to consumer interests. Physicians, for example, act both as suppliers of health care and demanders of patient services. When physicians are partners or stockholders in services, such as laboratories or radiographic facilities, they are more likely to order such tests, according to studies by the Department of Health and Human Services. Conversely, HMO or PPO physicians who receive incentives for not referring patients to specialists are less likely to do so.

Cost Efficiency Is Not Always a Motivator for Suppliers

Although businesses are expected to operate with cost-efficiency, others, particularly some nonprofit organizations, may be influenced by other factors. By law, nonprofits cannot keep or distribute profit or surplus of funds at the end of the fiscal year, but there is no law that dictates how they spend that money. Most nonprofits operate efficiently and at the lowest cost to consumers; others have been found to use their funds to provide amenities and perks for staff and board members, such as plush exercise facilities, all-expense-paid trips, or purchases of private boxes at sports stadiums.

Modified from Maurer FA: Financing of health care: context for community health nursing. In Smith C, Maurer FA, editors: *Community health nursing: theory and practice,* ed 2, Philadelphia, 2000, WB Saunders.

factors that reduce the efficient functioning of free-market economics in the health care market.

CURRENT METHODS OF PAYMENT FOR HEALTH CARE

There are four major methods of payment for health care in use today: personal payment, Medicare, Medicaid, and private insurance. Workers' compensation is an additional mechanism for financing some health care services. Each of these is briefly explained below.

Personal (Out-of-Pocket) Payment

Personal payment for health care services is the least common method. The last several years have seen an increase in personal payments resulting from rising costs in copayments and deductibles determined by insurers. Few people can afford **out-of-pocket payment** for more than the most basic health services. At today's prices, an illness or injury severe enough to require hospitalization can quickly exhaust a family's financial reserves, forcing them into bankruptcy. Generally, only those people without access to some form of private group insurance or public insurance rely on personal payment. It sometimes takes years to pay a single, large medical bill.

Medicare

Medicare, or Title XVIII of the Social Security Act, is a nationwide federal health insurance program established in 1965. Medicare is available to people aged 65 and over, regardless of the recipient's income. It also covers certain disabled individuals and people requiring dialysis or kidney transplants. Medicare has two separate but coordinated programs. The first, known as Part A, is a hospitalization insurance program. Part B is a supplementary medical insurance program that covers visits to physicians' offices and other outpatient services. Originally intended to be a no-cost or low-cost program for the elderly, the cost of participating in Medicare has risen steadily. By 2003, Part A required participants to pay a deductible of $840 for hospitalization, and Part B required an annual $100 deductible and a monthly premium of $58.70 (Medicare and You, 2003). Although the program was originally designed to be all-inclusive, many elderly people now find they cannot afford to participate in Medicare. Ironically, some elderly are so poor that they qualify for Medicaid assistance in paying their Medicare premiums.

In November 2003, Congress passed legislation creating major changes to Medicare. Highlights of these changes are itemized in Box 16-2.

Medicaid

Medicaid, or Title XIX of the Social Security Act, is a group of jointly funded federal-state programs for low-income, elderly, blind, and disabled individuals. It, too, was established in 1965. There are broad federal guidelines, but states have some flexibility in how they administer the program. People must meet eligibility requirements determined by each state. Eligibility depends on income and varies from state to state. Rates of payment also vary, with some states providing far higher payments than others. The amount the federal government contributes to Medicaid

| Box 16-2 | **Highlights of Changes to Medicare Program: The Medicare Prescription Drug Improvement and Modernization Act of 2003** |

Effective in 2004 and 2005

- Interim prescription drug discount card available for $30/year.
- Pharmacies and drug companies to provide discounts up to 25 percent of the cost of medications.
- Details on how the program will work not available at press time.

Effective in 2006

- Optional drug plan begins. Seniors pay $35/month with a $250 annual deductible.
- Medicare covers 75 percent of the first $2250 in drug costs.
- "Window" of noncoverage for the next $2850 in yearly drug costs.
- Catastrophic coverage pays 95 percent of all remaining drug costs (after out-of-pocket costs per senior reach $3600).

Effective 2010

- Private competition test program. Private health insurance companies will be allowed to compete with Medicare in six metropolitan test areas.
- Private companies will be compensated with a $12 billion subsidy during the test period.

Prevention Emphasis

- Medicare will pay for initial physical exam on all new enrollees.
- Automatic screenings for diabetes and heart disease.

varies from a minimum of 50 percent of total costs to a maximum of 76.8 percent. The differences in eligibility and payment rates lead to wide variations in the level of care provided to the poor in different states. In contrast to those on Medicare, people who receive Medicaid are not required to pay any fees to participate. Table 16-1 highlights the similarities and differences in the Medicare and Medicaid programs.

Private Insurance

Private insurance, also called voluntary insurance, is a system wherein insurance premiums are either paid by insured individuals or their employers or shared between individuals and employers. Periodic payments (**premiums**) are paid into the insurance plan, and certain health care benefits are covered as long as the premiums are paid. Early in the development of private insurance, many treatments were covered only if they were performed in an inpatient (hospital) setting. This was one of the features that tended to drive up the cost of services. Today most insurers stipulate that costs of hospitalization are reimbursable only if treatment cannot be performed on an outpatient basis.

Table 16-1 FACTS ABOUT MEDICARE AND MEDICAID

	Medicare	Medicaid
Funding	Federal government	Federal and state governments
Administration	Federal government	State governments
Eligibility	People over 65 and certain others	Selected poor and disabled (includes some elderly)
Level of benefits	Same nationwide	Varies from state to state
Payment by recipients?	Required	Usually not required; copayments may be required in Medicaid managed care
Coverage	Hospitalization; outpatient care; optional prescriptions; no custodial, nursing, or optical care	Comprehensive, including prescriptions and optical care

Modified from CMS: *Medicare and Medicaid statistical supplement, 2001,* Baltimore, MD, 2002, Health Care Financing Review, Centers for Medicare and Medicaid Services.

Workers' Compensation

Workers' compensation constitutes a small proportion of insurance coverage. The program varies from state to state but generally covers only workers who are injured on the job. It usually covers treatment for injuries and weekly payments during the time the worker is absent from work for injury-related causes. In the case of accidental death, the worker's family receives compensation. Companies are required by law to contribute to a compensation fund from which money is withdrawn when accidental injuries or deaths occur at work.

Figure 16-2 represents the proportion each of the major payment methods contributed to the funding of health care services in the United States in 2001.

HISTORY OF HEALTH CARE FINANCE

Before 1940, more than 90 percent of Americans either paid directly from their own pockets for health care or depended on charity care. Few had private health insurance. Public insurance programs, such as Medicare and Medicaid, did not exist. Following World War II, most industrialized countries began publicly financed health care systems that provided care for all citizens. The United States, however, did not adopt a public, universal access system, choosing instead to continue the private, fee-for-service system.

Growth of Private Insurance

In 1943, the Internal Revenue Service (IRS) ruled that health benefits paid by employers were not taxable as income. Employers began to offer health benefits as a reward to employees. States granted tax-exempt status to private insurance companies, such as Blue Cross and Blue Shield, and private insurers grew dramatically. By 1960, two thirds of nonelderly Americans had private health insurance, mostly paid for by employers.

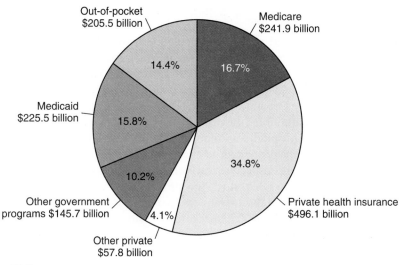

Figure 16-2
Funding sources for health care (2001) in billions of dollars (total $1424 billion). The category "Other private" included industrial health services, nonpatient revenues, and privately financed construction. (Data from Centers for Medicare and Medicaid Services, Office of the Actuary, National Health Statistics Group.)

Hill-Burton Act

In 1946, the U.S. Congress passed the Hospital Survey and Construction Act (the **Hill-Burton Act**). This law called for and funded surveys of states' needs for hospitals, paid for planning hospitals and public health centers, and provided partial funding for constructing and equipping them. The Hill-Burton Act spurred community hospital construction. With accessible, new, well-equipped hospitals in many towns and employer-paid health insurance a standard job benefit, the stage was set for increased consumer demand, leading to dramatic increases in the utilization of hospitals and health care services.

Rise of Public Insurance Programs

The problem of paying for health care for the unemployed and the elderly was not solved by the advent of private insurance, and many continued to receive inadequate care. In 1965, Congress responded by approving two public insurance programs to cover these groups: Medicare for the elderly and certain disabled people, and Medicaid for the poor. These programs were designed to ensure that citizens who were uninsured by employers and unable to afford their own private health insurance would be protected. At that point in time, a unique public-private partnership system of insurance that would care for all seemed to be in place. Unfortunately, that partnership has not lived up to anyone's expectations and, 40 years later, universal health care coverage for all Americans remains an elusive goal.

Retrospective Reimbursement

Originally, both public and private insurance plans were based on **retrospective** (after-the-fact) **reimbursement.** This meant that when Patient Doe went to the hospital with pneumonia, a request was sent to the insurer for reimbursement for whatever services were rendered (chest radiographs, blood work, physical examinations, and antibiotic therapy). Depending on the terms of Patient Doe's insurance policy and the level of her **deductible** (the portion she has to pay yearly before insurance coverage begins), the hospital was reimbursed for much, or even most, of the charges. **Copayments** (the percentage of charges the patient pays) were low, often as low as 10 percent. Using retrospective reimbursement, the cost of services to insured consumers of health care was extremely low or zero. Because neither the orderers of health care (physicians) nor the consumers (patients) were concerned about cost, the demand for health care services became virtually insatiable, driving costs up dramatically (Jacob and Rapoport, 2002).

Early Cost-Containment Initiatives

In the late 1960s, new federal legislation required states to develop comprehensive health planning. At least one agency per state was established and empowered to review the health care needs of communities in order to reduce costs **cost-containment** and duplication of service. A **certificate of need (CON)** had to be approved by the health planning agency before new construction, expansion of existing facilities, or major equipment purchases were permitted. Only projects that could demonstrate a real need were issued CONs. The result was a dramatic slowing in the construction and expansion of hospitals and public health facilities nationwide (Lampe, 1987).

By 1975, additional serious cost-containment efforts were under way, stimulated by the concerns of politicians, consumer groups, and employers about costs. Some states initiated rate setting, placing limits on reimbursement to health care providers for services. One important strategy was a move toward replacing retrospective payment for services to **prospective payment systems (PPS).** In prospective payment systems, providers, such as physicians and hospitals, receive payment on a per-case basis, regardless of the cost to the provider to deliver the services. Prospective payment systems were developed because of escalating costs in the Medicare and Medicaid programs. It became apparent that basic changes in payment mechanisms were needed. Box 16-3 contains information about the dramatic increases in costs to taxpayers of Medicare and Medicaid since they were implemented in 1967.

The passage of the Tax Equity and Fiscal Responsibility Act (TEFRA) in 1982 dramatically restructured the payment method for Medicare to a prospective payment system based on **diagnosis-related groups (DRGs),** which are described later in this chapter. Prospective payment was designed to create more competition and resulted in an emphasis on efficiency, cost-effectiveness, and financial accountability. It also stimulated competition among health care providers by awarding incentives to those who operated in a cost-effective manner. Because prospective payment has the potential to encourage providers to undertreat patients to reduce costs, quality management initiatives were implemented to protect consumers.

Box **16-3** Medicare and Medicaid Costs, 1967* and 2001

Medicare

1967	*2001*
$5 billion	$241.9 billion

- Those helped equal 95 percent of the elderly, regardless of family resources and persons receiving social security because of disability.

Medicaid

1967	*2001*
$2.3 billion	$205.3 billion

- Those helped in 1980 equal 65 percent of the poor.
- Those helped in 2000 equal 50 percent of the poor.
- Medicaid is the fastest-growing spending program in the United States.

*First full year of operation for Medicare and Medicaid.
Data from Organization for Economic Cooperation and Development: Health care expenditures and other data: an international compendium, *Health Care Financ Rev* (suppl):111-195, 1989; and CMS: *Medicare and Medicaid statistical supplement, 2001,* Baltimore, MD, 2002, Health Care Financing Review, Center for Medicare and Medicaid Services.

CONTINUED ESCALATION OF HEALTH CARE COSTS

Despite those early comprehensive cost planning efforts, health care costs continued to rise in the 1980s and 1990s. In addition to the imperfect operation of a market economy in health care, other factors have affected costs. Some of the most important ones are inflation, new technologies and drugs, increased demand for health care services, and the impact of fraud and abuse.

Inflation

Inflation generally affects all business sectors but has tended to escalate faster in health care than in other segments of the economy. Even during economic climates of low to moderate inflation, health care costs continue to consume a greater portion of the GDP, limiting what can be spent on other segments of the economy.

New Technologies and Drugs

Another reason for the rise in costs is related to the development of and demand for new technologies and new drugs. In fact, some believe this is the primary cause of increasing health care costs (Sultz and Young, 2001). Modern medical care depends on advanced technologies that were not even dreamed of a few decades ago. New equipment such as magnetic resonance imaging, and new procedures such as angioplasty and hip replacement are commonplace. New technologies are extremely costly: A single x-ray machine can cost up to $250,000, and more advanced types of diagnostic imaging machines can cost more than $2 million. Health care costs are also driven upward by new lifestyle drugs, such as Viagra, a male potency drug, and Zoloft, an antidepressant, which had revenues of $1.7 billion and $2.7 billion respectively in 2002 (Pfizer, 2003).

Increased Demand for Health Care Services

Demographics also play a role in escalating health care costs. The United States has experienced rapid growth in both the elderly and the uninsured nonelderly populations. Medicare and Medicaid have improved access for the poor and elderly, two groups that previously had limited access because of inability to pay. Because older persons are more likely to have chronic illnesses, their demand for health care services exceeds that of younger segments of the population. The elderly population is expected to continue to rise, thus increasing the demand for health care services. Although in 2001 only one in eight Americans was over 65 years of age, by 2020, this figure will increase to one in five, or 20 percent of the population (Statistical Abstract of the U.S. [Part 1], 2002). With the total population of the United States expected to reach 300 million in the next decade, overall population growth will continue to fuel the demand for health care services.

Fraud and Abuse of Payment Systems

Fraud and abuse of payment systems account for part of the problem as well. An estimated $75 billion of the United States' annual health expenditures may be due to fraud, including as much as 20 percent of all workers' compensation claims and up to 10 percent in Medicare losses.

Health care providers such as physicians, clinics, and hospitals are on the honor system, but some intentionally cheat the system. In response, the Department of Health and Human Services developed *Operation Restore Trust* in 1995 to combat fraud in the Medicare program. Originally a demonstration project for the five most populous states, *Operation Restore Trust* was expanded to include other states after its initial success. This program's stringent oversight of health care charges has reduced unnecessary costs by about half. In 1998, unnecessary charges were $12.8 billion as opposed to $23.2 billion in 1996 (Vice and Adams, 2000). Despite these efforts, problems continue.

In 2003, for example, Tenet Healthcare, a large national health corporation, agreed to pay $54 million to settle a U.S. Justice Department suit (Eichenwald, 2003). The federal government charged that Tenet physicians had conducted unnecessary heart procedures and operations on hundreds of patients. Tenet is under investigation in a case of increasing charges in order to inflate the amount Medicare would pay for enrollee health care services at some of its hospitals. In an example of Medicaid fraud, the U.S. Justice Department settled a $500 million charge against National Medical Care Inc. The company, one of the largest providers of dialysis products and services, had performed unnecessary tests on kidney dialysis patients and also paid kickbacks to laboratories for referrals (Vice and Adams, 2000).

The result of upwardly spiraling costs fueled by technology, demand for services, and fraud, is that health care costs accounted for an increasing portion of U.S. resources. Most economists believe that this trend cannot continue without damaging the nation's economy.

COST-CONTAINMENT MEASURES REVISITED

Both public and private health care entities have a vested interest in containing costs. The continuous escalation in health care costs during the 1980s and 1990s caused both public and private insurers to rethink past containment strategies and to institute a variety of newer measures designed to reduce costs. Sometimes alone, sometimes in tandem with one another, and frequently with one sector leading and the other following, new initiatives have been developed and older ones revitalized. Several cost-containment entities and legislative efforts of which students should be aware are described below.

Centers for Medicare and Medicaid Services (CMS)

The **Centers for Medicare and Medicaid Services (CMS),** formerly the Health Care Financing Administration (HCFA), is a federal cost-containment program. Its purpose is to establish standards and monitor care in both programs. It has the authority to enforce these standards for hospitals, nursing homes and other long-term care facilities, laboratories, clinics, and other health entities that care for Medicare and Medicaid patients. It is responsible for establishing regulation and oversight of any changes legislated by Congress to either program.

The CMS contracts private insurance agencies, such as Blue Cross and Blue Shield, to service the Medicare program. When patients or their families have questions about coverage or payments, nurses advise them to contact the insurer who administers the program in their area, not the CMS. While retaining oversight of the Medicaid program, the CMS has ceded administration of that program to the states. CMS publications are a good source of information on health care costs, government share of funding, descriptions of the populations served by both programs, and evaluations of program effectiveness *(www.cms.hhs.gov).*

Professional Review Organizations (PROs)

Professional review organizations (PROs) are designed to monitor the quality of care received by health care consumers and to ensure that care meets professional standards. The peer review process is a combined public and private effort. These organizations are usually private, but their functions in certain situations are a requirement of federal regulation. Peer review started as a voluntary review process that brought prestige to hospitals passing review.

Professional review organizations became mandatory as a result of Medicare regulations, which stipulated that all hospitals receiving Medicare payments had to submit to peer review. Medicare demanded those hospital admissions and lengths of stay be examined to ensure that a patient's health and treatment needs were best met in a hospital environment; as a result PROs expanded. If a patient is hospitalized unnecessarily or for a period of time longer than the PRO determines to be appropriate or if procedures are performed that the PRO determines are unnecessary, the hospital is denied Medicare reimbursement for the extra days and the unnecessary procedures. This causes hospitals to be careful about whom they admit, how long they allow patients to stay, and what procedures are performed while patients are hospitalized.

Professional review organizations first concentrated on care delivered in hospitals because that was Medicare's emphasis for peer review. Private sector insurance companies expanded the peer review process into other areas, such as outpatient and community-based services. In addition, **managed care organizations (MCOs)** developed a peer review process. The National Committee for Quality Assurance

(NCQA) developed a set of quality measurements (HEDIS) based on clinical outcomes and patient satisfaction (Thompson, Bost, Ahmed, et al., 1998). What started as a voluntary annual review process became a required protocol for Medicare, Medicaid, and private insurance reimbursement contracts (McGlynn and Adams, 2001).

Diagnosis-Related Groups (DRGs)

Diagnosis-related groups (DRGs) were developed as part of the reform of Medicare payments into a prospective payment system. They place diagnoses with similar resource consumptions and length-of-stay patterns into a single category. Diseases are grouped into 495 DRGs, or categories, for reimbursement purposes. For each DRG, the Medicare system has predetermined a fair price for hospital services based on averages. This represents the amount the hospital is paid by Medicare to treat patients in that particular DRG. If the hospital's costs exceed the pre-established reimbursement rate, it loses money. If the hospital is able to treat the patient successfully for less than the established reimbursement rate, it can keep the excess.

Private insurers have benefited from this cost-containment initiative because they tend to establish private reimbursement rates at the same level the federal government uses for reimbursing hospitals for Medicare DRGs.

Block Grants

Combined with the enactment of DRGs and prospective payment, federal reform efforts in the 1980s included block grants to states. Block grants changed the funding mechanism the federal government employed to supply monies for combined federal-state programs. Instead of sharing the expense of a program, such as matching a state's expenditures on Medicaid, the block grant program gave the state a set amount of money, depending on several factors, including caseload. The state government then decided how to spend the federal and state dollars on behalf of Medicaid patients.

Since inception, block grants have reduced the proportion of health program costs paid by the federal government, while the states' shares have increased. At the same time, states have been mandated by federal requirements to provide specific health services to Medicaid patients, such as poor children and the elderly. Block grants have dramatically increased the number of dollars state budgets have been required to expend on health care, thereby forcing either tax increases or reductions in other state-funded programs (Black and Kominski, 2001).

Reform proposals in the mid-1990s brought further reductions in federal block grants and frequent proposals to lower federal standards for mandated care, such as in nursing homes. There are added concerns for the Medicaid program. Since 2001, most states have experienced budget crises due to reduced tax revenues caused by the economic downturn. This adds to the ever-present strain on the states' abilities to fund the Medicaid program (Patel and Rushefsky, 1999; Gold and Mittler, 2000). Concerned health professionals believe that increased state budget constraints will leave the poor, especially children and the elderly, at greater risk for reduced access to care and lower quality of care.

Continued Expansion of Managed Care

Private insurers and employers have increasingly relied on the managed care concept to lower their health care costs. By 2001, managed care had become the largest provider of health care in the United States. Over 100 million Americans were enrolled either in private or public sector managed care programs (Statistical Abstracts of the United States, 2002). Managed care programs limit consumers' choices of treatment options or provider of care (or both) but are not intended to reduce quality of care. As reviewed in Chapter 14, they include **health maintenance organizations (HMOs), preferred provider organizations (PPOs), point-of-service (POS)** providers, and **health care networks**. Box 16-4 provides descriptions of various types of managed care organizations.

Federal attempts at health care reform, although unsuccessful, spurred the reliance on managed care in employer-provided health plans and the formation of large health networks. Business interests, determined to survive in the changing health care market, merged and consolidated assets into larger systems. For example, the Henry Ford Health System, a large nonprofit organization in Michigan, offers a comprehensive package of services including preventive services, primary care, specialty care, acute care, and long-term care. This system has purchased smaller health care systems and now manages health care for over 600,000 lives (Flasch, 2001). Coventry Health Care, a large for-profit company, recently acquired two smaller HMOs, Mid-America and New Alliance (Benko, 2002; Insurance Advocate, 2002). The company acquired 180,000 new enrollees in these purchases and now serves a total membership of 580,000.

Although the private sector initiated managed care, the public sector soon followed. The Medicare program has allowed seniors to use managed care organizations for some time and in 1998 unveiled several new health care options for seniors with a managed care emphasis. Federal legislation allowed states to pilot the use of managed care in the Medicaid program, and legislation in 1997 expanded that use to most of the clients in Medicaid programs. These two initiatives are discussed in detail in the next section.

RECENT LEGISLATIVE EFFORTS IN HEALTH CARE REFORM

Although the Clintons' plan for wholesale health care reform was rejected in 1993, several pieces of federal legislation designed to improve consumer access to health care services and reduce the federal share of health care costs were subsequently enacted. Two important measures are reviewed here briefly.

Health Insurance Portability and Accountability Act (HIPAA)

The **Health Insurance Portability and Accountability Act (HIPAA)** of 1996, administered by the Centers for Medicare and Medicaid Services, was designed to protect health insurance coverage for workers and their families when they change or lose their jobs. Its provisions placed new restrictions on insurance companies, including the following:

- Portability of health insurance for people who change jobs must be guaranteed.
- Exclusions for preexisting conditions are limited.

Box 16-4 Types of Managed Care Organizations

Health Maintenance Organizations

Networks or groups of providers who agree to provide certain basic health care services for a single predetermined yearly fee, called a **capitation** fee, constitute a health maintenance organization (HMO). The voluntarily enrolled participants in HMOs pay the same amount regardless of the amount and kind of services they actually receive. Health maintenance organizations have an incentive to promote health and prevent illness in the enrolled participants. They benefit financially when their patients stay well, because they receive the same fee whether patients use services or not.

Preferred Provider Organizations

Groups of physicians or institutions who contract with insurance companies to provide services at discounted prices characterize preferred provider organizations (PPO). Policy holders are provided a list of preferred providers from which to choose. If they choose to use providers not on the list, they usually must pay a larger share of the costs of care. Insurers save money through PPOs because services are provided at discounted rates.

Point-of-Service Organizations

A hybrid of the PPO concept, these groups have a provider network of physicians. The consumer selects a primary care physician who acts as a **gatekeeper** and makes decisions about clients' needs for specific health services and referrals. Consumers may seek care from other sources within or outside the provider network but may incur additional costs, unless they have the express permission of the primary care physician. Some plans do not pay for services not approved by the primary physician. Some may even pay physicians bonuses for reducing the number of services used by their patients. Insurers save money through providers by discounted services, reducing services, and eliminating unnecessary specialist referrals.

Health Care Networks

A corporation with a consolidated set of facilities and services intended to provide comprehensive health care to its consumers is a health care network. This is a private health care system. Referrals for almost all services are made within the network. Managed care and other cost-containment efforts are a significant part of any health network operation. A well-developed network* includes the following components:

- A major hospital
- Several small hospitals
- A long-term care facility
- A rehabilitation center
- A home health care agency
- A subacute center

*From Nornhold: What networks mean to you, *Nursing 95,* 25(1):49-50, 1995.

- Access to health insurance coverage for small employers and their employees is improved.

Although the act did limit insurers' use of "preexisting conditions" as justification for denying health insurance coverage to new workers who were covered in their previous jobs (Gabel, Jensen, and Hawkins, 2003), this legislation has had limited impact in the other areas addressed. The bill did not require employers to offer health insurance, and few small employers added coverage as a result of this legislation. Portability applied only to workers who moved from one job to another. If the new employer had an insurance plan, the new worker was covered immediately, eliminating waiting periods. If the employer did not offer insurance, the employee was forced to purchase an individual plan or do without. The bill did nothing to control the costs of individual plans. These plans can cost from $2,600 to $5,100 annually, with family plans ranging from $6,200 to $11,800. These prices make it difficult for most consumers to purchase individual coverage (Government Accounting Office, 1997, 1998). A recent ad for Kaiser Permanente, one of the lower-cost insurers, advertised a premium of $6480/year for a family of 3 or more whose oldest member was 35 to 39 years old. Even this is out of reach for many families.

As you will see in the discussion of uninsured Americans to follow, Congress' well-intentioned HIPAA has not stemmed the rising tide of the uninsured in this country.

Patient confidentiality

An additional provision of HIPAA required health care providers to exercise increased vigilance ensuring confidentiality of patient records. Although the legislation was passed in 1996, the confidentiality portion of the law did not take effect until April 2003 in order to allow providers time to prepare new privacy policies and procedures. Privacy regulations define who should have access to patient records. HIPAA requires providers to list the measures they take to ensure records remain inaccessible to anyone without authorized access. This regulation does nothing to prevent the sharing of health information among various departments and companies, who provide care, nor does it prevent the sharing of information by health insurance companies.

HIPAA's provisions for security and privacy of health data is discussed further in Chapter 20.

Balanced Budget Act (BBA) of 1997

A major piece of legislation, the Balanced Budget Act (BBA) of 1997, was enacted in hopes of saving $115 billion dollars over 5 years (Wilensky and Newhouse, 1999). It concentrated on Medicare reforms, although it did address several other issues. Among other features, the BBA:

- Provided a Medicare+Choice (Part C) program with new optional features, including a Medicare PPO, private contracts with physicians (outside Medicare regulations), medical savings accounts, and provider-sponsored organizations (PSO), a new hybrid form of managed care.
- Expanded the prospective payment system to include hospital outpatient, home care, and skilled nursing facilities.

- Adjusted capitation rates to reduce geographic variations.
- Shifted home visits from Medicare Part A to Medicare Part B.
- Funded new preventive measures.
- Established the Children's Health Insurance Program to increase access to health care for uninsured children.

Many of the reforms dictated by BBA were not operational until 1998 and 1999. They caused considerable turmoil in home care, skilled nursing facilities, and outpatient care, as well as with Medicare patients needing home care, who had to bear greater out-of-pocket expenses. Some nursing homes went out of business (Sultz and Young, 2001). Between 1995 and 1997, the number of nursing homes declined by 1500. By 1999, however, nursing home numbers had returned to their previous levels (Statistical Abstracts of the United States, 2002).

Children's Health Insurance Program (CHIP)

Part of the Balanced Budget Act of 1997, the Children's Health Insurance Program provided federal funds to states in an effort to increase health care services to at-risk children not previously covered by public or private health insurance. The program is believed to be responsible for part of the decline in the reported number of children living in poverty. From 1998 to 2001, the number of at-risk and uninsured children dropped from 11 million to 8.5 million (Statistical Abstract of the United States, 2002).

The Children's Health Insurance Program (CHIP or SCHIP) started as a 5-year pilot program with $24 billion in federal grants administered by the states. States could enroll at-risk children in Medicaid or establish a new health program. CHIP has resulted in increased health care access for children. In 2002 it provided care to 3.7 million children, at a cost of $2.8 billion dollars (Statistical Abstract of the United States, 2002; Smith and Rousseau, 2003). It is too early for a complete evaluation of CHIP, but preliminary data suggest enrollment efforts have not been vigorous enough to enroll many qualified children (Sultz and Young, 2001). A major concern is the funding mechanism and time limit set by the legislation. After the 5-year pilot funding ended, Congress continued the program indefinitely. Several questions remain unanswered—for example, "What will happen if Congress decides to stop federal funding?" and "Will the states be left with the decision to cover all costs or discontinue CHIPs?"

In summary, the full impact of these initiatives on consumers and providers of health care has not yet been determined. There is some concern that the BBA will merely shift the cost of services from the federal government to individual consumers, health care businesses, and state governments rather than actually saving dollars. The shifting of costs is illustrated in the accompanying Case Study.

CURRENT ISSUES OF CONCERN

Despite public sector efforts to improve health care access, a substantial group of people remain at risk. These individuals either have no health insurance or are in danger of losing employer-provided health coverage.

case study

The Changing Face of Health Care Finance—One Person's Story

Situation

- Mrs. Martin is an 80-year-old widow who lives alone. She has just returned home from a skilled nursing home, where she was transferred after her hospitalization and treatment for a fractured hip. She is hypertensive and diabetic and takes oral medications for these conditions, including a beta blocker. As the home health nurse, you visit Mrs. Martin to determine how she is adjusting.

Assessment

- Mrs. Martin is able to ambulate and perform all activities of daily living without difficulty.
- She is very upset, having just received notice that her Medicare health maintenance organization (HMO) will no longer cover her.
- She does not know what to do because she is on a fixed income, consisting of social security benefits of $600 per month ($8,388 per year), which is the average widow's social security benefit.
- Although Mrs. Martin changed to the current HMO because it included a prescription drug benefit and reduced her insurance paperwork, she is willing to change again to another HMO.
- Her prescription drugs will cost $125 per month ($1,500 per year) if she must pay out of pocket for them.
- Mrs. Martin's daughter lives in the area, but she is not financially able to assist with her mother's expenses.

Continued Assessment

After you leave Mrs. Martin's home, you investigate further and discover that no other HMO is willing to enroll her, and therefore, she will have to return to the basic Medicare program.

- She will need Medigap insurance to cover her Medicare deductibles and copayments.
- Her out-of-pocket expenses for basic health care costs, even if she has no other medical emergencies or hospitalizations, will be as follows: Medicare part A is free but requires a deductible per hospitalization or skilled nursing facility stay. Medicare part B equals $646 in yearly premiums, as well as copayments for service. Note: Premiums are expected to increase to $1,172 by 2006; prescription drugs are $1,500 annually; and Medigap policy costs $1,461* annually. The total is $3,607, or 43 percent of her total annual income.

  Mrs. Martin will not be able to pay this much for health care because she has to pay for food, clothing, and shelter. Even without the Medigap insurance, the cost would be 26 percent of her total annual income, and she would have no coverage for her copayments and deductibles if she has another sustained health care need.

Plan of Care

Your employer has restricted you from helping Mrs. Martin with her financial issues because they are not considered nursing services and the agency cannot bill Medicare for them. So you problem-solve with her during your regular follow-up visits for the hip fracture and medication assessments and establish a plan. You arrange to meet with Mrs. Martin's daughter and validate that she is unable to assist her mother financially. Then enlist her help in completing the following activities:

- Mrs. Martin must apply to Medicaid for assistance to low-income Medicare patients. If she is eligible, she will not need to purchase Medigap insurance. This will require much paperwork and waiting for approvals.
- Mrs. Martin should investigate the possibility that a pharmaceutical company might assist her in obtaining her medications at low or no cost. This will require many phone calls and more paperwork. As soon as they become available, she should apply for a drug discount card provided for in the Medicare Modernization Act of 2003.
- Mrs. Martin should contact her local Office on Aging. This agency may be able to provide additional financial assistance, some social work support to negotiate the Medicaid system, and transportation to various offices as needed.

---

*American Association of Retired Persons' Plan C rates.

Continuing Crisis: Uninsured Americans

The number of uninsured Americans continues to grow at an alarming rate. In 2002, an estimated 43.6 million adults and children, more than 1 in 7 Americans, had no health insurance (U.S. Census Bureau, 2003). When the temporarily uninsured are added to the count, the number of persons without health insurance is even greater. Between 1993 and 1996, 71.5 million Americans, or one of every 3.3 citizens, was uninsured for some or all of that period (Bennefield, 1998). The poor, near poor, foreign-born, and young adults (between 18 and 24) are in greatest danger of having no health insurance.

Because most nonelderly Americans are insured by job-related policies, they are at risk if they change or lose their jobs or if their employer chooses not to offer health insurance benefits. It is myth that people do not have health insurance because they do not work. Some uninsured people do not work, but most have part-time or full-time jobs. Feder and colleagues (2001) report that 72 percent of the uninsured are employed or are family members of employed individuals. Fifty-one percent of all poor workers are uninsured (U.S. Census Bureau, 2002). Ironically, poor workers are less likely to be insured than poor nonworkers, perhaps because many poor nonworkers may be eligible for government-sponsored health care such as Medicaid. Figure 16-3 depicts the typical characteristics of the uninsured in 2001 by age, income, and work status.

In addition to the uninsured, many Americans are *underinsured* because their insurance plan either requires unaffordable out-of-pocket expenses or limits coverage for catastrophic illnesses. There are no recent estimates, but in 1995 the size of this at-risk group was estimated at around 29 million people (Short and Banthin, 1995).

The number of uninsured Americans is expected to continue to rise. This should be a concern for all, because being uninsured affects the health and well-being of a major segment of our population. Studies have revealed major disparities in access to care between people with health insurance and those without. According to a 2003 Kaiser Foundation health insurance survey, 47 percent of the uninsured reported postponing care because of cost while 35 percent decided to forego care altogether. Not filling a prescription because of cost was reported by 37 percent of the uninsured. In addition, 36 percent of uninsured reported problems paying medical bills, and 23 percent had been contacted by collection agencies about their medical bills (Kaiser Foundation, 2003).

Serious consequences can arise for people who forgo care. Nearly 60 percent of uninsured respondents to the Kaiser Foundation survey reported suffering a painful temporary disability as a result of not getting care while 19 percent reported long-term disability. The Kaiser Commission on Medicaid and the Uninsured reviewed numerous population and research studies before making their report to Congress in October 2003. Their review of research by Hadley (2003) revealed that the uninsured:

- Use fewer preventive and screening services.
- Are sicker when diagnosed.
- Receive fewer therapeutic services.

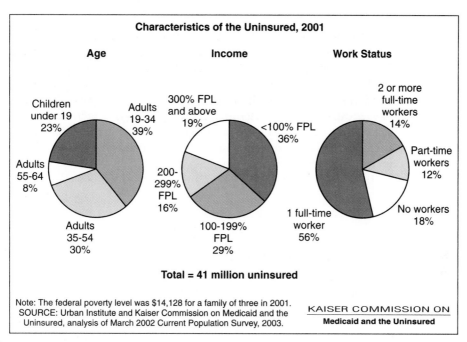

Figure 16-3
Characteristics of the uninsured, 2001. (From Health challenges facing the nation: statement before the Joint Economic Committee United States Congress, October 1, 2003. Reprinted with permission of the Kaiser Family Foundation, The Kaiser Commission on Medicaid and the Uninsured.)

- Have poorer health outcomes (higher mortality and disability rates).
- Have lower annual earnings because of poorer health.

The Commission concluded that "health insurance coverage remains one of the nation's most pressing and persistent health care challenges," and "... addressing our growing uninsured population ought to be among the nation's highest priorities" (Rowland, 2003, pp. 1, 17). The Commission's comprehensive review can be found online *(www.kff.org/content/2003/4144).*

Reduction or Elimination of Employer-Provided Health Insurance

A major reason for the growth of the uninsured population is change in employer-provided health insurance. Because of increased costs, some employers have left the system and insured their own employees (called **self-insurance**), scaled back or eliminated health benefits, limited the employees' choice of insurance plans, or passed more of the costs of insurance on to employees.

Employers led the charge to managed care, and now many employers limit their health insurance plan to managed care options. At the same time employers have increased the employee share of premium costs, making health insurance unaffordable to many workers. As health care costs increase, health insurance programs sponsored by employers continue to decline.

In 1979, 15.1 percent of workers did not have health insurance; by 2002, the number had risen to 38 percent (Kronich and Gilmer, 1999). Smaller firms, nonunionized work places, and service industries were more likely than other employers not to provide insurance. In 2002, only 39 percent of workers in firms with under 10 employees had employer-based health coverage, whereas 69 percent of workers in firms with at least 1,000 employees had health insurance (Kaiser/HRET, 2002).

Even when small business owners wish to provide their employees with health benefits, they can be victimized by sham insurance companies selling bogus insurance policies. News Note 1 describes this recurring type of fraud and its impact on small businesses and their employees.

news note 1

No Protection: Sham Health Insurance Is on the Rise, Leaving People With Big Bills They Thought Were Covered

Skyrocketing health care insurance premiums over the past few years have led to a fast-rising number of sham companies selling bogus policies. These scams lure in mostly small businesses with the promise of low premiums and few sign-up requirements. The sham insurers go in, collect premiums, and even pay some small claims—then stop when claims get high, leaving the businesses' workers stuck with expensive hospital bills.

This proliferation of phony health insurers "is one of the largest, most vicious, and damaging insurance swindles of the last 10 years," said James Quiggle, senior executive with the Washington, D.C.–based Coalition Against Insurance Fraud. "Hundreds of thousands of people have been swindled (out of) tens of millions of dollars in premiums and unpaid medical bills that they have to pay out of their own pockets when their insurance plan suddenly disappears."

A recent study by the Commonwealth Fund, a New York–based private research foundation, found an unprecedented outbreak of unauthorized insurers selling fake health plans across the country.

The report looked at four such plans, which, combined, left nearly 100,000 people around the country with $85 million in unpaid medical bills. The total impact of the phony plans is bound to be much larger: in December, the U.S. Department of Labor reported that it had 107 civil and 19 criminal investigations open nationwide. Some estimates have found that as many as 500,000 people across the country have been affected.

One of the companies that drew investigators' attention was Nevada-based Employers Mutual LLC, which was shut down in February 2002 after collecting $14 million in premiums in 10 months. The company paid $3 million in claims, but some 22,000 policyholders were left with an estimated $4.5 million in unpaid bills, according to the Labor Department.

The plans, which offer premiums as much as 60 percent lower than conventional insurers, appear when the cost of health insurance soars.

n e w s **note 1—cont'd**

According to Commonwealth, the last time health scams were common was in the late 1980s. Back then, according to the General Accounting Office, unauthorized plans left some 400,000 patients with $123 million in unpaid medical bills. That's also the last period when skyrocketing health care costs hammered Americans.

Health insurance costs are rising again. Premiums jumped 13.9 percent this year, the third straight year of double-digit hikes, according to the Kaiser Family Foundation.

Small companies get lured in by the phony plans because they're least able to cope with rising premiums. Companies selling fake plans promise low premiums and few requirements for participation, making them attractive to employers who want to save money but still provide good health coverage.

Many times, after the scam insurer gets caught, its assets are frozen, leaving employers and their workers to seek restitution through the courts by going after agents who sold the plans, a process that can take years.

Modified from Maze J: No protection: sham health insurance is on the rise, leaving people with big bills they thought were covered, Charleston, SC, *The Post and Courier*, October 13, 16-17E, 2003.

Retirees at Risk for Loss of Health Insurance

In an effort to cut costs, employers are dropping health care coverage for their retirees. This is particularly burdensome for young retirees, those under age 65. They are not yet eligible for Medicare and must either pay for individual health coverage, often only available at very high costs, or go without coverage. Between 1993 and 1996, approximately 1 in every 10 retirees were dropped from their employer-provided plan (Government Accounting Office, 1998). A change in company ownership or company bankruptcy also place retirees are risk. In 2003, for example, Bethlehem Steel Corporation declared bankruptcy, leaving 90,000 retirees without health insurance (Sementes, 2003).

IMPACT OF MANAGED CARE ON HEALTH SERVICES

During the 1990s, the rapid growth of HMOs and related managed care organizations raised concerns that quality of care might suffer. Care decisions, formerly based on the needs of the patient, were increasingly influenced by business interests. Physicians, hospitals, and other providers were being forced to provide services for less. These conditions created shock waves in the health care industry, resulting in limits on choice and services, a drive to expand managed care to vulnerable populations, and physician gags and financial incentives to limit services. Each will be discussed below.

Limits on Choice and Services

Since the mid-1990s, many employers have limited employees' choice of health plans. Some managed care plans increased the cost (copayments or deductibles) to consumers who used out-of-plan providers and services. Some plans refused to pay any part of out-of-plan services.

Managed care plans set stricter limits than other health insurance plans on the types of services covered. Expensive new therapies, such as bone marrow transplants for breast cancer and costly treatments for rare conditions were often denied, as were referrals, especially outside the plan (Studdert and Gresenz, 2003; Murray and Henriques, 2003). Routine services, such as hospitalization after childbirth, were also cut. News Note 2 describes congressional reaction to such cuts.

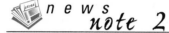

news note 2

Getting Tough on Drive-Through Delivery

Government intervention is necessary to stop insurers from forcing mothers and newborns from the hospital too soon after delivery, Kathryn Moore, director of government relations for the American College of Obstetricians and Gynecologists, said December 13 [1995].

Moore spoke at a panel discussion on the issue at a National Conference of State Legislatures meeting in Washington.

About half of the states have introduced or passed maternity-stay legislation since Maryland adopted the first such law earlier this year, Moore said. The trend is a reaction to so-called "drive-through" deliveries—a growing insurer practice of limiting maternity-stay coverage to 24 hours or less after delivery. The obstetrician/gynecologist group and the American Academy of Pediatrics recommend 48-hour stays following a normal vaginal delivery and 96 hours for a cesarean section.

"We have a situation of insurers limiting consumers' coverage, of insurers pressuring doctors, ignoring medical guidelines and not producing any conclusive data that their practice is safe," Moore said.

Getting Tough

In some cases, insurers are overruling physicians' decisions to keep women in the hospital longer than their coverage allows, she said. Some insurers also threaten to cut physicians from the insurance panel unless they release women and infants early, she added.

State maternity-stay laws are a reaction to market forces' inability to change insurer practices, Moore said. "Given all of these factors, government intervention is necessary," she said.

E. Neil Trautman, manager for health care policy for the U.S. Chamber of Commerce, disagreed. "If we encourage the marketplace to respond to

n e w s
note 2—cont'd   ■

consumer demands, we can do better," he said. The Chamber opposes insurance-benefit mandates, Trautman said. Each mandate makes insurance less affordable and could price health coverage out of some Americans' reach, he added.

Supporters of maternity-stay legislation maintain that its price would be low. According to Colleen Meiman, legislative assistant to Sen. Bill Bradley (D-NJ), maternity-stay legislation would only add $1.13 a year to insurance premiums. Bradley, along with Sen. Nancy Kassebaum (R-KS), sponsors federal maternity-stay legislation currently before Congress. Bradley is looking for a measure to attach the legislation to a vote. Kassebaum said she prefers to hold hearings on the measure first and then bring it before the Senate next year.

Like the Bradley/Kassebaum bill, most maternity-stay legislation requires that insurers follow national guidelines. Many measures, including the federal proposal, permit early discharges if the physician and woman approve, and if follow-up care is provided.

Maryland has had trouble enforcing its new law, which took effect October 1, 1995. Insurers are forcing doctors to discharge women early with follow-up care, rather than giving physicians and women a choice, said Maryland Delegate Marilyn Goldwater (D-Bethesda). State lawmakers are trying to close that loophole, she said.

Reprinted from Ashton G: Getting tough on drive-through delivery, *AHA News* 31(50):3, 1995. Copyright 1995, by Health Forum, Inc.

As managed care became widespread, concern also developed about managed care practices toward patients with psychiatric illnesses, as denials and limits on coverage for chronic problems became routine (Salkever, Shinogle, and Goldman, 1999; Wang, Demler, and Kessler, 2002).

Drive to Expand Managed Care to Vulnerable Populations

Federal and state initiatives to reduce costs have been designed to enroll large segments of the Medicare and Medicaid populations in managed care health plans. Critics voiced concern that these two vulnerable populations, who traditionally had poorer health status than employed adults, would not be well served by managed care. Pilot programs with Medicare HMOs reported that seniors were less satisfied and disenrolled more frequently than consumers covered by employer-provided managed plans (Zarabozo, 2002).

States experimenting with using managed care to control Medicaid expenses reported that some plans practiced fraud and misrepresentation in efforts to enroll Medicaid patients by overstating available benefits and services. In addition to abuses, there was some evidence that Medicaid patients had difficulty negotiating the gatekeeping process to access services. Patients often needed to call several times to succeed in getting an appointment or were given appointments at geographically inaccessible sites (Gold and Mittler, 2000).

By the late 1990s, many states required Medicaid patients to be enrolled in managed care. For Medicare clients, however, managed care was still optional. Many seniors liked the managed care option because prescription drugs were included and there was little or no paperwork associated with filing health insurance claims. By 2002 there were 5.5 million Medicare clients and around 22 million Medicaid clients in managed care programs (Hileman, Moroz, Wrightson, et al., 2002; Hurley and Draper, 2002).

At the end of the 1990s, a number of managed care organizations were reconsidering their participation in Medicare and Medicaid. Some, for example, Aetna/U.S. HealthCare, Humana, and Kaiser Permanente disenrolled Medicare clients in certain geographic areas. An estimated 2.3 million Medicare patients were involuntarily dropped from managed care between 1998 and 2002 because of cost (Pizer and Frakt, 2002).

In the meantime, managed care organizations with Medicaid clients complained of financial losses, slowed or eliminated their efforts to enroll Medicaid patients, and lobbied state and federal governments to increase capitation fees (McCue, Hurley, Draper, et al., 1999). Some of the financial difficulties experienced by managed care organizations with Medicaid and Medicare patients result from their increased usage rates. These patients need more medical services because of the health risks associated with poverty, near poverty, or advancing age.

Physician Financial Incentives to Limit Services

Managed care has made efforts to regulate information supplied to patients by their physicians. Physicians were sometimes discouraged or forbidden by their managed care contracts to mention treatment options that were expensive or not covered by a patient's managed care plan (Larson, 1996). These "gag" rules have been voluntarily discontinued because of intense negative publicity or, in some cases, by state regulation. Other influences to limit service persist.

Some managed care plans offered physicians bonuses for limiting services and referrals to other health care providers. Physicians were offered bonuses if they were able to reduce hospital stays, limit emergency department use, limit use of costly prescription drugs, and reduce referrals to specialists (Hillman, Pauly, Escarce, et al., 1999; Schweitzer and Comanor, 2001). Such bonuses placed physicians in conflict between the best interests of patients and their own economic best interests. Physicians who called attention to bonus plans or exceeded average costs for services could be terminated by the plans. These practices evoked concern by organized medicine, organized nursing, consumer groups, and the U.S. Congress.

Costs of Prescription Drugs

The rising cost of prescription medication is a concern, especially for seniors. The elderly use more prescription drugs than any other segment of the population. Before 2004, Medicare did not routinely pay anything for medications. Depending on a senior's financial situation, the cost of drugs can consume up to 40 percent of their income, even with a discount drugcard (Sambamoorthi, Shea, and Crystal, 2003).

Seniors have resorted to importing drugs from other countries, taking over-the-border bus trips to import medications, using less medicine than prescribed, or discontinuing medication altogether. One quarter of seniors report skipping doses so that medicine lasts longer (Safran, Newman, Schoen, et al., 2002).

Even with the passage of the Medicare Prescription Drug Improvement and Modernization Act in late 2003, significant relief from burdensome medication costs will not occur until the year 2006 or later.

Malpractice Costs and the Impact on Access to Care

Physicians and hospitals have experienced dramatic increases in the cost of malpractice insurance. In Florida, for example, malpractice insurance costs general surgeons an average of $174,368, and obstetricians/gynecologists pay $201,736 annually (Glabman, 2003). There is some concern these increases will limit access to health care services as physicians limit or discontinue practicing as a result of the financial burden of insurance.

The Government Accounting Office (GAO) conducted a study (2003) in response to access concerns. They measured the impact of rising malpractice costs on access in the nine states most affected. The GAO found no widespread access problems. It did find limited sporadic access problems in some rural and isolated communities. Unless the malpractice crisis becomes more widespread or severe, it appears malpractice costs will not endanger access to services for most people. Meanwhile, there is discussion of Congressional action on tort reform, which would limit the amounts juries could award in medical malpractice cases. This is vigorously opposed by consumer advocacy groups and trial attorneys' associations.

ECONOMICS OF NURSING CARE

Historically, nurses were unconcerned with the cost of care, believing all patients were entitled to high-quality nursing care regardless of ability to pay. Until fairly recently, few efforts were made to determine the actual cost of nursing care. The average hospital bill included the cost of nursing services in the general category of "room rate," just as housekeeping services are included in the room rate. In the past, the hospital census (number of patients) was used to determine the number of nurses needed. This worked fairly well when payment was retrospective. With the advent of prospective payment, however, it was imperative for hospitals to determine their staffing needs more efficiently.

It has long been recognized that different patients require different amounts of nursing time, depending in large part on how sick they are. The **patient classification system (PCS)** was developed to identify patients' needs for nursing care in quantitative terms in order to help hospitals determine the need for nursing resources. Patient classification systems have been developed that depend on patient **acuity,** or degree of illness, and the resulting amount and complexity of nursing care required.

Initiatives called *costing nursing services* have been used to determine precisely the cost of nursing care. Not knowing the exact costs of nursing services limits nurses' ability to determine what high-quality nursing care costs and to calculate the number of hours of nursing care it takes to provide service for each DRG. Determining the best **skill mix**—that is, the ratio of registered nurses to licensed practical nurses and nursing assistants in each hospital unit—is also impaired when the cost of nursing care is unknown.

In the past, it was assumed that the cost of nurses was a major part of hospital expenses. During tough economic times, the first cost reduction efforts were therefore aimed at nursing. Studies in the mid-1980s found that nursing accounted for only 20 to 28 percent of the costs of hospitalization for two thirds of the DRGs examined (McKibben, 1985). Costing nursing services and developing standardized reimbursements based on costs were expected to enhance the ability of nurse managers to control nursing resources and negotiate for a fair share of hospital financial resources.

There is some concern, however, that costing nursing services may not be beneficial to nursing. Costing strategies may make nursing more vulnerable to labor substitution efforts as hospital administrators experience increasing pressure to reduce costs. Isolating nursing costs might also lead to efforts to devalue nursing services by reducing wages or impeding salary increases (salary compression). In fact, there is some evidence to suggest that managed care and other cost-containment efforts have had a direct negative impact on nurse staffing and salaries (Buerhaus and Staiger, 1999; Gordon, 2001). The debate continues.

Impact of Cost Containment on Nursing Care

When the drive to provide high-quality nursing care meets the constraints of cost containment head-on, something has to give. What nurses hope, as both providers and consumers of health care, is that quality will not suffer because of the emphasis on "the bottom line." To many, this is a forlorn hope. Yet the financial realities that affect the institutions in which 59 percent of nurses practice—hospitals—cannot be ignored. To stay in business, hospitals must make at least enough money to pay personnel, maintain buildings and equipment, and pay suppliers of goods and services. One cost-reduction strategy has been to reorganize and restructure the delivery of hospital nursing services, reduce nursing personnel, and substitute unlicensed assistive personnel for registered nurses (Sochalski, 2002).

For a time, employment of nurses in community health settings increased as cost-cutting measures reduced hospital-based employment opportunities. It was thought that more cost-effective nursing care services would be offered in community settings, such as home health. However in the past 5 years, the home care market has also demonstrated a reduced demand for nursing services. Managed care appears responsible for a significant portion of the reduced demand. In areas where managed care organizations are more concentrated, employment rates and wage scales for nurses are lower than in areas with fewer of these care models (Gordon, 2001; Sochalski, 2002). Medicare's expansion of prospective payment systems into community-based settings such as home care and skilled nursing facilities is likely to increase pressure to reduce costs and may also adversely affect nurse : patient ratios.

The leadership of the American Nurses Association (ANA) has been outspoken in their assertion that overzealous cost-containment efforts have led to lower quality hospital care. In 1996, the ANA president called on professional nurses to inform family members, friends, and acquaintances about the "eroding quality in acute care" (Betts, 1996, p. 4). The ANA's "Every Patient Deserves a Nurse" campaign was a concrete step taken by the professional organization to educate the public about these concerns. News Note 3 elaborates on the effects of overemphasizing cost

news note 3

Who's Taking Care of Mama?

The delivery of health care in America has changed a great deal. Unless you are very young, you probably remember doctors making house calls. We knew our doctors quite well and the nurses who worked with them. Those days are long gone, and with them, it's sad to say, is much of the trust that we reposed in our health care delivery system. Now, we must all ask who's taking care of mama when she goes to the hospital?

Nursing's Proud History

As a child, I dreamed of being a professional nurse. Caring for others who were not able to care for themselves was a calling for me as it has been for generations of nurses. There is simply no reward like that received for serving another human being who is depending upon you for their recovery or even their life.

Through the years, I have witnessed changes in our nursing profession that are both exciting for the professional nurse and essential for our patients. Nursing has made strides educationally and professionally that have brought it to the forefront of the national health care debate. Every day, there is more evidence that the professional nurse is the key to successful and cost-effective health care delivery.

Research shows that when there are more nurses in a health facility, there will be lower mortality rates, shorter lengths of stay, lower costs and fewer complications. In addition to boosting health outcomes, professional nurse staffing levels are tied closely to a hospital's ability to provide care in the least costly, most highly effective means possible.

Opportunities Stifled

Despite this, changes in the health care community are stifling the opportunities that the professional nurse brings to health care delivery. Many external and internal forces, ranging from political and economic to social, are driving the health care industry to make sweeping but not yet fully evaluated changes in how, where and by whom health services are delivered.

These forces have been escalating rapidly over the past few years and include a heightened scrutiny by consumers and insurers about rising costs, pressure to move services to less expensive environments, and embarrassing public health statistics. In addition, continually tightening federal reimbursement guidelines

Continued

for Medicare and Medicaid have spawned a myriad of managed care networks that have resulted in even more changes.

I am disappointed to say that these forces have culminated in an institutional mentality in hospitals that is driven much more by the bottom line than by health outcomes. Health care facilities, in what they perceive as a scramble to survive, are borrowing cost-containment strategies utilized by other industries. These strategies include "downsizing" or "right-sizing" the work force to cut labor costs, and then crosstraining or "multi-skilling" remaining workers to maximize their productivity. Facilities are merging, closing and forming networks to better utilize existing services and resources—all in an effort to self-regulate and limit external controls and, perhaps, public accountability.

Dangers of Change

Professional nurses are greatly concerned about the implications of these changes in health care. Highest on the list of concerns is the impact on patient safety and quality of care and the current lack of data collection and sophisticated quality measurements to quantify these concerns. Nurses are concerned about the "deskilling" of nursing, the fragmentation of comprehensive care into a series of tasks and the assignments of these tasks to unlicensed individuals. When a hospital staff is diluted to a staff mix of as few as 50 percent registered nurses, the facility is risking increased mortality. When the hospital assigns more and more administrative functions to professional nurses, patient care also will suffer.

Hospitals have now reached the point that, in too many cases, the personnel tending its patients' needs are neither qualified nor trained adequately to perform the duties assigned to them. They are instead unlicensed employees who, while dressed appropriately, are not professional nurses at all. In some hospitals, professional nurses are told not to wear any identification indicating they are registered nurses (RNs) so that patients will not know the difference between the professional staff and the unlicensed, untrained staff. That is simply shocking!

Yet, these are exactly the kinds of changes that we are witnessing today, and it could not come at a more critical time in our history—a time when there is an increasing growth of an aging patient population that dictates an increased, rather than decreased, nursing service.

Consumer Education

As professional nurses, we feel obligated to tell our friends, families and the public that hospital care must be sought and procured with apprehension and diligence. No patient should be admitted to hospital care without an informed and active advocate, whether a relative or friend. Health care in America has changed dramatically and the public must change with it, or change it. Until then, America's professional nurse must educate consumers by issuing the warning that it is critical to ask: "Who's taking care of mama?"

Reprinted with permission of Morris EA: Who's taking care of Mama? *Am Nurse* 28(1):4, 1996.

reductions in hospitals and other health care facilities from the viewpoint of a professional nurse.

Quality of care is expected to become a more important competitive feature among managed care and health network providers. Polls show that nurses are favorably regarded as care providers when compared with other health professionals. Eighty percent of Americans believe nurses do a good job, whereas only 65 percent believe doctors and hospitals do, and only 34 percent believe that managed care organizations are doing right by the consumer (Blendon, Brodie, Benson, et al., 1998). To the extent that the nursing profession can link quality of care with nursing care, the demand for nursing services will continue to flourish (Buerhaus, 1995).

A strong boost to nursing's contention that the number and mix of nurses in a hospital makes a difference in patient outcomes came with the April 2001 release of a U.S. Department of Health and Human Services study. Conducted by the Harvard University School of Public Health, the study, *Nurse Staffing and Patient Outcomes in Hospitals,* was based on 1997 data from over 5 million patients discharged from 799 hospitals in eleven states. The study found

> a strong and consistent relationship between nurse staffing and five outcomes in medical patients—urinary tract infection, pneumonia, shock, upper gastrointestinal bleeding, and length-of-stay. A higher number of registered nurses was associated with a 3 percent to 12 percent reduction in the rates of adverse outcomes, while higher staffing levels for all types of nurses was associated with a decrease in adverse outcomes from 2 percent to 25 percent (U.S. Department of Health and Human Services, 2001).

According to the study, "reductions in the rates of adverse outcomes reduce hospital costs as well as significant financial and psychological costs to patients and their families."

A 2003 study published in the *Journal of the American Medical Association (JAMA)* demonstrated that nurses' educational levels were correlated with surgical patient outcomes. This study is discussed further in Chapter 21.

COST CONTAINMENT AND QUALITY MANAGEMENT

Most people agree that there is potential for disaster if cost reduction is the only outcome that matters in the health care system. The challenge is to balance the cost-effectiveness and quality of patient care. Concern for maintaining high-quality services in the face of cost constraints has led to the development of a health care initiative called **quality management.** As discussed in Chapter 13, this field is growing and changing rapidly and creating change within hospitals and other health care settings. The Interview on p. 444 with two nurses involved in quality management gives insights into the complexities and satisfactions of participation in quality management initiatives (Robertson, 1999; Alexander, 1999).

HEALTH CARE REFORM AND NATIONAL HEALTH INSURANCE

In 2003, the United States and South Africa were the only two industrialized nations not providing universal access to health care to all citizens. Despite the fact that 2002

At the time of this interview, JoAnn Alexander, MSN, RN, was chief operations officer, and Charlene Robertson, MSN, RN, was chief nursing officer, at a private not-for-profit hospital in a midsized city in the southeastern United States. Although the interview took place several years ago, it illustrates how quality improvement initiatives can maintain or even improve the quality of care while improving cost-effectiveness.

Interviewer: Tell me a little about the hospital—its size, services, and the number of nurses employed there.

Robertson: This is a 365-bed hospital. We have all services, including obstetrics, pediatrics, and behavioral health. There are 596 members on the nursing staff, which includes 464 RNs [registered nurses], 38 LPNs [licensed practical nurses], and 94 nursing assistants.

Interviewer: What specific cost-containment programs have been started here in the past few years that have influenced nursing care?

Robertson: Specific cost-containment programs began in 1992 with intensive education of physicians, nurses, and support staff on continuous quality improvement strategies, managed care strategies, and cost containment. The implementation of continuous quality improvement enhanced several multidisciplinary clinical groups to achieve good outcomes. For example:

- The pneumonia group reduced length of stay by 4 days and cost per discharge.
- A multidisciplinary CareTrac [clinical pathway] tool was implemented house-wide with physician support.
- A short-stay, one-stop unit for PTCA [percutaneous transluminal coronary angioplasty] patients was implemented. Patient care was also redesigned with a combination of an RN and cardiac tech who make up a "care pair." This approach has reduced cost by $1,400 per case, with high patient and physician satisfaction.

Interviewer: What has been done to relieve nurses of nonnursing tasks?

Robertson: Improvement in documentation comes immediately to mind, with charting by exception, bedside charting, computerized Kardexes and MAR, and the implementation of CareTracs, which has reduced redundant documentation. Other strategies include the formation of care pairs in the cardiac short-stay unit, cross-training in the operative suite, and implementation of the Pyxis system.

Interviewer: What is the goal of quality management?

Alexander: The focus of continuous quality improvement is to view our hospital system from our patient, physician, and family perspective. Multidisciplinary cross-functional teams identify barriers to service and systematically implement change using the PDCA [plan, do, check, and act] approach.

Interviewer: Who participates in quality management?

Alexander: All members of the health care team, including physicians, nurses, and support and clinical services associates participate in quality management. The cross-functional team allows all persons to have an active role. Customer service is everyone's responsibility.

interv i e w *with JoAnn Alexander, MSN, RN, and*
Charlene Robertson, MSN, RN—cont'd

Interviewer: How are nurses involved in quality management?

Robertson: About 5 years ago, we reorganized nursing and decentralized certain functions. The director of each unit has the responsibility of quality management and continuous quality improvement activities for that unit. When our hospital-wide and unit-specific quality monitoring programs reveal a problem, an action plan is developed either on the unit or by the nursing council. For example, the response on a hospital-wide patient satisfaction survey showed that patients felt that the call lights were not being responded to in a timely manner for pain medication or other needs. The nursing staff was apprised of this concern and, as a means of addressing this concern, a nurse pager system was implemented. Patient care needs are communicated immediately. The pager dials in directly to the nurse who provides that care. This response is monitored internally by placing a phone call to the patient after discharge, and the unit secretary completes periodic monitoring of actual time frames of nurse response to patient call lights. By increasing the sensitivity of the patient's need for immediate call-light response and by implementing the new pager system, the patient satisfaction in this area has greatly increased.

The hospital is organized around a service line structure. The chief nursing officer is accountable for nursing wherever nursing is practiced. Nursing leads some of the cross-functional teams and was involved with the development of the CareTracs. Most of the care managers are nurses who manage patients daily through the system and are starting to establish a method to manage across the continuum.

Interviewer: How does quality management affect the way nursing care is provided?

Alexander: The CareTracs eliminate the need for nurses to be mind readers of other disciplines involved in the care of the patient. It allows better dialogue with the disciplines and the patient. It makes the truly collaborative model easier to live with on a daily basis. It also gives nurses more objective outcome data to measure the effectiveness of their care.

Interviewer: What would you say about cost containment and quality management to students of professional nursing around the United States?

Alexander: It is important for nurses to adopt a philosophy of rather than finding fault, find a remedy. The public will not accept a continued escalation in cost, and nurses are in a good position to broaden their skills outside of the hospital and be primary care providers. I believe that the cross-functional team is the model that will provide productivity with time. Be a risk taker and have the initiative to try something different and remember that cost and quality can be measured.

Courtesy JoAnn Alexander and Charlene Robertson.

health care expenditures in this country averaged $5,035 per person, U.S. infant mortality ranked 24 of 29 industrialized countries. This low ranking indicates that our infant mortality rate was higher than that of many countries with far fewer national resources (Andersen and Pouiller, 2001; Levit, Smith, Cowan, et al., 2003). Two thirds of inner-city children under 4 years of age did not have the full series of immunizations that could protect them from preventable childhood diseases. There was no established minimum set of health services available to the entire population, and access to health care was not universal.

Concerns about health care in the United States are not new. In the 1992 presidential campaign, candidates in both political parties, as well as nonpartisan groups, advocated some type of health care reform. These groups included nursing organizations, the American Association of Retired Persons, labor unions, the American College of Physicians, the National Leadership Coalition for Health Care Reform, and members of the U.S. Congress. Most of these groups put forward specific plans for reform, including "Nursing's Agenda for Health Care Reform," mentioned in Chapter 4. Despite widespread public support for reform, the effort failed. Lack of legislation on health care reform was aided by powerful interest groups such as the pharmaceutical, health insurance, and health equipment industries, as well as the American Medical Association and the American Hospital Association.

Today, concerns about access to health care, the quality of care, and limits on consumer choice in managed care have fueled a new debate about health care in this country. There is the question about what to do with the millions of people who have no insurance and limited access to health care. In addition, growing concern exists about consumer choice restrictions in MCOs. A 2002 Harris Poll found 38% of respondents think health insurance companies do a bad job, and 45% think managed care companies do not serve patients well (Harris, 2002). A Patient's Bill of Rights has stalled in Congress every year since 1997. Many of its most vocal opponents are the same groups who opposed President Clinton's plan for health care reform.

In the present political climate, it seems unlikely that a systematic and comprehensive reform of the entire health care system is possible. Instead, we can expect to see incremental efforts to address specific issues of concern. Box 16-5 identifies some of the proposals under consideration in the year 2000 and beyond. Most experts agree that reform efforts must be projected to reduce, or at least not increase, the cost of health care if they are to be supported by Congress.

Guidelines for Evaluating Reform Proposals

Despite wide-ranging differences of opinion about the specifics of health care reform proposals, there are areas of general agreement. Some form of health care reform will ultimately be enacted. Some general questions to ask in evaluating reform proposals are the following:

1. Is there a uniform minimum set of benefits for all citizens, otherwise known as **universal care?**
2. Are coverage and benefits continuous and not dependent on where people live or work?
3. Are there mechanisms for controlling costs, especially administrative expenses?
4. Are provisions made for care to be provided by the most cost-effective personnel, taking quality issues and patient outcomes into consideration?

Employer-Provided Health Insurance

- Employers will be required to provide health insurance for all employees, including part-time workers (mandated insurance coverage).
- Employees might be given an allowance (a medical savings account, or MSA) and expected to purchase their own insurance. (Hawaii is the only state currently requiring health insurance coverage for all employees.)

Universal Health Insurance

- Every American will be covered by health insurance.
- Government will expand health insurance funding for all vulnerable populations, including those currently not covered.
- Employees will be covered by employer-provided plans.

Catastrophic Limits

- Catastrophic coverage will be part of every health insurance plan, and lifetime limits on costs of care will be increased or limits eliminated altogether.

Medicare

- Medicare payments for services will continue to decline.
- Copayments or deductibles will rise.
- Increased pressure to enroll all Medicare recipients in managed care plans is likely.
- Well-off seniors may be required to pay more in premiums than those who are less affluent. This is known as *means testing*.
- *Expansion to Medicare D, which will provide prescription drug coverage.
- *Interim Prescription Discount Program to provide seniors with discount cards for lower-priced drugs while waiting for Medicare D to take effect.
- Expand enrollment to young (under 65) retirees.

Medicaid

- Expansion of states requiring managed care enrollment for Medicaid recipients will occur.
- Changes in the standard set of health services paid for by the program will occur, with most likely reductions in services likely.
- Reduction in federal oversight will occur, freeing states to change eligibility standards for service.
- Some states might continue existing eligibility criteria; others might expand or reduce criteria.
- Minimal copayments for services in all states.

Block Grants

- Expect to see more federal funds distributed in block grants, with less federal oversight of funded programs and greater state autonomy in selection of services and populations served by federal funds.

Managed Care and Health Networks

- The proportion of the population covered by managed care will continue to expand.
- Health care providers will continue to merge into large health networks.

*Signed into law in December 2003.

Continued

Box 16-5 **Potential Health Care Reform Initiatives: Some Predictions Based on Anticipated Changes to Health Insurance Laws and Regulations—cont'd**

Managed Care and Vulnerable Populations

- All the cost savings of switching vulnerable populations to managed care have been realized.
- Managed care organizations (MCOs) are finding it difficult to care for Medicare and Medicaid populations for the established capitation fees and are disenrolling or declining new enrollments. This will continue and may accelerate.
- Studies indicate that MCOs have the healthiest of the Medicaid and Medicare populations; that is, seniors with few chronic conditions, young mothers, infants, and children (Braden, Cowan, Lazenby, et al., 1998; Government Accounting Office, 1999).
- If the government persists in continuing MCO enrollment of all (including the less healthy Medicare and Medicaid populations), capitation fees will increase, cost savings will disappear, health care costs for MCOs will increase, and the government will reduce the menu of benefits required of health care providers to keep costs down.

Managed Care and Legislation

- If federal legislation regulating MCO practices does not pass, states will pass more laws.
- Consumers will find regulations differ depending on the state in which they live. In 2002, 42 states had laws providing comprehensive consumer health protection, 22 banned financial incentives to physicians, 47 banned gag clauses in physician contracts, and 37 required direct access for consumers to obstetrics/gynecological services.

Patients' Bill of Rights

Various versions of patients' rights legislation have been considered by Congress every year since 1997. In whatever version ultimately passes, some provisions are expected to be:
- The right to sue your MCO.
- The right to go to the doctor of your choice.
- The right to see appropriate specialists outside the MCO.
- The right to use the emergency department for services any prudent layperson considers necessary.
- The right for expedited review of denials of health care services.
- The right to be provided with a list of all treatment options for your condition.
- The right to privacy of medical records to be expanded (sharing of health information limited to use for clinical decision making, not to be shared with other insurers).
- Protection for health care professional whistle-blowers from retaliation by employers.

Rationing

- Current rationing of care is by ability to pay; insurance coverage ensures care for most.
- Because for-profit structures dominate the health market, there may be additional curtailments on such items as expensive therapies, disputes between providers and payers about what constitutes "experimental procedures," and shortening of allowable hospital recovery times.
- Legislation may be necessary to compel care.
- Unless a minimum standard of care is established at the federal level, each state may need to take action separately to address each inequity. For example, some states have already passed legislation that ensures a new mother's right to extend postdelivery hospital stays to 48 hours. Insurers had been willing to pay for 24 hours or less.

Box **16-5** Potential Health Care Reform Initiatives: Some Predictions
Based on Anticipated Changes to Health Insurance Laws and Regulations—cont'd

Two-Tiered System of Health Care
- Health care services will be based on ability to pay.
- There will be a basic level of benefits established for those with public health insurance (similar to the Oregon Medicaid Plan).
- All other individuals will be free to purchase additional benefits based on ability to pay.
- Private employers might provide only the basic plan, or a range of plans, and employees will be free to chose more costly options and pay the premium difference out of pocket.

Sources: Association of Operating Room Nurses: Patient rights still hot topic in Congress and the states, *AORN J* 69(5):1031-1036, 1999; Braden BR, Cowan CA, Lazenby HC, et al: National health expenditures, 1997, *Health Care Financing Rev* 20(1):83-126, 1998; Government Accounting Office: *Medicare managed care: better risk adjustment expected to reduce excess payments overall while making them fairer to individual plans* (GAO/T-HEHS-99-72, February 25), Washington, DC, 1999, Government Printing Office; Black JT, Kominski GF: Medicaid reform. In Andersen RM, Rice TH, Komenski GF: *Changing the U.S. health care system,* San Francisco, 2001, Jossey-Bass, pp 406-435; and Davis K, Schoen C: Creating consensus on coverage choices, *Health Affairs Web Exclusives* W3-199-211, 2002.

5. Are the issues of adequate facilities and personnel to ensure access for all addressed?
6. Is there an emphasis on quality care?
7. Are there incentives for healthy lifestyles and preventive care?

A point of particular interest to nurses is the issue of cost-effectiveness of personnel. If care is to be provided by the most cost-effective personnel, it should mean an expansion of the role of nurses as primary care providers (Figure 16-4). Studies have shown that nurses are cost-effective caregivers and are well accepted by the public (Harrington and Estes, 1994; and Scott and Rantz, 1997; Sochalski, 2002). Organized medicine, however, actively opposes moves to give clinical autonomy to almost all non-physician providers (Feldstein, 1998). This is a conflict that must be resolved for true reform to occur, and nurses themselves must be active in its resolution.

Summary of Key Points
- Health care financing in the United States has changed dramatically from a system dominated by personal payment to one dominated by third-party payment.
- This change created basic economic disequilibrium in health care because people who do not pay directly for health care are not sensitive to the price of care.
- Medicare and Medicaid programs, begun in 1965, quickly created a serious financial drain on federal and state budgets that continues today. In response, cost-containment efforts were begun by the federal government in the 1970s and persist in various old and new forms.
- Initial cost-containment efforts were unsuccessful, so in 1982 more sweeping reforms were initiated. Retrospective payment was replaced by prospective payment.
- In the early 1990s, system-wide health reform efforts were supported by public opinion but failed to pass the U.S. Congress. Even without governmental action, many Americans have seen substantial changes in their health care plans, stimulated by business interests and employers.
- There has been a dramatic escalation in managed care plans and consolidation of health providers into larger health networks.

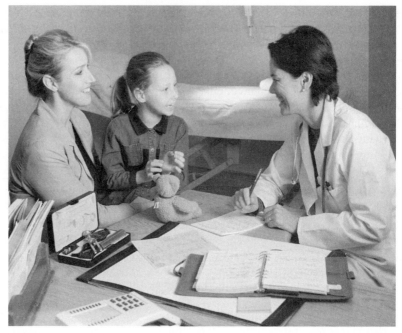

Figure 16-4
Cost-containment initiatives have strengthened the demand for nurse practitioners. Another result has been federal legislation requiring reimbursement of nurse practitioners who care for certain populations. Only sweeping reimbursement reform, however, will allow nurse practitioners, like this family nurse practitioner, to demonstrate their brand of high-quality, cost-effective, primary care and thereby contribute to the nation's efforts to contain health care costs. (Photo courtesy Hamilton Medical Center, Dalton, Georgia.)

- By the beginning of the twenty-first century, governmental action imposed some restrictions on health insurance practices, made an effort to improve health care for a limited number of at-risk children, and encouraged or mandated the enrollment of Medicaid and Medicare clients in managed care.
- The entire health care system, including nurses and nursing services, has been profoundly affected by these changes.
- Further changes are on the horizon. Most likely they will be *incremental,* rather than revolutionary. It remains to be seen whether these changes will improve access and maintain quality of health care for all Americans.

CRITICAL THINKING QUESTIONS
1. In your view, is access to health care a basic right? Who should pay for it? Be prepared to defend your opinions.
2. List the basic health care services that should be provided to all citizens. Compare your list with the lists of classmates and discuss the rationale for your priorities.
3. Should there be a limit on the percentage of national resources expended on health care? If so, how should the limit be established? Who should be responsible for determining the limit?

4. What process should be used to determine how health care resources are allocated? List criteria you would suggest to determine whether or not a person should receive a kidney transplant, a hip replacement, or a bone marrow transplant.
5. Should people with healthy lifestyles pay the same for care or insurance as those whose habits result in a greater likelihood of illness? How could such a differentiation be determined?
6. Should there be rationing of extremely expensive procedures, such as heart transplants, even if the patient is able to pay? Give a rationale for your answer.

REFERENCES

Andersen RM, Pouillier JP: Health spending, access, and outcomes: trends in industrialized countries. In Harrington C, Estes CL: *Health policy: crisis and reform in the U.S. health care delivery system,* ed 3, Boston, MA, 2001, Jones and Bartlett.

Ashton G: Getting tough on drive-through delivery, *AHA News* 31(50):3, 1995.

Association of Operating Room Nurses: Patient rights still hot topic in Congress and the states, *AORN J* 69(5):1031-1036, 1999.

Benko LB: Coventry buys New Alliance, *Mod Healthcare* 32(14):25, 2002.

Bennefield RL: Dynamics of economic well-being: health insurance, 1993-1996, *Current Population Reports,* Washington, DC, 1998, U.S. Census Bureau, pp 70-64.

Betts VT: 1996—Speak out for quality care, *Am Nurse* 28(1):4, 1996.

Black JT, Kominski GF: Medicaid reform. In Andersen RM, Rice TH, Komenski GF: *Changing the U.S. health care system,* San Francisco, 2001, Jossey-Bass, pp 406-435.

Blendon RJ, Brodie M, Benson JM, et al: Understanding the managed care backlash, *Health Aff* 17-17(4):80-94, 1998.

Braden BR, Cowan CA, Lazenby HC, et al: National health expenditures, 1997, *Health Care Financing Rev* 20(1):83-126, 1998.

Buerhaus PI: Economics and reform: forces affecting nurse staffing, *Nursing Policy Forum* 1(2):8-14, 1995a.

Buerhaus PI: Economic pressures building in the hospital employed RN labor market, *Nurs Econ* 13(3):137-141, 1995.

Centers for Medicare and Medicaid Services: National health care expenditures projections: 2001-2011, Online, August 12, 2003 *(www.cms.hhs.gov/statistics/nhe/projections-2001).*

Davis K, Schoen C: Universal coverage building on Medicare and employer financing, *Health Aff* 13(1):7-20, 1994.

Davis K, Schoen C: Creating consensus on coverage choices, *Health Affairs Web Exclusives* W3-199-211, 2002.

Eichenwald K: Tenet Healthcare paying $54 million in fraud settlement, *The New York Times,* August 7, 2003, A-1.

Feder J, Uccello C, O'Brien E: The difference different approaches make: comparing proposals to expand health insurance. In Harrington C, Estes CL: *Health policy: crisis and reform in the U.S. health care delivery system,* ed 3, Boston, MA, 2001, Jones and Bartlett.

Feldstein PJ: *Health care economics,* ed 5, West Albany, NY, 1998, Delmar.

Flasch HM: Provider-owned plan focuses on quality, growth, and new technology, *Healthcare Financ Manage* 55(12):30-34, 2001.

Gabel JR, Jensen GA, Hawkins S: Self-insurance in times of growing and retreating managed care, *Health Aff* 22(2):202-10, 2003.

Glabman M: Bare bones: as the cost of malpractice insurance skyrockets, doctors, hospitals and patients suffer, *Trustee* 56(3):8-13, 2003.

Gold M, Mittler J: Second-generation Medicaid managed care: can it deliver? *Health Care Financ Rev* 22(2):29-47, 2000.

Gordon S: "Nurse interrupted": the other health care crisis. In Harrington C, Estes, CL: *Health policy: crisis and reform in the U.S. health care delivery system,* ed 3, Boston, 2001, Jones and Bartlett.

Government Accounting Office: *Private health insurance: continued erosion of coverage linked to cost pressure* (GAO-HEHS-97-122, July 27), Washington, DC, 1997, Government Printing Office.

Government Accounting Office: *Retiree health insurance: erosion in retirement health benefits offered by large employers* (GAO-HEHS-98-110, March 10), Washington, DC, 1998, Government Printing Office.

Government Accounting Office: *Medicare managed care: better risk adjustment expected to reduce excess payments overall while making them fairer to individual plans,* Washington DC, 1999, Government Printing Office.

Government Accounting Office: *Medical malpractice: implication of rising premiums on access to health care* (GAO-03-836), Washington, DC, 2003, Government Printing Office.

Grimaldi PL: Medicare increases managed care's accountability, part 2, *Nurs Manage* 30(2): 10-11, 1999.

Hadley J: Sicker and poorer—the consequences of being uninsured: a review of the research on the relationship between health insurance, medical care use, health, work, and income, *Med Care Res Rev* 60(2S):3S-75S, 2003.

Hakin D: Their health costs soaring, automakers are to begin labor talks, *The New York Times,* July 12, 2003, C1, 2003.

Harrington C, Estes CL: Health policy and nursing: crisis and reform in the U.S. delivery system, Boston, MA, 1994, Jones and Bartlett.

Harris Poll 2002: The public's health—a matter of trust—trust and distrust, Retrieved online, Sept 5, 2003 *(www.hsph.harvard.edu/ccpe/Trust/trust_distrust.htm).*

Health Care Finance Administration: *Medicare and Medicaid statistical supplement,* Washington, DC, 1998, Government Printing Office.

Hileman GR, Moroz KE, Wrightson, et al: Medicare+Choice individual and group enrollment 2001–2002, *Health Care Financ Rev* 24(1):145-154, 2002.

Hillman AL, Pauly MV, Escarce JJ, et al: Financial incentives and drug spending in managed care, *Health Aff* 18(2):189-200, 1999.

Hurley RE, Draper DA: Medicaid confronts a changing managed care marketplace, *Health Care Financ Rev* 24(1):11-26, 2002.

Idelson C: Safe staffing law puts California nurses in the spotlight. In Harrington C, Estes CL: *Health policy: crisis and reform in the U.S. health care delivery system,* ed 3, Boston, MA, 2001, Jones and Bartlett.

Insurance Advocate: Coventry Health Care signs pact to acquire Mid-Atlantic HMO, *Insurance Advocate* 113(36):38, 2002.

Jacob P, Rapoport J: *The economics of health and medical care,* Sudbury, MA, 2002, Jones and Bartlett.

Kaiser Family Foundation: *Health insurance survey,* Menlo Park, CA, 2003, Kaiser Family Foundation.

Kaiser/HRET: *Employer health benefits, 2002 summary of findings,* Menlo Park CA, 2002, Kaiser Family Foundation.

Kronich R, Gilmer T: Exploring the decline in health insurance coverage, 1979–1995, *Health Aff* 18(2):30-47, 1999.

Lampe S: Costing hospital nursing services: A review of the literature. Washington, DC, 1987, U.S. Department of Health and Human Services.

Larson E: The soul of an HMO, *Time* 147(4):44-52, 1996.

Levit K, Smith C, Cowan C, et al: Trends in U.S. health care spending, 2001, *Health Aff* 22(1):154-164, 2003.

Maurer FA: Financing of health care: context for community health nursing. In Smith C, Maurer FA, editors: *Community health nursing: theory and practice,* ed 2, Philadelphia, 2000, WB Saunders.

Maze J: No protection: sham health insurance is on the rise, leaving people with big bills they thought were covered, Charleston, SC, *The Post and Courier,* October 13, 16-17E, 2003.

McCue MJ, Hurley RE, Draper et al: Reversal of fortune: commercial HMOs with the Medicaid market, *Health Aff* 18(1):223-230, 1999.

McGlynn EA, Adams JL: Public release of information on quality. In Andersen RM, Rice TH, Kominski GF: *Changing the U.S. health care system,* San Francisco, 2001, Jossey-Bass.

McKibben RC: *DRGs and nursing care,* Kansas City, MO, 1985, American Nurses Association Center for Research.

Medicare and You: Baltimore MD, 2003, Centers for Medicare and Medicaid Services.

Morris EA: Who's taking care of Mama? *Am Nurse* 28(1):4, 1996.

Murray ME, Henriques JB: Denials of reimbursement for hospital care, *Managed Care Interface* 16(4):22-27, 2003.

Nornhold P: What networks mean to you, *Nursing 95* 25(1):49-50, 1995.

Organization for Economic Cooperation and Development: Health care expenditures and other data: an international compendium, *Health Care Financ Rev* (suppl):111-195, 1989.

Patel K, Rushefsky ME: *Health care politics and policy in America,* ed 2, Armonk, NY, 1999, ME Sharpe.

Pfizer: Annual Report, 2002, Retrieved online, Sept 5, 2003 *(www.pfizer.com/are/investors_reports/annual_2002/p2002ar31c_32a.htm).*

Pizer SD, Frakt AB: Payment policy and competition in the Medicare+Choice program, *Health Care Financ Rev* 24(1):83-94, 2002.

Rowland D: *Statement before the joint economic committee United States Congress: health challenges facing the nation,* Menlo Park, CA, 2003, The Kaiser Commission on Medicaid and the Uninsured. Available online *(www.kff.org/content/2003/4144).*

Safran DG, Newman P, Schoen C, et al: Prescription drug coverage and seniors: how well are states closing the gap? *Health Affairs Supplemental Web Exclusives* W253-268, 2002.

Salkever DS, Shinogle MS, Goldman H: Mental health benefit limits and cost sharing under managed care: a national survey of employers, *Psychiatr Serv* 50(12):1631-1633, 1999.

Sambamoorthi U, Shea D, Crystal S: Total out of pocket expenditures for prescription drugs among older persons, *Gerontologist* 43(3):345-359, 2003.

Schweitzer SO, Comanor WS: Pharmaceutical prices and expenditures. In Andersen RM, Rice TH, Kominski GF: *Changing the U.S. health care system,* San Francisco, 2001, Jossey-Bass, pp 100-126.

Scott J, Rantz M: Managing chronically ill older people in the midst of health care revolution, *Nurs Admin Q* 21(2):55-64, 1997.

Sentementes GG: Steel union's leaders OK pact, *Baltimore Sun,* May 6, 2003, B-2, 2003.

Short PF, Banthin JS: New estimates of the underinsured younger than 65 years, *JAMA* 274:1302-1306, 2003.

Smith VK, Rousseau DM: *SCHIP program enrollment: December 2002 update,* Kaiser Commission on Medicaid and the uninsured, Menlo Park, CA, 2003, Kaiser Family Foundation.

Sochalski J: Nursing shortage redux: Turning the corner on an enduring problem, *Health Aff* 21(5):151-181, 2002.

Statistical Abstract of the United States, Washington, DC, 2002, Government Printing Office.

Statistical Abstract of the United States, Washington, DC, 1998, Government Printing Office.

Studdert DM, Gresenz CR: Enrollee appeals of preservice coverage denials at two health maintenance organizations, *J Am Med Assoc* 289(7):864-870, 2003.

Sultz HA, Young KM: *Health care USA: understanding its organization and delivery,* ed 3, Gaithersberg, MD, 2001, Aspen Publishers Inc.

The Hay Group: *Nursing shortage study,* Walnut Creek, CA, 1998, The Hay Group.

Thompson JW, Bost J, Ahmed F et al: The NCQA's quality compass: evaluating managed care in the U.S., *Health Aff* 17(1):152-158, 1998.

Tumulty K: Health care has a relapse, *Time* 159(10):42-44, 2002.

U.S. Census Bureau: *Health insurance coverage: 2001,* Washington, DC, 2002, Government Printing Office.

U.S. Census Bureau: *Current population survey, March 2002,* Washington, DC, 2003, Government Printing Office.

U.S. Department of Health and Human Services: HHS study finds strong link between patient outcomes and nurse staffing in hospitals, Online, 2001 *(www.newsroom.hrsa.gov/releases/2001%20Releases/nursestudy.htm).*

Vice DA, Adams L: Firm settles health care fraud case for $500 million, *The New York Times,* January 19, 2000, A16.

Wang PS, Demler O, Kessler RC: Adequacy of treatment for serious mental illness in the United States, *Am J Pub Health* 92(1):92-98, 2002.

Wilensky GR, Newhouse JP: Medicare: What's right? What's wrong? What's next? *Health Aff* 18(1):92-106, 1999.

Zarabozo C: Issues in managed care, *Health Care Financ Rev* 24(1):1-10, 2002.

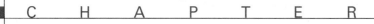

17

Illness and Culture: Impact on Patients, Families, and Nurses

Kay Kittrell Chitty

Acute Illness	Disease	Remission
Anxiety	Ethnocentric	Resilience
Chronic Illness	Exacerbation	Sick Role
Coping	Hardiness	Spirituality
Cultural Assessment	Illness	Stereotyping
Culturally Competent Care	Learned Resourcefulness	Stress
Culture	Parental Modeling	Stressor
Dependency	Personal Space	

Learning Outcomes

After studying this chapter, students will be able to:

- Differentiate between acute and chronic illness.
- Describe the stages of illness.
- Describe behavioral responses to illness.
- Identify internal and external influences on illness behaviors.
- Discuss the influence of culture on illness behaviors.
- Describe the characteristics of the culturally competent nurse.
- Describe the physical, emotional, and cognitive effects of stress.
- Discuss how family functioning is altered during illness.
- Explain the necessity of and strategies for self-care by nurses.

Although prevention and health maintenance activities are primary functions of nurses, many nurse-patient interactions center on the management of illness. A unique characteristic of nursing is the emphasis on viewing patients holistically. Nurses recognize that human beings are complex organisms with physical, mental, emotional, spiritual, social, and cultural components—all of which affect how a person responds when ill. The effective nurse takes each of these dimensions into consideration when planning nursing care. This chapter explores the stages of illness, illness behaviors, cultural factors that influence how people behave during illness, and the impact of illness and culture on patients and families. It also explores briefly the reasons why nurses need to develop balance in their lives and engage in self-care.

ILLNESS

Illness is a highly personal experience. It is differentiated from disease in that **disease** is an alteration at the tissue or organ level causing reduced capacities or reduction of the normal life span. **Illness** is usually considered a subjective state. One may feel ill in the absence of a disease. Conversely, one may be unaware of a disease, such as high blood pressure, and not feel ill.

Ellis and Nowlis (1994) discuss the concept of "illness with evidence." This means that there must be demonstrable evidence of an organic nature for an illness to exist. In other words, health care professionals may define a state of illness, such as hypertension, even in the absence of subjective symptoms in the ill person.

People's perceptions of change or loss play a major role in whether or not they see themselves as ill. People with mild arthritic changes who have no decrease in their activities and who need to use only over-the-counter analgesics such as aspirin may not consider themselves ill. To a radiologist looking at a radiography, however, arthritic changes indicating a disease process may be evident.

Whether the presence of illness is determined by the individual or by a health care provider, illness is experienced differently by individuals and their families. Culture plays a powerful role in health beliefs and behaviors; it also determines how individuals and families react to illness. The nurse's responses to patients must be defined in terms of these unique reactions.

Acute Illness

Illnesses can be classified as either acute or chronic. **Acute illness** is characterized by severe symptoms that are relatively short-lived. Symptoms tend to appear suddenly, progress steadily, and subside quickly. Depending on the illness, the patient may or may not require medical attention. The common cold is an example of an acute illness that does not usually require a health care provider's attention. Others, such as acute appendicitis, may be fatal without rapid medical intervention. Unless complications arise, people suffering from acute illness usually return rather quickly to their previous level of wellness.

Individuals with sudden, catastrophic injuries, such as a spinal cord injury, experience dramatic and extensive change. They face physical limitations, significant modifications in daily living, and changes in social roles. Daily, they must bear challenges that most people consider unbearable. Research Note 1 describes a study of how individuals with catastrophic illnesses and injuries cope with their disabilities (Dewar and Lee, 2000).

Chronic Illness

Chronic illnesses cannot usually be cured. They develop gradually, require ongoing medical attention, and may continue for the duration of the person's life. Hypertension, diabetes, and Parkinson's disease are examples of chronic illnesses.

RESEARCH note 1

Canadian nurse researchers Anne Dewar and Elizabeth Lee wondered how individuals with catastrophic illness and injury faced challenges that others consider unbearable and test the limits of human endurance. They conducted individual interviews with 28 men and women from 18 to 75 years of age. These interviewees had endured chronic conditions, such as spinal cord injuries, multiple sclerosis, or major burns, for time periods ranging from 3 to 25 years. The researchers analyzed subjects' responses using grounded theory methods, a qualitative research methodology. The theoretical framework selected by the researchers was *symbolic interactionism,* which seeks to determine the relationship between the individual and the social world in which he or she lives.

They found that these individuals experienced three phases in bearing their difficulties. The researchers termed these phases *finding out, facing reality,* and *managing reality.* They discovered that the individuals in their study did not progress through stages, as others have suggested, but instead the phases flowed together and were reexperienced continuously. These individuals used three enduring strategies in all phases, which the researchers termed *protecting, modifying,* and *boosting. Protecting* involved insulating oneself from further emotional pain by limiting requests for assistance and not sharing emotional distress with significant others. *Modifying* meant learning to manage the physical, emotional, and social aspects of a condition by learning new skills and diffusing their emotions to preserve their social support, that is, not "whining." *Boosting* meant efforts to enhance self-esteem, such as comparing themselves with others who were in worse condition.

Dewar and Lee concluded that "the burdens of chronic illness and injuries [are] exceedingly complex, as individuals are forced to rebuild an image of themselves, manage their daily lives, and preserve relationships with others. Social support is important but forces the sufferer to make modifications to meet the needs of others as well as his or her own" (p. 924). They recommended that nurses and other health care professionals "accept and support the individual's need to express emotions such as anger, sorrow, and despair in all phases of the illness" (p. 922).

Abstracted from Dewar AL, Lee EA: Bearing illness and injury, *West J Nurs Res* 22(8):912-926, 2000.

It is increasingly important for nurses to understand chronic illnesses and their impact, because they are one of the fastest-growing health problems in the United States. It is estimated that one third to one half of the U.S. population has one or more chronic illnesses. Factors such as sedentary lifestyles and the aging of the population are expected to contribute to a continued increase in the number of chronically ill Americans for the foreseeable future.

Chronic illnesses are caused by permanent changes that leave residual disability. They vary in severity and outcomes, but there is generally not an end point at which normal health is regained. Some chronic illnesses are progressively debilitating and result in premature death, whereas others are associated with a normal life span, even though functioning is impaired. Some chronic illnesses go through periods of **remission,** when symptoms subside, and **exacerbation,** when symptoms reappear or worsen.

Chronic illnesses are pervasive and life-altering. They lead to altered individual functioning and disruption of family life. Long-term medical management of chronic illness can create financial hardship as well. Patients with chronic illness need to make lifestyle changes, often many changes simultaneously. They must begin doing things they are not accustomed to doing and stop doing things they normally do. Patients with diabetes, for example, must begin monitoring their blood sugar levels and change their eating habits.

Being diagnosed with a chronic illness is often a major life crisis. The emotional reactions of the patient and family sometimes present a greater challenge than dealing with the physical aspects of the disease. Most medical and nursing attention, however, is focused on physical symptoms and the disease process rather than emotions (Cassidy, 1999). Box 17-1 describes how one patient experiences a chronic illness, lupus erythematosis, and describes its impact on her feelings, family responsibilities, and relationships.

STAGES OF ILLNESS

Adjustment to illness is a process. Although the behaviors are different for each person, people who are ill tend to progress through certain recognizable stages. Ellis and Nowlis (1994) have identified five stages: disbelief and denial, irritability and

---

Box 17-1 **Comments of a Patient With a Chronic Disease: Lupus Erythematosis**

If there is one thing I want to say to nurses who work with patients with chronic disease, it is "Be patient and understand our problems and feelings." When I go to the doctor's office or to the hospital, I usually leave feeling guilty because I have been impatient with everyone I saw. Guilt and anger are the two feelings I seem to have had since I was diagnosed with this disease. I alternate between being angry that I got lupus and feeling that I should be grateful for the fact that I have something I can at least live with when others are not so fortunate.

I guess the thing that bothers me most is that the nurses keep telling me what changes I need to make to take better care of myself. They never seem to understand that I am doing the best I can do. I can't possibly get the amount of rest they seem to think I need, and I can't avoid as much stress as they seem to think I should avoid. Both my husband and I work hard at our jobs, and I hate asking him and my sons to take over my responsibilities at home when I am sick, so I wind up compromising. I ask them to help some and I do more than I should. When I get the lecture from the nurses on how I should take better care of myself, I usually just nod and say that I will, even when I know that I probably won't be able to.

—Anonymous

anger, attempting to gain control, depression and despair, and acceptance and participation. Nurses encounter patients in each stage, so it is important to have some understanding of the types of behaviors associated with each. Remember that a person's culture affects how he or she responds to illness and that Ellis and Nowlis's studies were done with people of individualistic, Western cultures. Also remember that stage theories are convenient ways of conceptualizing and learning, but often human beings do not fit neatly into the identified stages.

Stage I: Disbelief and Denial

According to Ellis and Nowlis (1994), the first stage results from difficulty in believing that the signs and symptoms being experienced are caused by illness. Often, there is a belief that the symptoms will go away. Fear of illness often leads to the hope that the symptoms will subside without treatment.

Denial is a defense mechanism that people sometimes use to avoid the anxiety associated with illness. People who pride themselves on their vigor and health may downplay the significance of symptoms. If this occurs, they may avoid treatment or attempt inappropriate self-treatment. Extended denial can have serious results, because some illnesses, left untreated, may become too advanced for effective treatment.

Stage II: Irritability and Anger

As the ability to function is altered by illness, irritability results. Anger is directed toward the body because it is not performing as it should. With the current emphasis on wellness and prevention, anger may be directed inward, and guilt feelings may occur for failing to prevent the illness. Anger may also be directed toward others—spouse, family members, co-workers, or health care providers.

Stage III: Attempting to Gain Control

In this stage, people may try over-the-counter medications, folk practices, or home remedies. They are aware that they are ill and usually experience some concern or even fear about the outcome. These fears usually stimulate treatment-seeking behavior as a way of gaining control over the illness, but they may lead to further denial and avoidance. Family members may become involved, encouraging the person to seek treatment.

Stage IV: Depression and Despair

Depression is perhaps the most common mood that occurs with illness. The ability to work is altered, daily activities must be modified, and the sense of well-being and freedom from pain are lost. Illness results in many types of loss, and depression is a normal response. The severity of the depression varies according to the severity and length of the illness, as well as the individual's personality characteristics and coping abilities. Individuals with chronic illnesses often undergo cycles of depression as remissions and exacerbations occur.

Stage V: Acceptance and Participation

By the time this stage occurs, the patient has acknowledged the reality of illness and is ready to participate in decisions about treatment. Active involvement and the hope attached to pursuing treatment usually lead to increased feelings of mastery and serve to decrease depression.

Not all individuals go through every stage, and they do not necessarily go through them at the same rate or in the same order. Those with acute illnesses may progress through stages in a different way than those with chronic illnesses. As mentioned, culture plays a major role in how people respond to illness.

Illness Behavior and the Sick Role

Although illness is highly subjective and is experienced differently by each individual, a number of factors influence how a particular person will respond. One important factor is the cultural expectation about how people *should* behave when ill. Children learn the part they are expected to play as an ill person through **parental modeling**— that is, by observing how their parents respond to major and minor illnesses. Do their significant adult figures avoid work and other activities when ill, or do they forge ahead stoically, ignoring minor illness or pain?

Each culture generally requires that certain criteria be met before people can qualify as "sick." Talcott Parsons (1964), a renowned sociologist, identified five attributes and expectations of the **sick role** that guided the view of illness in Anglo-American society for decades. According to Parsons, the sick Anglo-American:

1. Is exempt from social responsibilities.
2. Cannot be expected to care for himself or herself.
3. Should want to get well.
4. Should seek medical advice.
5. Should cooperate with the medical experts.

In other words, Parson's definition of the sick role includes behavior that is dependent, passive, and submissive. For decades, Parson's sick role expectations were taught in medical and nursing schools and guided the way health care providers viewed patients' reactions to pain and illness for many years. In our multicultural society, however, this view is no longer adequate, because different cultures have differing sick role expectations.

The cultural makeup of the nation and the world are changing. By 2010, whites will be the smallest ethnic minority in the world. Nurses, regardless of their own cultural backgrounds, must strive to provide **culturally competent care** to patients of many diverse cultures. With over 66 different categories of race listed in the 2000 U.S. Census, this can seem like an overwhelming task. In fact, it is probably impossible for nurses to master the subtleties of every culture they encounter. Nurses can learn about their patients' culturally determined health care and illness beliefs, values, and practices, however, by consistently performing cultural assessments. These instruments will be discussed later in this chapter.

The current Anglo-American expectation is that people should accept responsibility for their own care rather than completely submit to health care providers; this is the consumer-oriented approach to health care. There is a presumption that ill people should want to get well and should behave in a way that leads to wellness.

This expectation that ill persons should want to get well and return to their normal activities as quickly as possible means that patients should cooperate in the treatment process and, to a great extent, become submissive and compliant, placing themselves in the hands of the caretakers. Persons who refuse to take medications as ordered or who refuse to perform prescribed activities, such as adhering to an exercise program or therapeutic diet, are viewed in a negative light. Their friends and family members may become irritated at their lack of participation in getting well again. Their caregivers call them "noncompliant." Often what is missing is an understanding of the patient's perception of the illness. Shifting from a focus of caring *for* patients to partnering *with* them is helpful in overcoming negative attitudes.

In caring for patients with acute and chronic illnesses, it is important for nurses to refrain from making judgments about patients' lifestyle choices. Emphasis should be on encouraging and reinforcing healthy behaviors. Education and support are important role functions for the nurse, especially in the management of patients with chronic disorders.

Working with patients with chronic illnesses can be particularly challenging for nurses. The inability of modern medicine to cure disease sometimes leads caregivers to feel hopeless and powerless. They may also feel overwhelmed and inadequate at times. Self-aware nurses recognize these feelings and do not allow them to interfere with the nurse-patient relationship.

Internal Influences on Illness Behavior

Although some behaviors are expected of sick people, there is also a wide variation in responses. Each person who is newly diagnosed with hypertension, for example, behaves somewhat differently from other people with the same condition. Both internal and external variables affect how an individual acts when ill. An ill individual's personality has a great deal of influence on the response to illness. Past experiences with illness and cultural background also influence illness behaviors.

Personality structure is an internal variable that determines, to a large extent, how one manages illness. Personality characteristics the nurse should consider when assessing the ill person are dependence/independence, coping ability, hardiness, learned resourcefulness, resilience, and spirituality.

Dependence and independence

Patients' needs for dependence are unrelated to the severity of their illnesses. Some patients adopt a passive attitude and rely completely on others to take care of them. Others deny they are ill or have problems with being dependent and try to continue living as independently as they did before becoming sick.

We have all encountered sick people who have expressed views such as, "I don't ask any questions—I know that my doctor and nurses know what is best for me, and I do what they tell me." Perhaps you also know someone who reacted to illness by saying, "They don't know what they are talking about. I don't need to be in bed, and I don't need to take that medicine." These two sentiments are at the opposite ends of the **dependency** continuum.

People who perceive themselves as helpless may be more willing to submit to health care personnel and do what they are told. Those who are used to being in charge and see themselves as independent may resent the enforced dependency of hospitalization and illness. These two different attitudes are illustrated in the following Case Study.

case study

Example 1: *Dependence*

Mrs. Johnson has been in the hospital for several days following major abdominal surgery. Even after she progressed to the point at which she could feed herself, turn over in bed, and go to the bathroom unaided, she continued to call for assistance when she needed to turn or to get out of bed. She now calls the nurse every few minutes, making some small request that she is quite capable of performing for herself. She is communicating to the nurse that she needs a great deal of assistance and is demonstrating overly dependent behavior.

Example 2: *Independence*

One hour ago Mr. Thomas returned to his room after surgery. The nurse found him trying to get out of bed by himself. He does not call to ask for assistance, although he is still groggy from anesthesia. He says that he is used to doing things for himself and feels uncomfortable asking the nurses for help. Mr. Thomas is demonstrating behavior that is too independent for his current physical status.

Both overly dependent and overly independent behavior can be frustrating to nurses, who sometimes become angry with patients who request help with activities they are capable of doing themselves. The patient who is too dependent requires assistance to assume gradually more responsibility. The patient who needs to be "in charge" may have problems turning control over to caregivers and is often too independent. This patient needs assistance in recognizing limitations and using available resources to get needs met.

Because nurses most often focus on promoting patient independence, they may react negatively to patients who are exhibiting dependent behavior. It is important for the nurse to be aware of personal feelings about dependent behaviors and to keep in mind that these behaviors may be the patient's way of signaling an increased need for security or support. Sometimes independence may not be the desired outcome. For patients with chronic illnesses who must rely on others for assistance in meeting their needs, too much independence may actually be dysfunctional (Whiting, 1994) as well as dangerous.

Coping ability

An individual copes with disease or illness in a variety of ways. **Coping** is the method a person uses to assess and manage demands. With an acute illness, coping is generally short-term and leads to a return to the preillness state. With chronic disorders, coping behaviors must be used continuously.

Sick people use coping methods to deal with the negative consequences of the disorder, such as pain or physical limitations. Each individual has a unique coping repertoire that is called into play to achieve a sense of control. With chronic health problems, there is a continuous need for adjustments to maintain well-being and prevent the feelings of despair that can result from high stress conditions (Bowsher and Keep, 1995).

Hardiness and learned resourcefulness

Hardiness and learned resourcefulness are two concepts that have received attention as personal characteristics related to coping. **Hardiness** is viewed as a function of resistance to stressful life events (Bowsher and Keep, 1995). The tendency to believe that one can influence the course of events, viewing change as a challenge, and feeling commitment to values or goals are seen as the interrelated dimensions of hardiness.

The person with high levels of hardiness is believed to be better able to manage the changes associated with illness and to have less physical illness resulting from stress. Hardy people are likely to perceive themselves as having some control over a situation, even when ill. This feeling can affect a person's sense of well-being and adaptation to acute and chronic health problems.

Zauszniewski (1995) has described the concept of **learned resourcefulness** as a characteristic useful in promoting adaptive, healthy lifestyles. Throughout life, individuals acquire a number of skills that enable them to cope effectively with stressful situations. The resulting attitude of self-control can be particularly helpful in reducing the feelings of depression and helplessness that often accompany the numerous stressors of chronic illness.

The nurse can enhance both hardiness and resourcefulness by teaching new coping skills. Stress inoculation and skills in self-regulation, problem solving, conflict resolution, and emotion control are examples of the types of educational interventions the nurse may implement.

Resilience

Scholars studying human behavior have often noted that some children did well in spite of difficult circumstances that defeated others. They attributed the differing reactions as a function of the phenomenon of **resilience.** Resilience is an aspect of coping that can be defined as "a pattern of successful adaptation despite challenging or threatening circumstances" (Humphreys, 2001). Resilient responses are thought to be due to three factors:

- Disposition (i.e., temperament, personality, overall health and appearance, and cognitive style)
- Family factors such as warmth, support, and organization
- Outside support factors, such as a supportive network and success in school or work

Resilience can be thought of as both a process and an outcome. It can develop over a person's lifetime and can be taught, modeled, and learned (Wolin, 1993).

The study of resilience has broadened to include adolescents and adults who face difficult, traumatic, or adverse circumstances. It has also been applied to adults with critical illness, battered women, survivors of sexual abuse, and others. You can expect to see much more about resilience as this phenomenon continues to be studied and better understood. A useful website to help you begin understanding the concept of resilience can be found online *(www.projectresilience.com).*

Spirituality

The concept of spirituality is receiving increased interest in society as a whole, as well as in nursing. **Spirituality** is defined as "inner strength related to belief in and sense of connectedness with a higher power" (Chilton, 1998). The degree of spiritual awareness varies from individual to individual. This awareness can be dormant, suppressed, or may be expressed through religious worship and prayer, although it is not necessarily manifested in overt religious practices (Cavendish, et al., 2000). Religion is a specific way of organizing rituals and beliefs to create meaning. Spirituality is a larger umbrella concept under which religion resides. Spirituality is less differentiated than religion and can include concepts and beliefs from many religions and philosophies.

Spiritual growth occurs over the life span and is a very internal process. Spiritual growth consists of increasing awareness of meaning, connectedness, purpose, and values in life (Cavendish, et al., 2000).

The role of spiritual beliefs in health and illness has only recently been formally investigated. A growing number of scholars and health professionals think that spiritual beliefs have psychological, medical, and financial benefits that can be and have been proved scientifically.

One of the leading proponents of the spirituality and healing movement in American medicine is Dr. Herbert Benson, a Harvard Medical School cardiologist and founder of the Mind/Body Institute. He originated the relaxation-response therapy to reduce stress in patients with hypertension, chronic pain, and other stress-related illnesses. According to Benson, many people use prayer as part of the relaxation response (Benson and Stark, 1996). The Mind/Body Medical Institute of Pathway Health Network in Boston has studied the effects of the relaxation response and asserts the following benefits (Larson, 1996):

- A 36 percent reduction in physician visits by chronic pain patients
- Significantly fewer postoperative complications in open heart surgery patients
- Lowered blood pressure and decreased use of medications in 80 percent of hypertensive patients
- A 50 percent reduction in health maintenance organization (HMO) visits by relaxation-response users

Another indication of the priority of meeting patients' spiritual needs in health care settings is the increase in chaplain presence in some inpatient and outpatient settings. More than 90 percent of the patients surveyed believed that having a chaplain available was helpful, and 60 percent were more likely to return to a hospital with a pastoral presence in an otherwise frightening and confusing environment (Larson, 1996).

Nurses can do more than call the chaplain. They can recognize the individuality and value of each patient's spiritual beliefs and encourage their use in coping with illness. Cavendish and colleagues (2000) identified eight ways nurses can help patients engage their spirituality:

- Assess human responses in the spiritual domain.
- Be present for patients.
- Allow patients to discuss beliefs in a higher power or the hereafter without introducing your own religious beliefs.
- Help patients explore what is meaningful and important in their lives.
- Value patients' inner strengths and motivations.
- Encourage patients to trust messages from an inner voice or divine providence.

- Understand that how nurses connect with patients affects patient outcomes.
- Go beyond caring for physical needs and recognize spiritual aspects of patients.

Nurses are participating in the use of spirituality in healing. St. Francis Hospital's Congregational Nurse Program in Evanston, Illinois, for example, is reaching 15,000 local families in an interfaith health project. Following training as congregational nurses, nurses spend approximately 20 hours weekly at churches and other places of worship providing classes, counseling, and referrals. They dovetail their efforts with the spiritual beliefs and customs of each congregation. As you learned in Chapter 5, the congregational/parish nurse concept is being implemented in numerous communities around the United States. By respecting and treating the whole person, these practitioners are affirming that a key dimension of health and healing is the spiritual dimension.

External Influences on Illness Behavior

External factors that bear on illness behaviors include past experiences and cultural group membership. Both directly influence how an individual perceives and responds to illness. The values that guide feelings about illness and steer a person toward particular methods of treatment are acquired primarily in the family of origin and in the culture.

Past experiences

Adults who were pampered during childhood illnesses may accept being ill fairly easily. Relying on others for care may not bother them, and they may settle into the sick role easily. Adults who received childhood messages such as "It is weak to be ill" or "One must keep going even when not feeling well" may have difficulty accepting illness and the restrictions that accompany it. Still other adults who experienced traumatic hospitalizations as children or who were threatened with injections for misbehaving may see hospitals and nurses as threatening. Clearly, these adults behave differently when ill.

Nurses should determine the patient's past experiences with illness and the health care system during a careful admission assessment. They can then use these findings to individualize care.

Culture

Culture is a pattern of learned behavior and values that are reinforced through social interactions, shared by members of a particular group, and transmitted from one generation to the next. Culture exerts considerable influence over most of an individual's life experiences, including illness. Meanings attached to illness and perceptions of treatment are affected to a large degree by a person's culture. Culture determines when one seeks help and the type of practitioner consulted. It also prescribes customs of responding to the sick. Culture defines whether illness is seen as a punishment for misdeeds or as the result of inadequate personal health practices. It influences whether one goes to an acupuncturist, an herbalist, a folk healer, or a traditional physician.

Beginning in the early 1970s, schools of nursing began including cultural concepts in their curricula. Increasing numbers of universities and colleges offered graduate programs in transcultural nursing. The Transcultural Nursing Society was legally incorporated in 1981, and in 1988 it began certifying nurses in transcultural nursing. Through oral and written examinations and evaluation of educational background and working experiences, a qualified nurse can become a certified transcultural nurse (CTN) (Andrews, 1992).

The Transcultural Nursing Society began publishing the *Journal of Transcultural Nursing* in 1989. By 1993, a resolution was adopted by the American Nurses Association's House of Delegates to identify and determine strategies to promote diverse and multicultural nursing in the workforce (Kirkpatrick and Deloughery, 1995). Changes in the nursing workforce are needed in order to deal more effectively with commonalities and differences in patients. Clearly, transcultural nursing is an important field of study, practice, and research and an essential one in today's increasingly diverse society.

Knowledge of a patient's culture directs the nurse in understanding behaviors and planning appropriate approaches to patient problems. Because culture may guide the patient's response to health care providers, and their interventions, it is necessary for the nurse to be knowledgeable about cultural influences. Understanding a patient's cultural background can facilitate communication and support establishing an effective nurse-patient relationship. Conversely, lack of understanding can create barriers that impede nursing care.

The shared values and beliefs in a culture enable its members to predict each other's actions. They also affect how members react to each other's behavior. When nurses work with patients from cultures about which little is known, they lack these familiar guidelines for predicting behavior. This can cause anxiety and feelings of distrust in both patient and nurse.

Stereotyping. In an effort to predict behavior, the nurse may resort to **stereotyping** patients from different cultures. It is important that nurses refrain from overgeneralizing and stereotyping members of cultures or ethnic groups that are different from their own. Individual assessment is always the best basis for care, whatever the patient's culture or ethnic group.

Communication. The nurse should keep in mind that patterns of communication are strongly influenced by culture. The Asian patient who smiles and nods may be communicating politeness and respect rather then agreeing or indicating understanding. Anglo-Americans tend to value a direct approach to problems, but in other cultures, subtlety and indirectness may be valued. Although Western culture values direct eye contact, some cultures view this as impolite, particularly direct eye contact between men and women.

Personal space and structure. The amount of **personal space** needed is another factor that varies depending on cultural experience. Some cultures use touch as a major form of communication; in others, touching between persons who are not considered family is disrespectful. Culture also has a primary influence on the type of stress its members experience at various points in their lives. Every society places stress on its members at one or more stages of development. For instance, Anglo-American adolescents are typically under great stress as they struggle with independence. Amish adolescents tend to experience less stress, because their behavior during this period of development is more rigidly prescribed by their culture.

Values. Values held by the nurse may come into conflict with patients' cultural values. In the Navajo culture, for example, great value is placed on keeping pain and discomfort to oneself. Letting others know how you feel is seen as weak. The nurse who expects patients to ask for medication when in pain may assume that the Navajo patient is comfortable when the opposite is actually the case. On the other hand, a nurse who values suffering in silence may underrate the discomfort of a patient who comes from a culture that promotes overt expression of discomfort.

Role expectations. The role expectations of nurses also vary from culture to culture. A common Anglo-American view of nurses is that they treat people as equals, are passive, and take direction from physicians. These patients feel free to ask questions of their nurses. Asians, however, may expect nurses to be authoritative, to provide directives, and to be expert practitioners who take charge. Out of respect for authority, they may not speak until spoken to and may verbally agree with anything nurses propose. The following patient case study illustrates a cultural difference between patient and nurse in expressing pain.

Cultural Expression of Pain

Mrs. L, a 42-year-old Asian woman, became ill and required surgery while visiting her daughter in the United States. Following surgery, she was placed on a patient-controlled analgesia pump (PCA). The nurse explained how she should self-administer medication when she felt pain. Mrs. L smiled and nodded her head when asked whether she understood the instructions. Much later the nurse noticed that this patient appeared to be in great pain. After talking with Mrs. L's daughter, the nurse realized that Mrs. L had not understood how to use the equipment but was unwilling to ask for additional instructions or complain of pain.

Ethnocentrism. Nurses respond to sick people based not only on their formal education but also on their own socialization and culture. All too often people are unaware of their own biases and tend to be **ethnocentric.** Ethnocentrism is the inclination to view one's own cultural group as superior to others and to view differences negatively. The nurse who identifies how personal beliefs and expectations can influence care is better able to recognize and deal with any prejudices that may impede patient care. Cultural assessment, therefore, begins with self-assessment.

To begin a cultural self-assessment, examine your own values. What behaviors do you expect from people who are ill? Toward what groups do you have prejudices or biases? The nurse who is frustrated by the difficulty of caring for a patient from a different culture may benefit from taking a few minutes to imagine what it would be like to be hospitalized in a foreign country. Candidly answering the questions in Box 17-2 will help you begin the important process of self-assessment.

Cultural assessment

An important step in meeting the challenge of providing nursing care to diverse patients is the **cultural assessment.** Cultural assessments are used to identify beliefs,

Box **17-2** **Sociocultural Self-Assessment**

Directions: Use your answers to these questions to understand your own social and cultural beliefs and expectations better.

1. To what groups do I belong? What is my cultural heritage? My socioeconomic status? My age-group? My religious affiliation?
2. How do I describe myself? What parts of the description come from the groups I belong to?
3. What kinds of contact have I had with persons from different groups? Do I assume that others have the same values and beliefs that I have?
4. What about my group affiliations do I feel proud of? Am I ethnocentric in my attitudes and behavior? What about my group affiliations would I change if I could? Why?
5. Have I ever experienced the feeling of being rejected by another group? Did this experience heighten my sensitivity to other cultures or cause me to denigrate others different from myself?
6. When I was growing up, what messages did I get from parents and friends about people from groups different from mine? Do these attitudes cause me any difficulty today?
7. What are the major stereotypes I hold about people from different groups? Do these biases help or hinder me in developing cultural sensitivity?
8. To work effectively with people from different cultural groups, what do I need to change about myself?

values, and health practices that may help or hinder nursing interventions. Dr. Madeleine Leininger, nurse anthropologist, nurse theorist, and founder of transcultural nursing, advocated that nurses routinely perform cultural assessments to determine patients' culturally specific needs. To demystify the process, it may be helpful to think of cultural assessment as "merely asking people their preferences, what they think, who we should talk to in making a decision" (Villaire, 1994, p. 138). There are numerous cultural assessment instruments available. Some of these instruments require in-depth interviews and comprehensive data gathering, which may require more time than is available in today's health care settings.

You can continue the process of becoming a culturally competent nurse by using the "Cultural Assessment Checklist" in Box 17-3. It was designed for use by home health nurses but is easily adapted for use in other settings. Its concise yet comprehensive nature takes into account the limited amount of time nurses may have to get to know new patients—but also recognizes the necessity of developing a culturally congruent plan of care if desired outcomes are to be achieved.

Culturally competent nurses take cultural differences into consideration, usually interpret patient behavior accurately, and recognize problems that need to be managed. They realize that cultural norms must be included in the plan of care to prevent conflicts between nursing goals and patient/family goals. They recognize that planning culturally congruent care is the most time effective way to achieve the

Box **17-3** **Cultural Assessment Checklist**

Patient-identified cultural/ethnic group _____
Religion _____

Etiquette and Social Customs

- Typical greeting. Form of address: Handshake appropriate? Shoes worn in home?
- Social customs before "business." Social exchanges? Refreshment?
- Direct or indirect communication patterns?

Nonverbal Patterns of Communication

- Eye contact. Is eye contact considered polite or rude?
- Tone of voice. What does a soft voice or a loud voice mean in this culture?
- Personal space. Is personal space wider or narrower than in the American culture?
- Facial expressions, gestures. What do smiles, nods, and hand gestures mean?
- Touch. When, where, and by whom can a patient be touched?

Client's Explanation of Problem

- Diagnosis. What do you call this illness? How would you describe this problem?
- Cause. What caused the problem? What might other people think is wrong with you?
- Course. How does the illness work? What does it do to you? What do you fear most about this problem?
- Treatment. How have you treated the illness? What treatment should you receive? Who in your family or community can help?
- Prognosis. How long will the problem last? Is it serious?
- Expectations. What are you hoping the nurses will do for you when we come?

Nutrition Assessment

- Pattern of meals. What is eaten? When are meals eaten?
- Sick [comfort] foods.
- Food intolerance and taboos.

Pain Assessment

- Cultural responses to pain.
- Patient's perception of pain response.

Medication Assessment

- Patient's perception of "Western" medications.
- Possible pharmacogenetic variations.

Psychosocial Assessment

- Decision maker.
- Sick role.
- Language barriers, translators.
- Cultural/ethnic community resources.

Reprinted with permission of Narayan MC: Cultural assessment in home healthcare, *Home Healthcare Nurse* 15(10):663-672, 1997.

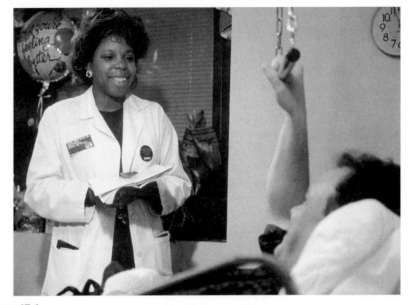

Figure 17-1
The culturally competent nurse recognizes that performing a cultural assessment is an increasingly important measure that improves the effectiveness of nursing care. (Photo by Wilson Baker.)

desired goals (Figure 17-1). In addition, being knowledgeable about other cultures promotes feelings of respect and enhances understanding of attitudes, behaviors, and the impact of illness. The accompanying Interview with Dr. Madeleine Leininger provides insights into her vast experience and strongly held beliefs about cultural competence in nursing.

IMPACT OF ILLNESS ON PATIENTS AND FAMILIES

Regardless of culture, illness results in a number of changes for both patients and families. Common experiences include behavioral and emotional changes, changes in roles, and disturbed family dynamics. Illness creates stress and other emotional responses. Factors affecting responses to illness include personality prior to illness; suddenness, extent, and duration of required lifestyle changes; individual and family resources for dealing with the stress of illness; the life-cycle stage of the patient and family; previous experiences with illness or crisis; and social support (Lewis, 1998). Religious faith also plays a role in responses to illness.

Severe illnesses that profoundly affect physical appearance and functioning are more likely to result in high levels of anxiety and extensive behavioral changes than are short-term, non–life-threatening illnesses. The impact of a chronic illness is significant and continues for the lifetime of the patient. When planning holistic nursing care, the nurse must take into consideration how the family both influences and is influenced by the illness of a family member.

Interviewer: Dr. Leininger, please tell us what you mean by the term "culturally competent."

Dr. Leininger: Culturally competent care has been defined as the culturally based knowledge with a care focus that is used in creative, meaningful, and appropriate ways to provide beneficial and satisfying care to individuals, families, groups, or communities or to help people face death or disabilities. I coined this term in 1962 as the goal of my theory of culture care diversity and universality. The term has caught hold today and is being used by many health care providers. It is now used as a requirement for JCAHO [Joint Commission on Accreditation of Healthcare Organizations] accreditation and with other organizations as essential to work effectively with cultures and their health care needs.

Interviewer: Please describe how a culturally competent nurse's patient care differs from that of one who is not culturally competent.

Dr. Leininger: A culturally competent nurse demonstrates the following attributes and skills: (1) Uses transcultural nursing concepts, principles, and available research findings to assess and guide care practices; (2) understands and values the cultural beliefs and practices of designated cultures so that nursing care is tailor-made or fits individuals' needs in meaningful ways; (3) knows how to prevent major kinds of cultural conflicts, clashes, or hurtful care practices; (4) demonstrates reasonable confidence to work effectively and knowingly with clients of different cultures and can also evaluate transcultural nursing care outcomes.

The nurse who is unable to demonstrate these culturally competent attributes often shows signs of being frustrated and impatient with people of different cultures. Moreover, the nurse who does not practice cultural competencies often shows signs of excessive ethnocentrism, biases, and related problems that impede client recovery and well-being.

Interviewer: How do patients respond differently when nurses take their cultural patterns into consideration when planning and implementing care?

Dr. Leininger: It is most encouraging to observe and listen to clients who have received culturally based nursing care. These clients often exhibit the following behaviors: (1) They show signs of being satisfied and very pleased with nurse's actions and decisions. (2) They make comments such as, "This is the best care I or my family members have received from health care providers." Frequently they say, "How did you know about my values, my culture and how to use these ideas in my care? You anticipated my needs well." (3) They appreciate the different ways the nurse incorporates their cultural needs. They express their gratitude to the nurse. (4) Clients appreciate respect for their culture shown by the nurse in care decisions and practices. (5) The clients do not experience racial biases and negative comments about their cultures or familiar lifeways.

Continued

interv i e w *with Dr. Madeleine Leininger,*
Founder of Transcultural
Nursing—cont'd

Interviewer: With so many cultural groups in this country, knowing all one needs to know about other cultures seems overwhelming. How do you advise nurses to begin the process of becoming culturally competent?

Dr. Leininger: The nurse should first enroll in a substantive transcultural nursing course to learn the basic and important concepts, principles and practices of transcultural nursing. This knowledge base is essential so the nurse becomes aware of common cultural needs and ways to work with a few cultures that are different. A few cultures are studied in-depth, focusing on common and unique cultural features. The most frequently occurring cultures in the nurse's home or local region are studied first and then one learns about other cultures over time, becoming sensitive and knowledgeable about these cultures. The nurse can greatly increase her or his knowledge of several cultures or subcultures by reading the literature, or by studying specific cultures when caring for people under transcultural mentors. Gradually, the nurse learns several cultures in a general way and a few in-depth. As the nurse becomes increasingly knowledgeable about several cultures, comparative knowledge and competencies become evident.

There is no expectation that professional nurses can know all human cultures, as this would be impossible. An open learning attitude and mind with a sincere desire to learn as much as possible about a few cultures will help the nurse in becoming culturally knowledgeable, competent, and sensitive.

Interviewer: What signs can students look for to determine whether their nursing programs are preparing them to provide culturally competent care?

Dr. Leininger: Nursing students will find they are able to provide culturally competent care when (or if) the following signs are evident:

- They consistently know, understand, and respect specific cultures and appreciate commonalities and differences among cultures.
- They feel a sense of confidence, creativity, and competence in their nursing care practices and see how their care fits specific cultures and accommodate cultural differences in meaningful and creative ways.
- They go beyond common sense to actual use of culture-specific knowledge in patient care as shown in the Sunrise Model (see Figure 11-2).
- They creatively use the clients' beliefs, values, and patterns along with appropriate professional knowledge and skills that meet clients' needs.
- They prevent racial discrimination practices in nursing and in other places; they avoid cultural imposition, ethnocentrism, cultural conflicts, cultural pain, and related negative practices.
- They value and know how to use Leininger's Culture Care Theory and basic transcultural care concepts, principles, and research findings in their nursing practices to provide culturally congruent care for people's health and well-being.

interv i e w *with Dr. Madeleine Leininger,*
Founder of Transcultural
Nursing—cont'd

- They appreciate a global perspective of nursing and value transcultural nursing to meet a growing and intense multicultural world.
- They markedly grow in their professional knowledge and sensitivities, developing a global worldview of transcultural nursing. They reach out to help cultural strangers in different living contexts.

Courtesy Dr. Madeleine Leininger.

Impact of Illness on Patients

Illness creates a variety of emotional responses. Among the more common responses are guilt, anger, anxiety, and stress.

Guilt

Individuals may experience guilt about becoming ill, particularly if the illness is related to lifestyle choices, such as smoking. Guilt may also be associated with the inability to perform usual activities because of illness. A mother who is unable to perform childcare tasks or a father who has to take a lower-paying job because of illness may experience considerable guilt. Some cultures view certain illnesses as shameful and people suffering from them as guilty of cultural transgressions. Nurses who identify and encourage patients to discuss guilt feelings may help prevent the depression that can be a consequence of illness-induced alterations in lifestyle.

Anger

Anger is another common emotional response to illness, particularly in the Anglo-American culture. When patients must make sacrifices to manage their illnesses, such as giving up favorite foods or activities, they may experience anger about the changes. At times, they may feel that their bodies have betrayed them, which results in self-directed anger. Anger may also be directed toward caregivers for their inability to produce a cure, reduce pain, or prevent negative consequences of the illness. Nurses must be prepared to accept such angry feelings, to refrain from rejecting or avoiding patients who express their fears through anger, and to encourage the adaptive expression of angry feelings.

Anxiety

Anxiety is a common and universal experience. It is also a common emotional response to illness and hospitalization. Anxiety is an ill-defined, diffuse feeling of apprehension and uncertainty (Ellis and Nowlis, 1994). Anxiety occurs as a result of some threat to an individual's selfhood, self-esteem, or identity.

A number of threats are associated with illness. Illness may alter the way people view themselves. Some illnesses result in a change in physical appearance. Often, ability to function is affected, altering relationships, work performance, and abilities to meet others' expectations. In addition, there may be concern about pain and discomfort associated with illness or treatment. Because of real and potential threats and changes arising from illness, nurses must develop skills that enable them to help patients recognize and manage anxiety.

Although the responses are similar, there is general agreement that anxiety and fear are different. Fear results from specific known causes, whereas with anxiety the cause of the feelings is unknown (Ellis and Nowlis, 1994). For example, if you are home alone at night and you hear an unusual noise outside, most likely, your heartbeat and respirations increase, your stomach tightens, and you perspire. The emotion in this situation is fear of an intruder. If you begin to have the same feelings but have heard no noises and cannot identify a source of fear, you are experiencing anxiety. Both emotions may be present at the same time. The patient who is in the hospital for an operation may experience anxiety about the unknown consequences of the surgery and fear of pain and disfigurement from the procedure itself.

Symptoms of anxiety. Nurses should be familiar with the numerous symptoms of anxiety. They are classified as physiological, emotional, and cognitive. Physiological symptoms include increased heart rate, respirations, and blood pressure; insomnia; nausea and vomiting; fatigue; sweaty palms; and tremors. Emotional responses include restlessness, irritability, feelings of helplessness, crying, and depression. Cognitive symptoms include inability to concentrate, forgetfulness, inattention to surroundings, and preoccupation.

Responses to anxiety. Responses to anxiety occur on a continuum. Peplau (1963) described four levels: mild, moderate, severe, and panic. A mild level is characterized by increased alertness and ability to focus attention and concentrate. There is an expanded capacity for learning at this stage.

A person with a moderate level of anxiety is able to concentrate on only one thing at a time. Frequently, there is increased body movement (restlessness), more rapid speech, and a subjective awareness of discomfort.

At the severe level, thoughts become scattered. The severely anxious person may not be able to communicate verbally, and there is considerable discomfort accompanied by purposeless movements such as handwringing and pacing.

At the panic level, the person becomes completely disorganized and loses the ability to differentiate between reality and unreality. There are constant random and purposeless movements. The individual experiencing panic levels of anxiety is unable to function without assistance. Panic levels of anxiety cannot be continued indefinitely, because the body will become exhausted, and death may occur if the anxiety is not reduced. Box 17-4 lists the characteristics of each level of anxiety.

Because anxiety is such a common response to illness and hospitalization, nurses often encounter patients who are experiencing mild or moderate anxiety and, occasionally, patients who are severely anxious. When interacting with an anxious patient, the nurse should carefully assess the level of anxiety before attempting to develop the plan of care.

According to Peplau (1963), anxiety is communicated interpersonally. In other words, it is "contagious." For this reason, it is crucial that the nurse be aware of and manage personal anxiety so that it is not inadvertently transferred to patients. Likewise, self-awareness is essential to prevent absorbing patients' anxiety.

Box **17-4** Levels of Anxiety

Mild Anxiety

- Increased alertness, increased ability to focus, improved concentration, expanded capacity for learning.

Moderate Anxiety

- Concentration limited to one thing, increased body movement, rapid speech, subjective awareness of discomfort.

Severe Anxiety

- Scattered thoughts, difficulty with verbal communication, considerable discomfort, purposeless movements.

Panic

- Complete disorganization, difficulty differentiating reality from unreality, constant random movements, unable to function without assistance.

Stress

Stress is another internal variable that affects patients. Stress is both a response to illness and an important factor in the development of illness. Because illness and hospitalization involve so many alterations in lifestyle, they tend to cause a great deal of stress.

Stress is an unavoidable and essential part of life. To survive and grow, individuals must cope adaptively with constantly changing demands. The stress related to examinations, for example, motivates most students to grow by studying and learning. Although stress is unavoidable, and even sometimes desirable, some control can be exerted over the number and types of **stressors** encountered, and responses to the stressors can often be managed.

Hospitalized patients are removed from their usual support systems. They lose much of their control because nurses and other care providers make decisions for them. Being ill often means that they are no longer able to perform activities as they did before the illness occurred. Some patients find themselves in the role of comforting other family members rather than being comforted to avoid increasing family members' distress. Stress is a common response to all these circumstances.

Differentiating between stress and anxiety. Stress and anxiety have some characteristics in common. The physiological responses are similar. Anxiety is a response to some real or perceived threat to the individual, whereas stress is an interaction between the individual and the environment. Stress includes all the responses the body makes while striving to maintain equilibrium and deal with demands. The following Case Study describes one example of stress and anxiety.

Internal, external, and interpersonal stressors. Selye (1956) defined stress as the nonspecific response of the body to any demand made upon it. He named this

Stress and Anxiety

Mary S is a 32-year-old single mother and a lawyer who was recently hired by an established law firm. One morning as she prepares to take her 2-year-old daughter to the child care center, she receives a call saying that the day care center owner was severely injured in an accident and will be closing the center indefinitely. Ms. S experiences both stress and anxiety in this situation. She has a number of demands placed on her from her workplace and from her family that lead to stress.

The additional demands caused by the sudden change in her plans results in even higher levels of stress. In addition, even though none of the male lawyers has responsibility for child care, Ms. S has placed the expectation on herself that she will perform her job exactly like the men in the firm. Being late or missing work as a result of making new arrangements for child care conflicts with her self-expectations and poses a threat to her self-esteem. This threat leads to feelings of anxiety.

response the *general adaptation syndrome* and identified three stages through which the body progresses while responding to stress.

Stressors trigger the body's stress response. Stressors are agents, or stimuli, that an individual perceives as posing a threat to homeostasis. Stressors may come from external, interpersonal, or internal sources. External stressors include such things as noise, heat, cold, malfunctioning equipment (such as a car that will not run), or organizational rules and expectations. Interpersonal sources of stress include the demands made by others and conflicts with others. Placing unrealistic expectations on oneself is an example of an internal stressor. In the example of Mary S, an internal stressor is her expectation that her child care responsibilities will not affect the hours she works. It is an unrealistic expectation for any single parent of a small child to expect that the child's needs will never interfere with work.

Responses to stress. Outward responses to stress are determined by the individual's perception of the stressor. Cognitive appraisal, or the way one thinks about a specific situation, determines the degree to which the situation is considered stressful. For example, adolescents may perceive loud music at a rock concert considerably less stressful than their parents do.

Another factor related to the assessment of threat is whether the individual feels capable of handling the threat, that is, whether the person exhibits hardiness. The person who feels capable can be expected to feel less stress than the person who does not generally feel competent.

Stress affects the physical, emotional, and cognitive areas of functioning just as anxiety does. Physically, there is a feeling of fatigue; muscles are tight and tense. There is an increase in heart rate and respiration. The person who is under prolonged stress may be unable to sleep or eat, or there may be excessive sleeping or eating in an attempt to avoid or cope with the stress.

Emotionally, people under stress feel drained and unable to care for themselves or others. This can result in social isolation and distancing from others. They experience difficulty with enjoying life. They may have feelings of hopelessness and of being out of control. Irritability and impatience often occur.

Cognitively, stress causes decreased mental capacity and problem-solving skills. Therefore, there is a tendency to have difficulty making decisions.

Stress and illness. It has been known for some time that stress plays a major role in the development of illness. More recent research has provided better understanding of the links between prolonged stress and body functioning.

The person who is under stress for long periods of time is at risk for a number of physical problems. The exhaustion that results from excessive, unmanaged stress leads to physiological breakdowns and predisposition to a number of problems. Disorders such as peptic ulcers, hypertension, and rheumatoid arthritis have been termed *stress-related diseases* because they frequently occur in individuals who have been severely stressed.

Stress has been found to be related to a reduction in the immune response, which can delay healing and result in greater susceptibility to infectious disorders such as colds and flu. Long-term studies of persons with medical illnesses revealed that the more stress people experienced in a given year, the more likely they were to develop physical illness.

Coping with stress. Nurses have a role in helping patients modify their stressors. They should assess patients' abilities to recognize symptoms of stress and their usual methods of coping.

Coping with stress can be direct or indirect. In assisting patients to use direct coping, nurses assist patients to identify those situations that can be changed and to take responsibility for changing them. The focus is on using problem-solving skills and planning to eliminate or avoid as many stressors as possible. It is important to realize that completely eliminating stress from one's life is neither possible nor desirable.

In helping patients use indirect coping, nurses' actions are aimed at reducing the affective (feelings) and physiological (bodily) disturbances resulting from stress. Patients are taught techniques such as deep breathing, muscle relaxation, and imagery, which help them cope more effectively with stress (Boxes 17-5 and 17-6).

To help patients to manage stress, nurses must be skilled in assessing and managing their own personal stress. Nurses who are feeling stressed themselves have difficulty

---

Box 17-5 **Breathing Exercises**

1. Sit comfortably with feet on the floor and eyes closed.
2. Inhale slowly and deeply through the nose and fill the lungs completely. As you breathe in, imagine the oxygen flowing to all your cells. Hold your breath while slowly counting to 4.
3. Slowly release all the air while thinking the word *calm.* As you breathe out, imagine the air taking all the tension out with it.
4. Repeat the cycle four times. Try to banish all thoughts except those related to your breathing, but don't fight them if other thoughts creep in.
5. When you have completed the exercise, open your eyes slowly and sit for a moment before resuming your regular activities.

| Box 17-6 | Relaxation Exercises |

Get into a comfortable position in a place where you will not be interrupted. First focus on slow, deep breathing. Close your eyes and begin to think about the muscle sensations in your body. Identify where you are feeling tense. Slowly inhale as you stretch like a cat; then exhale and allow the tension to flow out.

Neck and Shoulders

- Slowly bend your head forward and backward, then side to side three times. Bring your shoulders up as if you were trying to touch them to your ears. Slowly relax and feel the difference in tension.

Arms and Hands

- Make a tight fist in one hand and tighten the muscles throughout your arm. Slowly release the muscles from the shoulder to the hand. Repeat with the other arm and hand.

Head

- Make a wide smile and hold for a count of five. Slowly relax your face muscles and let your jaw go loose. Tightly close your eyes and feel the tension. Slowly give up the tension and allow your eyes to remain gently closed.

Stomach

- Make your stomach muscles tight by pushing them out as far as possible. Make your stomach hard and feel the tension. Slowly relax your muscles and notice the difference.

Legs and Feet

- Holding your leg still, curl your toes down to point to the floor. Do first one leg and then the other. As you tighten your muscles, feel the tension. Then slowly relax.

Sit quietly for a few moments and feel the relaxation in your body before you resume your activities.

assisting patients in dealing with similar problems. The questions in Box 17-7 can help you identify your own sources of stress and develop self-awareness so that you can be effective in helping patients deal with their stress. For further exploration of stress management approaches, complete the University of Chicago Hospitals' self-study module online *(www.nsweb.nursingspectrum.com/ce/ce88.htm)*.

Coping with stress through learning. Patient education is a major part of nursing practice, and nurses have a professional responsibility to ensure that their patients' learning needs are met. When patients are competent in the knowledge and skills they need to manage their illnesses, they tend to feel more masterful and less stressed.

Box **17-7** Personal Stress Inventory	Very Often	Sometimes	Rarely or Never

1. I feel tense and anxious and have some nervous indigestion.
2. People at home, school, or work make me feel tense.
3. I eat, drink, or smoke in response to tension.
4. I have tension or pain in my neck or shoulders.
5. I have headaches or insomnia.
6. I have trouble turning off my thoughts long enough to feel relaxed.
7. I find it difficult to concentrate on what I am doing because I worry about other things.
8. I use alcohol, tranquilizers, or other medications to relax or sleep.
9. I feel a lot of pressure at work or school.
10. I do not feel that my work is appreciated.
11. My family does not appreciate what I do for them.
12. I feel I do not have enough time for myself.
13. I have difficulty saying "no."
14. I wish I had more friends with whom to share experiences.
15. I do not have enough time for physical exercise.

Scoring: Give yourself 2 points for every check in the Very Often column, 1 point for every check in the Sometimes column, and 0 points for every check in the Rarely or Never column. Total the number of points. A score of 20 to 30 represents a high level of stress. If you scored in this range, you should take steps to reduce your stress level. A score from 10 to 19 means that you are experiencing midlevel stress. You should monitor your stress and begin relaxation exercises. A score of 9 or under means that you are experiencing relatively low stress at the present time.

Nurses can assist patients in acquiring new methods of coping with stressors through learning, but first they must identify factors that can create barriers to learning. One factor is anxiety. Mild anxiety improves learning by increasing the ability to focus on the task. As anxiety increases, however, the ability to listen, pay attention, and concentrate decreases. Information is not retained, and the patient is unable to make the cognitive connections required for learning to take place.

Physiological factors may also impede learning. For instance, visual or hearing deficits must be overcome. Unmet physiological needs, such as fatigue, shortness of breath, hunger, and thirst, decrease the patient's attention to learning. Pain dramatically impairs the ability to learn. Nurses who ensure that patients' physiological needs are met enhance their readiness to learn.

Culture also influences learning. This is especially true when patient and nurse have different languages and patterns of learning. When the nurse works toward an educational goal that is not seen as desirable by a patient of a different culture, their cultural values may be in conflict. Understanding the meaning of illness in the patient's culture is necessary. Communicating in language and with handouts that the patient can understand (written in the patient's native language and at an appropriate reading level) is important. Learning a few words of the patient's language and obtaining the services of an interpreter also show sensitivity to cultural differences.

Lack of motivation and readiness are often significant barriers to education. The patient may still be reeling from an unexpected adverse diagnosis and may not be able to focus on learning. The patient may not be motivated to learn what the nurse believes is important to teach. Often, nurses believe that simply pointing out what patients need to know is sufficient to motivate them. It is usually more effective to assist patients to make their own decisions about the knowledge they need. This approach may require greater effort initially, but it is ultimately more efficient to assess patient motivation and readiness first, before engaging in patient teaching.

The nurse who is preparing to teach should also assess and manage the environment. A setting that is private, comfortable, and free of distractions is beneficial to the learning process. Boxes 17-8 and 17-9 review several simple principles of adult learning and teaching-learning concepts that are useful in working with patients.

Impact of Illness on Families

Families are best understood as systems, which means that change in one member changes the functioning of the total family. It is important to remember that the

---

Box 17-8 | **Principles of Adult Learning**

- Prior experiences are resources for learning.
  Example: If the patient enjoys gardening, try to link health maintenance suggestions to preventive maintenance of indoor/outdoor plants.
- Readiness to learn is usually related to a social role or developmental task.
  Example: New parents are usually eager to learn how to care for their first infants.
- Motivation to learn is greater when the material is seen as immediately useful.
  Example: The same new parents are more motivated to learn care of the small infant than they are to learn about disciplining toddlers.
- The learning environment must be arranged to facilitate learning.
  Example: The room is quiet, kept at a comfortable temperature, with adequate lighting, privacy, and seating.
- Physical needs are met prior to teaching session.
  Example: The patient has his or her reading glasses and/or hearing aid, has been given the opportunity to toilet, and is relatively pain free.

Box **17-9** Basic Teaching Tips for Patients and Families

- There may be barriers to learning, such as anxiety or physical/mental impairments.
- It is important to evaluate what the patient and family already know.
- Frequent, short sessions work better than long ones.
- Goals for each session must be realistic.
- Be respectful of cultural differences—for example, in diet planning.
- The presentation should proceed from simple to complex concepts.
- Present complex concepts only after there is mastery of simpler ones.
- Patients learn best when they are actively engaged.
- Learning is enhanced when multiple senses are used: seeing, hearing, telling, and doing make the best combination.
- Practice, or frequent repetition, reinforces skill acquisition.
- Reinforce learning with return demonstrations of skills.
- When you give feedback, be sure to include positives, as well as negatives.
- Written materials should be at a fourth-grade reading level and, if possible, in the patient's native language to make reading easier for the patient.
- Evaluate patient's understanding of the information presented.
- Remember to document the teaching session and your evaluation of the outcome.

entire family system is affected by a member's illness. Whether the ill family member is hospitalized or cared for in the home, illness drastically increases stress in a family and disrupts usual family function.

The most important factor in how a family tolerates stress is the individual and group coping abilities. Families already experiencing difficulties may find that their problems are intensified to the point of disruption when acute or chronic illness occurs.

A sick family member has to give up responsibility to other family members. The family must continue to fulfill its usual functions while dealing with the alterations imposed by the illness or absence of a member. Family members who are able to shift and assume different roles, who can share their feelings, and who seek assistance can be expected to adjust to changes better than those who are inflexible.

Both acute and chronic illness cause changes in family functioning. Chronic illness can be particularly stressful because it is never completely cured. Families experience emotional highs and lows as the patient has remissions and exacerbations. Resentment may be experienced. Family members who must take over the sick person's responsibilities may be angry and then feel guilty about their anger. If they cannot deal with feelings of anger, they may displace them onto nurses by becoming critical and demanding. Similarly, patients may feel guilty about creating hardships for loved ones. They may become convinced that they are no longer essential because others are capably taking over their roles.

Family members sometimes withdraw from each other because they fear that their negative feelings may not be understood and accepted. This mutual withdrawal leads to feelings of isolation for both patients and family members.

Families are often confused or uncertain about how to treat the sick member. They may have problems accepting and responding appropriately to the patients' dependency needs. As discussed earlier, patients may react to illness with either overly dependent or overly independent behaviors. Nurses need to monitor whether family members foster dependence, thereby keeping the patient from becoming more independent. Nurses should also be aware that some families are uncomfortable with the ill person being in a dependent role and do not allow the necessary dependency for recovery. For example, if a man who is very much in control in a family has a heart attack and is in the coronary care unit, family members may have difficulty seeing the usually strong father in a helpless position. They may continue to bring family problems to him. Other families may find it difficult to shift responsibilities back to the formerly ill member as he or she becomes able to resume role functions, thereby fostering dependence. Research Note 2 shows how illness affects family roles.

The nurse needs to recognize the anxiety in the family and take steps to reduce it. Talking with family members, explaining what is happening and what to expect, and teaching them how to participate in their loved one's care can help the family considerably. Some families find that becoming active in seeking information, such as through the Internet, helps them manage their anxieties. Support groups

☀ RESEARCH note 2

Research on how illness affects family roles increases the knowledge base needed to develop effective nursing interventions to meet family needs. Johnson and colleagues undertook a study designed to identify the changes in family roles and responsibilities resulting from the hospitalization of a family member in a critical care unit. They also studied how these changes were affected by the passage of time.

The study involved 52 family members who visited patients in critical care units in a large Midwestern medical center. The subjects completed the Iowa ICU Family Scale each day during the first week and weekly thereafter as long as the patient remained in the unit. Family members were asked to describe changes in family roles and responsibilities. Approximately 59 percent reported that they experienced changes in family roles or responsibilities as a result of the hospitalization. Qualitative analysis of their responses identified seven themes: (1) pulling together, (2) fragmentation, (3) increased dependence, (4) increased independence, (5) increased responsibilities, (6) change in routine, and (7) change in feelings. The researchers recommended that further research be conducted to examine how family roles vary within family systems.

Adapted with permission of Johnson S, Craft M, Titler M, et al: Perceived changes in adult family members' roles and responsibilities during critical illness, *Image J Nurs Sch* 27(3):238-243, 1995. Copyright 1995 by Sigma Theta Tau International.

and chat rooms, where family members can express their concerns and hear from others with similar issues, are also helpful. Nurses can help family members use these adaptive coping activities effectively by assisting them to find credible websites and evaluate the information they find online. Box 17-10 lists seven "levels of evidence" within health care literature, ranging from least reliable and trustworthy to most reliable and trustworthy.

Other families find that activism helps them control their anxiety. The News Note on p. 484 tells how one man's activism has become a powerful force in the search for a cure for a rare form of abdominal cancer.

The nurse should assess family functioning and the ability of the family to provide support for the patient within the family's cultural context. Observe for feelings of anger, resentment, and guilt and assist the family in identifying adaptive methods of expressing these feelings. The nurse needs to determine the level of knowledge of the family members and assist them to identify concerns and make realistic plans. Providing information and including the family in the planning can result in increased support for the patient and in effective care.

Nurses must be prepared to accept the anger and distrust that often is directed toward care providers who are unable to cure disease or relieve the negative consequences of illness. Understanding that anger expressed by patients and families is not personally directed can enable nurses to assess patients objectively and respond to feelings expressed in a nondefensive manner.

Despite the numerous stresses and adjustments necessitated by illness of a family member, many families find that there are also positive experiences. Finding new activities to share and working together to meet challenges can lead to feelings of closeness that were not present before. Previously unrecognized individual strengths may be identified as new roles and responsibilities are assumed.

Box 17-10 Seven Levels of Evidence

Patients, families, and nurses must bear in mind that not all published material, including material found on the Internet, has merit. It may or may not be based on evidence. Listed below are seven levels of evidence, ranging from least reliable to most reliable.

- Level 1: Ideas, editorials, letters, and opinion papers.
- Level 2: Case reports, case studies, and reports of unusual happenings, such as adverse reactions.
- Level 3: Information based on laboratory studies.
- Level 4: Information based on animal studies.
- Levels 5 and 6: Studies involving human subjects with increasing levels of complexity, scope, and rigor (for example, systematic research reviews, research-based protocols, and clinical practice guidelines).
- Level 7: Clinical trials are the "gold standard," but many problems are not amenable to clinical trials.

Adapted from McKibbon A: *PDQ: evidence-based principles and practice,* Hamilton, Ontario, BC, 1999, Decker, pp 7-12.

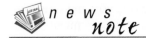

Norman Scherzer was compelled to look for help on the Internet following his wife Anita's diagnosis with abdominal cancer. In a patient-run chat room he discovered information about another, more aggressive type of cancer that seemed to match her symptoms more closely. This led the Scherzers to a physician who confirmed a different diagnosis: gastrointestinal stromal tumor (GIST). GIST, Mr. Scherzer learned online, is a rare but deadly cancer that seemed to show a positive response to the drug Gleevec, originally made to treat leukemia. He also learned on the Internet that a clinical trial of Gleevec with GIST patients was under way. Anita had not responded to conventional chemotherapy and her husband succeeded in getting her into the new clinical trial in August 2000. As a result her tumors shrank by 75 percent, and the Scherzers were able to celebrate their fortieth wedding anniversary in the Fall of 2001.

Mr. Scherzer went on to develop a website, newsletter, and establish a group he termed the *Life Raft Group (www.liferaftgroup.org)*. The group grew from three original members to over 125 GIST patients and their caregivers. They share information about Gleevec with each other, doctors, and the company that makes the drug, Novartis AG. The Life Raft Group studied side effects from the drug and presented their findings to Novartis. They also published the report on their website.

This is a prime example of how patient activists are using the Web in new ways to help others find reliable, comprehensive yet understandable health information online.

Modified from Landro L: The best way to get reliable health information, *The Wall Street Journal,* November 12, 2001, p R10.

New meanings for the entire family may emerge as values are reassessed and priorities are shifted.

IMPACT OF CAREGIVING ON NURSES

A caring attitude towards patients, their families, and colleagues begins with the caregiver—the nurse. Most nurses are not accustomed to caring for themselves, tending to put the needs of others before their own. Finding a balance between caring for others and self-care can be a challenging, lifelong pursuit.

Caring for Self While Caring for Others

Nurses often report that the needs of patients and families, as well as their own spouses and children, take priority over their own needs and they are left feeling stretched, overwhelmed, frustrated, unappreciated, and resentful. This has been termed *compassion fatigue* (Henry and Henry, 2004). Negative feelings interfere with the ability to maintain a caring attitude and drain caring out of our interactions with others. One nurse stated it well: "As a registered nurse, I try to connect with patients the best I can. Trust develops with personal rapport. When I'm busy and overworked, I become task oriented and don't have time to work on the trust building" (Roy, Turkel, and Marino, 2002, p. 10). Another used the empty pitcher analogy: "When I have given all I can give, I can't give any more until I get my own pitcher refilled" (Kelly, 2003).

Although the NANDA diagnosis *caregiver role strain* refers to family caregivers, not professional nurses, some of the defining characteristics of this diagnosis are the same for nurses: anger, stress, impatience, increased emotional lability, frustration, lack of time to meet personal needs, low work productivity, GI upset, difficulty performing/completing required tasks, lack of support, and insufficient time (NANDA, 2003, pp. 28-30). These descriptors could also be applied to nurses who feel overwhelmed with competing demands in their work and professional lives.

Nursing theorist Jean Watson referred to caring as the essence of nursing practice. Caregivers who are filled with stress and negativity cannot provide an atmosphere conducive to healing. The inescapable conclusion is that we must learn to care for ourselves in order to truly care for others. Diann Uustal (1997) refers to this as "creating a balanced life rather than merely maintaining a balancing act" (p. 19). She reminds us of the announcement heard before every airline departure, "… put on your own oxygen mask first, before assisting others who may need it" (p. 25). That announcement has a lot of relevance to our lives as professional caregivers. Just as airline passengers in an emergency depressurization need oxygen before they can help others, nurses need to meet their own needs so that they will have the physical and emotional energy to care for others.

There is probably no more stressful working environment for nurses today than the hospital. Because of the nursing shortage, nursing leaders in hospitals are focusing on retention, and they realize that the atmosphere can help nurses cope with stress in the workplace. One example can be seen in the initiatives designed to create a "Caring Practice Environment" at Hamilton Medical Center in Dalton, Georgia (Wisdom, 2003):

- Development of a caring vision, mission, and philosophy for the department of nursing, involving all the nurses through surveys, focus groups, and interviews.
- Implementation of Caring Groups, monthly meetings with trained facilitators to promote humor, stress reduction, conflict resolution, and focus on care for self and fellow nurses.
- A caring/healing room, open 24 hours a day, that offers massage therapy, paraffin treatments for hands and feet, aromatherapy, and soothing music. These services are available on a rotating and as-needed basis.
- Incorporation of new graduate nurses into a mentoring program with veteran nurses to help them integrate both clinically and socially into the world of nursing and to the caring environment.

Other activities are being planned.

The Magnet Recognition Program

Choosing to work in a milieu that supports professional nursing practice is another strategy to reduce the stress nurses feel while at work. The American Nurses Credentialing Center's Magnet Recognition Program formally recognizes health care organizations that have a proven level of excellence in nursing care. The Magnet program was developed by the ANCC "to recognize health care organizations that provide the very best in nursing care and uphold the tradition of professional nursing practice" (ANCC, 2003). Achieving Magnet designation demonstrates the importance of nursing and nurses to the entire organization. It recognizes the caliber of the nursing staff, which validates nurses for their hard work and elevates the self-esteem of the entire nursing staff.

As of March 2004, there were 101 Magnet-designated health care facilities in the United States. These facilities are "nurse friendly" and have low turnover and vacancy rates, demonstrating that they are desirable places for nurses to work. You can find out about Magnet facilities in your state at the ANCC's website *(www.nursingworld.org/ancc/magnet/facilities.html).*

Developing a Balanced Life

Keeping the balance between work and personal responsibilities takes conscious and continuous effort. Just as nurses use care plans to organize how they care for patients, they can also identify how to create balance in their own lives. Diann Uustal, in her book *Caring for Yourself, Caring for Others: The Ultimate Balance* (1997), recommends taking stock periodically using the guidelines listed in Box 17-11. This can be the beginning of a lifelong effort to maintain balance so that you can continue to be the caring person you want to be in all your life roles, personal and professional.

Summary of Key Points

- Illness is a highly personal experience.
- Reactions to illness are culturally determined.
- Sick people may progress through stages of disbelief and denial, irritability and anger, attempting to gain control, depression, and acceptance and participation.
- Although every culture has expectations about how sick people should behave, previous experience and personality characteristics also affect individuals' responses to illness.
- Culturally competent nurses perform cultural assessments to determine how best to work with patients and families.
- Because of the stress and anxiety involved with illness, it is important for the individual to have methods of coping.
- Coping ability is enhanced in people who exhibit personality characteristics of hardiness, learned resourcefulness, and resilience.
- Spiritual beliefs often play a role in stress reduction.
- Providing holistic care means that nurses must consider their patients' physical, mental, emotional, spiritual, social, cultural, and family strengths and challenges to personalize care.
- The family is a system in which a change in one member affects all the other members.
- Illness causes alterations in usual family functioning that can result in feelings of anger and guilt.
- The nurse needs to assess both how the family is influencing the patient and how they are being influenced by the member who is ill.

| Box **17-11** | **Create a Balanced Life Care Plan for Yourself** |

Read the following ideas and reflect on their practical application in your life.

- Taking personal responsibility for your health—physically, emotionally, intellectually, socially, and spiritually—is not easy, but it's the first step. Like it or not, there's no one who can do a better job of taking care of yourself than you.
- Start today with the changes you know are healthful. Make your choices one meal at a time or one day at a time. Don't beat yourself up if you don't always stick to the care plan.
- Balance. Try to stay in balance from a holistic perspective. What this means is different to each of us and different at various stages in our own lives.
- Increase your happiness quotient. Identify the things that bring you happiness and joy and enhance your quality of life. Try to do something pleasurable or satisfying each day.
- Identify and decrease the stressors in your personal and professional life. Develop strategies for decreasing the overall level of stress in your life. Some situations and habits can be corrected easily; others will take a real commitment and time to change.
- Make sure your goals and expectations are realistic. Unrealistic goals are self-defeating. Make sure the goals are measurable, manageable, and meaningful to you, not to please somebody else.
- Give yourself permission to relax and take some time for yourself each day. Learn to take "mental health breaks," no matter how brief. Enjoy the time without thinking about what you should be doing, so you can return refreshed.
- Prioritize your commitments based on your values. Make sure you give appropriate time and attention to the relationships that have stability and meaning over time.
- Learn to say "no" if you are pressured and overcommitted. Learn to say no without feeling guilty. Practice thinking that every problem is not your sole responsibility.
- Treat yourself like you treat your best friend. Do something special and "be-friend" yourself.
- Be a person of encouragement—to yourself. Be affirming to yourself. Don't "dump" on yourself or put yourself down.
- Make your physical fitness a priority. Commit to a balanced fitness program that includes stretching, aerobic exercise, and strength exercises. Sneak exercise into your daily life and exercise with a friend.
- Nutrition. Eat a balanced diet low in fat and cholesterol; take a multivitamin; drink lots of water and limit refined sugar intake. Practice portion control. If necessary, consult a dietitian.
- Sleep. Know how much you need and plan to get it. A pattern of too little sleep can injure your health. Avoid trying to be more productive by sleeping less. That can be counterproductive.
- Pay attention to your spiritual growth. Is your faith a first resort or a last resort when all else fails? What does it mean to be "spiritual?" Is being a part of a faith community important to you?

Continued

Box **17-11** Create a Balanced Life Care Plan for Yourself—cont'd

- Challenge yourself intellectually and develop your intellectual curiosity. Try to learn something new every day, no mater how small or insignificant it may seem.
- Stay connected with healthy people. Set time aside and plan for fun with people who can help you lighten up and enjoy some free time. Get out and do things you enjoy doing.
- Try a little "creative neglect" with the "basement people" (we all have them) in your life, especially when you are tired or handling too much. Spend as little time as possible with people who affect you negatively.
- Make sure you get enough "alone time." How much time alone each of us needs varies, so find out what's right for you. Most caregivers spend very little time alone. Check out your balance.
- Express your creativity through music, painting, needlework, sports, decorating, acting, or whatever lets you share yourself from the inside out.
- Don't be afraid to talk with a friend or a professional counselor to help you clarify your direction and put you back in balance again.

Reproduced from Uustal DB: *Caring for yourself, caring for others: the ultimate balance,* Jamestown, RI, 1997, Sea Spirit Press, Educational Resources in HealthCare, Inc., pp 113-116.

- An understanding of the cultural factors that affect behaviors associated with illness can provide a better framework for the delivery of nursing care that is both effective and satisfying to patients, families, and nurses.
- As nurses view responses to illness in a cultural context, they are better able to understand and accept the unique ways in which individuals and families react to illness, thereby providing more effective nursing care.
- Creating a balanced life, in which caring for self has a high priority, is the key to sustaining a caring approach to others.

CRITICAL THINKING QUESTIONS

1. Think of your most recent illness. Can you identify any benefits you gained from being ill? If this seems like a strange question, think about it some more.
2. If you or someone close to you has been hospitalized, how did the nurses encourage or discourage dependent behaviors? Independent behaviors?
3. Would it be easy or hard to allow yourself to be bathed and have other intimate needs met by nurses of the same gender? Of the opposite gender? Of your cultural group? Of a different cultural group? Identify the reasons for your comfort or discomfort.
4. If possible, identify your own cultural group's response to illness. What are your family's characteristic responses to illness of a member?
5. Interview someone from another cultural background to learn how he or she perceives illness. Prepare several specific questions to ask about the meaning, causes, treatment, and feelings engendered by both acute and chronic illnesses. How does his or her culture tend to view nurses?

6. Speculate about the potential changes in the family of a husband and father of four small children who has experienced a severe illness and will be unable to work for an extended period. What stresses is this family likely to encounter? How would these stresses be different if his wife (the mother of the four children) were the sick family member?

7. Working in a small group, design a nurse friendly work setting and present it to the entire class. Be prepared to give rationales for your choices.

REFERENCES

American Nurses Credentialing Center: ANCC magnet program: recognizing excellence in nursing services, Online, 2003 *(www.nursingworld.org/ancc/magnet.html)*.

Andrews MM: Cultural perspectives on nursing in the 21st century, *J Prof Nurs* 8(1):7-15, 1992.

Benson H, Stark M: *Timeless healing,* New York, 1996, Scribner.

Bowsher J, Keep D: Toward an understanding of three control constructs: Personal control, self-efficacy, and hardiness, *Issues Ment Health Nurs* 16(1):33-50, 1995.

Cassidy CA: Using the transtheoretical model to facilitate behavior change in patients with chronic illness, *J Am Acad Nurse Pract* 11(7):281-287, 1999.

Cavendish R, Luise BK, Horne K, et al: Opportunities for enhanced spirituality relevant to well adults, *Nurs Diagn* 11(4):151-163, 2000.

Chilton B: Recognizing spirituality, *Image J Nurs Sch* 30:400-401, 1998.

Dewar AL, Lee EA: Bearing illness and injury, *West J Nurs Res* 22(8):912-926, 2000.

Ellis J, Nowlis E: *Nursing: a human needs approach,* ed 5, Philadelphia, 1994, JB Lippincott.

Henry J, Henry L: Self-care begets holistic care, *Reflec Nurs Lead* 30(1):26-27, 2004.

Humphreys JC: Turnings and adaptations in resilient daughters of battered women, *J Nurs Schol* 33(3):245-251, 2001.

Johnson S, Craft M, Titler M, et al: Perceived changes in adult family members' roles and responsibilities during critical illness, *Image J Nurs Sch* 27(3):238-243, 1995.

Kirkpatrick SM, Deloughery GL: Cultural influences on nursing. In Deloughery GL, editor: *Issues and trends in nursing,* St. Louis, 1995, Mosby, pp 173-197.

Landro L: The best way to get reliable health information, *The Wall Street Journal,* November 12, 2001, p R10.

Larson L: Heaven and hospitals: the role of spirituality in healing, *AHA News* 32(1):7, 1996.

Leininger M: Personal communication, 1999.

Lewis KS: Emotional adjustment to a chronic illness, *Lippincotts Prim Care Pract* 2(1): 38-51, 1998.

McKibbon A: *PDQ: evidence-based principles and practice,* Hamilton, Ontario, BC, 1999, Decker.

NANDA: *Nursing diagnoses: definitions and classification, 2003-2004,* Philadelphia, PA, 2003, NANDA International.

Narayan MC: Cultural assessment in home health care, *Home Healthcare Nurse* 15(10): 663-672, 1997.

Parsons T: *The social system,* New York, 1964, Free Press.

Peplau H: A working definition of anxiety. In Burd SF, Marshall MA, editors: *Some clinical approaches to psychiatric nursing,* New York, 1963, Macmillan.

Roy MA, Turkel MC, Marino F: The transformative process for nursing in workforce redevelopment, *Nurs Admin Q* 26(2):1-14, 2002.

Selye H: *The stress of life,* New York, 1956, McGraw-Hill.

Uustal DB: *Caring for yourself, caring for others: the ultimate balance,* East Greenwich, RI, 1997, Educational Resources in HealthCare, Inc.

Villaire M: Toni Tripp-Reimer: crossing over the boundaries, *Crit Care Nurse* 14(3): 134-141, 1994.

Whiting SA: A Delphi study to determine defining characteristics of interdependence and dysfunctional independence as potential nursing diagnoses, *Issues Ment Health Nurs* 15(1):37-47, 1994.

Wisdom K: Personal communication, 2003.

Wolin SJ, Wolin S: *The resilient self: how survivors of troubled families rise above adversity,* New York, 1993, Villard.

Zauszniewski JA: Learned resourcefulness: a conceptual analysis, *Issues Ment Health Nurs* 16(1):13-31, 1995.

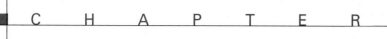

CHAPTER 18

Communication and Collaboration in Nursing

Kay Kittrell Chitty

Key Terms

Acceptance
Action Language
Active Listening
Appropriateness
Clarification
Communication
Congruent
Context
Efficiency
Empathy
Evaluation
False Reassurance
Feedback

Flexibility
Holistic Communication
Incongruent
Irrational Belief
Message
Nonjudgmental
    Acceptance
Nonverbal
    Communication
Nurse-Patient Relationship
Open-Ended Question
Open Posture
Orientation Phase

Perception
Professional Boundaries
Receiver
Reflection
Self-Awareness
Sender
Somatic Language
Stereotypes
Termination Phase
Transmission
Ventilation
Verbal Communication
Working Phase

Learning Outcomes

After studying this chapter, students will be able to:

- Describe therapeutic use of self.
- Identify and describe the phases of the traditional nurse-patient relationship.
- Explore the role self-awareness plays in the ability to use nonjudgmental acceptance as a helping technique.
- Identify their own communication strengths and challenges.
- Discuss factors creating successful or unsuccessful communication.
- Explain the concept of professional boundaries.
- Differentiate between therapeutic and social relationships.
- Evaluate helpful and unhelpful communication.
- Demonstrate components of active listening.
- Identify key prerequisites of collaboration.
- Explain the impact of gender and cultural diversity on nurse-patient and other professional relationships.

nterpersonal skills are important to professional nurses. Regardless of the settings in which they work and the roles they assume within those settings, most nurses interact with many people every day. The way in which they relate to patients, families, colleagues, and other professionals and nonprofessionals determines the level of comfort and trust others feel and, ultimately, the success of their interactions. This chapter includes information that can enhance the development of self-awareness, nonjudgmental acceptance of others, communication skills, and collaboration skills, all of which are essential components of effective interpersonal relationships in nursing.

THERAPEUTIC USE OF SELF

Hildegard Peplau first focused on the importance of the nurse-patient relationship in her 1952 book *Interpersonal Relations in Nursing*. She called using one's personality and communication skills to help patients improve their health status "therapeutic use of self."

The ability to use oneself therapeutically can be developed. Nurses develop this ability by acquiring certain knowledge, attitudes, and skills that assist them in relating effectively to patients, patients' families, co-workers, and other health care professionals.

The Nurse-Patient Relationship: The Traditional View

The nursing process can begin only after the nurse and patient establish their initial therapeutic relationship. Awareness of the three identifiable phases of the nurse-patient relationship helps nurses to be realistic in their expectations of this important relationship. Each of three phases—orientation, working, and termination—is sequential and builds on previous phases.

The orientation phase

The **orientation phase,** or introductory phase, is the period often described as "getting to know you" in social settings. Relationships between nurses and their patients have much in common with other types of relationships. The chief similarity is that there must be trust between the two parties for the relationship to develop. Nurses cannot expect patients to trust them automatically and to reveal their thoughts and feelings.

During the orientation phase, nurse and patient assess one another. Early impressions made by the nurse are important. Some people have difficulty accepting help of any kind, including nursing care. Putting the patient at ease with a pleasant, unhurried approach is important during the early part of any nurse-patient relationship.

During the orientation phase, the patient has a right to expect to learn the nurse's name, credentials, and extent of responsibility. The use of simple orienting statements is one way to begin: "Good morning, Mr. Davis. I am Jennifer Carter, and I am your nurse until noon today. I am responsible for your total care while I am here."

Developing trust. The orientation phase includes the beginning development of trust. Notice the use of the term *beginning development*. Full development of trust is slow and may take months of regular contact. A fact of contemporary nursing practice is that patient interactions may be brief, sometimes lasting only minutes. But even in the most abbreviated contacts, nurses must orient patients and help them feel comfortable and as trusting as possible.

Certain behaviors help patients develop trust in the nurse. A straightforward, nondefensive manner is important. Answering all questions as fully as possible and admitting to the limits of your knowledge also facilitate trust. Promise to find out the answers to all questions and report the information to the patient as soon as possible. Meet with patients at the designated times or make arrangements to let them know of a change in plans. Use active listening behaviors and accept the patient's thoughts and feelings without judgment.

Congruence between verbal and nonverbal communication is a key factor in the development of trust. Communicating in a congruent manner requires that nurses be aware of their own thoughts and feelings and be able to share those with others in a nonthreatening manner. The self-assessment of communication patterns in Box 18-1 is the type of activity that can help improve self-awareness.

Developing an initial understanding of the patient's problem or needs also starts in the orientation phase. Because patients themselves often do not clearly understand their problems or may be reluctant to discuss them, nurses must use their communication skills to elicit the information needed in order to make a nursing diagnosis. Communication skills are discussed later in this chapter.

Tasks of the orientation phase. By the end of a successful orientation phase, regardless of its length, several things will have happened. First, the patient will have

---

Box **18-1** **Communication Patterns Self-Assessment**

Directions: Answer the following true-or-false questions as honestly as possible; then review your answers and draw at least two conclusions about your habitual communication patterns. Check your conclusions for accuracy with a friend who knows your style of communicating well.
 1. I usually listen about as much as I talk.
 2. I rarely interrupt others.
 3. I pay close attention to what others say.
 4. I usually make eye contact with the person I am talking with.
 5. I can usually tell if someone is angry or upset.
 6. I would hesitate to interrupt someone to ask for clarification.
 7. People often tell me personal things about themselves.
 8. I find it is best to change the subject if someone gets too emotional.
 9. If I can't "make things better" for a friend with a problem, I feel uncomfortable.
10. I am comfortable talking with people much older or much younger than I am.
11. When there is conflict, I tend to:
    a. avoid.
    b. verbally attack.
    c. give in.
    d. become autocratic.

developed enough trust in the nurse to continue to participate in the relationship. Second, the patient and nurse will see each other as individuals, unique from all others and worthy of one another's respect. Third, the patient's perception of major problems and needs will have been identified. And fourth, the approximate length of the relationship will have been estimated, and the nurse and patient will have agreed to work together on some aspect of the identified problems. This agreement, whether formalized in writing or informally agreed upon, is sometimes called a "contract." An example of a contract that might emerge from the orientation phase of the relationship with a patient newly diagnosed with diabetes is an agreement to work together on his ability to calculate and inject his daily insulin requirement.

The working phase

The second phase of the nurse-patient relationship is called the **working phase,** because it is during this time that the nurse and patient tackle tasks outlined in the previous phase. Because the participants now know each other to some extent, there may be a sense of interpersonal comfort in the relationship that did not exist earlier.

Nurses should recognize that in the working phase patients may exhibit alternating periods of intense effort and periods of resistance to change. Continuing the example of the patient with diabetes, the nurse can anticipate that he will experience some degree of difficulty in accepting the life changes the illness causes. He may show progress in learning to give himself insulin one week but not be able to demonstrate injection technique the next week. Nurses who become frustrated when patients' progress toward self-care is not smooth and sustained must realize that regression is an ego defense mechanism that occurs as a reaction to stress and that regression often precedes periods of positive behavioral change.

It is difficult to make and sustain change. Patience, self-awareness, and maturity are required of nurses during the working phase. Continued building of trust, use of active listening, and other helpful communication responses facilitate the patient's expression of needs and feelings during the working phase.

The termination phase

The **termination phase** includes those activities that enable the patient and the nurse to end the relationship in a therapeutic manner. The process of terminating the nurse-patient relationship begins in the orientation phase when participants estimate the length of time it will take to accomplish the desired outcomes. This is part of the informal contract.

As in any relationship, positive and negative feelings often accompany termination. The patient and nurse feel good about the gains the patient has made in accomplishing goals. They may feel sadness about ending a relationship that has been open and trusting. People tend to respond to the end of relationships in much the same way they have responded to other losses in life. Feelings of anger and fear may surface, in addition to sadness.

Feelings evoked by termination should be discussed and accepted. Summarizing the gains the patient has made is an important activity during this phase. The importance of the relationship to both patient and nurse can be shared in a caring manner.

The giving and receiving of gifts at termination has different meanings for different people. The meaning of such behavior should be explored in a sensitive manner, and the agency's policies on gifts should be consulted.

Because termination is often painful, participants are sometimes tempted to continue the relationship on a social basis, and requests for addresses, phone numbers and e-mail addresses are not uncommon. The nurse must realize that professional relationships are different from social relationships. It is not helpful to stay in touch with patients following termination of a professional nurse-patient relationship. Several other differences between social and professional relationships are outlined in Box 18-2.

During the course of a professional career, every nurse will experience countless nurse-patient relationships, each with its own meaning and duration. If nurses can view each new relationship both as an opportunity to assist another human being to grow and change in a positive, healthful way and as a challenge to grow and change themselves, the rewards of nursing will be rich indeed.

Developing Self-Awareness

Awareness of oneself, called **self-awareness,** is basic to effective interpersonal relationships, especially the nurse-patient relationship. Robert Burns, the eighteenth-century Scottish poet, described the rarity of true self-awareness in his poem "To a Louse": "Oh wad some Power the giftie gie us/To see oursels as ithers see us!" (Barke, 1955).

As Burns knew, few people have the innate capacity to recognize their own emotional needs, biases, and blind spots, as well as their impact on others. With practice, however, most can become more effective in doing so, thus improving self-awareness.

Box 18-2 **Differences in Social and Professional Relationships**

Social
- Evolve spontaneously.
- Not time-limited.
- Not necessarily goal-directed; broad purpose is pleasure, companionship, sharing.
- Centered on meeting both parties' needs.
- Problem solving is rarely/occasionally a focus.
- May or may not include nonjudgmental acceptance.
- Outcome is pleasure for both parties.

Professional
- Evolve through recognized phases; use planned and purposeful interactions.
- Limited in time with termination date often predetermined.
- Goal-directed; systematic exploration of identified problem areas.
- Centered on meeting patient needs; does not address nurse's needs.
- Problem solving is a primary focus.
- Includes nonjudgmental acceptance.
- Outcome is improved health for patient.

An important guideline in professional nursing is this: nurses should get their own emotional needs met outside of the **nurse-patient relationship.** When nurses' strong unmet needs for **acceptance,** approval, friendship, or even love enter into their relationships with patients, professionalism is lost, and relationships become social in nature. Becoming aware of one's needs and making conscious efforts to meet those needs in private life make professional, therapeutic relationships with patients possible. As discussed earlier and summarized in Box 18-2, there are important differences in social and professional relationships.

The subject of professional boundaries is explored in a brochure published by the National Council of State Boards of Nursing (1996). It defines professional boundaries as "the spaces between the nurse's power and the client's vulnerability. The power of the nurse comes from the professional position and the access to private knowledge about the client" (p. 1). Boundary violations occur when "there is confusion between the needs of the nurse and those of the client" (p. 2).

According to the NCSBN brochure, nurse-patient relationships can be plotted on a continuum of professional behavior that ranges from *underinvolvement* (distancing, disinterest, neglect) through a *zone of helpfulness* to *overinvolvement* (excessive personal disclosure by the nurse, secrecy, role reversal, or sexual misconduct). Both underinvolvement and overinvolvement can be detrimental to patient and nurse (p. 3). Box 18-3 describes a case in which a nurse was disciplined by his

---

Box 18-3 Legal Note: Nurse's Relationship With Patient Results in Disciplinary Action

Tapp v. Board of Registered Nursing, 2002 WL 31820206 P.2d -CA

This case involved a California registered nurse at a psychiatric facility in Fresno who was accused of having sexual relations with his former patient following her discharge. The patient was hospitalized for emotional problems related to sex. She was hospitalized on a unit where the nurse worked the night shift. They became friendly; he brought her small gifts, gave her his telephone number, and called her during his off-work hours. After she was discharged, they spoke often by telephone and he began to visit her at her apartment. On one occasion, the nurse gave her a tablet of a controlled substance.

One week following her discharge, they began a sexual relationship that lasted for 2 weeks. Shortly after the relationship ended, the patient was readmitted, "suffering adverse effects from the affair" (p. 4). The California Board of Registered Nursing initiated disciplinary proceedings for "acts of unprofessional conduct." An administrative law judge heard testimony, made a determination of misconduct, and recommended that the nurse's license be revoked, but stayed the revocation and recommended that the nurse be placed on probation for 5 years on multiple conditions. The California Board of Registered Nursing disagreed and ordered the revocation of his license. There were subsequent appeals, dismissals, and further appeals.

Nurses must realize that there can be no socialization between themselves and patients, particularly sexual in nature. Not only was this nurse's behavior with this patient during her hospitalization "highly improper, but his socialization with the patient after her discharge from the hospital, not to mention the fact that he provided the patient with a controlled substance, was ample reason to impose strict disciplinary action" (p. 5).

Abstracted from Nurse's Relationship with Patient Results in Disciplinary Action: *Nursing Law's Regan Report* 43(8):4-5, 2003.

| Box 18-4 | **Principles for Determining Professional Boundaries** |

1. The nurse is responsible for delineating and maintaining boundaries.
2. The nurse should work within the "zone of helpfulness."
3. The nurse should examine any boundary crossing, be aware of its potential implications, and avoid repeated crossings.
4. Variables such as the care setting, community influences, client needs, and the nature of therapy affect the delineation of boundaries.
5. Actions that overstep established boundaries to meet the needs of the nurse are boundary violations.
6. The nurse should avoid dual relationships in which the nurse has a personal or business relationship, as well as the professional one.
7. Post-termination relationships are complex because the client may need additional services, and it may be difficult to determine when the nurse-client relationship is truly terminated.

Reprinted with permission from National Council of State Boards of Nursing: Professional boundaries: a nurse's guide to the importance of appropriate professional boundaries, Chicago, 1996, NCSBN, Online (www.ncsbn.org/pdfs/expectnurse.pdf).

state board of nursing for failing to honor the **professional boundaries** between a nurse and patient.

Box 18-4 contains seven "guiding principles to determining professional boundaries and the continuum of professional behavior" (p. 4) from the excellent NCSBN brochure. The brochure can be viewed online or downloaded in PDF format from the NCSBN website.

Nurses care for a diverse array of patients whose values, beliefs, and lifestyles may challenge the nurses' own. Patients sometimes are attractive or repellant to nurses. Sometimes nurses find themselves meeting their own needs to be liked or needed through relationships with patients. Nurses who have emotional reactions to patients, positive or negative, sometimes feel disturbed or guilty about these feelings. Part of self-awareness is recognizing one's feelings and understanding that although feelings cannot be controlled, behaviors can. Effective nurses control their behavior to prevent their own prejudices, beliefs, and needs from intruding into nurse-patient relationships.

Avoiding Stereotypes

Stereotypes are prejudices and attitudes developed through interactions with family, friends, and others in each individual's social and cultural system. It is not uncommon for even well-educated professionals to have stereotypical expectations of groups of people different from themselves. These stereotypes are established through childhood experiences and affect relationships with people in the stereotyped group. Because stereotypes and prejudices tend to persist despite contrary experiences, they are **irrational,** or illogical, **beliefs.**

The subtle intrusion of stereotyped expectations into the nurse-patient relationship can cause disturbed patterns of relating. For example, the expectation that all elderly people are irritable and demanding may cause the nurse to avoid all elderly patients or to treat their complaints as unimportant.

Professional nurses deliver high-quality care to all patients regardless of ethnicity, age, gender, religion, lifestyle, or diagnosis. The *Code of Ethics for Nurses* (see inside back cover of this text) calls upon nurses to do this. Nurses are not without stereotypes and prejudices, however, and must strive to be aware of their own irrational feelings toward patients. Every professional nurse's goal is to accept patients as individuals of dignity and worth who deserve the best nursing care possible.

Becoming Nonjudgmental

Acceptance is not always easy, because prejudices are strong and are often outside our awareness. This means that judging others as "good" or "bad" may occur automatically. It is important to remember that acceptance conveys neither approval nor disapproval of patients, their personal beliefs, habits, expressions of feelings, or chosen lifestyles. **Nonjudgmental acceptance** means that nurses acknowledge all patients' rights to be different and to express their "differentness."

Therapeutic use of self begins with the ability to convey acceptance to patients and requires self-awareness and nonjudgmental attitudes on the part of nurses. Ongoing examination of attitudes toward others is both a lifelong process and an essential part of self-awareness and interpersonal growth.

Reconceptualizing the Nurse-Patient Relationship: Theory of Human Relatedness

The kind of nurse-patient relationship (NPR) discussed in the previous section is the traditional model taught and practiced since the middle of the twentieth century. It is based on several assumptions that no longer hold true in many settings where nurses practice in today's fast-paced health care system. These assumptions are as follows (Hagerty and Patusky, 2003):

- The NPR is linear and proceeds through several phases, each building on the preceding one.
- Building trust is essential during early phases of the NPR.
- Time and repeated contacts are required to establish an effective NPR.
- Patients desire relationships with nurses, wish to receive services from them, and will cooperate and comply with those nurses.

Although the traditional, time-honored NPR is still appropriate in many settings, the assumptions on which it is based are being challenged by today's health care realities. The reality is that patients today are more acutely ill, nurses' workloads have increased, and the time nurses spend with patients may be quite limited, sometimes to only one or two contacts. Are these more limited NP contacts therefore doomed, or can we rethink the NPR and find ways to modify it to suit today's streamlined caregiving contexts?

Hagerty and Patusky (2003) proposed reconceptualizing the NPR using the *theory of human relatedness* as a framework. They recommended approaching each nurse-patient contact as an opportunity for connection and goal achievement rather than as one step in a lengthy relationship-building process. They also recommended that nurses approach their patients with a sense of the patient's autonomy, choice, and participation (p. 147), putting the relationship on a more equitable basis than the traditional nurse-patient relationship, which gives much of the power to the nurse. Research into these concepts continues.

These ideas can form the basis for classroom discussion and provide "new insights and opportunities for assessment, intervention, and research toward positive, hopeful, and efficacious nursing care" (Hagerty and Patusky, p. 149).

COMMUNICATION THEORY

Communication is the exchange of thoughts, ideas, or information and is at the heart of all relationships. Communication is a dynamic process that is the primary instrument through which change occurs in nursing situations. Nurses use their communication skills in all phases of the nursing process. These skills are vital to effective nursing care and to effective interaction with others in health care.

Jurgen Ruesch (1972, p. 16), a pioneer communications theorist, defined communication as "all the modes of behavior that one individual employs, conscious or unconscious, to affect another: not only the spoken and written word, but also gestures, body movements, somatic signals, and symbolism in the arts."

Communication begins the moment two people become aware of each other's presence. It is impossible not to communicate when in the presence of another person, even if no words are spoken. Even when alone, people routinely engage in "self-talk," which is an internal form of communication.

Levels of Communication

Communication exists simultaneously on at least two levels: verbal and nonverbal. **Verbal communication** consists of all speech and represents part of communication. Much communication is **nonverbal communication,** which consists of grooming, clothing, gestures, posture, facial expressions, tone and volume of voice, and actions, among other things (Figure 18-1). Words can be used to hide feelings, but individuals tend to exercise less conscious control over nonverbal communication than verbal communication. Therefore, nonverbal component is considered a more reliable expression of feeling. Certainly nurses must pay as much attention to nonverbal messages as they do to verbal ones.

Consider this example: a nurse who is preparing a patient for a breast biopsy notices that the patient keeps her head turned away and will not look at the nurse. When the nurse says, "Is there anything you want to talk about or ask?" the patient responds, "No, I'm fine." The wise nurse would pay more attention to her nonverbal communication than to the spoken word. If the nurse pays attention only to the patient's words, her underlying feelings would be ignored. The nurse's job in evaluating this patient's needs is made more difficult by the incongruence between her verbal and nonverbal messages.

When **congruent** communication occurs, the verbal and nonverbal aspects match and reinforce each other. In **incongruent** communication, the words and nonverbal communication do not match. Incongruent communication creates confusion in receivers, who are unsure to which level of communication they should respond. Nurses should be alert to incongruent communication for clues to patients' unexpressed feelings.

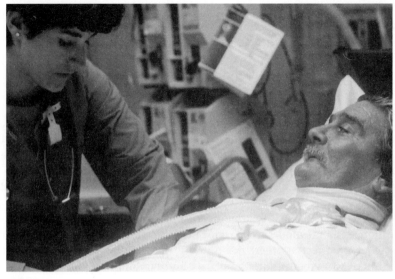

Figure **18-1**
Nonverbal communication consists of grooming, clothing, gestures, posture, facial expressions, tone and volume of voice, and actions. Nonverbal communication is particularly important to patients whose ability to speak is impaired. (Courtesy Medical University of South Carolina.)

Elements of the Communication Process

Ruesch identified five major elements that must be present for communication to take place: a sender, a message, a receiver, feedback, and context. The **sender** is the person sending the message, the **message** is what is actually said plus accompanying nonverbal communication, and the **receiver** is the person receiving the message. A response to a message is termed **feedback.** The setting in which an interaction occurs—including the mood, relationship between sender and receiver, and other factors—is known as the **context.** All of these elements are necessary for communication to occur.

Consider the classroom situation. During a lecture, the professor is the sender, the lecture is the message, and students are the receivers. The professor (sender) receives feedback from the students (receivers) through their facial expressions, alertness, posture, and attentiveness. The atmosphere in the classroom is the context. If the atmosphere is a relaxed one of give-and-take between students and professor, the feedback is quite different from feedback in a more formal context. Figure 18-2 shows the relationships among the five elements of communication.

Operations in the Communication Process

In addition to the five elements of communication, Ruesch also identified three major operations in communication: perception, evaluation, and transmission.

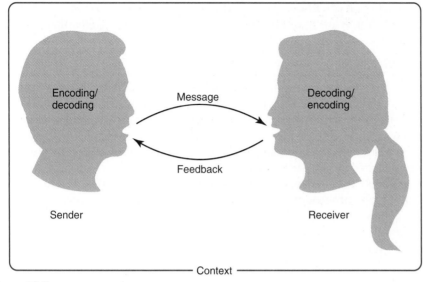

Figure **18-2**
Elements of the communication process.

Perception

Perception is the selection, organization, and interpretation of incoming signals into meaningful messages. In the classroom situation just described, students select, organize, and interpret various pieces of the professor's message or lecture. Each student perceives the information differently, based on factors such as personal experience, previous knowledge, alertness, sensitivity to subtleties of meaning, and sociocultural background.

Evaluation

Evaluation is the analysis of information received. Is the content of the professor's lecture useful? Is it important or relevant to the students' needs? Is it likely to be on the next test? Each student evaluates the message in a different manner.

Transmission

Transmission refers to the expression of information, verbal or nonverbal. While the professor is transmitting his verbal message to the students, his or her nonverbal behavior of excitement about his subject matter also transmits a message to the class.

Factors influencing perception, evaluation, and transmission

Perception, evaluation, and transmission are influenced by many factors. The gender and culture of the sender and receiver; the interest and mood of both parties; the value, clarity, and length of the message; the presence or absence of feedback; and the atmosphere of the context all are powerful influences. Also involved are individuals' needs, values, self-concepts, sensory and intellectual abilities or deficits, and sociocultural conditioning. Given the variety of factors involved, it is clear that communication is a complex human activity worthy of nurses' attention.

HOW COMMUNICATION DEVELOPS

Humans learn to communicate through a certain developmental sequence, which begins in infancy. Infants use **somatic language** to signal their needs to caretakers. Somatic language consists of crying; reddening of the skin; fast, shallow breathing; facial expressions; and jerking of the limbs. The sequence progresses to action language in older infants. **Action language** consists of reaching out, pointing, crawling toward a desired object, or closing the lips and turning the head when an undesired food is offered. Last to develop is verbal language, beginning with repetitive noises and sounds and progressing to words, phrases, and complete sentences.

If a child's development is normal, any one or combination of these forms of communication can be used. Somatic language usually decreases with maturity, but because it is not under conscious control, some somatic language may persist past childhood. A familiar example is facial blushing when embarrassed or angry. The development of communication is determined by inborn and environmental factors. The amount of verbal stimulation an infant receives can enhance or retard the development of language skills. The extent of a caretaker's vocabulary and verbal ability is therefore influential. Some families engage in lengthy discussions on a variety of issues, thereby providing intense verbal stimulation, whereas others are less verbal.

Nonverbal communication development is similarly influenced by environment. Some families communicate through nonverbal gestures such as touch or facial expressions, which children learn to "read" at young ages. Other families ascribe to the adage "Children should be seen and not heard," thus discouraging verbal expression and increasing dependence on nonverbal cues for communicating. The ability to communicate effectively is dependent on a number of factors. Primary among these are the quantity and quality of verbal and nonverbal stimulation received during early developmental periods.

CRITERIA FOR SUCCESSFUL COMMUNICATION

Everyone has had the experience of being the sender or receiver of unsuccessful communication. A simple example is arriving for an appointment with a friend at the wrong time or wrong place because of a communication mix-up. Unsuccessful communication creates little harm when done under social circumstances. In nursing situations, however, accurate, complete communication is vitally important. Nurses can achieve successful communication on most occasions if they plan their communication to meet four major criteria: *feedback, appropriateness, efficiency,* and *flexibility*.

Feedback

When a receiver relays to a sender the effect of the sender's message, feedback has occurred. Feedback was identified as one of Ruesch's five elements necessary for communication (see Figure 18-2). It is also a criterion for successful communication.

In making the social appointment mentioned previously, if the receiver of the message had said, "Let's make sure I understand you. We'll meet at 12:30 on Tuesday at Cafe Al Fresco," that feedback could have led to successful communication.

In a nurse-patient interaction, a nurse can give feedback to a patient by saying, "If I understand you correctly, you have pain in your lower abdomen every time you stand up." The patient can then either agree or correct what the nurse has said: "No, the pain is there only when I arise in the morning." Effective nurses do not assume that they fully understand what their patients are telling them until they feed the statement back to the patient and receive confirmation.

Appropriateness

When a reply fits the circumstances and matches the message, and the amount is neither too great nor too little, **appropriateness** has been achieved. In day-to-day conversation among acquaintances passing on the street, most people recognize the question "How are you?" as a social nicety, not a genuine question. The individual who launches into a detailed description of how his morning has gone has communicated inappropriately. The reply does not fit the circumstances, and the quantity is too great. An appropriate response is, "Fine, and how are you?"

If a patient asks, "When is my lunch coming?" just after having eaten lunch, the nurse will be alert to other inappropriate messages by this patient that may signal a variety of problems. In this instance, the inappropriate message does not match the context.

Efficiency

Using simple, clear words that are timed at a pace suitable to participants meets the criterion of **efficiency.** Explaining to an adult that she will have "an angioplasty" tomorrow morning probably will not result in successful communication. Telling her she will have "a procedure in which a small balloon is threaded into an artery and inflated to open up the vessel so more blood can flow through" will more likely ensure her understanding. This message would not be an efficient one for a small child, however. Messages must be adapted to each patient's age, verbal level, and level of understanding.

Some examples of patients who require special assistance in evaluating and responding to messages are young children, the mentally ill, some people with neurological deficits, and those recovering from anesthesia. For efficient communication to occur, nurses must recognize patients' needs and adjust messages accordingly.

Flexibility

The fourth criterion for successful communication is **flexibility.** The flexible communicator bases messages on the immediate situation rather than preconceived expectations. When a student nurse who plans to teach a patient about diabetic diets enters the patient's room and finds her crying, the nurse must be flexible enough to change gears and deal with the feelings the patient is expressing. Pressing on with the lesson plan in the face of the patient's distress shows a lack of compassion as well as inflexibility in communicating.

Nurses can learn to use these four measures of successful communication to enhance their effectiveness with patients. The continuing absence or malfunction of any of these four criteria can create disturbed communication and hamper the implementation of the nursing process.

BECOMING A BETTER COMMUNICATOR

People are not born as good communicators. Communication skills can be developed if you are willing to put forth a moderate amount of time and energy. Becoming a better listener, learning a few basic helpful responding styles, and avoiding common causes of communication breakdown can put you on the path to becoming a better communicator.

Listening

A requirement of successful verbal communication in any setting is listening, but too often we hear without listening. **Active listening** is a method of communicating interest and attention. Fostering an unrushed manner and using such signals as good eye contact, nodding, and "mumbles" ("mm-hmm") and encouraging the speaker ("Go on" or "Tell me more about this") help to communicate interest. Facing the speaker squarely with an inviting facial expression and using an **open posture** (arms uncrossed) also communicate interest. Bend or stoop to place your eye level at that of the patient and repeat (reflect) what you hear, including feelings, checking to be sure you heard correctly. These indications of interest and active listening will help you focus on patients and tune into the meanings behind their words (listening with the "third ear").

Having someone listen to concerns, even if no problem solving takes place, is considered therapeutic. **Ventilation** is the term used to describe the verbal "letting off steam" that occurs when talking about concerns or frustrations. The experience of feeling "listened to" is becoming so rare in contemporary American society that a columnist for *The Christian Science Monitor* was prompted to write about it (see News Note).

> *news*
> *note*
>
> **Where Did All the Listeners Go?**
> When everybody learned how to tune out their machines—blabbing-off radio and television ads, hanging up on computer phone calls, and so on—they also learned how to tune out other people.
>
> During the talkiest era ever, nobody listens. Or so it is assumed. In his new novel, *A Tenured Professor*, Harvard economist John Kenneth Galbraith puts it nicely: "By long custom, social discourse in Cambridge is intended to impart and only rarely to obtain information. People talk; it is not expected that anyone

will listen. A respectful show of attention is all that is required until the listener takes over in his or her turn."

But wait. Just as it seems that the glazed-over eye and the numbed ear typify the Age of the Non-Listener, there is heartening news.

In Milwaukee, the Roman Catholic Archdiocese is sponsoring six "listening sessions" to give Catholic women a chance to express their feelings about abortion.

The first session, held last month in a college gymnasium in Fond du Lac, Wisconsin, drew 100 women. While participants gathered in small groups to discuss the volatile issue, Archbishop Rembert Weakland, who organized the event, moved from table to table, listening and reportedly saying little.

Archbishop Weakland, considered one of the more liberal Catholic leaders, has been criticized within his church for his gesture. But as he explained to a reporter, "The polarization about this issue has become so great that I had to admit we needed dialogue about it within the Catholic community."

It is one thing for equals to listen to equals, or for subordinates to listen to those in authority. But it is a high tribute when individuals in power listen to those below them.

Once upon a time, being a "good listener" was considered a social grace. At least 51 percent of the world were "good listeners." They were also called women. A young woman learned by example that her gender role was to listen to what others—especially men—were saying. Her mouth was primarily for smiling at what she heard, with an occasional rhythmic "uh-huh."

Today that "uh-huh" is increasingly likely to come from a stranger. Lending an ear has become a paid profession. As if to signify a national hunger for "listening sessions," an entire industry has sprung up.

Eight-year-olds phone latchkey hotlines for after-school comfort and conversation while Mom—the original "good listener"—is off at work. Bereaved dog and cat owners call on pet grief counselors for animal-loving shoulders to cry on. Even technology offers an ear, this one electronic, as answering machines and voice mailboxes do more and more of the listening.

Then of course there is the biggest listening post of all, the talk show. What does it say about the desperate yearning for an audience, any audience, that guests are willing to bare their souls and share their most intimate secrets not with close friends but with Oprah, Phil, Geraldo—and millions of TV viewers?

Is this what it takes to get a word in edgewise in the late 20th century?

Outside the TV studio, other cameras reveal that finding a "good listener"—or any listener at all—can be a tricky business in classrooms as well, especially for women.

Catherine Krupnick, a researcher at the Harvard Graduate School of Education, videotaped thousands of hours of college classes. She discovered that even when male students made up just one tenth of a class, the men would do one

Continued

quarter of the talking. Other studies over the past two decades confirm Ms. Krupnick's findings, showing that professors are more likely to call on men.

The philosopher Mortimer Adler has called listening "the untaught skill." Those like Archbishop Weakland may be thought of as pioneers in retraining. But the changeover from mouth to ear won't come easily. The thing about listening is that it takes more time and, in fact, more thought than merely talking.

When a reporter, after one of the "listening sessions" in Wisconsin, asked the Archbishop what he thought, he gave the right answer: "I'm still listening."

—Marilyn Gardner

Gardner M: Where did all the listeners go? This article first appeared in *The Christian Science Monitor* on April 27, 1990, and is reproduced with permission. Copyright 1990, The Christian Science Publishing Society. All rights reserved.

Nurses may have difficulty listening for a variety of reasons. They may be intent on accomplishing a task and be frustrated by the time it takes to be a good listener. They may be planning their own next response and not hear what the patient is saying. They may be distracted by a vibrating pager or announcement. Similar to other people, nurses have their own personal and professional problems that sometimes preoccupy them and interfere with effective listening. Nurses must remember that no verbal message can be received if the receiver (the nurse) is not listening.

Three common listening faults include interrupting, finishing sentences for others, and lack of interest. It is important for nurses to remember that what the patient is saying is just as important as what the nurse wishes to say.

Being listened to meets the patient's emotional need to be respected and valued by the nurse. Listening can help avert problems by letting people ventilate about the pressures they feel. Hospitalized patients particularly may feel that their lives are out of control and that they are isolated or invisible. They may need to discuss those feelings with someone who will listen without becoming defensive (Figure 18-3).

Nurses at all levels find listening a useful and rewarding skill. Nurse managers often use listening as a tool for dealing with staff members' problems and concerns and find that no other intervention is required. Listening is a talent that can be developed; properly used, it can be an essential part of a nurse's communication repertoire.

Using Helpful Responding Techniques

There are many helpful responding techniques nurses can use to demonstrate respect and encourage patients to communicate openly. Helpful responses that have already been discussed in this chapter include being nonjudgmental, observing body language, and active listening. Other useful responses include empathy, open-ended questions, giving information, reflection, and silence. Each will be explained.

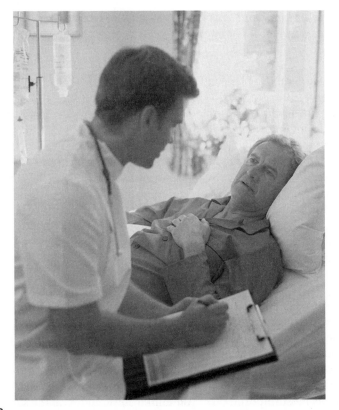

Figure **18-3**
Being an active listener is an important part of communication. (Courtesy Hamilton Medical
Center, Dalton, Georgia.)

Empathy

Empathy consists of awareness of, sensitivity to, and identification with the feelings
of another person. Nurses can empathize with patients even if they have not experienced an event in their own lives exactly like the one the patient is experiencing.
If nurses have had a similar or parallel experience, empathy is possible. For example,
the feeling of loss is familiar to most nurses, even though they may not personally
have lost a close family member.

Empathy is different from sympathy in that the sympathetic nurse enters into the
feeling with the patient, whereas the empathic nurse appreciates the patient's feelings but is not swept along with the feelings. "You seem upset about the upcoming
procedure" is an example of a nursing statement that demonstrates empathy.

Open-ended questions

An **open-ended question** is one that causes the patient to answer fully, giving more
than a "Yes" or "No" answer. Open-ended questions are very useful in data gathering and in the opening stages of any nurse-patient interaction. For example, asking

a patient, "Are you in pain?" may elicit only a confirming "Yes." Saying to him, "Tell me about your pain" is more likely to elicit information about the site, type, intensity, and duration of the pain, therefore making the nurse-patient interaction more useful.

Giving information

An essential part of nursing is providing information to patients and their significant others. Giving information includes sharing knowledge that the recipients are not expected to know. Nurses provide information when they tell patients what to expect during diagnostic procedures, inform them of their rights as patients, and teach them about their conditions, diets, or medications.

An important distinction every nurse needs to make is the difference between providing information and giving opinions. While providing information is a helpful aspect of the nursing role, giving opinions is considered unhelpful. Instead, nurses should encourage patients to consider their own values and opinions as primary in importance. The nurse's opinion is irrelevant.

Reflection

The nurse using **reflection** is serving as a mirror for the patient. Reflection is a method of encouraging patients to think through problems for themselves by directing patient questions back to the patient. Reflection implies respect because the nurse believes the patient has adequate resources to solve the problem without outside assistance. In response to the patient's question, "Do you think I should go through with this surgery?" the nurse can reflect the question: "*Your* thinking on this question is most important. Do *you* think you should have the surgery?"

Silence

Although silent periods in social conversations often feel uncomfortable, using silence in nurse-patient relationships can be a helpful response. Using silence means allowing periods of reflection during an interaction without feeling pressure to "fill the gap" with conversation or activity. For example, when a patient has just been given upsetting news, sitting quietly without making any demands for conversation may be the most therapeutic response a nurse can make at that time. "Being with" patients is often just as valuable as "doing for" them. Professional nurses learn to use both of these tools and find time in their busy schedules to be with patients.

There are many more helpful responding styles nurses can use in their interactions with patients. The five discussed here can be a foundation upon which to build.

Culturally Competent Communication

Since communication is the means by which people connect, nurses must take cultural differences into consideration when planning and implementing care. No hard and fast rules can be given because communication practices are unique for each individual and vary widely for people from the same cultural backgrounds. Various elements to assess include dialect, style, volume, use of touch, emotional tone, gestures, stance, space needs, and eye contact (Davidhizar, Dowd, and Giger, 1998).

Culturally competent nurses recognize that even when individuals speak the same language, sender and receiver may perceive different meanings because of unique life experiences. Patients may be unwilling to share certain information with nurses because of cultural taboos. Nurses may inadvertently offend patients or family members by violating cultural norms concerning touch, space, and eye contact.

Later in this chapter, Box 18-5 provides guidelines for communicating effectively with co-workers of different cultural backgrounds. It is easily adapted for use with patients and provides strategies for promoting cross-cultural communication.

Avoiding Common Causes of Communication Breakdown

Just as there are many factors influencing successful communication, unsuccessful communication can occur for many reasons. A sender may send an incomplete or confusing message. A message may not be received, or it may be misunderstood or distorted by the receiver. Incongruent messages may cause confusion in the receiver. In nursing situations, there are several common causes of communication breakdown. These include failing to see each individual as unique, failing to recognize levels of meaning, using value statements, using false reassurance, and failing to clarify unclear messages.

Failing to see the uniqueness of the individual

Failing to see the uniqueness of each individual is a frequent cause of communication breakdown. This failure is caused by preconceived ideas, prejudices, and **stereotypes,** illustrated by the following interchange between a patient and a nurse:

Patient: "My back is really hurting today. I can hardly turn over in bed."

Nurse: "I guess we have to expect these little problems when we get older."

This nurse has pigeonholed the patient in a mental group, "old people," and therefore does not react to the patient as an individual. The nurse could have promoted continued communication by responding to the patient as an individual:

Nurse: "Tell me exactly how your back hurts, Mrs. Jameson."

Failing to recognize levels of meaning

When nurses recognize no level of meaning other than the obvious ones, communication breakdown can occur. Patients often give verbal cues to meanings that lie under the surface content of their verbalizations:

Patient: "It's getting awfully warm in here."

Nurse: *(Responding only to surface meaning)* "I'll adjust the air conditioning for you."

This response does not help the patient express himself fully. A different type of response focuses on the symbolic level of meaning:

Nurse: "Perhaps the questions I am asking are making you uncomfortable."

Although it takes a lot of experience to know when and how to respond to symbolic communication, nurses should be aware of its existence.

Using value statements and clichés

Using value statements and clichés is another communication problem. The use of clichés, which are trite, stereotyped expressions, is common in social conversation. Consider the prevalence of the cliché "Have a good day." This statement has come to have little real meaning. This common error can cut off communication by showing the patient that the nurse does not understand the patient's true feelings.

Patient: "My mother is coming to see me today."

Nurse: "How nice. Do you want to put on a fresh gown?"

This nurse has failed to verify whether the patient actually wishes to see her mother. In fact, the patient and her mother may have a difficult relationship, and the patient may dread the impending visit. By assuming otherwise, the nurse has contributed to communication breakdown. This patient probably will not attempt to discuss her relationship with her mother any further with this nurse. A more helpful response would be:

Nurse: "How do you feel about her visit?"

This allows the patient to ventilate her feelings about her mother's visit, whether positive or negative. The nurse has conveyed a genuine interest in the patient's true feelings.

Giving false reassurance

Using **false reassurance** is another communication pitfall. It may help the nurse feel better but does not facilitate communication and help the patient.

Patient: "I'm so afraid the biopsy will be cancer."

Nurse: "Don't worry. You have the best doctor in town. Besides, cancer treatment is really good these days."

For a fearful patient, this type of glib reassurance does not help. This nurse has no way of knowing that the patient's concerns are not legitimate. She may indeed *have* cancer. A more sensitive response would be:

Nurse: "Why don't we talk about it?"

This kind of response keeps the lines of communication open between patient and nurse.

Failing to clarify

Failing to clarify the patient's unclear statements is a fifth common communication pitfall.

Patient: "I've got to get out of the hospital. They have found out I'm here and may come after me."

Nurse: "No one will harm you here."

This nurse has responded as if the patient's meaning was clear. A clarifying response might be:

Nurse: "Who are 'they,' Mrs. Johnson?"

Confused patients or those with psychiatric illnesses often communicate in ways that are difficult to understand. It is reassuring to patients to know that nurses are trying to understand them, even if they are not always successful. Communication is facilitated by **clarification** responses.

Practicing Helpful Responses

Nurses can practice using helpful responses and avoiding common communication pitfalls with family members, friends, and co-workers, as well as in patient contacts. Being a good communicator takes practice and usually feels unnatural at first.

Any new behavior takes time to integrate into habitual patterns. By continuing to practice, nurses soon find themselves feeling more natural. They find that these newly acquired skills are beneficial both professionally and personally. The accompanying Critical Thinking Exercise compares different responses in a nurse-patient interaction.

CRITICAL THINKING *Exercise*

Helpful and Unhelpful Responding Techniques

Directions: Critique both interactions, identifying the helpful and unhelpful responses used by the nurse. Describe how you imagine the patient might feel at the close of each interaction. Identify what the nurse has accomplished in each instance.

Mr. Goodman has been admitted to the hospital for coronary bypass surgery. During the admission process, the following interactions might take place.

Interaction One

Nurse: Mr. Goodman, I am Mrs. Scott. Can I get some information about you now?
Patient: Okay.
Nurse: You're here for bypass surgery?
Patient: Yes, that's what they tell me.
Nurse: (Taking blood pressure) Do you have any allergies to foods or medications?
Patient: Not that I know of. I've never been in a hospital before.
Nurse: Well, your blood pressure looks good. (Silence while patient has thermometer in mouth.) This is a really nice room—just remodeled. I know you'll be comfortable here. Will your wife be coming to see you tonight? (Removes thermometer)
Patient: My wife is sick. She hasn't been able to leave home for 2 years. I don't know what will happen to her while I am here.
Nurse: Gosh, I'm so sorry to hear that. I guess having you back home healthy is what she wants though, isn't it? And you've got a great surgeon. Well, I've got to run now. Check on you later.

Interaction Two

Nurse: Good afternoon, Mr. Goodman. I'm Mrs. Scott, and I'll be your nurse this evening. If this is a good time, I'd like to ask you some questions and complete your admission process.
Patient: Okay.
Nurse: First, I'll get your temperature and blood pressure, and then we'll talk. (Silence while nurse takes vital signs.) Everything looks good. Do you have any allergies to foods or medications?
Patient: Not that I know of. I've never been in a hospital before.
Nurse: Hospitals can be a little overwhelming, especially when you've never been a patient before. Now, would you please tell me in your own words why you are here?
Patient: Well, the doc tells me I have a clogged artery, and I need a bypass. I guess they'll open up my heart.
Nurse: What exactly do you know about the surgery?
Patient: Not too much, really. He told me yesterday that I need it right away—and here I am.

Continued

CRITICAL THINKING *Exercise—cont'd*

Helpful and Unhelpful Responding Techniques

Nurse: It sounds like you need some more information about what will happen. Later this evening I will come back, and we'll talk some more. Are you expecting to have visitors tonight?

Patient: No, my wife can't leave home. I don't know what she will do without me while I'm here. This came up so suddenly.

Nurse: I can see that this is a serious concern for you. We can explore some possibilities when I come back this evening. I'll plan to come around 7:15, if that suits you.

Patient: Sure, I can use all the help I can get.

Caring Through Holistic Communication

Holistic communication is "the art of sharing emotional and factual information. It involves letting go of judgments and appreciating the patient's point of view" (Klagsbrun, 2001, p. 116). Think about those words; how reassuring would it be to you right now to have someone who, without judgment, appreciated *your* point of view? Virtually all nurses begin their professional lives wanting to give patients that kind of attention. But the reality of too many patients and too little time often reduces communication to its barest essentials. The holistic view of communication speeds the healing process, whereas functional communication, which ignores all but instructions and quick responses, inhibits it.

Some nurses fear that holistic communication will take too much time. But when patients are listened to in this way, their anxiety decreases, they complain less, call for attention less often, feel more understood and valued, and "are more likely to comply with their treatment plan" (Klagsbrun, p. 116).

Holistic communicators actively *attend* to their patients through such intentional gestures as an accepting facial expression, warm eye contact, turning toward the patient with open posture, and encouraging expression of concerns. They show a willingness to listen to whatever issues the patient needs to share by asking simple, open-ended questions such as "Are you OK?"

Holistic communicators use the principles of active listening—that is, listening to the whole person and paying "gentle, compassionate attention to what has been said or implied" (Klagsbrun, p. 116). This kind of *being present with* patients means avoiding analyzing, judging, or problem solving. It means avoiding defensiveness, even when the patient is critical of you or your co-workers. And it has a beneficial effect on the well-being of nurses and patients.

COMMUNICATION WITH PROFESSIONAL COLLEAGUES

This chapter has focused on nurse-patient communication as the core of the nursing process and foundation of the therapeutic use of self. In addition to patients and their families, however, nurses must also communicate effectively with a variety of professional and unlicensed personnel such as physicians, other nurses, and nursing assistants. Health care delivery suffers when the members of the health care team experience communication breakdown.

As a general rule, nurses can use with colleagues the same communication skills that have been discussed as part of nurse-patient communication. The attitude of respect for others, regardless of position, is essential. Active listening, acceptance, and nonjudgmentalism are key elements, as are the conscious use of feedback, appropriateness, efficiency, and flexibility.

Communication in Today's Multicultural Workplace

Sensitivity to cultural differences in communication is essential in today's culturally diverse workplace. The composition of the health care workforce is being rapidly transformed by the population demographics of the nation. Diversity in age, race, gender, ethnicity, country of origin, sexual orientation, and disability is present, creating opportunities for nurses to develop skill in transcultural communication.

As discussed in earlier chapters, culture is the lens through which all other aspects of life are viewed. Culture determines an individual's health beliefs and practices. It also affects profoundly the meaning individuals attribute to work. Different cultures view caring for the sick in widely varying ways, such as a divine calling, a religious vocation, or an occupation for the lower classes.

The meaning of work in a given culture also affects how people of that culture communicate. Andrews (1998) pointed out that verbal or nonverbal communication issues are often at the root of conflict in the multicultural health care setting. According to Andrews, the decision to speak directly with someone, send a memorandum, make a phone call, or not to communicate at all should be made only after taking the receiving staff member's cultural preferences into consideration. Strategies for promoting effective cross-cultural communication in the workplace are found in Box 18-5.

Wise nurses do not leave their communication skills at the patient's bedside but use them throughout their personal and professional lives. Using clear, simple messages and clarifying the intent of others constitute a positive goal in all personal and professional communication. As with patients, trust must exist before communication with co-workers can be effective.

COLLABORATION SKILLS

Collaboration is a complex process that is related to communication. An often-misunderstood concept, collaboration in health care settings is far more than simply cooperation or compromise. Henneman and colleagues analyzed collaboration to understand its complexities better. They asserted that collaboration implies working jointly with other professionals, all of whom are respected for their unique knowledge and abilities, to benefit a patient's wellness or illness needs or to solve an organizational problem. It involves sharing knowledge and authority and is non-hierarchical. For collaboration to occur, a variety of human and organizational factors must be in place (Henneman, Lee, and Cohen, 1995).

Human Factors in Collaboration

Although it may seem obvious, all collaborating parties must be willing to work together if the collaboration is to be successful. They must have attained a level of

Box **18-5** **Strategies to Promote Effective Communication in the Multicultural Workplace**

- Pronounce names correctly; when in doubt, ask for the correct pronunciation.
- Use proper titles of respect (e.g., doctor, reverend, mister). Be sure to ask for the person's permission to use his or her first name or wait until you are given permission to do so.
- Be aware of gender sensitivities. If uncertain about the marital status of a woman or her preferred title, it is best to refer to her as "Ms." (pronounced *miz*) initially, then at the first opportunity, ask her what she prefers to be called.
- Be aware of subtle linguistic messages that may convey bias or inequality— for example, referring to a white male as "Mr." while addressing an African-American female by her first name.
- Refrain from Anglicizing or shortening a person's given name without his or her permission. For example, calling a Russian American "Mike" instead of Mikhael, or shortening the name of Italian American Maria Rosaria to Maria. The same principle applies to the surname.
- Call people by their proper name. Avoid slang such as "girl," "boy," "honey," "dear," "guy," "fella," "babe," "chief," "mama," "sweetheart," or similar terms. When in doubt, ask whether a particular term is offensive.
- Refrain from using slang, pejorative, or derogatory terms when referring to persons from particular ethnic, racial, or religious groups.
- Identify people by race, color, ethnic origin, religion, or physical handicap/ disability only when necessary and appropriate.
- Avoid using words and phrases that may be offensive to others. For example, "culturally deprived" or "culturally disadvantaged" implies inferiority, and "nonwhite" implies that white is the normative standard.
- Avoid clichés and platitudes, such as, "Some of my best friends are Mexicans" or "I went to school with African-Americans."
- In communications, use language that includes all staff.
- Do not expect a staff member to know all the other employees of his or her background or to speak for them. They share ethnicity, not necessarily the same experiences, friendships, or beliefs.
- Refrain from telling stories or jokes demeaning to certain ethnic, racial, age, or religious groups. Also avoid those pertaining to gender-related issues or to persons with physical or mental disabilities.
- Avoid remarks that suggest to staff from diverse backgrounds that they should consider themselves fortunate to be in the organization. Do not compare their employment opportunities and conditions to people in their country of origin.
- Remember that communication problems multiply in telephone communications because important nonverbal cues are lost and accents may be difficult to interpret.

Adapted with permission from Andrews MM: Transcultural perspectives in nursing administration, *JONA* 28(11):34, 1998.

readiness to collaborate through education, maturity, and prior experience (Henneman, Lee, and Cohen, 1995). They must know what knowledge and expertise they bring to the table and have confidence in the worth of their contributions. They must understand their own limits and their discipline's boundaries while respecting what other professions and professionals can contribute. Above all, they must communicate effectively, trust one another, and be committed to working together (Henneman, Lee, and Cohen, 1995).

Organizational Factors in Collaboration

Just as the people involved must have certain attributes that facilitate collaboration, the organization in which the collaboration takes place also must be supportive. According to Henneman and colleagues, factors supporting collaboration include a flat, as opposed to a multi-tiered, organizational structure; encouragement and support of individuals to act autonomously; recognition of team accomplishments, as opposed to individual accomplishments; cooperation as opposed to competition; and valuing of knowledge and expertise rather than titles or roles. Collaborative organizations have values that support equality and interdependence rather than status and pecking orders. Creativity and shared vision are also valued (Henneman, Lee, and Cohen, 1995).

Outcomes of Collaboration

Collaboration is a positive process that benefits the people involved, as individuals and as a group; the organization in which they work; and health care consumers. Henneman and colleagues identified increased feelings of self-worth, a sense of accomplishment, esprit de corps, enhanced collegiality and respect, and increased productivity, retention, and employee satisfaction as positive benefits of collaboration. They suggested that patient outcomes are also improved by collaboration among health care professionals (Henneman, Lee, and Cohen, 1995).

Nurse-Physician Collaboration

Among the most problematic relationships that nurses encounter during practice are those with physicians. Despite rising male enrollments in nursing schools and even more dramatic female enrollments in medical schools, practicing physicians are predominantly male and practicing nurses overwhelmingly female. This leads to differences in styles of communicating and behaving that can cause challenges in collaborative relationships.

During female-dominated nursing school experiences, most nurses are encouraged to view physicians as teammates and to collaborate with them whenever possible. Male-dominated medical schools, however, tend to instill in their graduates a hierarchical model of teamwork with the physician at the top of the hierarchy. These two divergent cultures, when combined with gender differences in communication and teamwork patterns, further complicate the relationship between the two professions. Too often, gender differences are interpreted as professional differences, leading to further misunderstanding.

People realize that there are differences in communication styles and behavior among individuals of different cultures. What too few people recognize is that gender is a type of culture, because men and women grow up learning different lessons about what is appropriate adult behavior. From birth, boy babies and girl babies are dressed differently, given different toys, praised for different types of behavior, and socialized to gender-appropriate behavior in dozens of more subtle ways. Teachers treat boys and girls differently; authors of children's books and television scripts depict men and women differently (Heim, 1995). Is it any wonder that as adults, men and women may have differing expectations of professional relationships?

According to Heim, women tend to treat other people as equal, regardless of their position in the organizational hierarchy. They spend time chatting with others, building and maintaining relationships, and frequently make friends at work. Even when in management roles, they tend to tell people what to do indirectly. In general, they come to meetings expecting to discuss the issues and make decisions depending on the outcome of the discussion. They value the process aspects of decision-making as much as the outcome (Heim, 1995).

Men tend to see other workers as above, below, or parallel to them in the organizational structure and to treat them accordingly. They chat less, are friendly but tend not to become friends with co-workers, and are likely to tell subordinates what to do directly. In general, they come to meetings already having discussed the issues, make decisions beforehand, and line up the votes they need to get their decisions approved. They are more goal-oriented and pay less attention to process than to outcome (Heim, 1995).

Differences in gender cultures create challenges in all aspects of personal and professional life if they are not understood. For insight into how gender culture may affect your working relationships, take the gender culture self-assessment in Box 18-6 and discuss it in a small group composed of both genders.

Collaboration With Assistive Personnel

Relationships between registered nurses and unlicensed assistive personnel, formerly known as nurse's aides or nursing assistants, affect the quality of care given to hospitalized patients. All too often, mutual respect and cooperation are missing in these important relationships, and both groups feel frustrated and unappreciated. In many areas, ethnic and cultural differences complicate the relationship between nurses and unlicensed personnel. Language is often a barrier as are nonverbal and other culturally determined behaviors, such as the value placed on punctuality. Differences in beliefs, values, perceptions, and priorities create conflict, result in poor teamwork, reduce job satisfaction, and ultimately have a negative impact on patient care (Grossman and Taylor, 1995).

Hayes (1994) reported on team building sessions with registered nurses and unlicensed personnel on three general hospital units. The purpose was to identify and align the needs of work-related relationships in both groups with the needs of the nursing unit. This is a key step in team building, which was the model chosen to encourage collaboration between the two groups.

Teams were defined as groups of workers with a fairly stable composition. They worked interdependently and "shared a common purpose" (Hayes, 1994, p. 52). To emphasize that the nurses and unlicensed personnel needed to work cooperatively,

Box **18-6** Gender Culture Self-Assessment

Directions: For each of the paired statements, select the one that most accurately expresses your experiences or feelings.

Column One

I prefer to compete to win.

I like to work where I know the hierarchy so that I know what is expected of me.

When I lead a meeting, I prefer to sit in front of the group or at the head of the table.

In arriving at a decision, I study the options, select one, and move ahead with it.

I define a "team player" as someone who follows orders, supports the leader unquestioningly, and does what is needed no matter how he or she feels.

I can disagree or even argue with my friends and not allow it to affect the friendship.

In the workplace, competent people don't worry about being nice.

I spend little time in getting to know my co-workers personally.

Column Two

I prefer to find win-win solutions.

I like to work in situations where power is equally shared.

When I lead a meeting, I prefer to sit with the group or in a circle.

In arriving at a decision, I usually ask several other people for their opinions.

I define a "team player" as someone who shares ideas, listens even when they disagree, and works collaboratively.

I expect my friends to side with me in disagreements and tend to take it personally if they don't.

In the workplace it is possible to be both competent and nice.

It is worthwhile to spend time getting to know my co-workers on a personal level.

Scoring instructions: If most of your checks were in Column One, you have a traditionally male gender style. When you work with women, you can anticipate some challenges because of differences in behavior and conversational styles. These challenges can be overcome.

If most of your checks were in Column Two, you have a traditionally female gender style. When you work with men, you can anticipate some challenges because of differences in behavior and conversational styles. These challenges can be overcome.

If your checks were about equally balanced between Column One and Column Two, you have a combination of male and female gender styles. You should be able to work easily with both men and women.

researchers asked each group questions, such as the following: "What do you need from each other to make your day go better?" "What is important for you to have in the way of working relationships on this nursing unit?" "What do you need from the registered nurses?" and "What do you need from the nursing assistants?" (Hayes, 1994, p. 52).

Unlicensed personnel reported needing to feel welcome, appreciated, and respected but instead reported feeling unwelcome, unrecognized, and unappreciated. They did not realize that registered nurses were expected to plan, supervise, and evaluate the work of unlicensed personnel. The registered nurses expressed the need to feel competent as managers and to have unlicensed personnel comply with requests and give feedback about assigned activities. Some registered nurses reported that they preferred to complete work themselves rather than experience embarrassment when unlicensed personnel failed to comply with their requests.

> **Box 18-7** Colleagues Learn What They Live
>
> If a colleague lives with criticism, s/he learns to condemn.
> If a colleague lives with hostility, s/he learns to fight.
> If a colleague lives with ridicule, s/he learns to be shy.
> If a colleague lives with shame, s/he learns to feel guilty.
> If a colleague lives with tolerance, s/he learns to be patient.
> If a colleague lives with encouragement, s/he learns confidence.
> If a colleague lives with praise, s/he learns to appreciate.
> If a colleague lives with fairness, s/he learns justice.
> If a colleague lives with security, s/he learns to have faith.
> If a colleague lives with approval, s/he learns to like her/himself.
> If a colleague lives with acceptance and friendship, s/he learns to find satisfaction in professional nursing.

Adapted with permission of Uustal DB: *Values and ethics in nursing: from theory to practice,*
East Greenwich, RI, 1985, Educational Resources in Nursing and Wholistic Health.

Team-building sessions centered around identifying problematic feelings and misperceptions and correcting them. For example, in response to the unlicensed personnel's belief that their contributions to patient welfare were unappreciated, the registered nurses replied, "We could not run the unit without you" and "What you do makes the difference in how comfortable the patients feel" (Hayes, 1994, p. 53).

During team building with these groups, Hayes reported that misperceptions were aired and discussed and expectations were clarified. Registered nurses' legitimate authority and legal responsibility for unlicensed personnel were clarified. The result was an increase in mutual respect and understanding.

To stress the importance of positive working relationships, Diann B. Uustal, clinical ethicist and consultant, adapted the familiar poem, "Children Learn What They Live" to apply to colleagues (Box 18-7). It reminds us that professional co-workers, as much as patients, deserve respectful concern.

Summary of Key Points

- The "therapeutic use of self" means using one's personality and communication skills effectively while implementing the nursing process to help patients improve their health status.
- Phases in the traditional nurse-patient relationship include the orientation phase, the working phase, and the termination phase. Short-term patient contacts in today's streamlined care delivery system also present opportunities for connection and goal achievement.
- In long-term nurse-patient relationships, each phase has specific tasks that should be accomplished before progressing to subsequent phases.
- Acceptance of others' values, beliefs, and lifestyles is important in nursing.
- Developing awareness of biases can help nurses to prevent the intrusion of these biases into nurse-patient relationships.

- Communication is the core of all relationships and is the primary instrument through which desired change is effected in others.
- Communication is both verbal and nonverbal and consists of a sender, a receiver, a message, feedback, and context.
- Perception, evaluation, and transmission are the three major operations in communication.
- Communication develops sequentially, beginning with somatic language and progressing to action language and then to verbal language.
- Communication may be successful or unsuccessful. Successful communication meets four major criteria: feedback, appropriateness, efficiency, and flexibility.
- Active listening is a key factor in holistic communication.
- Unsuccessful communication is caused by a variety of factors that can be identified and eliminated.
- In addition to communicating well with patients, nurses use communication skills to collaborate effectively with physicians, other nurses, unlicensed personnel, and other members of the health care delivery team.
- Professional nurses must be sensitive to sociocultural factors such as ethnicity and gender that can affect communication and collaboration.

CRITICAL THINKING QUESTIONS

1. Explain what is meant by the term "therapeutic use of self."
2. List the phases of the traditional nurse-patient relationship and the tasks of each.
3. Identify ways nurses can quickly "connect" with patients and help them move toward wellness during short-term opportunities.
4. Explain why nonverbal communication may be more revealing than verbal communication.
5. List as many factors as you can that influence the communication process.
6. Identify a recent interaction you have had in which communication was incongruent. Analyze the effect of the incongruence on the communication. When are people most likely to use incongruent communication?
7. Think of a person with whom you have experienced difficult communication. Identify which of the barriers to successful communication are functioning in that person's communication with you and analyze your responses to that person.
8. Describe a collaborative experience you have had. What factors differentiated it from cooperation or compromise?

REFERENCES

Andrews MM: Transcultural perspectives in nursing administration. *JONA* 28(11):30-38, 1998.

Barke J, editor: *Burns' poems and songs*, London, 1955, Collins.

Davidhizar R, Dowd S, Giger JN: Recognizing abuse in culturally diverse clients, *Health Care Supervisor* 17(2):10-20, 1998.

Gardner M: Where did all the listeners go? *Christian Science Monitor*, April 27, 1990, 14.

Grossman D, Taylor R: Cultural diversity on the unit, *Am J Nurs* 95(2):64-66, 1995.

Hagerty BM, Patusky KL: Reconceptualizing the nurse-patient relationship, *J Nurs Sch* 35(2):145-150, 2003.

Hayes PM: Team building: Bringing RNs and NAs together, *Nursing Management*, 25(5): 52-55, 1994.

Heim P: Getting beyond "she said, he said," *Nurs Admin Q* 19(2):6-18, 1995.

Henneman EA, Lee JL, Cohen JI: Collaboration: a concept analysis, *J Adv Nurs* 21(1):103-109, 1995.

Klagsbrun J: Listening and focusing: holistic health care tools for nurses, *Nurs Clin N Am* 36(1):115-130, 2001.

National Council of State Boards of Nursing: *Professional boundaries: a nurse's guide to the importance of appropriate professional boundaries*, Chicago, 1996, NCSBN, Online *(www.ncsbn.org/public/resources/res/expectnurse.pdf)*.

Nurse's Relationship with Patient Results in Disciplinary Action: *Nursing Law's Regan Report* 43(8):4-5, 2003.

Peplau H: *Interpersonal relations in nursing*, New York, 1952, GP Putnam's Sons.

Ruesch J: *Disturbed communication: the clinical assessment of normal and pathological communicative behavior*, New York, 1972, WW Norton.

Uustal DB: *Values and ethics in nursing: from theory to practice*, East Greenwich, RI, 1985, Educational Resources in Nursing and Wholistic Health.

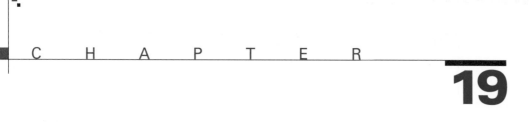

CHAPTER 19

Nursing Ethics

Pamela S. Chally and M. Catherine Hough

Key Terms

Advance Directives
Autonomy
Beneficence
Bioethics
Code of Ethics
Double Effect
Deontology

Ethical Decision Making
Ethics
Fidelity
Justice
Moral Development
Morals
Nonmaleficence

Patient Rights
Personal Value System
Respect for Persons
Utilitarianism
Veracity
Virtue Ethics

Learning Outcomes

After studying this chapter, students will be able to:

- Differentiate between morals and ethics.
- Discuss the importance to nursing of having a code of ethics.
- Identify basic theories and principles central to ethical dilemmas and moral development.
- Describe ethical dilemmas resulting from conflicts between patients, health care professionals, and institutions.
- Describe a model for ethical decision making.
- Discuss the impact of ethical issues on nurses and other health care professionals.

Nurses, by the very nature of the work they do, face ethical dilemmas daily. As indicated in Box 19-1 ("Letter to Nursing Students From a Nurse Practitioner"), nurses must decide how to allocate scarce resources, what information to share with patients and their families, how to manage low-functioning colleagues, and how to resolve conflicts between patient wishes and institutional policies. Preparing to deal with these and other issues requires an understanding of ethical theories and principles and the ability to use an ethical decision-making model that works for the individual nurse in the context of his or her own value system.

Box **19-1** **Letter to Nursing Students From a Nurse Practitioner**

Dear Nursing Student,

As you begin your nursing education, your focus may be on competently performing tangible clinical skills that require psychomotor dexterity. Knowledge of ethical decision making skills and encountering ethical dilemmas may seem to be near the end of a long list of overwhelming responsibilities. However, a solid ethical decision making foundation will long outlast the initial anxiety associated with learning new psychomotor skills.

In your nursing career, regardless of your chosen practice location, you will routinely be faced with opportunities to develop your ethical decision making skills. What are some points to consider when developing these skills?

Take a critical look at yourself. Identify your values and beliefs. Are these values and beliefs firmly entrenched, or are you easily swayed toward change by outside pressure? Are you willing to take a firm advocacy stance on an issue you believe is correct? Are you just as willing to admit if you are wrong and learn from your experience? Are you comfortable with sensitive or confidential information placed in your possession? When necessary, can you take a neutral stance and avoid the temptation to give advice? Can you comfortably accept both personal praise and constructive criticism?

Like many of these questions, ethical dilemmas cannot always be answered by a simple "yes" or "no." Ethical dilemmas may occur at the individual, group or community level. Many of you will face these dilemmas on a routine basis. Some situations will be more obviously dramatic than others. You may be involved in supporting a patient or family through a "do not resuscitate" decision, the decision to terminate life support systems in a nonviable patient, or organ donation decisions. You may encounter a suicidal or homicidal patient who confides in no one else. You may encounter a chemically or otherwise impaired health care provider.

As you mature in your nursing experience, encountering and resolving ethical dilemmas to the best possible outcome, can prove to be a personally rewarding experience for both you and those who benefit from your abilities. Do not avoid these ethical dilemmas. Instead, meet these challenges with confidence and professionalism using the principles of ethical decision making.

Best wishes as you continue your nursing education and in your future nursing career.

—Sandra H. Carr, MN, ARNP

Courtesy Sandra H. Carr.

To understand ethics and its relationship to health care, the terms *morals, ethics,* and *bioethics* must first be clarified. It is important to recognize that philosophers and scholars have conflicting viewpoints on how to define these terms. For the purposes of this textbook, we have chosen to use the following definitions. **Morals** are established rules in situations in which a decision about right and wrong must be made. Morals provide standards of behavior. These standards guide the behavior of an individual or social group. Morals reflect the *is* or reality of how individuals or groups behave. An example of a moral standard is "Good people do not lie."

Morals reflect the *is* of human behavior, whereas **ethics** is a term used to reflect the *should* of human behavior. Ethics identify what *should* be done for individuals to live in relative harmony with one another. Ethics are process-oriented and involve critical analysis of actions. If ethicists, people who study ethics, reflected on the moral statement "One should not lie," they would clarify definitions of lying and explore whether or not there are circumstances under which lying might be acceptable.

Despite the fact that differences between ethics and morals are noted by several authors (Burkhardt and Nathaniel, 2002; Davis, Aroskar, Liaschenko, et al., 1997; Volbrecht, 2002), in everyday speech the terms are often used interchangeably (Johnstone, 1999).

The application of ethical theories and principles to problems in health care is called **bioethics.** Bioethics as an area of ethical inquiry came into existence around 1970, when health care began to shift its focus from curing disease toward concern for the total patient (Husted and Husted, 1995). The term, *clinical ethics,* is increasingly being used.

Advances in medicine, science, and technology, while solving some problems, can create ethical dilemmas. For example, people can now be kept "alive" even when there is no higher brain activity. Should they be kept alive under these circumstances just because we now have the technology to do so? This kind of issue mandates that nurses be concerned with what should be done for patients under their care. It is important that actions be critically analyzed for their appropriateness because health care professionals possess a good deal of power over those in their care.

Within this context, nurses need to study codes of ethics, ethical theories and principles, moral development, ethical dilemmas, and ethical decision-making models. Such knowledge increases nurses' ability to participate in the resolution of ethical dilemmas. The accompanying Interview of respected ethicist Mila Aroskar, RN, EdD, FAAN, highlights some of the reasons why professional nurses need ethical decision-making skills.

NURSING CODES OF ETHICS

As discussed in Chapter 6, an essential characteristic of professions is that they have a **code of ethics.** A code of ethics is an implied contract through which the profession informs society of the principles and rules by which it functions.

Ethical codes help with professional self-regulation. They serve as guidelines to the members of the profession, who then can meet the societal need for trustworthy, qualified, and accountable caregivers. It is important to remember that codes are useful only if they are known and upheld by the members of the profession.

American Nurses Association's *Code of Ethics for Nurses*

The *Code of Ethics for Nurses with Interpretive Statements* is the nursing profession's expression of its ethical values and duties to the public. The need for a code of ethics was expressed by the Nurses' Associated Alumnae (forerunner of the American

🐚 interv i e w *with Mila A. Aroskar, Associate Professor,*
School of Public Health, University of
Minnesota, Minneapolis, Minnesota

Interviewer: Who most influenced your thinking about ethics and why?

Aroskar: The foundations were laid by my parents who were wonderful role models for learning personal responsibility, respect for living beings, and concern for the good of the community. Before entering nursing school at Columbia University, I completed a degree in religion at Wooster College in Wooster, Ohio. My professors taught and modeled respect for persons and reflective thinking about significant issues that affected individuals, groups, communities, and nations. Several individuals who have contributed to the field of bioethics over the past three decades have influenced my thinking and work in ethics and nursing. Early influences include the writings of philosophers such as Daniel Callahan, cofounder of The Hastings Center, who writes about priorities and goals of health care, end-of-life decision making, and societal obligations to the elderly; Sissela Bok's writings on lying and truth-telling in the context of individual moral choices and consequences for community; and theologian Paul Ramsey, who wrote about health professionals' obligations to patients and issues in genetics decades before today's Human Genome Project. I am grateful to numerous others working in bioethics who have contributed to my thinking and writing about professional and applied ethics over the past two decades.

Interviewer: Why is ethical decision making so important for nurses?

Aroskar: The societal obligation of the nursing profession is caring for the sick, the healthy, and the worried well. In their professional roles and relationships, nurses offer a holistic perspective of human beings and their health needs in health care and other organizations. Respect for persons, avoiding harm, providing benefits of nursing care for all in need, and promotion of justice in health care are foundational obligations in the practice of nursing as found in the American Nurses Association's *Code for Nurses* (American Nurses Association, 1976, 1985). These ethical principles and values have been and are currently challenged by the power, administrative, and payment structures found in health care institutions and systems. These are not new challenges but put nursing values in even more serious jeopardy with the current emphasis on cost containment in health care. Learning skills in reflective thinking that incorporate consideration of ethical principles and obligations are critical for nurses to be able to respond to the ethical dilemmas and challenges they face at the bedside and in efforts to influence the development of institutional and public policy for health care funding and delivery of services that are accessible to all. Nurses are and can be superb advocates for the health needs of all human beings, including their own physical, psychological, emotional, and spiritual health needs. An ongoing challenge is to maintain a level of energy and commitment to doing so as nurse staffing is reduced as a major cost cutting measure in so many settings.

interv i e w *with Mila A. Aroskar, Associate Professor,*
School of Public Health, University of
Minnesota, Minneapolis,
Minnesota—cont'd

Interviewer: How can nurses prepare to deal with ethical dilemmas?
Aroskar: First, all nursing education programs should include learning opportunities in nursing and health care ethics—to identify ethical issues/problems in practice and learn the skills necessary to respond to these issues in a thoughtful and reasoned way that incorporates attention to the nurses' employment settings, their political and power aspects. There are many excellent workshops and seminars available locally and nationally that enrich nurses' decision making and practice from an ethical perspective. The American Nurses Association and many state nurses associations have an ethics and human rights committee or other resources such as position statements on ethical issues in nursing that help nurses in dealing with ethical concerns in practice. Participation as members of institutional ethics committees, attending their educational programs, and using their consultation resources are other avenues for dealing with ethical practice dilemmas. Nursing journals and bioethics publications contain articles dealing with ethical issues in nursing practice, health care, and organizational ethics. Literature searches via the Web are an additional resource for nurses who do not have easy access to some of the other resources identified here. Visit Evolve WebLinks related to the content of this chapter: **http://evolve.elsevier.com/Chitty/professional/.**

Nurses Association [ANA]) as early as 1897 (Veins, 1989). A written code was first adopted in 1950. During the 53-year interval between 1897 and 1950, nursing was emerging as a profession in its own right.

The 1950 *Code* consisted of 17 short, succinct statements depicting the nurse in action (e.g., "The nurse accepts ...," "The nurse sustains ...") (Veins, 1989). Even in 1950, the broad-spectrum role of the nurse—in illness, prevention, and health promotion—was stressed. In addition, this *Code* encouraged nurses to participate in lifelong learning activities. Minor revisions to the first *Code* were agreed on by delegates to the ANA's conventions throughout the 1950s.

In 1958, the ANA's Committee on Ethical Standards began reviewing the entire *Code*, and in 1960, major revisions were suggested (Veins, 1989). The 1960 *Code* also contained 17 statements, but new statements were added and others deleted. The new statements addressed nurses' responsibilities to participate in the professional organization and the necessity of identifying and upholding professional standards. Another new statement addressed nurses' participation in negotiating terms of employment. This opened the way, in later years, for the ANA to function as a collective-bargaining agent for nurses. An earlier statement, describing nurses' obligations to physicians, was eliminated from the 1960 *Code* (Veins, 1989).

The next major revision of the *Code*, completed in 1976, resulted in 11 statements. The emphasis of the 1976 *Code* was the nurse's relationship to the client.

No longer was the word *patient* used. *Client* was adopted in the belief that it was a more inclusive term than *patient*. All gender-related language was eliminated. A paragraph dealing with consequences of breaking the *Code* was also added. Accordingly, the nurse who violated the *Code* could be censured, suspended, or expelled from the ANA. Any violations of civil law would subject the nurse to legal action as well (American Nurses Association, 1976). Clarifying statements were added to each point in the *Code* in the 1976 revision. These interpretations provided definitions of key terms and elaborated on the meaning of each statement.

In 1985, the *Code* was again reviewed. All 11 statements remained the same, but the interpretations were updated. In particular, more emphasis was placed on clients' rights. In 1996, a task force was appointed to review the *Code*. The revised *Code* went through several reviews and was adopted in 2001 by the ANA House of Delegates.

The *Code of Ethics for Nurses with Interpretive Statements* is the latest version of nursing's ethical code. The *Code of Ethics for Nurses* (American Nurses Association, 2001) can be found on the inside back cover of this text. Interpretive statements can be found online *(www.nursingworld.org/ethics/code/ethicscode150.htm)*. The *Code* is reviewed periodically to ensure that it reflects both the constancy and change in the nursing profession (Fowler, 1999). Modification of the *Code* is necessary to meet the ever-changing demands of health care and society.

International Council of Nurses Code of Ethics for Nurses

The International Council of Nurses (ICN) (1973) also has published a code of ethics for the profession. This document discusses the rights and responsibilities of nurses related to people, practice, society, co-workers, and the profession. The ICN first adopted a code of ethics in 1953. Its last revision (2000) represents agreement by more than 80 national nursing associations that participate in the international association. Inherent in the *International Council of Nurses Code for Nurses* is nursing's respect for the life, dignity, and rights of all people in a manner that is unmindful of nationality, race, creed, color, age, sex, political affiliation, or social status. The ICN's most recent revisions were adopted in 2000. You can view the *ICN's Code for Nurses* online *(www.icn.ch/ethics.htm)*.

ETHICAL THEORIES

There is no single ethical theory ascribed to by all philosophers or ethicists. Numerous theories have been developed. In this section, we discuss three of the primary ethical theories that nurse ethicists have identified as useful: deontology, utilitarianism, and virtue ethics.

Deontology

The major proponent of **deontology** was Immanuel Kant (1724–1804). Kant believed that the rightness or wrongness of an action depended on the inherent moral significance of the action ([1959] 1985). He believed that an act was moral if it originated from good will. Ethical action consisted of doing one's duty. To do one's duty was right; not to do one's duty was wrong. According to Brannigan and Boss (2001), there is a duty to do what is right for its own sake. The moral agent must do what is right and refrain from what is wrong. Beyond this, nothing is ethically relevant. The outcomes or consequences of an action can be desired or deplored, but they are not relevant from an ethical perspective.

Deontology can be further divided into act deontology and rule deontology. Act deontologists determine the right thing to do by gathering all the facts and then making a decision. Much time and energy is needed to judge each situation carefully in and of itself. Once a decision is made, there is commitment to universalizing it. In other words, if one makes a moral judgment in one situation, the same judgment will be made in any similar situation.

Rule deontologists, on the other hand, emphasize that principles guide our actions. Examples of rules might be "Always keep a promise" or "Never tell a lie." In all situations, the rule is to be followed. Deontologists are not concerned with the consequences of adhering to certain rules or actions. If the principle believed in is "Always keep a promise," the deontologist will keep promises, even if circumstances have changed. For example, if a father has promised that he will take his son to a baseball game and then a close family member becomes critically ill, the baseball game promise will be kept regardless of the changed circumstances.

In nursing, there are many rules and duties that nurses follow. One such rule is "Do no harm" (**beneficence**). Another justifiable rule is "The patient should be allowed to make his or her own decisions" (**autonomy**). Consider the situation of a severely depressed young man who wishes to end his life by committing suicide and asks for the nurse's assistance. Clearly, the rule about doing no harm conflicts with allowing the young man to make his own decisions. You can see that dilemmas cannot always be resolved using theoretical approaches alone.

Utilitarianism

Utilitarianism is one of many consequentialism theories based on a fundamental belief that the moral rightness of an action is determined solely by its consequence. Utilitarianism theory was first described by David Hume (1711-1776) and was developed further by many notable philosophers, including Jeremy Benthal (1748-1832) and John Stuart Mill (1806-1873). Mill had a significant influence on utilitarian ethics as we know it today.

According to Mill, writing in 1863, a "right action" conforms to the "greatest happiness principle" (Mill, 1985). In other words, it is right to maximize the greatest good for the happiness or pleasure of the greatest number of people. Utilitarian ethics calculates the effect of all alternative actions on the general welfare of present and future generations. Thus, this position is also referred to as "calculus morality" (Davis, Aroskar, Liaschenko, et al., 1997).

The utilitarian approach to ethics assumes that it is possible to balance good and evil. The goal is that most people experience good rather than evil. Benefits are to be maximized for the greatest number of people possible. In this approach, each individual counts as one.

Professional health care providers employ utilitarian theory in many situations. The concept of triage, in which the sick or injured are classified by the severity of their condition to determine priority of treatment, is an example of utilitarianism.

In triage, those who are so gravely ill or injured that they cannot possibly recover are not treated until all other patients have been treated. Although this seems cruel, when there are many more sick and wounded than available facilities to care for them, triage is accepted worldwide as an ethical basis for determining treatment.

Frequently, utilitarianism is the basis for deciding how health care dollars should be spent. For example, money is more likely to be spent on research for diseases that affect large numbers of people than for research on diseases that affect relatively few. A difficulty of this approach is that although the appeal is made to the happiness of the majority, the interest of the individual or minority, who also deserve help, may be overlooked.

Virtue Ethics

Virtue ethics was first noted in the works of Plato, Aristotle, and early Christians. According to Aristotle, virtues are tendencies to act, feel, and judge that develop through appropriate training but come from natural tendencies. This suggests that individuals' actions are built from a degree of inborn moral virtue (Burkhardt and Nathaniel, 2002).

Recently, bioethics literature has emphasized the character of the decision maker. Virtues refer to specific character traits, including but not limited to honesty, courage, kindness, respectfulness, and integrity. These virtues become obvious through one's behaviors and are expressions of specific ethical principles. Truthfulness, for example, embodies the principle of veracity. Virtues are beneficial assets that positively affect moral decision making (Volbrecht, 2002).

Central to the mission of **virtue ethics** is the formation of character. Descriptions of character portray a way of being, rather than the process of decision making. From one's way of being flows a way of acting in both one's personal and professional life (Davis, Aroskar, Liaschenko, et al., 1997). A certain mental set does not guarantee right behavior, but it may predispose to right behavior.

Scott (1995) described how the ethical dimension serves as a foundation for nursing practice, since both nursing and ethics are concerned with the nature of persons relating to one another. It has been recognized that nurses' ways of being and acting are essential to the integrity of nursing practice and patient care. Nurses often practice in challenging circumstances in which they must rely on their own integrity to ensure that care is given conscientiously and consistently. Virtues may be what separates the competent nurse from the exemplary nurse. Table 19-1 summarizes the major points of these three ethical theories.

ETHICAL PRINCIPLES

Respect for persons is the most fundamental human right (Aroskar, 1995). It requires that each person be respected as a unique individual equal to all others. This means valuing every aspect of a person's life, not just the parts that are easy to value because they are congruent with one's own values. Respect for persons is the foundation of the six ethical principles discussed in this section: justice, autonomy, beneficence, nonmaleficence, veracity, and fidelity.

Table 19-1 PRIMARY ETHICAL THEORIES

Deontology	Moral rules are absolute and apply to all individuals.
	Concept of obligation overrides consequences of action.
	Duty must occur prior to value.
	Includes some religious traditions.
Utilitarianism	Moral rightness of actions are determined by their consequences.
	Basis found in the doctrine of psychological hedonism and the principle of utility that maximizes pleasure and minimizes pain.
	Interested in the greatest good for the greatest number.
Virtue Ethics	Introduces the character of the individual.
	Individual moral actions are based on innate moral virtue.
	Based on cardinal virtues (faith, hope, charity, wisdom).
	Focal virtues* as related to bioethics are compassion, discernment, trustworthiness, and integrity.

*Focal virtues identified by Beauchamp TL, Childless JF: *Principles of biomedical ethics*, ed 4, New York, 2001, Oxford University Press.

Justice

The principle of **justice** states that equals should be treated the same and that unequals should be treated differently (Beauchamp and Childless, 2001). In other words, patients with the same diagnosis and health care needs should receive the same care. Those with greater or lesser needs should receive different care.

In health care, the most common concern about justice relates to allocation of resources. How much of our national resources should be appropriated to health care? What health care problems should receive the most financial resources? What patients should have access to health care services? According to the principle of justice, the answer to these questions is based on treating all individuals equally.

Numerous models have been developed for distributing health care resources. These models include the following:

1. To each equally.
2. To each according to merit (this may include past or future contributions to society).
3. To each according to what can be acquired in the marketplace.
4. To each according to need (Jameton, 1984).

All of these suggestions for distribution have merit and make it difficult to decide who should be treated and for what condition. Ideally, all patients would receive all available treatment and resources for their health needs. Unfortunately, this is not possible because of costs and limited supplies, such as transplantable organs.

Justice as a principle often leaves us with more questions than answers. It raises our consciousness about making ethical decisions but certainly does not determine what the answer should be.

Autonomy

The principle of autonomy is based on the assertion that individuals have the right to determine their own actions and the freedom to make their own decisions.

Autonomy refers to the control individuals have over their own lives. Respect for the individual is the cornerstone of this principle.

Autonomy applies both to decisions and actions. Autonomous decisions are based on (1) individuals' values, (2) adequate information, (3) freedom from coercion, and (4) reason and deliberation. Autonomous actions result from autonomous decisions.

The concept of autonomy has featured prominently in ethics and philosophy since the time of the ancient Greeks. Philosophers and lawyers agree that people have a right to make decisions for themselves. Case law established more than 90 years ago that health care professionals should not act against the wishes of an adult human being of sound mind (*Schoendorf v. Society of New York Hospital*, 105 N.E., 92, 1914).

It is difficult to disagree with autonomy. Autonomy is a basic principle of the U.S. Constitution. Throughout the history of the United States, people have fought and died for the right of individual autonomy for themselves and others. Disregard for autonomy, however, is glaringly evident in the health care system.

Health care professionals often take actions that profoundly affect patients' lives without adequate consultation with the patients themselves. Incorporating the principle of autonomy in all health care situations is difficult, if not impossible. Patients cannot always make their own choices. Examples of those unable to participate in decisions include infants or small children, mentally incompetent patients, and unconscious patients. Other patients may be unable to participate in decision making because of external constraints, such as financial limitations, lack of necessary information, or the norms of their culture.

Beneficence

Beneficence is commonly defined as "the doing of good." According to Frankena (1988), beneficence involves four duties: (1) not to inflict harm or evil (**nonmaleficence**), (2) to prevent harm or evil, (3) to remove harm or evil, and (4) to promote or do good.

The first duty—not to inflict harm—takes priority over the three following duties. Even so, all four duties are obligations that must be taken into account. Virtually everyone would agree that causing good and avoiding harm are important to all human beings—and certainly to health care professionals. It may seem surprising, therefore, how often conflicts center around this principle. Additional considerations may take precedence when there is conflict about the appropriate course of action. For example, a surgical procedure inflicts harm on the body but potentially has long-term benefits. The procedure may be lifesaving, or it may diminish pain or increase mobility. In this sense, even though it inflicts harm in the short term, it is justified because of the long-term good that results.

In addition to consideration of both short-term and long-term benefits, the principle of beneficence conflicts with other ethical principles. Consider the elderly patient who has just broken her hip for the second time and refuses to eat. Should she be allowed to decide autonomously not to eat even though it will harm her? The principles of autonomy and beneficence are in conflict in this example.

Nonmaleficence

Nonmaleficence is defined as the duty to do no harm. This principle is the foundation of the medical profession's Hippocratic Oath; it is likewise critical to the nursing profession. Inherent in the *Code of Ethics for Nurses* (American Nurses Association, 2001), the nurse must not knowingly act in a manner that would intentionally harm the patient. Although this point appears straightforward, Chulay, Guzzetta, and Dossey (1997) argue that there are some situations in which it is necessary for the nurse to inflict potential harm in an effort to achieve a greater good for the patient. The concept that justifies inflicting harm is referred to as the principle of **double effect.**

The principle of double effect considers the intended foreseen effects of actions by the professional nurse. The doctrine states that as moral agents we many not intentionally produce evil. It is ethically permissible, however, to do what may produce an evil or undesirable result if the intent was to produce an overall good effect (Beauchamp and Childress, 2001).

According to Chulay, Guzzetta, and Dossey (1997), four conditions must be present to justify the use of the double effect principle:

1. The proposed action, independent of its consequences, must be good or at least morally neutral.
2. The nurse must intend only the good effects; the bad effect can be foreseen but not intended.
3. The unintended or bad effects cannot be a means to the end or good effect.
4. The good effects must proportionately outweigh the bad effects.

A classic example of double effect is found in administering medication for pain to the terminally ill as they near death. The proposed action of administering the medication to relieve pain is intrinsically good. Although the nurse intends only the good effect (relief of pain), a bad effect (depression of respiration) may result. The patient and family must be made aware that an undesired and unintended outcome may occur that could further compromise the patient and possibly result in hastening death. In this example, the good effects of pain relief outweigh the risks, as well as the prolonged pain that would occur if the medication were withheld.

Veracity

Veracity is defined as "telling the truth." Truth telling has long been identified as fundamental to the development and continuance of trust among human beings. Telling the truth is expected. It is necessary to basic communication, and societal relationships are built on the individual's right to know the truth.

All communication between individuals has the potential to be misleading. It is easy for information to be misunderstood, misinterpreted, or not comprehended. Usually, these misunderstandings are unintentional. Intentional deception, however, is considered morally wrong.

Despite this well-established fact, much intended deception occurs between health professionals and people seeking health care. Persons seeking health care often are not completely truthful when giving their health histories. For example, they may not reveal the extent of their use of drugs or alcohol.

At the same time, health care professionals are not always truthful in responding to patients' questions. They may choose to answer only part of a question, rather than giving all the known facts. A long tradition of a double standard in truth telling exists in health care (Tschudin, 1993). Health care professionals are not responsible for false information given to them by their patients. They are responsible, however, for information that they give *to* patients.

A number of reasons have been proposed to justify deception by health care professionals. For the most part, these justifications are related to the idea that patients would be better off not knowing certain information or that they are not capable of understanding the information. Based on these justifications, health care professionals often believe they have the right to decide what people should and should not know about their illnesses. However, if both patient and health care provider are respectful of each other as individuals, it is difficult to accept that deception is ever justified.

Fidelity

The principle of **fidelity** refers to faithfulness. The nurse is required to remain faithful in seriously considering all ethical mandates related to the practice of the profession. Through the process of licensure, nurses are granted the right to practice. The licensure process is intended to ensure that only a qualified nurse can practice nursing. When the nurse accepts licensure and becomes a part of the profession, it is mandated that he or she accept certain responsibilities as part of the contract with society. Burkhardt and Nathaniel (2002) state that nurses must be faithful in keeping their promises of respecting all individuals, upholding the *Code of Ethics for Nurses* (American Nurses Association, 2001), practicing within the scope of nursing practice, continuing competence in nursing, abiding by the policies of the employing institution, and keeping promises to patients. Being faithful entails meeting reasonable expectations in all these areas.

Fidelity is also the basis of the nurse-patient relationship. It suggests that one is faithful to the promises, agreements, and commitments made. This faithfulness creates the trust that is essential to any relationship. Most ethicists believe there is no absolute duty to keep promises, however. In every situation, the harmful consequences of the promised action must be weighed against the benefits of promise keeping (Burkhardt and Nathaniel, 2002).

THEORIES OF MORAL DEVELOPMENT

How does a person develop morality and thereby the ability to make decisions about right and wrong? Answering this question moves us into the realm of **moral development.** Moral development describes how a person learns to deal with moral dilemmas from childhood through adulthood. Two major theorists who have worked at understanding this area of human development are Lawrence Kohlberg (1973, 1986) and Carol Gilligan (1982, 1987).

Kohlberg's Levels of Moral Development

Kohlberg (1976, 1986) proposed three levels of moral development: (1) preconventional, (2) conventional, and (3) postconventional. In the preconventional level, the individual is inattentive to the norms of society when responding to moral problems. Instead, the individual's perspective is self-centered. At this level, what the individual wants or needs takes precedence over right or wrong. Kohlberg saw this level of moral development in most children under 9 years of age, as well as in some adolescents and adult criminal offenders.

The conventional level is characterized by making moral decisions that conform to the expectations of one's family, group, or society. When confronted with a moral choice, people functioning at the conventional level follow family or cultural group norms. According to Kohlberg, most adolescents and adults generally function at this level.

The postconventional level involves more independent modes of thinking than previous stages, so that the individual is able to define his or her own moral values. People at the postconventional level may ignore both self-interest and group norms in making moral choices. They create their own morality, which may differ from society's norms. Kohlberg believed that only a minority of adults achieve this level.

Each of Kohlberg's levels is subdivided into two stages. Progression through the stages occurs over varying lengths of time, but the stages are sequential and each stage is characterized by a higher capacity for logical reasoning than the preceding stage.

Kohlberg (1976) suggested that certain conditions may stimulate higher levels of moral development. Intellectual development is one necessary characteristic. Individuals at higher levels intellectually are generally more advanced in moral development than those operating at lower levels of intelligence.

An environment that offers people opportunities for group participation, shared decision-making processes, and responsibility for the consequences of their actions also promotes higher levels of moral reasoning. Further moral development is stimulated by the creation of conflict in settings in which the individual recognizes the limitations of present modes of thinking. Students have been stimulated to higher levels of moral reasoning through participating in courses on moral discussion and ethics (Kohlberg, 1973).

Gilligan's Levels of Moral Development

Gilligan (1982) was concerned that Kohlberg did not give adequate acknowledgment to the experiences of women in moral development. She recognized that Kohlberg's theories had largely been generated from research with men and boys. When women were tested using Kohlberg's levels of moral development, they scored lower than men.

Gilligan believed that this was due not to inadequate moral development in women but to the fact that women's identities are largely dependent on relationships with others. Because of the basic difference in the way men and women feel about relationships, Gilligan believed that Kohlberg's theory was inadequate to explain women's moral development.

She suggested that women view moral dilemmas in terms of conflicting responsibilities. The sequence she described included three levels and two transitions, with each level representing a more complex understanding of the relationship of self and others and each transition resulting in a crucial reevaluation of the conflict between selfishness and responsibility. Gilligan's levels of moral development are (1) orientation to individual survival, (2) a focus on goodness as self-sacrifice, and (3) the morality of nonviolence.

The moral person is one who responds to need and demonstrates a consideration of care and responsibility in relationships. Gilligan described a moral development perspective focused on care. This perspective differed from the orientation toward justice described by Kohlberg (1973, 1976).

More recent work by Gilligan and Attanucci (1988) has attempted to define the relationship between the two moral orientations of justice and care. They determined that both perspectives were present when people faced real-life moral dilemmas, but people generally tended to focus on one set of concerns and paid only minimal attention to the other perspective. As expected, the care focus was more often exhibited by women, and the justice focus was more often exemplified by men.

The justice and care perspectives in themselves are not competing theories but are two separate moral perspectives that organize thinking in different ways (Chally, 1990). The justice perspective strives to treat others fairly, whereas the care perspective is strongly based on relationships with others.

Gilligan, Brown, and Rogers (1988) described a combined care/justice perspective that incorporates both viewpoints as moral deliberations are made. Moral development theory must incorporate all perspectives, some of which may not yet be identified. Analysis of interviews of nurses suggest that nurses at times combine the care/justice perspective when forced to make ethical decisions (Chally, 1995). The accompanying Research Note explores how a preceptor can support ethical decision making by critical care nurses.

UNDERSTANDING ETHICAL DILEMMAS IN NURSING

Ethical dilemmas, as discussed in the Research Note, occur frequently in nursing practice. This is to be expected because nurses focus on life-and-death issues involving human beings. Many ethical dilemmas arise in nursing because of conflicts between patients, health care professionals, and institutions. In the following section, we will explore the major issues involved in these conflicts: (1) personal value systems, (2) peers' and other professionals' behaviors, (3) patients' rights, and (4) institutional and societal issues.

Role of Personal Value Systems

Values are important preferences that influence the behavior of individuals. Value systems are learned beliefs that help people choose among difficult alternatives.

As discussed in Chapter 9, each person has a value system. This value system has a beginning foundation in the beliefs, purposes, attitudes, qualities, and objects that are important to a child's early caregivers. In time, individuals develop their own value systems. A **personal value system** is a rank ordering of values with respect to their importance to one another.

Value systems vary among individuals. Something important to one person may hold greater or lesser significance to someone else. For example, a clean, neat home holds more value to some individuals than others.

Variations in value systems become highly significant when dealing with critical issues such as health and illness or life and death. Value systems enable

RESEARCH note

Critical care nurses are key care providers in critical care units, environments in which ethical dilemmas frequently occur. M. C. Hough, a doctoral student at Florida State University, wondered what factors might assist critical care nurses in ethical decision making. She designed a study to explore and describe ethical decision making in a critical care nursing practice.

A qualitative study design utilizing ethnographic methods was used to accomplish this goal. Data triangulation was accomplished by using three techniques of data collection: (1) open-ended, in-depth semistructured interviews and probes; (2) participant observation, and (3) document analysis.

Fifteen critical care nurses with various experience and education levels were interviewed to ensure a representation similar to that found in typical clinical practices. Verbatim transcriptions of each tape-recorded interview were analyzed for content using The Ethnograph, a computer software program. Participant observation was conducted with a hospital ethics committee; the researcher attended monthly business meetings and requested copies of all ethics consultations for a 12-month period. Informal short interviews were used to clarify, explain, or describe relevant issues as the researcher attempted to learn what role the ethics committee played as a nontraditional form of education with critical care nurses in the area of ethical decision making.

Document analysis was also conducted. This consisted of examination of written records of ethics committee consultations over a 12-month period prior to beginning the research study.

The findings indicated that nurses who had the advantage of an experienced preceptor or coach, particularly during orientation, had the most focused reflection and the least difficulty with sound, systematic, ethical discourse and decision making. Nurses who did not have this coaching had the greatest difficulty identifying and resolving ethical dilemmas in clinical practice. While difficulty was more often seen with nurses with less than 5 years of experience, the lack of a coach or mentor caused even more senior nurses to experience difficulty with focused reflection.

Hough concluded that institutions could benefit from developing programs to educate critical care nurses about ethical decision making. Such programs would be enhanced by training preceptors to function as coaches during critical care orientation.

From Hough MC: Walking the line: a qualitative study of critical care nursing and the importance of experiential learning in ethical decision making in clinical nursing practice, PhD dissertation, Florida State University, 1998, Dissertation Abstracts.

Research update: Hough is currently (2004) conducting a 3-year research study, funded by the Brook's Foundation, that builds on her dissertation work. This multiphased research study will test the focused reflection model of ethical decision making that has evolved from her research. The model is being tested along with different educational modes of instruction including traditional classroom instruction and audiostreamed PowerPoint instruction and the use of ethics case studies utilizing the Internet and Blackboard technology. The research is looking at ethical decision making in nursing practice. Participants in the study consist of nursing students at the University of North Florida and Queen's University Belfast in Northern Ireland and experienced nurses at a medical center in Jacksonville, Florida. A quasi-experimental design utilizing pretesting and posttesting is being used.

people to resolve conflicts and decide on a course of action based on a priority of importance. In professional nursing, it is not enough to recognize and act on one's personal values. In addition, one must determine whether the value system is ethical. Only after careful reflection can nurses take action based on their personal or professional values.

Identifying your personal value system and its influence on decision making helps you understand your behavior more clearly. In addition, it gives you clues as to why other people's choices are different from your own. The "Childhood Value Messages" exercise in Box 19-2 can help you identify values learned as a child that may still influence you today.

Box 19-2 Childhood Value Messages

By the time we are about 10 years old, most of our values have already been "programmed." Values are taught to us by family members and friends, through the media, in churches and schools, and by watching other people. What are the value messages you learned as a child?

Recall as many values as you can remember hearing as a child and write them in the blanks provided below. Here are a few examples to get you thinking:

"Nothing worthwhile ever comes easy."
"Life is fatal—you're eternal."
"You can accomplish almost anything you want to if you persevere."
"Clean your plate; there are starving children in China!"
"You are your brother's keeper—reach out to others."
"Tell me the truth, and I won't punish you!"
"Get your work done first; then you can play."

Now it's your turn to write some of your childhood values. How many of these values still influence the way you think and act today? Which ones influence you professionally? If you want to explore further:

1. Next to each value on your list, write the person's name who taught or modeled that value.
2. Put a star next to those messages that are still your values today.
3. Put a check mark next to those messages that you need to alter.
4. How are some of these values still influencing you today? Is this a positive or negative influence?

1. _____
2. _____
3. _____
4. _____
5. _____
6. _____
7. _____
8. _____

Reprinted with permission of Uustal DB: *Clinical ethics and values: issues and insights in a changing health care environment,* Jamestown, RI, 1993, Sea Spirit Press Educational Resources in Health Care, Inc.

To see how value conflicts can affect health care delivery, consider the following patient-centered situation:

Mrs. Hamid has recently relocated to the United States from Iran. It is important in her religious faith that men not be present during labor and delivery or at anytime when a woman's body is exposed. A female midwife is delivering Mrs. Hamid, but complications develop. Her baby's heart rate drops abruptly, and a cesarean delivery is indicated. The only obstetrical surgeon available for this emergency surgery is a man. What action should the nurse take to show sensitivity to Mrs. Hamid's personal value system?

Dilemmas Involving Peers' and Other Professionals' Behavior

All practicing nurses participate as members of the health care team. This involves cooperation and collaboration with other professionals. As is true in all situations involving human beings, conflicts can easily develop, particularly in stressful circumstances. These conflicts may be between two nurses, the nurse and physician, the nurse and agency policies, or the nurse and any other health care professional.

As discussed previously, conflicts can evolve because of differing value systems. A nurse may believe that assisting with abortions is wrong, whereas the institution in which he or she is employed routinely performs abortions. This creates a conflict between the nurse's value system and the institution's practices.

Some conflicts develop because individuals are not respectful of the human rights of other individuals. Conflicts in human rights often center around one of the ethical principles discussed earlier: justice, autonomy, beneficence, or veracity. In some circumstances, the ethical dilemma may result from a violation of even more basic human rights, those guaranteed by the U.S. Constitution.

At times, health care workers may be incompetent or their actions unethical (Fry, 1997). An incompetent worker may suffer from physical or mental impairment or may be ignorant of standards of care. Unethical actions result when health care workers break basic norms of conduct toward others, especially the patient, whatever the reason.

A serious issue today is the large number of nurses and other health care professionals impaired by drug dependence or other addictions. Deciding how and when to confront a suspected drug user may result in an ethical dilemma. Fortunately, some employers and state nurses associations have developed plans to assist impaired nurses in getting the help they need and make provisions for them to return to the profession once they are far enough along in their recovery process. Your state nurses association can provide information on specific programs for impaired nurses in your state.

To understand the ethical dilemmas that can result from conflict between peers, consider the following nurse-centered situation:

Miss Corbin, RN, works on a surgical floor. She has just assisted in the transfer of Mr. Hudson to his room from the postanesthesia unit after surgery and noticed that he was resting comfortably. Miss Corbin sees a nurse colleague drawing up a pain medication. The nurse colleague returns to the medicine room 10 minutes later with an empty syringe. Miss Corbin asks, "Who needed pain medication?" The colleague replies, "Mr. Hudson. He was in pain after surgery." Confused, Miss Corbin checks Mr. Hudson's room and learns from his wife that he has not asked for or received pain medication. What should Miss Corbin do now?

Conflicts Regarding Patients' Rights

Years ago, health professionals, particularly physicians, were considered "all-knowing" experts. Few patients questioned the physician, let alone demanded their basic human rights. Now consumers of health care are increasingly demanding to have a say in matters affecting their health care. A number of specialty groups have developed published lists of **patient rights.** Examples include *Declaration of the Rights of Mentally Retarded Persons, Dying Person's Bill of Rights, Pregnant Patient's Bill of Rights, Rights of Senior Citizens,* and the *United Nations Declaration of the Rights of the Child.* As consumers have become more aware of their rights, conflicts between patients, health care professionals, and institutions have developed. Many of the rights demanded by consumers are not only their moral rights but also their legal rights and have been upheld by the judicial system.

It is beyond the scope of this chapter to discuss all rights due patients. Some that have been identified are informed consent, the right to die, privacy, confidentiality, respectful care, and information concerning medical condition and treatment. In addition, patients have the right to be informed if any aspect of treatment is experimental. Based on that knowledge, patients have the right to refuse to participate in research projects.

PATIENT SELF-DETERMINATION ACT

Another safeguard for patients, the Patient Self-Determination Act, gives patients the legal right to determine how vigorously they wish to be treated in life or death situations. This Act forces individuals to think about the type of medical and nursing treatment they would want if they were to become critically injured or ill. When questions arise, the patient is often unconscious or too sick to make decisions or communicate personal wishes.

The Patient Self-Determination Act, which went into effect in December 1991, calls for hospitals to abide by patients' advance directives. **Advance directives** are legal documents that indicate the wishes of individuals in regard to end-of-life issues. The Patient Self-Determination Act specifies that any organization receiving Medicare or Medicaid funds must inform patients of state laws regarding directives, document the existence of directives in the patient's medical record, and educate the community about directives.

Advance directives are designed to ensure individuals the rights of autonomy, refusal of medical intervention, and death with dignity (Norman and Pinkham, 1994). Critically ill individuals can remain in charge of their own end-of-life decisions if their advance directives are carried out.

Families should talk about how each member wants critical situations to be handled. Individual preferences can then be understood, and ideally, family members, caregivers, and courts will not need to make decisions for the patient. Often the first time a patient learns about advance directives is upon admission to a health care facility. The question then arises as to who is responsible for discussing this sensitive issue with the patient. The ideal time for patients to make difficult end-of-life decisions is well in advance of the need (Figure 19-1).

Advance directives have not been without controversy. One problem is that states have passed different legislations, and there is no guarantee that one state will honor another's advanced directives. Another problem may arise when a person is designated as the proxy to decide about medical treatment if the patient cannot do so. In some situations, persons have been named as proxies without their knowledge. Some family members have vehemently disagreed with or refused to follow the directives of a parent or spouse. Conflict also sometimes arises among caregivers in honoring certain advance directives.

The following case illustrates a conflict related to patients' rights:

A 28-year-old quadriplegic man is admitted to the hospital with pneumonia and severe pressure ulcers. He asks not to be given antibiotics and to be allowed to die with dignity. At the insistence of the hospital administration, the physician orders intravenous antibiotics. What is the nurse's responsibility?

More information about patient rights and the Patient Self-Determination Act can be found in Chapter 20.

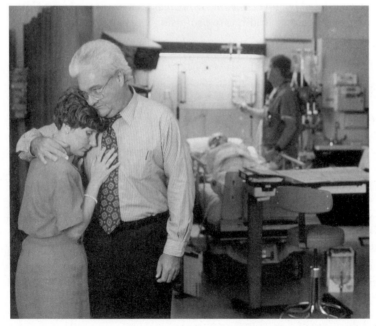

Figure **19-1**
To avoid unwanted, life-prolonging interventions, patients must make end-of-life decisions early, discuss them with family members and caregivers, commit them to writing in advance directive documents, and periodically review and renew them. (Courtesy Memorial Hospital, Chattanooga, Tennessee.)

Conflicts Created by Institutional and Societal Issues

Nurses experience ethical dilemmas when they disagree with the policies of their institution; conflicts can thus develop. Controversial health care policies at the local, state, or national level can also interfere with the nurse's ability to implement care safely and effectively.

Grave concerns over health care have centered around its cost. The rising cost of health care over the past 35 years has prompted worry by individuals, groups, and communities as well as governmental officials. All health care agencies must stress cost-containment measures to survive. At times, cost-containment policies conflict with the value system of the nurse, whose goal is to provide high-quality, individualized patient care.

Other institutional and societal concerns can result in ethical dilemmas for the nurse whose personal value system does not support the policies set forth by those in authority. Examples include policies concerning access to health care for the elderly, children, and persons with acquired immunodeficiency syndrome (AIDS).

Nurses today work in many settings. The scope and complexity of nursing actions vary significantly from large multiservice medical complexes to small clinics or offices. All organizations, however, that receive governmental funds are subject to public scrutiny and accountability. Ethical dilemmas between nurses and the organizations that employ them may develop over policies dictated by the organizations or mandated by governmental agencies. This chapter's News Note describes one family's conflict with health care professionals regarding end-of-life decisions.

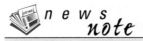
news note

It May Be a Family Matter, but Just Try to Define *Family*

The life of Terri Schiavo, however narrowly it has been lived in the 13 years since a heart attack left her severely brain-damaged at 26, is at its core a story of a family divided. Ms. Schiavo's husband believes she has no hope of recovery and chose to remove the feeding tube that keeps her alive. Her parents disagreed. Last week, the Florida Legislature gave Governor Jeb Bush the power to intervene; he ordered the tube replaced.

While the courts have been the main battleground, the case is fundamentally one of emotional, rather than legal, combat. It concerns the lengths to which love will go, the families people choose versus those they are born into and the question of who has the more valid claim to someone's destiny. Society's fears and suspicions collect around the stereotypes in play: a disloyal husband, overprotective parents.

"The case has been mischaracterized as the case of a woman who is disabled being starved to death," said Dr. Daniel Sulmasy, a Franciscan friar, medical doctor and the chairman of the ethics committee at St. Vincent's Hospital in Manhattan. "But the real moral issue is these sort of thorny disagreements that occur in the settings of real families."

n e w s
note—cont'd

Dr. Sulmasy, who regularly consults with relatives making life-or-death decisions within complicated family relationships, said it is easy for an ethicist to forget that people drag the flotsam of the past behind them.

"Is what's going on here just a history of suspicion that these in-laws have had against their son-in-law from the beginning?" he asked. "Or did he rescue her from a family that was always smothering and they now feel that they have to continue to care for her the way they always have?"

Overwhelmingly, state laws and courts have granted the spouse the first right to make life-or-death decisions. Next come the children, and then the parents. In a system focused on nuclear families, this reflects the view that spouses are far better equipped to make proxy decisions because they share responsibilities and have known each other intimately in their adult lives, rather than in childhood.

Parents, on the other hand, must contend with generational asymmetry, the idea that caring flows down the family tree more strongly than it climbs up.

While children may nurse a permanent ambivalence toward their parents, said Janna Malamud Smith, a clinical social worker and the author of "A Potent Spell: Mother Love and the Power of Fear," parents want nothing more than to have their children outlive them.

"Whatever your gratitude and deep love for a parent who raised you, you don't have this ongoing mandate for this creature that 'no matter what, I will protect you,'" Ms. Smith said.

In any case, the idea that the spouse knows best does not prove to be uniformly true. In a study that Dr. Sulmasy calls "the bioethics version of 'The Newlywed Game,'" health care questions were posed to people and their proxies to compare their answers. Faced with situations like whether to turn off a ventilator or withdraw a feeding tube, they did not agree 20 percent of the time.

It did not make a difference whether the proxy was related by blood, Dr. Sulmasy said. The best results came when the person explicitly told the proxy what he or she would want beforehand.

Ms. Schiavo may or may not have done that; her husband, Michael, has said that she had expressed a desire not to be kept on life support.

But even if she had not, the Florida Legislature has stripped Mr. Schiavo of his right to make choices for his wife for the time being. The marital intimacy that is normally inviolable even by parents or children, not to mention politicians or those whose stated aim is to protect family values, has been breached.

"In a sense that movement rests on a sentimental version of family—that whether or not blood is thicker than water, blood is somehow better," Ms. Smith said.

It is difficult for estate lawyers to think of a time when so much effort has been put into overriding a spouse's prerogatives. "Maybe in this post–Laci Peterson world, people are more skeptical of spouses and their motives," said Herbert E. Nass, a probate lawyer and the author of "Wills of the Rich and Famous."

Continued

n e w s note—cont'd

The very idea of pulling the plug conjures up a lurking fear, said Laura Kipnis, the author of *Against Love: A Polemic.* "There's a sort of undercurrent of mistrust and suspicion underlying the state of marriage these days," she said, "the idea that a spouse may leave you or try to murder you or have a secret life with someone else."

Mr. Schiavo is now living with another woman; they have a child and are expecting another. Ms. Schiavo's parents, Bob and Mary Schindler, point out that Mr. Schiavo won a million-dollar malpractice judgment to pay for his wife's care, which he would inherit if she died. Mr. Schiavo's lawyer argues that it has been 10 years since that settlement. And with a wife in a "vegetative state" for 13 years, doesn't a husband—or anyone, for that matter—have the right to walk away?

The Schindlers accuse Mr. Schiavo of having abused their daughter, and even of possibly causing her injury; doctors say she suffered a heart attack caused by a potassium deficiency. The Schindlers say that their daughter had told them she wanted a divorce and that Mr. Schiavo has denied her medical treatment that might help her. And, they claim, their daughter smiles and responds to their presence.

In the end, what is missing is not so much consensus as any sense of trust that both parties—the chosen companion and the birth family—want what is best for Ms. Schiavo.

"The people who oughtn't to be involved are the barbers and bankers and real estate agents that make up the Legislature, and the governor of Florida," said Thomas Lynch, a funeral director and author of two books of essays on themes of life and death. "It should have been an intimate conversation, not a big conversation. It should have been an intimate decision, not a public decision."

The struggle over the feeding tube is so compelling because it is so easy to agonize with both the parents and the husband. And, for that matter, with Ms. Schiavo herself, at the mercy of people for whom there is no obvious right choice.

Reflecting on the case, Cathleen Schine, a novelist whose most recent book, *She Is Me,* presents three generations of women from one family, offered her best answer: get a living will.

"Because otherwise," she said, "everybody's got their own version of you and what you would want."

Reprinted with permission from Dewan SK: It may be a family matter, but just try to define *family, The New York Times,* October 26, 2003, Section 4, p 1.

Ethics committees were created to assist with ethical dilemmas in institutional settings. These committees are multidisciplinary groups charged with the responsibility of providing consultation and emotional support in situations in which difficult ethical choices are necessary. Cases needing consideration are referred to the committee by those desiring help, usually clinical caregivers such as physicians and nurses.

The following vignette illustrates an ethical conflict between a nurse and the employing institution:

> Jennifer McLeod is a nurse working in a critical care unit. All beds in the unit are full. For the past 2 days, Ms. McLeod has been assigned to care for a 92-year-old woman critically ill with heart failure. The patient has no financial resources of her own, and no family member has seen her since she was admitted from a nursing home. She remains in very critical condition. Suddenly, orders come for the elderly woman to be transferred to a bed on a regular nursing unit. As she is being moved out of the critical care unit, a state senator's son in a diabetic coma is admitted to her recently vacated bed. What is the nurse's responsibility?

ETHICAL DECISION MAKING

Nurses encounter situations daily that require them to make professional judgments and act on those judgments. The judgments or decisions are often made in conjunction with other persons involved in the situation: patients, families, and other health care professionals. When an ethical decision is made, everyone must respect and value the perspectives held by others. Through respectful collaboration, the best decision can be reached in even the most difficult dilemma. Notice that it is suggested that the *best* decision will be made. In an ethical dilemma, there is not a right or wrong answer. Instead, we search for the best answer.

Ethical Decision Making Model

Whether involved in a collective or individual decision, nurses need to be knowledgeable about the steps in **ethical decision making,** listed in Table 19-2. Various models of ethical decision making have been developed. Each model is unique to some degree, but they share commonalities. Although the models all have steps,

Table 19-2 COMPARISON OF NURSING PROCESS AND ETHICAL DECISION-MAKING MODEL

Nursing Process	Ethical Decision-Making Model
Assess	Clarify the ethical dilemma
	Gather additional data
Analyze	Identify options
Plan	Make a decision
Implement	Act
Evaluate	Evaluate

they are not intended to be rigid processes for decision making. Instead, ethical decision making is a process in which ideas are thoroughly examined to determine the best solution to a difficult situation.

The following steps can be used in ethical decision making.

1. Clarify the ethical dilemma

What is the specific issue in question? Who owns the problem and should actually make the decision? Who is affected by the dilemma? Determine the ethical principle or theory related to the dilemma. Are there value conflicts? What is the time frame for the decision?

2. Gather additional data

After clarifying the ethical dilemma, in most instances more information needs to be gathered. It is important to have as many facts as possible about the situation. Make sure you are up-to-date on any legal cases related to the situation because ethical and legal issues often overlap.

3. Identify options

Most ethical dilemmas have multiple solutions, some of which are more feasible than others. The more options that are identified, the more likely it is that an acceptable solution can be identified. Brainstorm with others and consider every possible alternative.

4. Make a decision

To make a decision, think through the options that are identified and determine each option's impact. Ethical principles and theories may help determine the significance of each option. When confronted with an ethical dilemma, a decision should be made. Refusing to make a decision is not a responsible professional behavior.

5. Act

Once a course of action has been determined, the decision must be carried out. Implementing the decision usually involves working collaboratively with others.

6. Evaluate

Unexpected outcomes are common in crisis situations that result in ethical dilemmas. It is important for decision makers to determine the impact an immediate decision may have on future ones. It is also important to consider whether a different course of action might have resulted in a better outcome. If the action accomplished its purpose, the ethical dilemma should be resolved. If the dilemma has not been resolved, additional deliberation is needed.

Consider these six ethical decision-making steps in the context of the following case study:

1. Clarify the ethical dilemma. The specific issue is the patient's right of autonomy versus your duty related to beneficence (to do good) and nonmaleficence (to do no harm). Mr. Johnson clearly owns the problem and appears alert enough

Administration of Pain Medication

Mr. Joe Johnson is a 56-year-old white male admitted with the diagnosis of acute myocardial infarction (MI) and cardiogenic shock. He has a history of severe coronary artery disease (CAD) and has suffered several MIs over the past 3 years. The patient has an advance directive and a do-not-resuscitate (DNR) order on his chart. When the nurse assesses the patient, he is short of breath and diaphoretic with a blood pressure of 69/36 and heart rate of 162. His respirations are labored and rapid at 42. Mr. Johnson is mentally alert and states he is having crushing midsternal chest pain radiating into his jaw and down his left arm. He is crying and requesting that the nurse give him something for the pain. There is an order for IV morphine sulfate, 2 to 10 mg for pain every 1 to 2 hours as needed. The nurse on the off-going shift refused to give the IV morphine because of the patient's compromised status and the fear of further depressing his respiratory and cardiac status. After receiving the report from his evening nurse, you enter the patient's room and find his wife and one of his sons. They are upset and demand you administer the IV pain medication immediately. **What do you do?**

to make a decision. Obviously, his wife and son are also affected by Mr. Johnson's pain, as is anyone who provides care to him. The dilemma needs to be resolved quickly because of the extent of the pain.

2. Gather additional data. A review of the medical record indicates that the patient has a do-not-resuscitate order. One of your experienced colleagues tells you about the double effect doctrine and the condition that must be met to justify its use. You realized that giving the medication to relieve the chest pain may further compromise the patient's already critical condition.

3. Identify options. Options include (1) asking someone else to care for Mr. Johnson with intention of avoiding the dilemma; (2) refusing to medicate Mr. Johnson and let him continue in pain; (3) medicating Mr. Johnson with 2 to 10 mg of morphine sulfate; and (4) asking for an order for a medication with fewer side effects.

4. Make a decision. You determine that to allow your patient to be in severe pain is unacceptable. Morphine sulfate is without question the drug of choice. You think through the principle of double effect and realize the proposed action of administering the medication to relieve pain is intrinsically good. You only intend the good effect (relieving pain) but realize there is potential for the undesired and unintended effect (premature death) from giving the morphine sulfate. You discuss the situation with the patient and his family, indicating both positive and negative consequences of giving the pain medication. You are honest enough to indicate that the morphine sulfate may cause him to stop breathing. Mr. Johnson, his family, and you decide that it is appropriate to administer the medication.

5. Act. You proceed to administer the diluted IV morphine sulfate slowly over a 10-minute period, frequently checking Mr. Johnson's blood pressure. After a total of 6 mg of morphine is given, he states that the pain has been relieved.

6. Evaluate. It would be important to determine whether the intended effect was achieved and also to identify any unintended effects. The patient's and family's satisfaction with the decision are also important. (*Note:* This situation is based on a real-life case. The patient lived for another 5 hours free of pain. He and his family visited throughout these remaining hours of his life and reminisced about past family memories. The patient, his wife, and son all expressed much appreciation for the relief of pain. You can read the nurse's verbatim account of this ethical dilemma in Box 19-3.)

Box 19-3 | Verbatim Account of Ethical Dilemma: Administration of Pain Medication

This case clearly shows the struggle of the critical care nurse, one of the chapter authors, as she decided whether or not to medicate Mr. Johnson. The nurse decided to medicate this patient for his pain despite his unstable hemodynamic condition. She gave the following verbatim account:

When I came out of report, I can remember walking into that room. I walked up to the bed; I introduced myself. He was ice cold. He looked at me and said, "I know I'm dying; my family knows I'm dying. Please give me something for the pain. I just can't stand it." His heart rate was 162. His blood pressure was 68/30 and I'm thinking, "I'm going to have to give him something for the pain, and the real strong possibility here is the guy is going to die when I give him something for the pain."

When I was up to 3 mg of morphine, I remember his blood pressure dropped down to the mid 50s, and I'm sitting there thinking in the back of my mind that I have the training and the skills and I have the technology sitting just 5 feet away from the door, and I could just run out and grab some atropine. Instead I looked at him and said, "Joe are you still having chest pain?" He said "Yes, please give me some more; I can't stand it." (Oddly enough, I remember thinking about the perspiration on my upper lip and the beads beginning to form on my forehead and thinking should I take time to wipe it off.) So I pushed another 0.25 mg of morphine, and I looked up at his monitor, and his heart rate was beginning to drop; his color was gray anyway. I sat there with him pushing the IV morphine slowly until I had given him about 6.5 mg. I remember checking his pressure, and it was about 46/20. We just sat there for about 4 or 5 minutes, and I asked him how he was feeling. He said that he was feeling a little bit better and the chest pain wasn't as bad. Gradually his pressure came up and about 10 minutes later his blood pressure was up to about 90/60 and he was pain free.

I can remember it was probably about three o'clock in the morning and I went in and was talking with him, and I asked him if he was having any pain. He said he wasn't having any pain. I put the blood pressure cuff on his arm. As it was coming down, I lost his pressure. I looked up at his monitor and his heart rate, which had gone back up to 130-140, was down to 90 and his blood pressure was about 70/50. I pumped it back up to recheck and his pressure was 65/30. I can remember looking at him, looking up at the monitor, and his heart rate was in the 60s. I looked up at the monitor, and then I looked down at Joe, and he had this look in his eyes. He just nodded his head to me. I reached over and touched his wife's hand. I just looked at her and said, "It's time!" I looked over at the son and said, "You had better get the rest of the family and bring them in." I checked Joe's blood pressure one last time. I think I heard it once in the mid 30s. His heart rate was below 40. I can remember stepping back and motioning for his son to come in. They started telling him how much they loved him, what a great father he was, and what a wonderful husband he was, just reminiscing. Actually, they had been reminiscing throughout the entire night, talking about baseball games and growing up, and family times.

By now I'm feeling kind of like an interloper, and I'm trying to back out of the room to give the family some privacy. Just when I was about to back out, Joe looked over and said, "Katie, come here," so I walked over to the bed. I had my stethoscope hanging from my neck. Joe reached up, he was very weak by this point, and grabbed my stethoscope and he pulled it and he pulled my head down and whispered in my ear, "Thank you for taking the time and sharing this with us. You don't know how much it means to all of us," and then he kissed my cheek. Needless to say, by now I'm crying, the entire

| Box **19-3** | **Verbatim Account of Ethical Dilemma: Administration of Pain Medication—cont'd** |

family is crying, Joe is crying. I remember as I stood up Joe just looked at me and said "Good-bye." Then each one of his children, his daughter-in-law, and his sister said good-bye to him and they all leaned down and kissed him. I remember he turned and looked at his wife and she said, "Joe, I love you so much," and he said, "Give me a kiss." She stood up, leaned over, and kissed him—and his heart stopped—he died.

The family had been glancing up at the monitor, and they saw the straight line and they all looked at me for conformation. I nodded my head and said, "Yes, he's gone." The youngest son turned with tears streaming down his face ... he walked over to me and put his arms around me and kissed me on the cheek and thanked me. Then every member of the family did the same thing.

It's been 9 years since this happened, but it seems like it was yesterday. It was one of those moments in your professional career that just touches your life so dramatically that I don't think I will ever forget it.

There is stress working in critical care, and a great many technical decisions and much expertise that you have to possess when you're making life-and-death decisions all the time. When something like this happens, it makes it all worthwhile. There are very few professions—in fact, I can't really think of any others—in which professionals have the privilege of sharing something like this with a family: being present when a human life ends.

I was placed in a situation where I had to make a decision. I had to weigh the possible ramifications that decision was going to have. Would I let this man continue to be in excruciating pain, having his life extended maybe 3 or 4 more hours and him die, and having that family remember his pain for the rest of their lives, or go ahead and give him the medication that was ordered with the chance that it might end his life? I can remember as I was walking over to the narcotic cabinet thinking that allowing the man to be in that much pain was certainly not ethical. I can remember when I finally made the decision to medicate him was when I was able to rationalize to myself that I wouldn't be giving him the medication to end his life, but I would be giving him the pain medication to end the pain, and that was an ethical decision!

With this scenario it really had a positive outcome. Joe lived for about 5 more hours, but the last 5 hours he was pain free. His family was in and out; they reminisced about the past. They had good memories, not memories of pain and suffering.

Obviously, this type of scenario does not occur every single shift when working in critical care, but it is a fairly common occurrence. It is these types of things that you have to deal with all the time. It can be very stressful, but it can also be very rewarding.

Courtesy Catherine ("Katie") Hough.

Summary of Key Points
- The terms *morals* and *ethics* are often used interchangeably. Technically, however, morals reflect what is done in a situation, whereas ethics are concerned with what should be done.
- It is important that nurses are familiar with ethical theories and principles, moral development, and decision-making models to participate actively in resolving ethical dilemmas that occur frequently in health care settings.

- Codes of ethics, developed by the profession's members, are important to the development of the profession.
- The ANA's *Code of Ethics for Nurses* (2001) serves as a guideline for nurses regarding ethical behavior.
- The history of the *Code of Ethics for Nurses* is reflective of nursing's history as a profession.
- Ethical dilemmas occur in all areas of nursing practice.
- Dilemmas often occur because of conflicts between personal value systems, patients, health care professionals, institutions, and society.
- Ethical decision-making models are helpful in determining the best action to take concerning an ethical dilemma.

CRITICAL THINKING QUESTIONS

1. What is the difference between morals and ethics? Give an example of each from your own value system.
2. How can the American Nurses Association's *Code of Ethics for Nurses* be used by the bedside nurse?
3. Compare the American Nurses Association's *Code of Ethics for Nurses* with the *International Council of Nurses Code of Ethics for Nurses.* How are they similar, and how are they different?
4. Select an ethical theory or principle that is most congruent with your approach to ethical dilemmas. Use it as a basis for resolving the ethical dilemmas in this chapter. How well does it hold up under these test conditions?
5. Discuss your reactions to the following questions in a small group:
   a. Mrs. Otto has recently undergone extensive surgery for gynecological cancer. The day after surgery, she asks for more pain medication than the physician has prescribed. You call for an order to increase the pain medication dosage, but she still complains every 2 hours that she cannot tolerate the pain. What should be done?
   b. Mrs. Loriz suffers from severe chronic pain, the cause of which has not been definitely diagnosed. Her husband has brought her into the emergency department for the fifth time this month asking for narcotic relief from the pain. In tears she states, "A shot of Demerol is the only thing that takes the edge off." She threatens suicide if she is sent home without some help. The physician has ordered a placebo. What is the nurse's responsibility?
   c. Mr. Nelson, age 87, suffered a serious stroke. His wife of 65 years keeps a constant vigil at his bedside. After 4 weeks, he remains totally unresponsive and develops pneumonia. A tracheotomy is performed and a feeding tube inserted. Mrs. Nelson feels agreeing to a "do-not-resuscitate" order is letting her husband down but recognizes he has no quality of life. How should the nurse counsel Mrs. Nelson?
   d. Emily and Michael Mills are parents of a young child dying of Tay-Sachs disease. Emily recently found out she was pregnant and wants to know whether their second child is affected with the same disease. Mrs. Mills undergoes genetic testing of the embryo and to the parents' extreme dismay, finds that their second child also has Tay-Sachs disease. How would the parents go about making a decision regarding the second pregnancy?

6. Answer the following questions, basing your answers on identified ethical principles:
   a. When is it acceptable to refuse an assignment?
   b. What is the nurses' duty when a patient wants to do something harmful to him or her self?
   c. Is health care a right?

REFERENCES

American Nurses Association: *Code for Nurses with interpretive statements,* Kansas City, MO, 1976, American Nurses Association.

American Nurses Association: *Code for nurses with interpretive statements,* Kansas City, MO, 1985, American Nurses Association.

American Nurses Association: *Code of ethics for nurses with interpretive statements,* Washington, DC, 2001, American Nurses Publishing.

Aroskar MA: Envisioning nursing as a moral community, *Nurs Outlook* 43(3):134-138, 1995.

Beauchamp TL, Childress JF: *Principles of biomedical ethics,* ed 4, New York, 2001, Oxford University Press.

Brannigan MC, Boss JA: *Healthcare ethics in a diverse society,* Mountain View, CA, 2001, Mayfield Publishing Company.

Burkhardt MA, Nathaniel AK: *Ethics and issues in contemporary nursing,* ed 2, Albany, NY, 2002, Delmar.

Chally PS: Theory derivation in moral development, *Nurs & Health Care* 11(6):302-306, 1990.

Chally PS: Nursing research: Moral decision making by nurses in intensive care, *Plast Surg Nurs* 15(2):120-124, 1995.

Chulay M, Guzzetta C, Dossey B: *Critical care nursing,* Stamford, CT, 1997, Appleton & Lange.

Conte C: A troubling death: Wishes of terminally ill patients are often ignored, new study says, *AARP Bulletin* 37(1):4-5, 1996.

Davis AJ, Aroskar MA, Liaschenko J, et al: *Ethical dilemmas and nursing practice,* ed 4, Stamford, CT, 1997, Appleton & Lange.

Fowler MD: Relic or resource? The Code for Nurses, *Am J Nurs* 99(3):56-57, 1999.

Frankena WK: *Ethics,* ed 2, Englewood Cliffs, NJ, 1988, Prentice-Hall.

Fry ST: Protecting patients from incompetent or unethical colleagues: an important dimension of the nurse's advocacy role, *J Nurs Law* 4(4):15-22, 1997.

Gilligan C: *In a different voice: psychological theory and women's development,* Cambridge, MA, 1982, Harvard University Press.

Gilligan C: Moral orientation and moral development. In Kittay E, Meyers D, editors: *Women and moral theory,* Totowa, NJ, 1987, Rowman & Littlefield, pp 19-33.

Gilligan C, Attanucci J: Two moral orientations: gender differences and similarities, *Merrill-Palmer Q* 34(3), 223-231, 1988.

Gilligan C, Brown L, Rogers A: *Psyche embedded: a place for body, relationships, and culture in personality theory* (Monograph No. 4), Cambridge, MA, Harvard University, 1988, Laboratory of Human Development.

Hough MC: *Walking the line: a qualitative study of critical care nursing and the importance of experiential learning in ethical decision making in clinical nursing practice,* PhD dissertation, Florida State University, 1998, Dissertation Abstracts.

Husted GL, Husted JH: *Ethical decision making in nursing,* ed 2, St. Louis, 1995, Mosby.

International Council of Nurses: *International Council of Nurses code for nurses,* Geneva, Switzerland, 2000, International Council of Nurses.

International Council of Nurses: *International Council of Nurses code for nurses,* Geneva, Switzerland, 1973, International Council of Nurses.

Jameton A: *Nursing practice: the ethical issues,* Englewood Cliffs, NJ, 1984, Prentice-Hall.

Johnstone M: *Bioethics: a nursing perspective,* ed 3, Philadelphia, 1999, Harcourt Sanders.

Kant I: The categorical imperative. In Feinburg J, editor: *Reason and responsibility: readings in some basic problems of philosophy,* ed 6, Belmont, CA, 1985, Wadsworth, pp 540-547.

Kant I: *Foundations of the metaphysics of morals,* Indianapolis, 1959 (reprint), Bobbs-Merrill, pp 31-49 (translated by LW Beck).

Kohlberg L: A current statement on some theoretical issues. In Modgil S, Modgil C, editors: *Lawrence Kohlberg: consensus and controversy* Philadelphia, 1986, Falmer Press, pp 485-546.

Kohlberg L: Moral stages and moralization: the cognitive developmental approach. In Lickona T, editor: *Moral development and behavior,* New York, 1976, Holt, Rinehart & Winston, pp 31-53.

Kohlberg L: Continuities and discontinuities in childhood and adult moral development revisited. In Kohlberg L, editor: *Collected papers on moral development and moral education,* Cambridge, MA, 1973, Moral Education Research Foundation.

Mill JS: Utilitarianism. In Feinburg J, editor: *Reason and responsibility: readings in some basic problems of philosophy,* ed 6, Belmont, CA, 1985, Wadsworth, pp 503-515 (originally published in 1863).

Norman EM, Pinkham DB: Advance directives: understanding their impact on care. In Strickland OL, Fishman DJ, editors: *Nursing issues in the 1990s,* Albany, NY, 1994, Delmar, pp 267-279.

Scott PA: Aristotle, nursing, and health care ethics, *Nurs ethics* 2(4):279-285, 1995.

Tschudin V, editor: *Ethics: nurses and patients,* London, 1993, Scutari Press.

Uustal DB: *Clinical ethics and values: issues and insights in a changing healthcare environment,* East Greenwich, RI, 1993, Educational Resources in HealthCare, Inc.

Veins DC: A history of nursing's code of ethics, *Nurs Outlook* 37(1):45-49, 1989.

Volbrecht MR: *Nursing ethics: communities in dialogue,* Upper Saddle River, NJ, 2002, Prentice Hall.

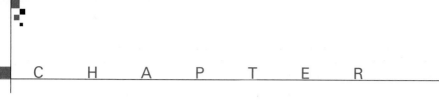

Legal Aspects of Nursing

Virginia Trotter Betts

Key Terms

Administrative Law
Advance Directive
Assault
Battery
"Captain of the Ship" Doctrine
Civil Law
Common Law
Competency
Confidentiality
Criminal Law
Delegation
Documentation
Duty of Care
Duty to Report

Expert Witness
Informed Consent
Law
Legal Authority
Licensure
Licensure by Endorsement
Malpractice
Managed Care Plans
Mutual Recognition Model
National Practitioner Data Bank
Negligence
Nurse Licensure Compact
Nurse Practice Act
Patient Self-Determination Act

Prescriptive Authority
Privileged Communication
Proximate Cause
Quality Improvement
Respondeat Superior
Risk Management
Standard of Care
Standard of Nursing Practice
State Board of Nursing
Statutory Law
Tort
Unlicensed Assistive
    Personnel
Voluntariness

Learning Outcomes

After studying this chapter, students will be able to:

- Describe the components of a model nurse practice act.
- Discuss the authority of state boards of nursing.
- Explain the conditions that must be present for malpractice to occur.
- Identify nursing concerns related to delegation, assault and battery, informed consent, and confidentiality.
- Describe strategies nurses can use to protect their patients, thereby protecting themselves from legal actions.

P rofessional nurses have many complex and intertwined relationships with the law that are important to identify and understand. The legal aspects of nursing is an area that is both extremely important and constantly changing. Therefore nursing education programs sometimes offer required or elective courses in law as applied to nursing. "Nursing and the law" is also one of the most popular continuing education topics for nurses. This chapter highlights key legal issues that affect professional nurses. It is essential to maintain a working knowledge of the law as it relates to professional nursing practice. Nurses who do not understand and stay abreast of the regulations that govern nursing practice may find themselves involved in disciplinary measures, fines, or litigation (Gaffney, 1998).

AMERICAN LEGAL SYSTEM

The purpose of the law in the United States is found in the Preamble to the U.S. Constitution: to ensure order, protect the individual person, resolve disputes, and promote the general welfare. To achieve these broad objectives, the law concerns itself with the legal relationships between persons and the government.

All law in the United States flows from the U.S. Constitution and must conform to its principles. The Constitution provides for division of powers through the establishment of three branches of government: judicial, executive, and legislative. The chief functions of the *judicial branch* are to resolve legal disputes, interpret statutory laws, and amend the common law. The *executive branch* implements laws through governmental agencies. The *legislative branch* may delegate authority to governmental agencies to create rules, regulations, and programs to meet the intent of a statute. The legislative branch makes statutory laws and speaks most directly for the people. Figure 20-1 depicts the sources of law in the United States.

The word **law** is defined as the sum total of man-made rules and regulations by which society is governed in a formal and binding manner (Hemelt and Mackert, 1982). Law encompasses the actions of the legislative branch in enacting statutes,

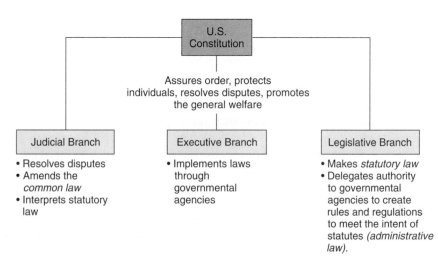

Figure **20-1**
Sources of law in the United States.

the executive branch in administering the statutes through rules, and the judicial branch in interpreting statutes and rules.

Three major types of laws govern American society: common law, statutory law, and administrative law. United States law evolved from centuries-old English **common law.** Common law is decisional or judge-made law. Every time a judge makes a legal decision, the body of common law expands.

In addition to common law, there are **statutory laws,** which are laws established through formal legislative processes. Every time the U.S. Congress or a state legislature passes legislation, the body of statutory law expands.

Administrative laws result when the legislative branch of a government delegates authority to governmental agencies to create laws that meet the intent of a statute. Both federal and state administrative laws have the force and effect of statutory law.

As important as it is to understand the sources and types of law, it is equally important to know how laws can be violated. A necessary distinction is the difference between civil and criminal law. **Civil law** involves issues between individuals, such as disputes over legal rights or duties of individuals in relation to one another (Gaffney, 1998). In civil cases, the party judged responsible for the harm may be required to pay compensation to the injured party. In contrast, **criminal law** involves public concerns against an individual's unlawful behavior that threatens society. Someone breaks a law and faces trial in the criminal court system. The convicted criminal pays through the loss of some degree of his or her freedom, ranging from probation to imprisonment or through payment of monetary fines. Violations of administrative law result when a person violates the regulations and rules established by administrative law, such as when a nurse practices without a valid license. Punishment may involve having a license revoked or suspended or being placed on probation.

Professional nurses need to be aware of a wide array of legal issues. Nurses must be particularly aware of the statutory authority governing nursing practice, executive authority of state boards of nursing, the civil law areas of torts, privacy rights, and the evolving common law related to health care. The remainder of this chapter focuses on these key areas.

NURSING AS A PRACTICE DISCIPLINE

The practice parameters of disciplines such as nursing, medicine, dentistry, law, and many others are established by state legislation and are regulated by the individual states through regulatory agencies and boards. These boards are established by state legislation and are given statutory authority by state legislatures to enforce professional practice acts. The practitioners of these disciplines cannot legally practice without a license.

The purpose of licensing certain professions is to protect the public health, safety, and welfare. The statute that defines and controls nursing is called a **nurse practice act.** All 50 states and several U.S. territories have nurse practice acts. They are administered and enforced through regulatory bodies known as **state boards of nursing.**

Statutory Authority of State Nurse Practice Acts

Nurses, as health care providers, have certain rights, responsibilities, and recognitions through various state laws, or statutes. The nurse practice act in each state does at least four things:

1. Defines the practice of professional nursing
2. Sets the minimum educational qualifications and other requirements for licensure
3. Determines the legal titles and abbreviations nurses may use
4. Provides for disciplinary action of licensees for certain causes

In many states, nurse practice acts also define the responsibilities and authorities of the **state board of nursing.** Thus, the nurse practice act of each state is the most important statutory law affecting nurses (Figure 20-2).

Once the law regarding nursing practice is legislatively established, the legislative branch delegates authority to an executive agency, usually the state board of nursing. State boards of nursing are responsible for enforcing the nurse practice acts in the various states. The state board of nursing promulgates rules and regulations that flesh out the law. The statutory law plus the rules and regulations promulgated by the state board of nursing give full meaning to the nurse practice act in each state.

Nurse practice acts are revised from time to time to keep up with new developments in health care and changes in nursing practice. State nurses associations are usually instrumental in lobbying for appropriate updating in nurse practice acts.

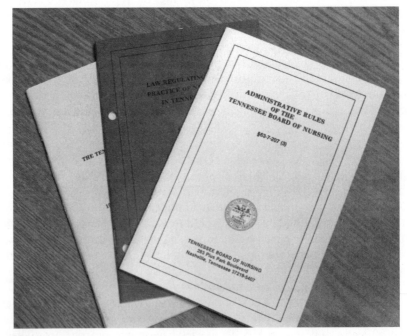

Figure 20-2
The nurse practice act and other state rules and regulations are vital documents that affect the legal practice of nursing. Every professional nurse should have current copies of these documents and be familiar with their contents. (Photo by Fielding Freed.)

Because of the importance of practice acts to professional nurses, both the American Nurses Association (ANA) and the National Council of State Boards of Nursing (NCSBN) have developed suggested language for the content of state nurse practice acts. The ANA's *Model Practice Act* was published in 1996 to guide state nurses associations seeking revisions in their nurse practice acts (American Nurses Association, 1996a). The guidelines encourage consideration of the many issues inherent in a nurse practice act and the political realities of each state's legislative and regulatory processes. Through this document, the ANA recognizes the great importance of the nurse practice act and urges that the following content be included:

1. A clear differentiation between advanced and generalist nursing practice
2. Authority for boards of nursing to regulate advanced nursing practice, including authority for prescription writing
3. Authority for boards of nursing to oversee unlicensed assistive personnel
4. Clarification of the nurse's responsibility for delegation to and supervision of other personnel
5. Support for mandatory licensure for nurses while retaining sufficient flexibility to accommodate the changing nature of nursing practice

The ANA document provides a broad definition of the practice of professional nursing and appropriate professional practice activities. It incorporates aspects of technical nursing practice and identifies technical activities (American Nurses Association, 1996a).

The model nurse practice act guidelines recognize the baccalaureate degree with a major in nursing (bachelor of science in nursing, or BSN) as the minimum educational credential for the professional nurse. There has been extensive debate about the need to change the minimum educational qualifications for professional nursing practice. In the early 1980s and again in 1995, the ANA reaffirmed its long-standing position that the baccalaureate degree should be the minimum educational qualification for professional nursing practice and the associate degree the minimum educational qualification for technical nursing practice.

Although a number of states support the BSN as the minimum entry into practice requirement, no states currently require it. Many constituent member (state nurses) associations, however, consider such changes a priority for future nurse practice act modifications. For 15 years the state of North Dakota pioneered by being the only state to require the BSN for licensure as a registered nurse. In 2003, this requirement was removed from North Dakota's nurse practice act. You can read a summary of the forces that led to that change in Chapter 21 (see Box 21-1).

The NCSBN's model nurse practice act (2003), still under review as this textbook went to press, is a very comprehensive document. It can be reviewed online *(www.ncsbn. org/public/regulation/nursingpractice_nursing_practice_model_practice_act.asp)*.

Executive Authority of State Boards of Nursing

Both federal and state laws provide for the executive branch of government to administer and implement laws. The state executive, or governor, generally delegates the responsibility for administering the nurse practice act to an executive agency, the state board of nursing. In most states, the state board of nursing consists of registered nurses (RNs), licensed practical nurses (LPNs), and consumers (members of the general public), all of whom are generally appointed to the board by the governor.

The state board of nursing's authority is limited. It can adopt rules that clarify general provisions of the nurse practice act, but it does not have the authority to enlarge the law.

State boards of nursing usually have three functions:

1. Quasiexecutive—authority to administer the nurse practice act
2. Quasilegislative—authority to adopt rules necessary to implement the act
3. Quasijudicial—authority to deny, suspend, or revoke a license or to otherwise discipline a licensee or to deny an application for licensure

Each of these functions is as broad or as limited as the state legislature specifies in the nurse practice act and related laws.

State boards of nursing may be independent agencies in the executive branch of state government or part of a department or bureau such as a department of licensure and regulation. Some state boards have authority to carry out the nurse practice act without review of their actions by other state officials. Others must recommend action to another department or bureau and receive approval of the recommendation before the decision is finalized.

Licensing powers

The **licensure** process is a police power of the state that, through the legislative branch, determines what groups are to be licensed and the limitations of such licenses. Licensure laws may be either mandatory or permissive. A mandatory law requires any person who practices the profession or occupation to be licensed. A permissive law protects the use of the title granted in the law but does not prohibit persons from practicing the profession or occupation if they do not use the title. All states now have a mandatory licensure law for the practice of nursing.

Just as the state has the power to issue a nursing license based on established criteria, so does it retain the power to discipline a licensee for performing professional functions in a manner that is dangerous to patients or the general public. Discipline may include sanctions such as license suspension or revocation arising from unsafe, uninformed, or impaired practice by the nurse licensee.

Historically, the nursing profession has demonstrated a commitment to the rehabilitation of nurses whose practice is below standard because of impairment by psychological dysfunction or substance abuse and misuse. In 1990, the ANA published suggested state legislation that included a Nursing Disciplinary Diversion Act (American Nurses Association, 1990). This publication recommended a diversion procedure, such as a peer assistance program to combat substance abuse, as a voluntary alternative to the traditional disciplinary actions of suspension or revocation of a license. In 2002, 40 state boards of nursing had nondisciplinary alternative programs (disciplinary diversion processes) to assist impaired nurses to return to safe nursing practice. Additionally, 24 boards also provided alternative programs for psychiatric and mental health problems (National Council of State Boards of Nursing, 2003).

In most states, state boards of nursing have the authority to enforce minimum criteria for nursing education programs. The practice act usually stipulates that an applicant for licensure must graduate from a state-approved nursing education program as a prerequisite to being admitted to the licensure examination.

State approval is generally less stringent than from national accreditation; many nursing education programs achieve accreditation by nationally recognized accrediting bodies. Although many other professions and occupations require graduation from a nationally accredited educational program as a prerequisite of licensure, only state approval is currently required in nursing.

Licensure examinations

Since 1944, most state boards of nursing have participated in a cooperative effort to assist in the interstate mobility of nurses, both registered nurses and licensed practical nurses. Because nurse licensure examinations are national examinations, they facilitate this system, called **licensure by endorsement.** Endorsement means that registered nurses or licensed practical nurses or licensed vocational nurses (LVNs) can move from state to state without having to take another licensing examination. If they submit proof of licensure in another state and pay a licensure fee, they can receive licensure in the new state by endorsement. Licensure by endorsement is not available to all practice disciplines. Nursing's plan serves as a national model for other licensed professions and occupations.

Until 1978, the national nursing licensing examination was developed by the ANA's Council of State Boards of Nursing, and the National League for Nursing served as the testing service. In 1978, the National Council of State Boards of Nursing (NCSBN) was established and continued the activities of the ANA Council of State Boards. Through the NCSBN, each state still participates in the licensing process through test development and adoption of a minimum passing score.

The nurse licensure examinations are now called the National Council Licensure Examination for Registered Nurses (NCLEX–RN) and the National Council Licensure Examination for Practical Nurses (NCLEX–PN). The test was traditionally administered by paper and pencil; however, the state boards of nursing and the NCSBN began administering them by computerized adaptive testing (CAT) in 1994. The test plan for the NCLEX–RN licensure examination, which is updated periodically, provides for the examination to measure critical thinking and nursing competence in all phases of the nursing process.

Trends in licensure: nurse licensure compact

As society has become more mobile, need for a new regulatory approach to promote mobility of nurses while still protecting the public health, safety, and welfare has been identified. In response to this mobility, the increase in travel nursing, the increasing practice of telehealth (being physically present in one state while providing nursing care to a patient in another state through electronic means), and other regulatory pressures, the National Council of State Boards of Nursing developed and promoted a **mutual recognition model** for nursing licensure. The mutual recognition model allows a registered nurse to have one license (in the state of residency) yet practice in other states without additional licenses. While practicing in another state, the nurse is subject to that state's laws, scope of practice, and discipline. According to the NCSBN, "the vision of the **Nurse Licensure Compact** is a state nursing license recognized nationally and enforced locally" (2000, p. 8).

Each state that wishes to participate must pass legislation to allow the board of nursing to enter into the interstate Nurse Licensure Compact. Utah was the first state to adopt the compact on March 14, 1998 (NCSBN, 2000). By March 2004 legislative session, 17 states had enacted this legislation and 3 more had enacted the Nurse Licensure Compact but had not yet implemented it (NCNSB, 2004). Nurses licensed in any state that has implemented the Compact can practice in their own states, as well as in any other Compact states, without applying for licensure by endorsement. Updated information about the status of states in relation to the Compact can be found online *(www.ncsbn.org/nlc/rnpvncompact_mutual _recognition_state.asp)*.

SPECIAL CONCERNS IN PROFESSIONAL NURSING PRACTICE

Nurses make decisions daily that affect the well-being of their patients. Because they must know personal information about patients and participate with them in difficult times, they are in positions of great responsibility and trust. Several areas of nursing practice—in particular, delegation, informed consent, and confidentiality—are fraught with legal risk, including charges of malpractice and assault and battery. In this section, we will discuss each of these areas of concern.

Malpractice

Malpractice lawsuits are on the rise and more nurses are being named defendants in these lawsuits (NPDB, 2001). **Malpractice** is the greatest legal concern of health care practitioners. To understand malpractice, nurses must first understand the legal concepts of torts and negligence. **Torts** are civil wrongs against a person and may be either intentional or unintentional. For a tort to exist, there must be harm resulting from the action, but the harm may be physical, emotional, or economic. An intentional tort refers to willful acts that violate another person's rights or property.

Negligence is the failure to act as a reasonably prudent person would have acted in specific circumstances. For example, if in burning yard debris on a windy day, a man sets fire to his neighbor's garage, the neighbor may charge negligence. A reasonably prudent person would not have started a yard fire on a windy day, and an injury (the burned garage) can be shown to be a direct result of his failure to act prudently. The differences between negligence and intentional torts are summarized in Table 20-1.

Malpractice is negligence applied to the acts of a professional. In other words, malpractice occurs when a professional fails to act as a reasonably prudent professional would have acted under specific circumstances. Malpractice is classified as an unintentional tort. This means that it is not necessary to prove that the professional intended to be negligent. In malpractice, legal action may be based on the accused person *doing* things that should not have been done (commissions) and *not doing* things that should have been done (omissions).

When a patient brings a malpractice claim against a nurse defendant, evidence is presented to the jury to determine whether the elements of liability are present. At question is whether the nurse met the prevailing **standard of care.** The nursing standard of care is what the reasonably prudent nurse, under similar circumstances,

Table 20-1 DIFFERENCES BETWEEN NEGLIGENCE AND INTENTIONAL TORTS

Negligence	Intentional Torts*
INTENT	
May occur without any intent to act.	Requires an intent to interfere with another's rights; a hostile motive not required.
PROOF OF DAMAGES	
Requires proof of a specific injury.	Proof of actual injury not required.
DUTY OR STANDARDS OF CARE	
Relevant; usually involves expert witnesses.	Not needed.
CONSENT	
Not necessarily a defense.	Always may be a defense.

*Examples of intentional torts include defamation (libel or slander), invasion of privacy, assault and battery, false imprisonment, and intentional infliction of emotional distress.
From Aiken: *Legal, ethical, and political issues in nursing,* Philadelphia, 2004, FA Davis.

would have done. It is a peer standard of care that reflects not excellence but a minimum standard of "do no harm." The nursing standard of care is decided by a jury on a case-by-case basis and is developed through use of **expert witness** testimony; documents, including national **standards of nursing practice;** the patient record; and other pertinent evidence such as the direct testimony of the patient, the nurse, and others.

The prerequisite of a malpractice action is twofold: The defendant (nurse) has specialized knowledge and skills and through the practice of that specialized knowledge causes the plaintiff's (patient's) injury. For a plaintiff patient to prove that the nurse defendant is liable for the injury, all elements of a cause of action for negligence must be proved. These elements, the same for any professional accused of malpractice, are as follows:

1. The professional (nurse) has assumed the **duty of care** (responsibility for the patient's care).
2. The professional (nurse) breached the duty of care by failing to meet the standard of care.
3. The failure of the professional (nurse) to meet the standard of care was the **proximate cause** of the injury.
4. The injury is proved.

Setting forth all elements of a malpractice action requires a high degree of proof. Monetary damages are awarded when a patient plaintiff prevails. These awards are based on proven economic losses, such as time missed from work or out-of-pocket health care costs and on remuneration for pain and suffering caused by the injury. In the case of a death, the next of kin can become the plaintiff on behalf of the deceased patient.

In the past, some malpractice lawsuits involved nurses, but the physician or hospital defendants were traditionally called on to pay damages even when the substandard care was provided by nurses. In these instances, physicians were implicated through the **"captain of the ship" doctrine.** This doctrine implies that the physician is ultimately in charge of all patient care and thus should be responsible financially. Hospitals were implicated through the legal theory of **respondeat superior** (from Latin, meaning "let the master answer"), which attributes the acts of employees to their employer. However, as nurses have obtained more credentials and their expertise, autonomy, and authority for nursing practice have increased, direct liability for nursing care has correspondingly risen.

Croke (2003) conducted a review of "more than 350 trial, appellate, and supreme court case summaries" (p. 56) from a variety of legal research sources and analyzed 253 cases that met the following criteria: A nurse was engaged in the practice of nursing as defined by his or her state's nurse practice act; a nurse was a defendant in a civil lawsuit as the result of an unintentional action (no criminal cases were considered); and a trial was held between 1995 and 2001.

Croke's analysis revealed, not surprisingly, that the largest number of cases of reported negligence occurred in acute care hospitals (60%). Other settings included nursing homes/rehabilitation/transitional care units (18%), psychiatric settings (8%), home health settings (2%), in physician offices (2%), and by care of advanced practice nurses (9%).

Croke's review identified six major categories of negligence resulting in malpractice lawsuits against nurses: failure to follow standards of care, failure to use equipment in a responsible manner, failure to communicate, failure to document, failure to assess and monitor, and failure to act as a patient advocate. More details of her analysis are presented in Box 20-1.

Some examples of malpractice that involved professional nurses were covered in the popular press. One such highly publicized case involved a number of nurses at a Massachusetts hospital who carried out a physician's faulty order and gave two different cancer patients overdoses of chemotherapy (Trossman, 1999). Another example is an operating room nurse who failed to follow well-established hospital policy for identifying and preparing patients for surgery. This breach of procedure resulted in the removal of one patient's only functioning kidney (*Holbrooks v. Duke Hospital, Inc.*, 305 SE[2] 69, 1983). Although physicians and facilities were also involved in both of these cases, the nurses were named as codefendants because they too fell below the standard of care, and "but for" their actions, these serious injuries would not have occurred.

The lesson to be learned from such malpractice cases is that professional nurses must carefully consider the legal implications of practice and be willing and capable of conforming to professional standards and all legal expectations. Among factors leading to the increase in the number of malpractice cases against nurses is delegation.

Delegation

Delegation—that is, "empowering one to act for another"—is an issue that carries great legal and safety importance in nursing practice. The ability to delegate has

| Box 20-1 | **Six Major Categories of Negligence That Result in Malpractice Lawsuits** |

Failure to follow standards of care, including failure to:
- Perform a complete admission assessment or design a plan of care.
- Adhere to standardized protocols or institutional policies and procedures (for example, using an improper injection site).
- Follow a physician's verbal or written orders.

Failure to use equipment in a responsible manner, including failure to:
- Follow the manufacturer's recommendations for operating equipment.
- Check equipment for safety prior to use.
- Place equipment properly during treatment.
- Learn how equipment functions.

Failure to communicate, including failure to:
- Notify a physician in a timely manner when conditions warrant it.
- Listen to a patient's complaints and act on them.
- Communicate effectively with a patient (for example, inadequate or ineffective communication of discharge instructions).
- Seek higher medical authorization for a treatment.

Failure to document, including failure to note in the patient's medical record:
- A patient's progress and response to treatment.
- A patient's injuries.
- Pertinent nursing assessment information (for example, drug allergies).
- A physician's medical orders.
- Information on telephone conversations with physicians, including time, content of communication between nurse and physician, and actions taken.

Failure to assess and monitor, including failure to:
- Complete a shift assessment.
- Implement a plan of care.
- Observe a patient's ongoing progress.
- Interpret a patient's signs and symptoms.

Failure to act as a patient advocate, including failure to:
- Question discharge orders when a patient's condition warrants it.
- Question incomplete or illegible medical orders.
- Provide a safe environment.

Reprinted with permission from Croke EM: Nurses, negligence, and malpractice: an analysis based on more than 250 cases against nurses, *Am J Nurs* 103(9):54-63, 2003.

generally been reserved for professionals because they hold licenses that sanction the entire scope of practice for a particular profession. Professional nurses, for example, may delegate independent nursing activities and delegated medical functions to other nursing personnel. State nurse practice acts do not give delegatory authority to licensed practical or vocational nurses.

It is critical to understand that professional nurses retain accountability for acts delegated to another person and are responsible for determining that the delegated person is competent to perform the delegated act. Likewise, the delegate is responsible for carrying out the delegated act safely. The professional nurse remains legally liable, however, for the nursing acts delegated to others unless the delegate is also a licensed professional whose scope includes the assigned act.

Delegatory acts must also be considered from the standpoint of their ethical implications. The ANA's *Code of Ethics for Nurses* states, "The nurse is responsible and accountable for individual nursing practice and determines the appropriate delegation of tasks consistent with the nurse's obligation to provide optimum patient care" (American Nurses Association, 2001, Section 4.4). An important related point is that nurses are ethically bound to refuse to perform acts that are not within their area of expertise, even if a physician or hospital authority requests that they perform them.

Delegation is an important liability and one not fully appreciated by many practicing nurses. The professional nurse's primary legal and ethical consideration must be the patient's right to safe, effective nursing care. Box 20-2 contains an excerpt from the *Code of Ethics for Nurses* pertaining to delegation (ANA, 2001, Section 4.4).

Recognizing that registered nurses are ethically and legally accountable during acts of delegation, the National Council of State Boards for Nursing (NCSBN) published *Five Rights of Delegation* (1995). These five rights are:

1. Right task: The task is appropriate for delegation and is identified in the delegate's job description.
2. Right circumstances: The appropriateness of the patient's health status, care delivery setting, complexity of the activity and delegate's competency, available resources, and other relevant factors are considered.
3. Right person: The nurse can verify that the delegates' competencies match the individual patient needs.
4. Right direction/communication: Clear, specific instructions are given, including the objective of the task, time frames, and expected results.
5. Right supervision/evaluation: Supervision and evaluation of the patient and the performance of the task are accomplished by the delegating nurse or other licensed nurse (NCSBN, 1995).

Additional information on delegation can be found on the National Council of State Boards of Nursing website *(www.ncsbn.org)*. Enter the search term *delegation* to download useful documents in PDF format.

Assault and Battery

Assault and battery is an intentional tort that is often the basis for legal action against a nurse defendant. **Assault** is a threat or an attempt to make bodily contact with another person without the person's consent. Assault precedes battery; it causes the person to fear that battery is about to occur. **Battery** is the assault carried out, the impermissible, unprivileged touching of one person by another. Actual harm may or may not occur as a result of assault and battery.

Box **20-2** **American Nurses Association's Code of Ethics for Nurses**

Section 4.4 Delegation of Nursing Activities

Since the nurse is accountable for the quality of nursing care given to patients, nurses are accountable for the assignment of nursing responsibilities to other nurses and the delegation of nursing care activities to other health care workers. While delegation and assignment are used here in a generic moral sense, it is understood that individual states may have a particular legal definition of these terms.

The nurse must make reasonable efforts to assess individual competence when assigning selected components of nursing care to other healthcare workers. This assessment involves evaluating the knowledge, skills, and experience of the individual to whom the care is assigned, the complexity of the assigned tasks, and the health status of the patient. The nurse is also responsible for monitoring the activities of these individuals and evaluating the quality of the care provided. Nurses may not delegate responsibilities such as assessment and evaluation; they may delegate tasks. The nurse must not knowingly assign or delegate to any member of the nursing team a task for which that person is not prepared or qualified. Employer policies or directives do not relieve the nurse of responsibility for making judgments about the delegation and assignment of nursing care tasks.

Nurses functioning in management or administrative roles have a particular responsibility to provide an environment that supports and facilitates appropriate assignment and delegation. This includes providing appropriate orientation to staff, assisting less experienced nurses in developing necessary skills and competencies, and establishing policies and procedures that protect both the patient and the nurse from the inappropriate assignment or delegation of nursing responsibilities, activities, or tasks.

Nurses functioning in educator or preceptor roles may have less direct relationships with patients. However, through assignment of nursing care activities to learners, they share responsibility and accountability for the care provided. It is imperative that the knowledge and skills of the learner be sufficient to provide the assigned nursing care and that appropriate supervision be provided to protect both the patient and the learner.

Reprinted with permission of American Nurses Association: *Code of Ethics for Nurses With Interpretive Statements*, Washington, DC, 2001, American Nurses Publishing, Section 4.4.

If, for example, a nurse threatens a patient with a vitamin injection if he does not eat his meals, the patient may charge assault. Actually giving the patient a vitamin injection against his will leaves the nurse open to charges of battery, even if there is a physician's order. It is important to remember that patients have the right to refuse treatment, even if the treatment would be in their best interest. Both by common law and by statute, **informed consent** is required in the health care context as a defense to battery (*42 United States Code* 1395 cc., 1990).

Informed Consent

All patients should be given an opportunity to grant informed consent before treatment unless there is a life-threatening emergency. Three major conditions of informed consent are:

1. Consent must be given voluntarily.
2. Consent must be given by an individual with the capacity and competence to understand.
3. The patient must be given enough information to be the ultimate decision maker.

   Informed consent is a full, knowing authorization by the patient for care, treatment, and procedures and must include information about the risks, benefits, side effects, costs, and alternatives. Consumers of health care need a great deal of information and should be told everything that they would consider significant in making a treatment decision (*Canterbury v. Spence*, 464 F^2 772, 1972).

   For informed consent to be legally valid, elements of completeness, competency, and voluntariness are evaluated. Completeness refers to the quality of the information provided. **Competency** takes into account the capability of a particular patient to understand the information given and make a choice. **Voluntariness** refers to the freedom the patient has to accept or reject alternatives. In the case of patients who are minors, or who are under the effects of drugs or alcohol (including preoperative medications), or who have other mental deficits, it is questionable that competency to consent exists.

   The role of nurses in informed consent, unless they are themselves primary providers, is to collaborate with the primary provider, most often a physician. A nurse may witness a patient's signing of informed consent documents but is not responsible for explaining the proposed treatment (Figure 20-3). The nurse is not responsible for evaluating whether the physician has truly explained the significant risks, benefits, and alternative treatments. Professional nurses are responsible for determining that the elements for valid consent are in place, providing feedback if the patient wishes to change consent, and communicating the patient's need for further information to the primary provider.

Confidentiality

Confidentiality is both a legal and an ethical concern in nursing practice. Confidentiality is the protection of private information gathered about a patient during the provision of health care services. The *Code of Ethics for Nurses* states, "… the nurse has a duty to maintain confidentiality of all patient information. … Only information pertinent to a patient's treatment and welfare is disclosed, and only to those directly involved with the patient's care. The nurse safeguards the client's right to privacy by judiciously protecting information of a confidential nature" (American Nurses Association, 2001, Section 3.2).

   The *Code* acknowledges exceptions to the obligation of confidentiality. These include discussing the care of patients with others involved in their direct care, quality assurance activities, legally mandated disclosure to public health authorities, and information required by third-party payers (American Nurses Association, 2001). The *Code* also recognizes the need to disclose information without the

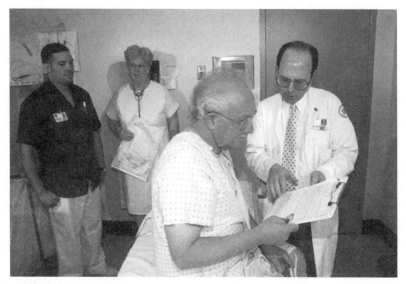

Figure **20-3**
Professional nurses may be called on to witness a patient's signing of informed consent documents. The primary provider, however, is responsible for providing necessary information to the patient or legal guardian. (From Leahy JM, Kizilay PE: *Foundations of nursing practice*, Philadelphia, 1998, WB Saunders.)

patient's consent when the safety of innocent parties is in question (*Tarasoff v. Board of Regents of the University of California*, 551 P² 334, 1976).

The principle of confidentiality is protected by state and federal statutes, but there are exceptions and limitations. Although some professions have statutorily protected **privileged communication,** nurses are usually not included in such statutes. Thus nurses may be ordered by a court to share information without the patient's consent. It is essential for the professional nurse to understand these legal limitations.

In certain situations, through statute and common law, the antithesis of confidentiality has developed—the **duty to report** or disclose. These laws require nurses and other health professionals to report child abuse, gunshot wounds, certain communicable diseases, and threats toward third parties. These laws vary by state and may be the responsibility of institutions providing health care services and not of an individual practitioner.

The Health Insurance Portability and Accountability Act of 1996 (HIPAA)

The Health Insurance Portability and Accountability Act of 1996 (HIPAA) is the first-ever federal privacy standard governing protection of patients' medical records. The privacy provisions in the act began as a 337-word guideline, but as the final regulations were written, the provisions swelled to 101,000 words (Parker, 2003). HIPAA was designed, in part, to reinforce the protection of patient information as it is transmitted electronically, but the final Act goes far beyond that goal.

The new regulations protect medical records and other individually identifiable health information, whether on paper, in computers, or communicated orally.

HIPAA requires all health care providers, including doctors, hospitals, health plans, pharmacies, public health authorities, insurance companies, billing agencies, information systems sales and service providers, and others to ensure the privacy and confidentiality of patients. Although passed in 1996, the confidentiality regulations were not implemented until April 2003 in order to give providers time to prepare the necessary safeguards and documents and to train workers in their use.

HIPAA regulations require several major patient protections:

- Patients are able to see and obtain copies of their medical records, generally within 30 days of their request, and to request corrections if they detect errors. Providers may charge patients for the cost of copying and mailing the records.
- Providers must give patients written notice describing the provider's information practices and explaining patients' rights. Patients must be asked to agree to these practices by signing or initialing the notice.
- Limitations are placed on the length of time records can be retrieved, what information can be shared, where it can be shared, and who can be present when it is shared.

A number of other protections are provided in this comprehensive federal legislation. The document can be viewed online *(www.hhs.gov/news/facts/privacy.html)*.

In the early months following implementation of HIPAA requirements, doctors, nurses, hospitals, and other providers experienced confusion about which disclosures were allowed. Since the Act makes provision for civil and criminal penalties, including stiff fines, for entities that misuse personal health information, health care professionals were understandably reluctant to talk to others about a patient, even when the other person was a family member or caregiver with a genuine need to know (Landro, 2003). This confusion is expected to decrease as providers become more knowledgeable about and comfortable using the regulations. The Department of Health and Human Services, which was delegated the role of developing the regulations and rules of this law, provides extensive outreach, guidance, and technical assistance to providers online *(www.hhs.gov/ocr/hipaa)*.

EVOLVING LEGAL ISSUES AND THE NURSE

Because of the dynamic nature of nursing and health care, legal issues affecting nursing practice are also evolving. Specific legal issues that illustrate the changing nature of nursing practice are related to role changes, supervision of assistive personnel, payment mechanisms, and issues associated with the implementation of the Patient Self-Determination Act. Each of these issues is briefly discussed in the following sections.

Role Changes in Health Care

Just as a nurse's knowledge base and the nurse's accountability for nursing practice have increased over time, so has the need to expand the **legal authority** for nursing practice. Even though the definitions and parameters of nursing outlined in nurse practice acts may seem to be an issue of concern only to nurses, this is not the case.

Nurses have found that as they worked through their constituent member (state nurses) associations to modify and update these acts, they met significant political resistance. This is due, in part, to the defensiveness of organized medicine, which often views an expansion of nurses' domain as a diminishment of physicians' roles or as a threat to physicians' economic base.

Professional nurses realize that it is important for a state nurse practice act to reflect nursing practice accurately and to keep up with changes in health care delivery as they occur. Otherwise, nurses have questionable legal basis for practice and are open to prosecution. Health care is becoming more specialized, so nursing specialties and subspecialties are increasing. Advanced practice nurses set the pace for evolving nursing practice, and the nurse practice act must support their ability to offer nursing services to consumers in various settings. Many functions defined as advanced practice have been absorbed into the statutory scope of professional nursing practice.

Historically, in some states, nurses in advanced practice, such as nurse-midwives, nurse practitioners, and nurses in private practice, have not been supported by timely changes in the nurse practice act. For example, nurses in a women's health practice in Missouri were sued for practicing medicine without a license. After intense litigation, their practice was supported by the Missouri Supreme Court. The court found "legislative intent" in the nurse practice act not to limit nursing practice except to protect the public. The nurses in question were well credentialed and were practicing with the knowledge and support of the Missouri Board of Nursing and the Missouri Nurses Association, so the safety of the public was not in question (*Sermchief v. Gonzales*, 660 SW[2] 683, 1983).

This is only one example of the legal exposure nurses face when their state's nurse practice act is not updated periodically to support explicitly an expanded scope of practice. Working within the constituent member (state nurses) association to expand the evolving scope of nursing practice appropriately ensures the growth of the profession and increases the number of primary care providers needed by the public. Professional nurses must support their professional associations, which led the development of legislation that accurately reflects current nursing practice at all levels.

Prescriptive authority

An important role addition for advanced practice nurses is prescriptive authority. **Prescriptive authority** is defined as the legal acknowledgment of prescription writing as an appropriate act of nursing practice. The ANA, the American Academy of Nurse Practitioners, and others support prescriptive authority for advanced practice nurses (APNs), as distinguished from generalist registered nurses.

Nurses should consider several questions about prescriptive authority: Does the state recognize prescriptive authority for nurses? If so, is the state board of nursing the state regulatory authority for this practice? Does the law require physician collaboration or supervision or written protocols? What are the parameters for prescribing controlled substances, if any?

In 2003, advanced practice nurses had some type of prescriptive authority in all 50 states. This authority ranged from completely independent authority with no collaborative requirements in 12 states (Alaska, Arizona, Iowa, Maine, Montana, New Hampshire, New Mexico, Oregon, Utah, Washington, Wisconsin, and Wyoming) and in the District of Columbia, to 5 states (Alabama, Florida, Kentucky, Missouri, Texas) where nurse practitioners can prescribe (excluding controlled substances) with some degree of physician involvement or delegation of prescription writing (Pearson, 2003). In the remaining states, nurse practitioners can prescribe (including controlled substances) with some degree of physician involvement or delegation of prescription writing (Pearson, 2003).

Both generalist and advanced practice nurses must understand prescriptive authority of advanced practice in their states. Generalist nurses must know from whom they can accept medication orders, and APNs must stay within their legal scope of practice.

Supervision of unlicensed assistive personnel

Another evolving legal issue is the continued role expansion of **unlicensed assistive personnel** or limited licensed (licensed practical/vocational nurses) personnel within health care institutions. Nurse aides (i.e., unlicensed assistive personnel) are increasingly being substituted for nurses, thus creating greater risks to patients and enlarging the liability of nurses, who supervise their work. Studies such as the one described in the accompanying Research Note indicate that lack of professional nurse supervision and the educational level of nurses themselves pose significant risks to patients, institutions, and nurses alike (Institute of Medicine, 1996; Buerhaus, Needleman, Mattke, et al., 2002; Aiken, Clarke, Cheung, et al., 2003).

The substitution of unlicensed personnel for registered nurses is a strategy used by health care facilities to hold down costs. Such substitution is ill advised because it jeopardizes quality of care and places the registered nurse at increased risk for patient injury liability because of acts performed or omitted by unlicensed assistive personnel. It is questionable whether, in the long term, professional nursing care is actually more expensive than care provided by unlicensed personnel, who are less likely to do patient teaching and recognize complications.

The ANA first issued a Position Statement on Registered Nurse Utilization of Unlicensed Assistive Personnel in 1992. It was supported in 1997 by the addition of definitions of key terms. These statements indicate that the ANA recognizes that unlicensed assistive personnel provide support services that assist the registered nurse in providing nursing care (American Nurses Association, 1992, 1997). The statement identifies the need to clarify the activities that should be in the domain of the registered nurse and those that can be safely delegated. Additional materials were developed by the ANA to provide registered nurses and health care facilities guidance on utilization of unlicensed assistive personnel in the workplace (American Nurses Association, 1996b). The ANA's position statement, *Registered Nurse Utilization of Unlicensed Assistive Personnel,* can be found in its entirety online *(www.nursingworld.org/readroom/position/uap/uapuse.htm).*

Historically, organized nursing has opposed the licensure or legal recognition of nurse aides, nursing assistants, and home health aides. This position needs further

RESEARCH note

An interdisciplinary group of Pennsylvania researchers, led by Linda Aiken, a doctorally prepared nurse from the University of Pennsylvania, was concerned about nurse understaffing and the resulting threats to patient safety in hospitals. The group members decided to study the educational composition of registered nurses (RNs) in relation to patient outcomes. Their objective was "to examine whether the proportion of hospital RNs educated at the baccalaureate level or higher is associated with risk-adjusted mortality and failure to rescue (deaths in surgical patients with serious complications)" (p. 1617).

The researchers analyzed outcome data for 232,342 general, orthopedic, and vascular surgery patients discharged from 168 nonfederal adult general Pennsylvania hospitals between April 1, 1998, and November 30, 1999. These figures were linked to data on educational composition, staffing, and other characteristics.

The percentage of RNs with a bachelor's or higher degree ranged from 0 percent to 77 percent in the various hospitals in the study. "After adjusting for patient characteristics and hospital structural characteristics (size, teaching status, level of technology), as well as for nurse staffing, nurse experience, and whether the patient's surgeon was board-certified, a 10 percent increase in the proportion of bedside nurses holding a bachelor's degree was associated with a 5 percent decrease in both the likelihood of patients dying within 30 days of admission and the odds of failure to rescue" (p. 1617).

These researchers concluded that significantly lower mortality and failure to rescue rates were found in hospitals with higher proportions of baccalaureate-prepared nurses. They recommended that investments in public funds be made to increase the number of baccalaureate nurses in order to substantially improve the quality of care in the nation.

Aiken LH, Clarke SP, Cheung RB, et al: Educational levels of hospital nurses and surgical patient mortality, *J Am Med Assoc* 290(12):1617-1623, 2003.

study, however, following congressional action mandating training and state registration of nurse aides in Medicaid-certified and Medicare-certified nursing facilities and Medicare-certified home health agencies. In spite of these mandates, in 2002, only 13 state boards were actively licensing assistive personnel. A variety of other agencies, such as state departments of health/human services, the American Red Cross, and other state agencies were also licensing assistive personnel. In three states, Alaska, Idaho, and Minnesota, assistive personnel are not licensed at all (National Council of State Boards of Nursing, 2003).

The licensure or state approval of assistive personnel is a complex and confounding issue that has relevance for registered nurses because professional nurses are legally responsible for the tasks performed by assistive personnel they supervise. Having nationally standardized education and training for these workers would assure nurses of a minimum level of competence in their co-workers.

Whatever their preparation, it remains the responsibility of professional nurses to know the limitations of the assistive personnel under their supervision.

Payment mechanisms for nurses

As discussed in Chapter 5, nurses are increasingly practicing in nontraditional roles and settings. Many professional nurses are both capable of and interested in offering nursing services as private practitioners, but payment mechanisms may limit such activities. Nurses are concerned about offering services for which consumers are unable to obtain reimbursement from their insurance carriers, and third-party reimbursement has traditionally been limited to care provided by physicians.

Over the years, nurses and their professional associations have supported state and federal legislation to provide direct and indirect payments to nurses for nursing services rendered. A major legislative victory in the 8-year fight to obtain direct reimbursement of advanced practice nurses came with the passage of the 1997 Balanced Budget Act. This legislation authorized nurse practitioners and clinical specialists, beginning in January 1998, to bill the Medicare program directly for nursing services furnished in any setting. It remains a regulatory challenge to devise a fair and equitable payment system for advanced practice nurses, whose scopes of practice vary from state to state.

This federal legislation became a model for commercial insurers. During the 1990s, changes in state insurance laws were enacted in many states to achieve direct payment for nursing services from private insurance companies. This means that consumers of health care may choose to receive services from physicians, nurses, or other qualified health professionals and receive insurance reimbursement for the chosen professional's fees. Nurses are concerned that these changes are often not implemented or that nurses are paid less for services similar to those provided by other health care professionals who are paid at a higher rate.

Laws are often passed that are not implemented. This occurs when the group affected by the law (for example, the insurance industry) is unwilling to implement the changes and no "watchdog" agency is created to ensure that changes occur. For example, federal legislation was enacted requiring state Medicaid agencies to pay certain nurses (nurse practitioners, nurse-midwives, and nurse anesthetists) directly for services provided to Medicaid recipients. As with the laws affecting private insurers, these requirements have not been implemented in every state. Nurses may need to seek legal remedies to require implementation of policies mandated by federal law (*Nurse Midwifery Associates v. Hibbett*, 918 Fed[2] 605, 1990).

Following the failed 1994 efforts to overhaul the entire health care system, health care finance nevertheless underwent dramatic changes. One change, discussed in Chapter 16, was from fee-for-service provider reimbursement to capitation. Additionally, many individual and group insurance plans changed from indemnity plans to **managed care plans,** such as health maintenance organizations (HMOs) and preferred provider organizations (PPOs). As of 2002, 57 percent of the nation's Medicaid recipients were enrolled in some form of managed care plan (Centers for Medicare and Medicaid Services, 2002). In a demonstration project in 20 states that began on January 1, 2003, 73,794 Medicare beneficiaries signed up for managed care plans in the first 9 months (Centers for Medicare and Medicaid Services, 2003).

These shifts have posed new challenges for nurses, because they are often not included on HMO and PPO provider panels. As a result of these new challenges, the ANA and constituent member (state) associations are working to ensure that nurses are included on managed care panels, in "any willing provider" clauses, and in all federal insurance programs as appropriate providers of basic plan services.

Patient Self-Determination Act

Although the **Patient Self-Determination Act** (PSDA) became effective in 1991, more than 10 years later there remain many problems in its implementation. Nurses are in a position to help patients and families understand this law and how it can assist them to have the end-of-life care they prefer.

As mentioned in Chapter 19, this act applies to acute care and long-term care facilities that receive Medicare and Medicaid funds. It encourages patients to consider which life-prolonging treatment options they desire and to document their preferences in case they should later become incapable of participating in the decision-making process. Written instructions recognized by state law that describe an individual's preferences in regard to medical intervention should the individual become incapacitated is called an **advance directive.**

This act was passed partly in response to the U.S. Supreme Court's decision in *Cruzan v. Director Missouri Department of Health* (110 Supreme Court 2841, 1990), which was viewed as limiting an individual's ability to direct health care when unable to do so. The PSDA requires the health care facility to document whether the patient has completed an advance directive.

The PSDA's basic assumption is that each person has legal and moral rights to informed consent about medical treatments with a focus on the person's right to choose (the ethical principle of autonomy). The act does not create any new rights, and no patient is required to execute an advance directive.

According to the PSDA, acute care (hospitals) and long-term care facilities must:
1. Provide written information to all adult patients about their rights under state law.
2. Ensure institutional compliance with state laws on advance directives.
3. Provide for education of staff and the community on advance directives.
4. Document in the medical record whether the patient has an advance directive.

The Agency for Health Care Policy Research reported that even when patients had advance directives in place, the directives were not guiding end-of-life care as legislators and advocates had anticipated. This was due to several factors: the patients were not considered hopelessly ill, the family members were either not available or too overwhelmed to implement the patient's wishes, and the advance directive itself was not specific enough or did not cover pertinent clinical issues (Ditto, Danks, and Smucker, 2001).

In addition to these problems, there have been a number of widely publicized cases wherein families and providers disagreed about whether to terminate life support mechanisms (see Chapter 19's News Note). Widespread education of the public about advance directives should result in fewer such legal and ethical dilemmas in the future. Documentation of the existence of advance directives and use of them in planning care is an important patient advocacy role for nurses and is a legal requirement that needs careful implementation in clinical settings.

PREVENTING LEGAL PROBLEMS IN NURSING PRACTICE

Although the range of potential "hot spots" for health care litigation may seem enormous, there are a number of effective strategies that professional nurses can use to limit the possibility of legal action.

Practice in a Safe Setting

To be truly safe, facilities in which nurses work must be committed to safe patient care. The safest situation is one in which the agency:

1. Employs an appropriate number and skill mix of personnel to care adequately for the number of agency patients at all levels of acuity.
2. Has policies, procedures, and personnel practices that promote **quality improvement.**
3. Keeps equipment in good working order.
4. Provides orientation to new employees, supervises all levels of employees, and provides opportunities for employees to learn new procedures consistent with the level of health care services provided by the agency.

In addition to an active quality improvement program, each health care organization should have a **risk management** program. Risk management seeks to identify and eliminate potential safety hazards, thereby reducing patient and staff injuries. Common areas of risk include patient falls, failure to monitor, failure to ensure patient safety, improper performance of a treatment, failure to respond to a patient, medication errors, failure to follow hospital procedure, improper technique, and failure to supervise treatment (Aiken, 2004).

Crossing the Quality Chasm: The IOM Health Care Quality Initiative

In 1996, the Institute of Medicine (IOM), an arm of the nonprofit National Academy of Science, launched "a concerted, ongoing effort focused on assessing and improving the nation's quality of care" (IOM, 2003). The IOM defines quality as, "the degree to which health services for individuals and populations increase the likelihood of desired health outcomes and are consistent with current professional knowledge" (IOM, 2003).

The first phase of this initiative documented a serious and pervasive quality problem in the nation's health care delivery system through an intensive review of the literature conducted by RAND. The second phase identified a vision for transformation of the health care system to "close the chasm between what we know to be good quality care and what actually exists in practice" (IOM, 2003). Two reports were released during the second phase: *To Err Is Human: Building a Safer Health System* and *Crossing the Quality Chasm: The IOM Health Care Quality Initiative.* These reports stressed complete reform of the health system, not just "reform around the margins." *To Err Is Human* described how "tens of thousands of Americans die each year from medical errors and effectively put the issue of patient safety and quality on the radar screen of public and private policymakers" (IOM, 2003). *Crossing the Quality Chasm* described "broader quality issues and defined six aims—care should be safe, effective, patient-centered, timely, efficient and equitable" (IOM, 2003).

The third phase of the IOM effort focuses on operationalizing the vision of the *Quality Chasm* report. The IOM, working in conjunction with representatives of many other professions, including nursing, hopes to create a more patient responsive twenty-first century health system. During this phase two specific reports of interest to nurses will be published: *Redesigning Care Delivery*, a report that will recommend ways to redesign nursing care delivery to improve patient safety, and *Health Professions Education: A Bridge to Quality*, which promotes reform of health professions education to improve quality.

These efforts, when combined with those of each professional nurse and each setting where nurses work, should create a safer, more effective health care system in which quality and safety have a high priority. Legal problems in nursing practice will thereby be minimized.

Communicate With Other Health Professionals, Patients, and Families

The professional nurse must have open and clear communication with nurses, physicians, and other health care professionals. Safe nurses trust their own assessments, inform physicians and others of changes in patients' conditions, and question unclear or inaccurate physicians' orders. A key aspect of communication essential in preventing legal problems is keeping good patient records. This written form of communication is called **documentation.**

The clinical record, particularly the nurse's notes, provides the core of evidence about each patient's nursing care. No matter how good the nursing care, if the nurse fails to document it in the clinical record, in the eyes of the law the care did not take place. Be sure to document accurately, in a timely manner, and concisely. Know the charting policies of your agency and your unit, particularly the acceptable abbreviations.

Current and descriptive documentation of patient care is essential, not only to provide quality care but also to protect the nurse. Assessments, plans, interventions, and evaluation of the patient's progress must be reflected in the patient's clinical record if malpractice is alleged. Nurses must also document telephone calls with patients, family members, physicians, and other health care providers.

If a patient is angry, noncompliant, or complaining, nurses should be even more careful to document thoroughly. Professional nurses recognize that establishing and maintaining good communication and rapport with patients and their families not only is an aspect of best practice, it also protects from lawsuits.

Meet the Standard of Care

The most important protective strategy for the nurse is to be a knowledgeable and safe practitioner and to meet the standard of care with all patients. Meeting the standard of care involves being technically competent, keeping up-to-date with health care innovations, being aware of peer expectations, and participating as an equal on the health care team.

Nurses must familiarize themselves with the policies and procedures of the agency in which they work and must not deviate from those policies. They must know how to use equipment properly and to know when that equipment is malfunctioning and in need of repair. They must keep up with trends in their area of practice through reading the professional literature and attending continuing education conferences and workshops. Professional nurses must use national standards of practice as parameters for care giving, care planning, and care evaluation. The ANA has promulgated generic and specialty standards of nursing practice and published these in the document *Nursing: Scope and Standards of Practice* (2003). These national standards can be used by quality improvement programs in individual hospitals in establishing their own "local" standards of nursing care.

Continued competence is an issue the nursing profession has not uniformly addressed. As you will recall from the discussion in Chapter 2, different states have different requirements for continuing education as a prerequisite for license renewal. The wise nurse recognizes that continuing education and maintaining competence is essential to safe practice, whether or not it is a state requirement.

In the final analysis, the best protection a nurse can have is to know the limits of his or her own education, expertise, and nurse practice act. Staying within those limits may sometimes require nurses to enlist assistance from more experienced nurses in order to meet the standard of care. This should be viewed as a learning opportunity and an indication of maturity rather than a failure or evidence of incompetence.

Carry and Understand Professional Liability Insurance

Despite the efforts of dedicated professionals, sometimes mistakes are made and, unfortunately, patients are injured. It is essential for nurses to carry professional liability insurance to protect their assets and income in case they are required to pay monetary compensation to an injured patient. Nursing students should also carry insurance, and most nursing education programs require that they do so. In addition to carrying the insurance, nurses must read and understand the provisions of their malpractice coverage to avoid unpleasant surprises.

Professional liability insurance policies vary. Generally, they provide up to $2 million coverage for a single incident and up to $4 million total. The amount of coverage depends on the nurse's specialty. Nurse-midwives, for example, pay much higher liability insurance premiums than do psychiatric nurses because a nurse-midwife's potential for being sued is greater. Look for a policy that has portable coverage and make sure that it covers court judgments, out-of-court settlements, legal fees, and court costs. Furthermore, a good policy covers incidents occurring anytime—as long as the incident took place while the policy was in force, even if you no longer carry the insurance (occurrence policy).

Professional liability insurance is available through most state nurses associations, nursing students associations, and private insurers. Group policies, such as those available through professional associations, are usually less expensive than individual policies and are an important benefit of association membership. Box 20-3 provides information about the two main types of professional liability policies.

Liability and the National Practitioner Data Bank

The Health Care Quality Improvement Act (Public Law 100-177) was passed by Congress in 1986. It established a **National Practitioner Data Bank** (NPDB) to encourage identification and discipline of health care practitioners who engage in unprofessional behavior. An additional purpose was to restrict the ability of those

| Box **20-3** | Basic Types of Professional Liability Insurance Policies |

Occurrence Policies

Cover injuries that occur during the period covered by the policy, whether or not the policy is still in effect at the time the suit is brought.

Claims-Made Policies

Cover injuries only if the injury occurs within the policy period and the claim is reported to the insurance company during the policy period or during the "tail." A tail is an uninterrupted extension of the policy period and is also known as the extending reporting endorsement.

practitioners to move from state to state without disclosing problems of damaging or incompetent practice. The act requires that the following be reported to the National Data Bank:

- Any malpractice payments made to any licensed health practitioner
- Any licensure action taken by a licensing body
- Any clinical privilege suspension or revocation by a health care facility
- Any clinical society censorship action

The NPDB is maintained by the U.S. Department of Health and Human Services, Bureau of Health Professions, Division of Practitioner Data Banks. It affects nurses in two major ways:

1. Malpractice payments made on behalf of a nurse are reported to the NPDB and copied to the state board of nursing.
2. An inquiry to the NPDB is required when nurses apply for hospital privileges and is required every 2 years for renewal of hospital privileges.

According to the NPDB, "malpractice payments for nurses are relatively rare" (National Practitioner Data Bank, 2002, p. 19). In 2001 the NPDB annual report stated that over the history of the database, registered nurses have been responsible for only 3,614 malpractice payments. This constitutes only 1.7 percent of all malpractice payments made. Slightly less than two thirds of those payments were for nonspecialized registered nurses. Just over one third of the claims were for advanced practice nurses. This includes nurse anesthetists, who were responsible for 22.7 percent of all nurse payments, and nurse-midwives, who were responsible for 8.2 percent of all nurse payments. Nurse practitioners accounted for 5.2 percent of all nurse payments.

The NPDB reported that problems with the monitoring of patients, implementing treatments, and medication problems have been responsible for the majority of payments for nonspecialized nurses, followed by obstetrical and surgical problems. In 2001, the median malpractice payment for all types of nurses was $125,000, and the mean was $288,618 (National Practitioner Data Bank, 2002).

Promote Positive Interpersonal Relationships

Even in the face of untoward outcomes from a health care provider, it is usually only the disgruntled patient that sues. Therefore the best strategy for the professional nurse is prevention of legal actions through positive interpersonal relationships.

Box 20-4 **Guidelines for Preventing Legal Problems in Nursing Practice**

- Practice safely in a safe setting.
- Communicate with other health professionals, patients, and—with patient's permission—family members. Document fully, carefully, and in a timely manner.
- Delegate wisely, remembering the five "rights" of delegation.
- Meet or exceed the standard of care by staying on top of new developments and skills.
- Carry professional liability insurance and know the specifics of the policy.
- Promote positive interpersonal relationships and a nondefensive manner while practicing caring, compassionate, holistic nursing care.

Prevention includes giving personalized, concerned care; including the patient and the family in planning and implementing care; and promoting positive, open interpersonal relationships that communicate caring and compassion. When confronted with angry patients or family members, wise nurses avoid criticizing or blaming other health care providers and maintain a concerned and nondefensive manner.

The professional nurse who is clinically competent and caring, communicates openly with patients, and acknowledges the holism of the patient is likely to prevent most legal problems. Box 20-4 summarizes the important steps nurses can take to avoid legal problems in professional practice.

Summary of Key Points

- Nurses must recognize that the law is a system of rules that governs conduct and attaches consequences to certain behavior.
- Consequences include civil or criminal action or both.
- Nursing practice is limited by the definition of practice in the state nurse practice act and the qualifications for licensure to practice nursing in that state.
- The law is dynamic and must be responsive to society's needs.
- Broadening the scope of nursing practice has increased the possibility for legal actions involving nurses.
- Technological advances have increased concern about informed consent and patients' right to direct the care they choose to receive or refuse.
- Many nurses possess inadequate knowledge of legal issues that affect nursing practice every day. These issues deserve increased attention by nurses in all areas of practice.

CRITICAL THINKING QUESTIONS

1. Using your state's nurse practice act, describe the scope of practice of the registered nurse. When was the last time the law was modified? Does it accurately reflect current nursing practice?
2. Read the section of the nurse practice act relating to advanced practice. What differences are identified between the scope of practice of the registered nurse and that of the advanced practice nurse?

3. If a physician writes an order for an unusually high dose of a medication, what should the nurse do?
4. What are the liability issues for a nurse who fails to raise the side rails on a post-operative patient's bed if the patient is injured in a fall?
5. Explain the Patient Self-Determination Act to your family and friends. What questions do they have about an advance directive? Find out what the laws regarding advance directives are in your state.
6. When you are interviewing for a position, what questions should you ask to determine whether it is a legally safe setting in which to practice?
7. Under what circumstances can a nurse who administers a medication causing an allergic reaction be found negligent?
8. Discuss the legal and ethical issues for a nurse who is asked by a nurse manager to help clear up a backlog of paperwork by postdating forms and signing off on inspections that were not performed as required.

REFERENCES

Aiken LH, Clarke SP, Cheung RB, et al: Educational levels of hospital nurses and surgical patient mortality, *J Am Med Assoc* 290(12):1617-1623, 2003.

Aiken T: *Legal, ethical and political issues in nursing,* Philadelphia, 2004, FA Davis.

American Association of Nurse Attorneys: *Demonstrating financial responsibility for nursing practice,* Baltimore, MD, 1984, American Association of Nurse Attorneys.

American Nurses Association: *Suggested state legislation: nurse practice act, nursing disciplinary diversion act, prescriptive authority act,* Kansas City, MO, 1990, American Nurses Association.

American Nurses Association: *Position statement on registered nurse utilization of unlicensed assistive personnel,* Washington, DC, 1992, American Nurses Publishing.

American Nurses Association: *Analysis and comparison of advanced practice recognition with medical reimbursement and insurance reimbursement,* Washington, DC, 1995a, American Nurses Publishing.

American Nurses Association: *Capital update, vol 13 and 14,* Washington, DC, 1995b, American Nurses Publishing.

American Nurses Association: *Model practice act,* Washington, DC, 1996a, American Nurses Publishing.

American Nurses Association: *Registered professional nurses and unlicensed assistive personnel,* ed 2, Washington, DC, 1996b, American Nurses Publishing.

American Nurses Association: Definitions related to ANA 1992 position statements on unlicensed assistive personnel, Online, 1997 *(www.nursingworld.org/readroom/position/uap/uapuse.htm).*

American Nurses Association: *Code of ethics for nurses with interpretive statements,* Washington, DC, 2001, American Nurses Publishing.

American Nurses Association: *Nursing: scope and standards of practice,* Washington, DC, 2003, American Nurses Publishing.

Buerhaus PI, Needleman J, Mattke S, et al: Strengthening hospital nursing, *Health Affairs* 21(5):123-132, 2002.

Centers for Medicare and Medicaid Services: *Medicaid managed care enrollment as of December 31, 2002,* Baltimore, MD, 2002, Centers for Medicare and Medicaid Services.

Centers for Medicare and Medicaid Services: *Medicare preferred provider organization demonstration.* Unpublished report given September 30, 2003, at the Managed Care Enrollment and Payment Conference, Baltimore, MD.

Crawford L: Regulation of registered nursing: the American perspective, *Reflect Nurs Leadersh* 27(4):1-3, 2001.

Ditto PH, Danks JH, Smucker WD: Advance directive as acts of communication, *Arch Intern Med* 161:421-430, 2001.

Gaffney T: Regulation of nursing practice. In Shinn LJ, editor: *Take control: a guide to risk management,* Chicago, 1998, Kirke-Van Orsdel.

Hemelt M, Mackert ME: *Dynamics of law in nursing and health care,* Reston, VA, 1982, Reston Publishing.

Institute of Medicine: *Nursing staff in hospitals and nursing homes: is it adequate?* Washington, DC, 1996, National Academy Press.

Institute of Medicine: Crossing the quality chasm: the IOM health care quality initiative, Online, 2003 (*www.iom.edu/focuson.asp?id=8089*).

Landro L: Health-privacy act poses problems, *The Wall Street Journal,* April 24, CCXLII(44):D-3, 2003.

National Council of State Boards of Nursing: *The five rights of delegation,* Chicago, 1995, National Council of State Boards of Nursing.

National Council of State Boards of Nursing: *Mutual recognition: frequently asked questions,* Chicago, 1999, National Council of State Boards of Nursing, Online (*www.ncsbn.org/files/mutual/mrfaq.asp*).

National Council of State Boards of Nursing: *Annual report, 1999-2000,* Chicago, 2000, National Council of State Boards of Nursing.

National Council of State Boards of Nursing: *Profiles of member boards—2002,* Chicago, 2003, National Council of State Boards of Nursing.

National Council of State Boards of Nursing: State by state map of nurse licensure compact, Chicago, 2004, National Council of State Boards of Nursing, Online (*www.ncsbn.org/rnlpvncompact_mutual_recognition_state.asp*).

Parker L: Medical-privacy law creates wide confusion, *USA Today,* October 17:1A-2A, 2003.

Pearson L: Fifteenth annual legislative update: how each state stands on legislative issues affecting advanced nursing practice: the nurse practitioner, *Am J Prim Health Care* 28(1):26-32, 2003.

Trossman S: ANA, MNA support Dana-Farber nurses facing disciplinary action, *Am Nurse* 31(2), 1999.

Nurses and Political Action

Judith Kline Leavitt and Virginia Trotter Betts

Key Terms

Balance of Power
Electoral Process
Executive Branch
Expert Power
General Election
Judicial Branch
Latent Power
Legislative Branch
Nurse Activist

Nurse Citizen
Nurse Politician
Pay Equity
Policy
Policy Outcomes
Political Action
   Committees (PACs)
Politics
Position Power

Power
Power Grabbing
Power Sharing
Powers of Appointment
Primary Election
Professional
   Outcomes
Referendum
Separation of powers

Learning Outcomes

After studying this chapter, students will be able to:

- Differentiate between politics and policy.
- Explain the concept of personalizing the political process.
- Cite examples of sources of both personal and professional power.
- Describe how nurses can become involved in politics and policy development at the levels of citizen, activist, and politician.
- Explain how organized nursing is involved in political activities designed to strengthen professional nursing and influence health policy.

Have you ever known a nurse member of Congress? Or a nurse mayor? Did you know that a nurse was responsible for developing the federal system for health care financing? Nurses have served as heads of the Social Security Administration and Planned Parenthood of America and as chief of staff for the majority leader in the U.S. Senate. Nurses have held major leadership roles in local, state, and federal government, professional and community organizations, and the workplace. This chapter discusses the policy process, describes how nurses can influence policy decisions and become politically active, and explains some of the ways in which nurse leaders have achieved positions of power and influence.

POLICY AND POLITICS: WHAT THEY ARE AND WHAT THEY ARE NOT

Policy and politics are more than what is happening in Washington, D.C. They encompass what happens to us daily in the workplace, as well as in government, and in our communities, as well as in organizations. Politics, the art of influencing decisions, is part of every aspect of our lives, both personal and professional. People often speak of politics with negative overtones. In fact, politics is neither good nor bad. It is the *outcome* of the political process that may be judged as positive or negative.

Policy is defined as principles that govern actions directed toward given ends; policy statements set forth a plan, direction, or goal for action. Policies may be laws, regulations, or guidelines that govern behavior in the public arena, such as in government, or in the private arena such as in workplaces, schools, organizations, and communities. Health policy refers to public or private rules, regulations, laws or guidelines that relate to the pursuit of health and the delivery of health services. Policy reflects the choices that an entity (government or workplace) makes regarding its goals and priorities and how it will allocate its resources.

Policy decisions (e.g., laws or regulations) reflect the values and beliefs of those making the decisions. As values and beliefs change, so do policy decisions (Mason, Leavitt, Chaffee, 2002). For instance, laws limiting smoking in public buildings or private restaurants were nonexistent 30 years ago because smoking was considered to be "cool" and sexy. The harmful effects of smoking were not as well known as they are today. As the public became more aware of the dangers of smoking, the values about smoking changed and so too did the laws. Laws limiting smoking and the sale of tobacco products became common. Elected officials responded to the changing values of the public and recognized that the public supported the passage of such laws.

Politics is the process of influencing the allocation of scarce resources. Policies are the decisions; politics is the influencing of those decisions. For example, the federal government is responsible for Medicare because it is a federal program of health care for the elderly and the disabled. In every congressional session, legislation is proposed to expand the program. Legislation has included expanding coverage to include long-term care, which (as of this date) is not part of the Medicare program. There are multiple groups (stakeholders) trying to influence members of Congress to either expand coverage (because of the high cost of long-term care) or limit coverage (because it will cost employers more). The elderly want expanded coverage; health plans, who pay part of the cost, want to limit coverage. The influence they exert to support their position reflects the politics of the policy process.

Public policy has significant impact on the practice of nursing. The ability of the individual nurse to provide care is affected by innumerable public policy decisions. Yet too few nurses are aware of the importance of their role in influencing such policy outcomes, because they miss the connection between their own practice and the world of public policy.

As discussed in Chapter 20, state licensure of a registered nurse (RN) derives from legislation that defines the scope of nursing practice. The defined scope determines what a nurse legally can and cannot do. For example, giving intravenous medication and performing physical assessments are now accepted as actions within the scope of nursing practice. Thirty years ago, such activities were within the scope of the medical practice act rather than the nursing practice act. As a result of changes in education and clinical practice, nursing influenced legislators to change state nurse practice acts to reflect what nurses were qualified to do (Box 21-1).

Regulations that are developed to implement legislation also affect practicing nurses and their work environments. For example, the rules for administering and documenting the administration of narcotic drugs are promulgated by a regulatory agency of the federal government, the Federal Drug Administration, under the Department of Health and Human Services. The way in which such regulations are written can greatly affect nurses' ability to practice. If nurses do not actively participate in developing regulations, policy outcomes are likely to restrict rather than enhance nursing authority for regulated activities.

Box **21-1** Politics Gone Wrong: A Painful Lesson for Nurses

An unfortunate event that dramatically illustrates how politics can influence policy occurred in the state of North Dakota in 2003. For about 15 years, North Dakota was the only state requiring the baccalaureate degree as the minimum educational requirement for registered nurse licensure. When a group of well-intentioned nurses attempted to get the oversight of nursing education moved from the Board of Nursing's jurisdiction to the Board of Higher Education's jurisdiction, those opposed to the mandatory BSN lobbied hard for a reversal. Community colleges were opposed to the BSN and representatives of long-term care agencies, long opposed to the BSN requirement, testified that they "needed the economic benefit that would result from having a lesser-educated nursing work force" (Mooney, 2003, p. 9). Unfortunately, nurses were divided and testified on both sides, confusing legislators. "Opponents to higher standards for nursing education used the dissent in the ranks of nurses to fuel their agenda and achieve their goals" (Mooney, p. 9).

As a result, the bill that ultimately passed and was signed into law removed the requirement for the baccalaureate degree, among other provisions. North Dakota's strong history of support for nursing education and high-quality health care ended with a very painful lesson for the nurses of the state and the rest of the nation lost a role model. Those with vested interests aligned against a divided nursing profession—and nursing lost. According to a professor at the North Dakota State University Department of Nursing, nurses must "strengthen the bonds of trust among ourselves, disagree without being disagreeable, discern which fights to keep in the family and which to advance to the public forum, and hone the political and negotiation skills of our future leaders" (Mooney, p. 9).

From Mooney MM: Hog-housed! *Reflect Nurs Leadersh* 29(4):8-9, 2003.

Another example involves advanced practice nurses, such as nurse practitioners, and certified registered nurse anesthetists (CRNA), who have been working hard at both state and federal levels against rules that have restricted their reimbursement. A November 2001 federal ruling from the Centers for Medicare and Medicaid Services (CMS) requires that CRNAs must practice under the "supervision" of a surgeon or anesthesiologist in order to receive Medicare reimbursement. This change limits what many states had previously allowed nurses to do—practice "collaboratively" rather than "under the supervision of." CRNAs are working with governors in each state to get an exception (known as an "opt-out") and enable previous state laws to take precedence (American Association of Nurse Anesthetists, 2001). Without such political involvement, CRNAs will have their practices, and their reimbursement, restricted.

Broader issues affecting the nursing profession are also political in nature. Issues of **pay equity,** or equal pay for work of comparable value are of concern to nurses, because they have historically been underpaid for their services. One of the earliest cases demonstrating the inequality of nursing salaries involved public health nurses in Colorado. They brought a case against the city of Denver, stating that they were paid considerably less than city tree trimmers and garbage collectors. The nurses demanded just compensation for their work by demonstrating that nursing requires more complex knowledge and is of greater value to society than these other occupations.

As a result of this suit, recognition of nursing's low pay was brought to public attention; this in turn mobilized public support for increasing nursing salaries. This is an example of political action by nurses that resulted in both **policy outcomes** (regulations that expanded comparable pay issues to other jobs) and **professional outcomes** (salary increases for the individual nurse). More recently, the nursing shortage has caused concern amongst the public that the number of nurses available to provide care in hospitals and other agencies is inadequate. Nurses in California mobilized the public and other constituency groups to get the first legislation requiring specific nurse-to-patient ratios passed in 1999. Other states are expected to follow suit.

"The Personal Is Political"

Women involved in the feminist movement in the 1960s coined the phrase "The personal is political." This statement recognized that each individual—woman or man—could use personal experience to understand and become involved in broader social and political issues. This concept enabled individuals who did not consider themselves political to gain insight into what needed to be changed in society and how they could help bring about the change. It gave power to each individual and resulted in people becoming involved in the political process—usually for the first time.

This premise of personalizing the political process has become a fundamental activity for organized nursing. Nurses at the grassroots level become involved in advocating for legislation and supporting candidates for elective office because they understand the relationship between public policy and their professional and personal lives. The American Nurses Association (ANA) is actively involved in federal legislation, regulation, and electoral politics. The ANA and many of its Constituent Member Associations (CMAs) have government relations experts on staff who analyze policy and lobby policymakers. In fact most health organizations, such as the American Association of Colleges of Nursing, the American Hospital

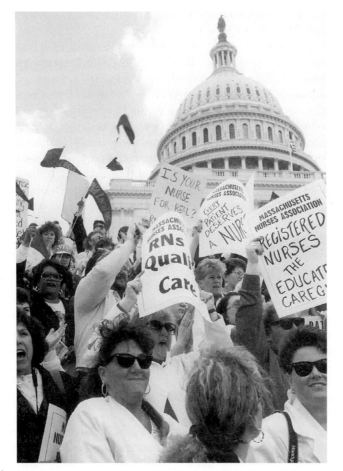

Figure **21-1**
Nurses gathered on the grounds of the Capitol building in Washington, D.C., for the historic
Nurses' March on Washington—March 25, 1995. Issuing a wake-up call to consumers and
lawmakers, the 25,000 nurses rallied and marched through Washington in a display of nursing
unity. (Courtesy the American Nurses Association.)

Association, and numerous specialty nursing organizations engage in lobbying to
advocate for the professional concerns of their members (Figure 21-1). Contemporary
nursing leaders recognize that "being political," both through professional associations and as individuals, is a professional responsibility essential to the practice and
promotion of the nursing profession.

POLITICS AND POWER

Politics connotes power. **Power** is the ability to make something happen. Without
power, there cannot be influence. To be effective in influencing the outcome of

decisions, an individual must ask, "Who has the power?" "How is it used?" "How can it be mobilized?"

There are different types of power. **Position power** is that which is inherent in a position such as that belonging to a dean, vice-president for nursing, or chief executive of a company. **Expert power** comes from the knowledge a person has that can influence an outcome. Nurses have expert power because of their knowledge about health care. There is power in numbers; a group is almost always more influential than an individual. There is power related to wealth. Wealth itself is a resource and provides access to other significant resources. Also, there has always been power accorded to whoever belongs to the dominant race, gender, or class in a community or nation.

Latent power is power that is untapped and underused. As the largest group of health care providers, nurses have had latent power. Although there are more than 2.7 million nurses in the United States, nurses are only recently recognizing the potential power that such numbers suggest. Of all women voters in the United States, 1 in 44 is a nurse. Imagine how influential nursing could be if that power were used collectively. Nurses could be pivotal in getting laws passed to improve health care and getting policymakers elected to office who would support nursing's agenda. The power of nursing knowledge has also been underused. No other group of health care providers spends as much time as nurses in direct patient contact. Nurses know what patients need, and they can use this knowledge to develop workplace and community policies. More nurses than ever are using their expertise to participate in the development of health policy, by sharing knowledge with legislators and regulators. In addition, they are using nursing research to substantiate the need for public policies that have been shown to affect positive health outcomes and provide needed public health services.

Power, like politics, is neither good nor bad; how it is used gives it value. If, for example, nurses use the power of persuasion to motivate patients to take prescribed medication, they are using the power of position and knowledge positively.

Power is not given; it must be taken. The taking of power converts latent power into action. Nurses are beginning to recognize that to have power they must want it, and they must use it. Use of power is a hallmark of political activity.

There are differences in the way women and men have traditionally used power. The traditional male model of power has been described as **power grabbing.** It involves hoarding power and control, taking it from others, or wielding it over others. Women more often use **power sharing,** which is a process of equalizing resources, knowledge, or control. Again, it is important to recognize that these two ways of using power are neither good nor bad. The most effective power brokers are those who can use both methods and know which is most effective in a given situation.

The Power of the Media

The Woodhull Study on Nursing and the Media (Sigma Theta Tau, 1997), described in Chapter 3, analyzed more than 2,000 health-related articles from 16 major news publications. Recognizing that communication media are the most effective ways in which to send a message to a large audience, this study recommended that the nursing profession be proactive in promoting and establishing ongoing dialogue with representatives of these media. Effective utilization of media is a powerful political tool for influencing both the public and those who hold elective offices (Sigma Theta Tau, 1997). The *American Journal of Nursing* has the largest circulation of any health professional journal in the world. Many of their research articles are picked up in the national press. Such media coverage is critical for nurses' expertise to be recognized by the public and ultimately by the policymakers who make the laws and regulations that affect nursing practice.

Different media provide different ways to influence opinions. For example, talk radio has proven to be very influential. Talk radio hosts advocate certain opinions, often with little factual information. By controlling who gets to talk, these radio hosts can control the kind of information and the values expressed by callers and eliminate those that are in opposition to the host. Prior to the 1994 elections, when the Republican Party took control of both houses of Congress, the majority of talk radio supported the Republican agenda. It is believed that their collective messages influenced the outcomes of the elections. More recently, the Internet has become a powerful medium to generate support for political candidates. Howard Dean mobilized his campaign as a Democratic presidential candidate in 2003 largely through donations and information from his website. In fact, most candidates for state and federal offices have websites to garner financial contributions as well as to mobilize voters.

Television can be a forceful medium for visual influence, particularly political advertisements. In 1994, the demise of President Clinton's national health care reform efforts was directly affected by television ads sponsored by the health insurance industry. Despite initial support for national health care reform by Fortune 500 companies, health professional organizations, and major industries, the "Harry and Louise" advertisements were forceful enough to create a climate of fear and distrust about legislating health care. The power of those ads was partially credited with the defeat of federal health care legislation.

The print media are also effective in disclosing information about health issues. For example, the nursing shortage became major news in 1999 when numerous articles about the absence of qualified nurses appeared in major newspapers throughout the country. The public grew alarmed by inadequate nurse staffing in hospitals and other facilities and wanted policymakers and others to ensure that there would be a qualified and adequate workforce. Both the private and public sectors responded with ad campaigns and public funding to recruit more people into nursing. Johnson & Johnson, the giant health care company, gave over $25 million in public service announcements and created community coalitions to sponsor nursing scholarships *(www.discovernursing.com)*. State legislatures allocated increased funding for nursing scholarships and loan repayment programs, and the federal government passed legislation, the Nurse Reinvestment Act, to increase funding for baccalaureate and graduate education. The media response, as well as a downturn in the economy, resulted in a significant increase in applicants to nursing programs. Through support of private foundations, such as the Robert Wood Johnson Foundation and funding from state legislatures, many states established centers to study workforce issues and collect data about workforce needs. The media was a significant factor in getting legislators to support the efforts. The power of the media affects both legislators and the public. It is a tool that nurses must use to affect public policy.

A LESSON IN CIVICS COMES ALIVE

It is essential that nurses and other health professionals clearly understand how government works before they can successfully influence the process. Americans have the greatest system of democracy in the world; yet too few appreciate how vital it is to participate. In the last decade, less than 50 percent of registered voters participated in presidential elections.

The importance of how one vote can make a difference in the outcome of a presidential race was made clear in the 1996 and 2000 presidential elections. In 1996 President Bill Clinton won only 49 percent of the popular vote but won a majority of the electoral votes. The 2000 presidential election between Republican George W. Bush and Democrat Albert Gore, Jr., resulted in the closest and most bizarre vote count in the country. Although Democrat Al Gore won the popular vote with 50,996,582 votes over the Republican Bush's 50,456,062, that was not the final say in who won the election. After the Democrats charged that votes were undercounted and miscounted (the so-called "hanging chads" in Florida), the case went to the Florida Supreme Court, which ordered a recount of undercounted districts (Posner, 2001). However, the U.S. Supreme Court reversed the decision and refused to allow any recounts. As a result, Republican George Bush was declared the winner in Florida by 537 votes out of 6 million cast. The election was not decided until January 6, 2001, when the Electoral College votes were officially counted and Bush and Cheney were declared the winners with 271 votes compared with 267 for Gore and Leiberman (Eagleton Institute of Politics, 2000).

Imagine if you were one of the people who did not vote in Florida. Think how much your vote might have changed the outcome of the electoral votes and thus the outcome of the Presidential election. Who says one vote doesn't count?

Three Branches of Government

The framers of the U.S. Constitution had a major objective—the **separation of powers**—to prevent the aggregation of power in any one person or branch of government. Thus they set up a government with three branches—legislative, executive, and judicial—along with a mechanism of checks and balances for each. As intended by the founding fathers, U.S. history reveals a waxing and waning of the powers of each branch, depending on the personalities of incumbents, contemporary social problems, and world events.

Under the Constitution, each branch of the federal government has separate and distinct functions and powers. The function of the **legislative branch,** which includes the House of Representatives and the Senate, is to deliberate and enact laws. Examples of legislative powers include setting and collecting taxes, overseeing commerce, declaring war, defining criminal offenses, coining money, and amending the Constitution. The legislative branch, particularly the House of Representatives, is assumed to be the government's closest link to the people and more susceptible to change through social pressure (see Figure 20-1 on p. 552).

The chief function of the **executive branch** of government is to administer the laws of the land. At the federal level, power is vested with the president, who has a wide variety of governmental departments (the Cabinet) and employees (the bureaucracy) to carry out executive functions. The president has extensive **powers of appointment** (judges, ambassadors, agency heads) and is commander-in-chief of the armed forces. The president recommends legislation, gives the State of the Union report, and approves or vetoes the legislation of Congress, contributing to the **balance of power.**

The role of the **judicial branch** is to adjudicate, or decide, "cases or controversies" of particular matters. The judicial branch is divided into the federal and state court systems. The greatest power of the courts is to provide judicial review over governmental activities to uphold the privileges of the Constitution. The Supreme Court is the ultimate legal authority of the land and reviews decisions from lower courts.

The balance of power among the three branches of government is illustrated in Figure 21-2. Notice that all three branches are involved in the legislative process.

Three Levels of Government

Government in the United States is organized at federal, state, and local levels. The Constitution established the relative powers of federal and state governments and the rights of the individual. The Constitution identified specific powers of the federal government as matters of national interest needing uniform policies and reserved all other powers for the states. States, in turn, have developed their own constitutions and delineated power relationships with local communities and between branches of state government.

Exclusive powers of the federal government include declaring war, making treaties, administering public health services, and developing relationships with foreign powers. State and local governments maintain internal order, regulate domestic relationships, and protect the people. Currently, both the federal and the state governments can tax and spend and promote health. In times of shrinking resources, programs that are considered to be costly, such as health services, may be shifted to state control, calling into question the federal government's role in ensuring uniform access to health services throughout the United States.

All levels of government are expected to maintain their activities within the parameters of the Constitution. The Bill of Rights serves to promote and protect the rights of the individual from governmental intrusion.

Electoral Process

The process of electing public officials to office is known as the **electoral process.** Governmental elections for the most part focus on selecting local, state, and federal legislators and executive branch leaders such as the president, governor, and mayor. Federal judges are appointed, although in some states, the people elect judges.

In recent elections the American public appeared to be skeptical of politicians, the traditional political parties, and the entire electoral process. This was clearly shown in 1992 when Ross Perot of the United We Stand America Party (subsequently The Reform Party) received 19 percent of the votes cast for president. This was the highest percentage received by an independent or third-party candidate since the

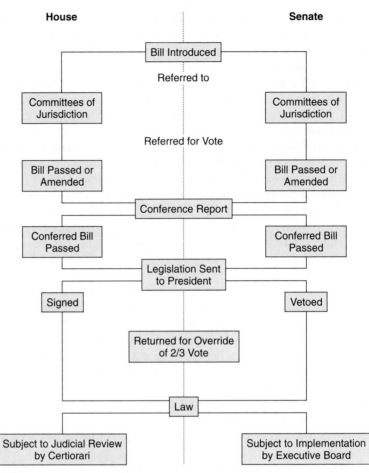

Figure 21-2

This flow chart shows how a bill progresses through the legislative process to become a law. Notice that both sides of Congress (the House of Representatives and the Senate) and the executive branch (the President) are involved and that laws are subject to judicial review. We call this involvement of all three branches of government the "balance of power."

early 1900s (Congressional Quarterly, 1993). In the 2000 presidential election the third-party candidate, Ralph Nader, received 2.7 percent of the vote (Presidential Race, 2000), because it was such a close presidential vote, many people saw the third party candidate as a spoiler. Others thought it was a message to long-term politicians and the traditional parties that they were not in touch with voters outside Washington, D.C.

During the 1994 election, members of third parties, such as United We Stand America, not only affected the outcome of the elections but also shaped the issues that were discussed as part of a "change agenda." Up until this point, the process of getting elected to office had occurred primarily through the two major parties—the Democratic and Republican parties. Third parties have become active in different regions at different times. Besides the Reform Party (formerly United We Stand America), some of the more familiar third parties are the Right to Life, Conservative, Green, Socialist, Communist, and Rainbow Coalition parties. At the state level in 1994, a third-party organization, the Reform Party, was successful. Their candidate, former professional wrestler Jesse Ventura, won a gubernatorial campaign in Minnesota in 1998 with a voter turnout of 61 percent. However, Ventura served only one term, primarily because he lost the support of the public.

In most states until recently, citizens declared a party affiliation when they registered to vote. This has begun to change, however, and fewer states are requiring people to declare a party affiliation when registering. Registered voters may participate in three major types of elections: primary and general elections and referendums.

Primary elections are those in which a party is choosing among several party-affiliated candidates for a particular office. The outcome of primary elections is the selection of a party's candidate for a particular office. Voters may vote only in the primary of the party in which they are registered. For those states that do not require a party designation, voters can choose which party's primary ticket to support. There is no obligation to vote for the same party in the next primary election.

In **general elections,** all registered voters may vote. They are not required to vote a "straight party ticket"—that is, the voter can choose a candidate from any party on the ballot. Unless there is a tie or a challenge to the general election, the outcome of the general election is usually the candidate with the highest number of votes. However, some states require a majority for elected office and may have a run-off between the two highest vote getters if a majority is not achieved. Length of service as an elected official depends on the office. For example, U.S. senators serve 6-year terms, and members of the House of Representatives serve 2-year terms; most governors and state legislators serve 4-year terms.

A **referendum** occurs when registered voters are asked to express directly their preferences on a policy issue. Usually, these issues are referred to the public either by a legislative body or by civic activists who have gathered enough signatures to require a vote. For example, a county commission may seek a referendum on raising property taxes to support school reform. Activist groups may seek a state referendum on gay rights, assisted suicide, or other controversial issues. The 2003 recall election of Governor Gray Davis of California occurred because of a referendum to oust him for his unpopular fiscal and energy policies.

Working on a campaign, raising money for a candidate, and running for office require strict adherence to election laws. Rules vary from locality to locality and from state to federal elections. In recent years, Congress has passed legislation to tighten rules for individuals, businesses, labor unions, organizations and political action committees (PACs) to fund candidates running for office. Running for election is a very expensive process. The different election laws for local, state and federal elections require candidates to file financial reports indicating how much money they receive and spend for elections. The purpose is to prevent any one individual or organization from "buying" an election and to inject fairness for all candidates. As new fundraising ideas emerge in response to election reform, so too does the creative response of political fundraisers to test new approaches.

Information about election regulations can be accessed in each state through the Secretary of State and for federal elections through the Federal Election Commission.

HEALTH CARE LEGISLATION AND REGULATION

Many issues facing nursing professionals can best be addressed through public policy, which requires that nurses influence government. The key questions for nurses to ask when seeking governmental intervention to improve nursing practice and health care are "Where can we play?" and "Where can we win?" The options to consider are the judicial, regulatory, or legislative arenas.

There are local, state, and federal courts, all of which require standing (a material interest in the outcome of a case) to seek a judicial remedy. In the executive branch there are mayors, governors, presidents, and their staffs and department heads who make key decisions about how to implement (or not implement) rules and regulations. Most often, nurses have focused on legislative remedies to change health policy and have learned to be effective with legislative branch relationships. The nursing profession has now broadened its focus to use the regulatory and the judicial branches more effectively.

There have been three major eras in health policy development in the United States. As you learned in Chapter 16, the era extending from post-World War II through the 1960s served to increase health services dramatically and expand health delivery capacity. The 1970s and 1980s focused on enhanced research, technology development, and concerns about escalating costs in acute care. During the 1990s, several different issues were predominant, including comprehensive health care reform addressing access, cost, and quality of health care. When attempts at comprehensive reform were unsuccessful, a dramatic restructuring of the health care payment and delivery systems to decrease aggregate health care costs followed. Between 2000 and 2003 the focus continued to be on stemming rising costs, as well as attempts to make the private sector the arena for health policy change. For example, the rise in the cost of health insurance for employers has led employers to decrease their share of the cost and increase the cost to the employee. This is true even for public programs like Medicaid and Medicare. The result has been a rapid rise in the number of those without insurance, from 38 million in 1999 to over 41 million by 2003 (Issue Spotlight, 2003).

Unfortunately, the nursing profession was not well organized politically during the time of expanding health care capacity and access in the early 1960's. Despite being the only health provider group in favor of the Medicare/Medicaid programs in the 1960s, nurses were not included as reimbursable providers. Times have changed. Nurses have increased their political savvy. Through the well-orchestrated efforts of the ANA, other professional organizations, constituent member associations, and **political action committees (PACs),** nurses are now participating much more effectively in both governmental and electoral politics. Nursing PACs raise and distribute money to candidates who support the organization's stand on certain issues. Nurses' endorsements of candidates have become a valued political asset for many local, state, and federal candidates.

Influencing Public Policy

Nurses can make a difference in health policy outcomes. Through the political process, nurses influence policy by identifying health problems as policy problems, by formulating policy through drafting legislation with legislators and providing formal testimony, by lobbying governmental officials in the executive and legislative branches to make certain health policies a priority for action, and by filing suit as a party or as a *friend of the court* to implement health policy strategies on behalf of consumers.

Capitol Update, an online newsletter published by the ANA, reports on the progress of nursing influence with the president, members of Congress and their staffs, and the regulatory agencies that set policy for health programs *(www.capitolupdate.org/newsletter/).* Such activity reflects the work of both ANA members and staff. The ANA's political activity in Washington, D.C., is mirrored throughout the United States by other nursing organizations and by ANA constituent member associations conducting similar work with their state governments.

Nurses Strategic Action Teams (N-STAT) is ANA's grassroots network of nurses from across the country who keep elected representatives in Congress informed about issues of concern to patients and nurses. By notifying members of the network, ANA can mobilize nurses to lobby their federal representatives to support or oppose particular legislation and/or rules and regulations. Through the use of telephones, fax, email and regular mail, NSTAT members can respond by sending well-timed, well-targeted messages to members of Congress.

Organized activity in identifying, financially supporting, and working for candidates who are committed to nursing and "nurse-friendly" issues has dramatically increased since the early 1990s. The electoral process is an essential function of the professional association. No better example of the interrelationship of nursing, public policy, and political action exists than the 1992 presidential election and its aftermath. In August 1992, the ANA-PAC endorsed the Clinton/Gore ticket at a nationally televised rally in California. Thousands of nurses were present along with patients and their families. The ANA became the first national health care organization to support Clinton's candidacy publicly, and nurses throughout the United States worked visibly and diligently during the campaign.

That early and visible political support meant that nursing enjoyed unprecedented access to the White House during the Clinton/Gore administration. Nurses were involved significantly in the development of the president's Health Security Act of 1993, and nurses were included as qualified providers in that historic federal proposal. Despite the failure of the 103rd Congress to pass comprehensive health reform legislation in 1994, nursing achieved visibility, influence, and inclusion as a force in national health policy. As nursing united through the development of Nursing's Agenda for Health Care Reform, the latent power of nursing became evident to the public, to policymakers, and to nurses themselves. Nursing has continued to exert national influence through the American Nurses Association, specialty organizations, and labor unions. The Nurse Reinvestment Act, passed in 2002, was the culmination of work by many national organizations and individual nurses who lobbied for the federal legislation to ease the nursing shortage (Figure 21-3).

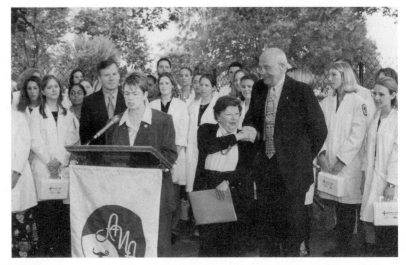

Figure **21-3**
A press conference was held during National Nurses Week, May 7, 2002, to announce the passage of the Nurse Reinvestment Act. Pictured are ANA past president Mary Foley, Senator Tim Hutchinson (R-AK), Senator Barbara Mikulski (R-MD), and Senator John D. Dingell (D-MI, 16th). (Courtesy American Nurses Association.)

The legislation provides loan repayment programs and scholarships for nursing students, public service announcements to encourage people to enter nursing, grants to schools to encourage nurses to enter gerontology, and repayment of loans for nurses to pursue careers in teaching.

Nurses working at the state level are also making their presence felt. In 2003 there were 79 nurses elected to state legislatures. Many hold important positions as leaders on health policy issues. For instance, Judy Robson is Chair of the Senate Health Committee in Wisconsin, and Paula Hollinger is Chair of the Health Committee in the Maryland Senate. In their leadership roles they have been critical in passing legislation around such issues as prohibiting mandatory overtime and authorizing nurse practitioners and clinical nurse specialists to prescribe medications.

Individual nurses can make a difference in policy development and elections. Either by election or by appointment, nurses need to be *making* health policy decisions, not just influencing them. Getting elected or appointed requires visibility, expertise, energy, risk taking, and a belief that policy and politics are critically important in achieving nursing's goals.

Getting Nurses Appointed

How does one get appointed to a powerful position in government? The chief executive of a city, county, state, or the nation makes appointments. Such appointments are to regulatory agencies, such as a state Board of Nursing, or to specific taskforces or committees focused on particular health issues. Appointments are usually the result of the expertise and visibility of the individual appointee and of the power and influence of that appointee's membership in an organization that supported the elected official.

Nurses at the national level have been appointed to a variety of significant national policymaking positions, often because of ANA's federal appointment project. To get appointed, a nurse needs to be known to organizations with considerable political influence. Because ANA worked intensively to help get President Clinton elected, there were more nurses appointed to office during his administration than in any previous administration. For example, during the Clinton/Gore administration's first term, Dr. Kristine Gebbie was appointed as the first national AIDS policy coordinator, Dr. Shirley Chater was appointed as director of the Social Security Administration, and Pat Montoya and Pat Ford-Roegner became regional directors of the Department of Health and Human Services.

In the 1996 election, ANA-PAC again endorsed the Clinton/Gore ticket and continued a close working relationship on health care and health care workplace safety. During President Clinton's second term Dr. Beverly Malone, ANA president from 1996 to 2000, and Marta Prado were appointed to the President's Advisory Commission on Consumer Protection and Quality in the Health Care Industry (1998), from which the Patient's Bill of Rights concept was developed; Dr. Mary Wakefield was also appointed to the Advisory Commission, as well as to the Medicare Payment Advisory Commission; and Catherine Dodd was appointed regional director of the Department of Health and Human Services. In 1998, the role of senior advisor on nursing and policy to the Secretary and Assistant Secretary was created within the Department of Health and Human Services. Virginia Trotter Betts, ANA president from 1992 to 1996, was the first to be appointed to this key position. The political activism of these nurses, along with the support of ANA and other national organizations, helped secure these and other important federal appointments of nurses.

During the administration of President George W. Bush, there have been few nurses appointed. One exception was the appointment of three nurses to the Federal Advisory Committee on Regulatory Reform for the Center on Medicare and Medicaid Services (CMS). The three, Karen Utterback, an executive in home health, Judith Ryan, an executive in long-term care, and Patricia Shafer, active in advocacy organizations, had all been very active in ANA or in their constituent member associations and thus were known to ANA, who endorsed their appointments.

The same process for appointments occurs at the state level. The governor makes appointments to many boards, commissions, and key government positions. Thus, gubernatorial elections are of critical importance to constituent member (state) associations. Qualified nurses who have supported the election of the governor and are known to their constituent member association are encouraged to seek appointments to regulatory bodies such as state boards of nursing. As previously discussed, state boards of nursing, through rules and regulations, make definitive health policy and are highly important to issues related to nursing practice. For most nurses, appointments at the state level are more attainable than national posts. It is vital that the executive director of the state organization knows the nurse, since they are often consulted in the appointment process.

GETTING INVOLVED

To get involved, a nurse must begin to understand the connections between individual practice and public policy. Once that happens, it is easy to get started. Three levels of political involvement in which nurses can participate are as nurse citizens, nurse activists, and nurse politicians.

Nurse Citizens

A **nurse citizen** brings the perspective of health care to the voting booth, to public forums that advocate for health and human services, and to involvement in community activities. For example, budget cuts to a school district might involve elimination of school nurses. At a school board meeting, nurses can effectively speak about the vital services that school nurses provide to children and the cost-effectiveness of maintaining the position.

Nurses tend to vote for candidates who advocate for improved health care. Here are some examples of how the nurse citizen can be politically active:
- Register to vote.
- Vote in every election.
- Keep informed about health care issues.
- Speak out when services or working conditions are inadequate.
- Participate in public forums.
- Know your local, state, and federal elected officials.
- Join politically active nursing organizations.
- Participate in community organizations that need health experts.
- Join a political party.

Once nurses make a decision to become involved politically, they need to learn how to get started. One of the best ways is to form a relationship with one or more policymakers. Box 21-2 contains several pointers for influencing policymakers.

Nurse Activists

The **nurse activist** takes a more active role than the nurse citizen and often does so because an issue arises that directly affects the nurse's professional life (Figure 21-4). The need to respond moves the nurse to a higher level of participation. For example, a nurse in private practice who has difficulty getting insurance companies to honor patients' claims for reimbursement of nursing services may become active in lobbying state legislators for changes in insurance regulations.

Nurse activists can make changes by:
- Joining politically active nursing organizations.
- Contacting a public official through letters, emails, or phone calls.
- Registering people to vote.
- Contributing money to a political campaign.
- Working in a campaign.
- Lobbying decision makers by providing pertinent statistical and anecdotal information.
- Forming or joining coalitions that support an issue of concern.
- Writing letters to the editor of local newspapers.

Box **21-2** **Communication Is the Key to Influence**

Cultivate a relationship with policymakers from your home district or state.
Communicate by visits, telephone, email, and letters. Letters need these elements:
- Use personal stationery.
- State who you are (a nursing student or registered nurse and a voter in a specific district).
- Identify the issue by a file number, if possible.
- Be clear on where you stand and why.
- Be positive when possible.
- Be concise.
- Ask for a commitment. State precisely what action you want the policymaker to take.
- Give your return address, email address, and phone number to urge dialogue.
- Be persistent. Follow up with calls or letters.
- If you plan to visit your policymaker on a specific issue, be sure to make your appointment in advance in writing and indicate what issue you are interested in discussing.
- Be quick to thank and praise policymakers when they do something you like.

- Inviting legislators to visit the workplace.
- Holding a media event to publicize an issue.
- Providing or giving testimony to legislators and regulatory bodies.

Box 21-3 on p. 597 includes some pointers on how to make a difference in health policy development.

Nurse Politicians

Once a nurse realizes and experiences the empowerment that can come from political activism, he or she may choose to run for office. No longer satisfied to help others get elected, the **nurse politician** desires to develop the legislation, not just influence it.

As of 2003, there are three nurses serving in Congress. In 1992, Congresswoman Eddie Bernice Johnson (D-TX) was the first nurse elected to the U.S. House of Representatives. She has been repeatedly reelected since. The second nurse, Carolyn McCarthy (D-NY), an LPN, was elected in 1996 as a result of her stance on gun control. Her husband was killed, and her son critically injured after a lone gunman with a 9-mm semiautomatic pistol walked through a train on the Long Island Railroad and killed 25 people and wounded 19 others. Carolyn was suddenly thrown into the national spotlight when she challenged the incumbent congressman, running for office, on his stand supporting a repeal on a ban for assault rifles. Her ability to speak passionately about the issue led to her campaign against the incumbent and her election to his seat. She has been a leader in the House of Representatives on gun control, as well as on nursing issues (Mason, Leavitt, Chaffee, 2002). In 1998, Congresswoman Lois Capps (D-CA) became the third nurse to be elected to the

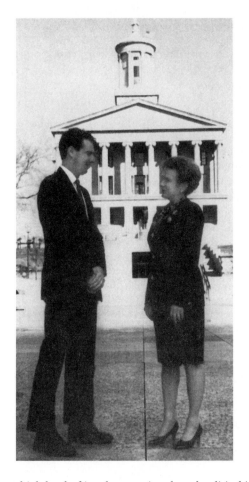

Figure **21-4**
This nurse activist has a high level of involvement in selected political issues. Here she visits with one of her state legislators at the state capitol. (Courtesy Tennessee Nurses Association. Photograph by Chip Powell).

House of Representatives. Congresswoman Capps was a long-time leader in health care and a school nurse. After her election to Congress, she drew on her extensive health care background to co-chair the House Democratic Task Force on Medicare Reform, and in 2003, she founded the Bipartisan Congressional Caucus on Nursing and the Bipartisan School Health and Safety Caucus.

The success and respect garnered by these three nurses as leaders on health care has encouraged other nurses to run for national office. In 2003, there were 79 nurse legislators elected to state legislatures, numerous nurses elected as local mayors and city council members, and hundreds of nurses appointed to governmental regulatory agencies.

Nurse politicians use their knowledge about people, their expertise about health, their ability to communicate effectively, and their superb organizational skills in

Box 21-3 **Key Questions for Nurses Who Want to Make a Difference in Health Policy**

1. Know the system. Is it a federal, state, or local issue? Is it in the hands of the executive, legislative, or judicial branch of government?
2. Know the issue. What is wrong? What should happen? Why is it not happening? What is needed: leadership, a plan, pressure, or data?
3. Know the players. Who is on your side, and who is not? Who will make the decision? Who knows whom? Will a coalition be effective? Are you a member of the professional nursing organization?
4. Know the process. Is this a vote? Is this an appropriation? Is this a legislative procedure? Is this a committee or subcommittee report?
5. Know what to do. Should you write, call, arrange a lunch meeting, organize a petition, show up at the hearing, give testimony, demonstrate, or file a suit?

running for office. Because the public places a high value on nurses, nurse politicians tend to be trusted. If nurses know how to run a campaign and can raise money, they stand a good chance of being elected.

Once nurses are elected, they can sponsor legislation that reflects their professional experiences. Many of the laws that expand reimbursement for nursing services, funding for services to women and children, occupational safety and health issues, and research on women's health have been sponsored by nurse legislators and supported by nurses working as key legislative staff members.

Political life can be grueling, and the nurse politician must be ready to sacrifice a regular schedule and personal privacy. In addition, adequate financial resources are critical to a successful campaign for office. Fortunately, more nurses are willing to make this commitment because they believe in their own power and ability to enhance the well-being of the public. Individual nurses and nurse-specific PACs are increasingly willing and able to support nurse candidates financially at all levels of government.

The nurse politician can:

- Run for an elected office.
- Seek appointment to a regulatory agency.
- Be appointed to a governing board in the public or private sector.
- Use nursing expertise as a front-line policymaker who can enhance health care and the profession.

WE WERE ALL ONCE NOVICES

In general, nurses who have achieved success as leaders started with no knowledge of the political process and no expectations of the greatness they would achieve. Instead, they became involved because some issue, injustice, or abuse of power affected their lives. Instead of complaining or feeling helpless, they responded by taking an active role in bringing about change.

The mark of a leader is the ability to identify a problem, have a goal, and know how to join others in reaching that goal. A leader must ask the right questions, analyze the positive and restraining forces toward meeting the goal, and know how to obtain and use power. A leader must know how to ask for help and how to give support to those who join the effort. These are the marks of nursing leaders who have been political experts.

A NURSE WHO KNEW HOW TO USE POLITICAL POWER

As discussed in Chapter 1, Florence Nightingale, the founder of modern nursing, was the consummate political woman. Her story tells how she learned to use her skills and power to bring about revolutionary change in health care in the nineteenth century. She never anticipated that she would achieve greatness, especially as a nurse—a lifestyle Victorian society considered demeaning to a woman of her social standing.

Nightingale achieved incredible achievements through her own intellect and determination and the use of the political influence of powerful friends in government. She was a strong-willed person with social and financial power. She had an excellent education and used theoretical knowledge, as well as practical experience, to learn about care of the sick. She developed and nurtured connections to powerful men (since there were few powerful women at the time other than Queen Victoria). She sought their support and, in turn, supported them when they needed her help.

Nightingale's goals changed as new problems arose because she recognized that being adaptable was a characteristic of leadership. In essence, she used her public support, her connections to people in powerful positions, and her intellectual skills to reach an unparalleled position of leadership. As a result, she was able to gain personal and professional power to move nursing and health care into the modern era. Thus Nightingale was the first nurse politician.

NURSING AWAITS YOUR CONTRIBUTION

You can apply the skills discussed in this chapter. Look to teachers, family, friends, and community leaders whom you admire. What are the qualities they possess that you wish to have? These individuals can offer inspiration and serve as role models for you to imitate.

You may also choose to form a relationship with a political mentor. A mentor not only serves as a role model but also actively teaches, encourages, and critiques the process of growth and change in the learner. All nurses who have become political leaders have found mentors along the way to guide and support their growth. Your mentor could be a faculty member, such as the adviser to the nursing student organization or honor society, who can teach you leadership skills. Ask for help in running for a class office or student council president. If elected office does not appeal to you, use your political skills to develop a school or community project with other nursing students.

You may have a relative or friend involved in a political campaign who could help you learn about the political process. You might find a problem during a clinical experience that inhibits your ability to provide necessary care or the level of care that you wish to provide. Seek a faculty member or nurse in a clinical facility who can guide you through the process of change.

Watch the communication skills of your role models or mentors. How does your own behavior compare with theirs? What enhances or impedes your progress? Get your friends and peers to join your activity. Seek their help and support. Always thank them and be ready to offer your help and support when they need it.

Summary of Key Points

- Professional organizations and professional nurses have much to offer in formulating policy decisions at federal, state, and local levels and in each branch of government.
- Nursing, once called "the sleeping giant of the health care industry," has awakened.
- Today, organized nursing is involved in politics at many levels in promoting (1) the principles for comprehensive health reform; (2) reimbursement for professional nurses at federal, state, and local levels and through all reimbursement mechanisms; (3) expanding the scope and authority of nursing practice in every jurisdiction; (4) protection of the civil and privacy rights of patients—for example, in the areas of reproductive rights, human immunodeficiency virus/acquired immunodeficiency syndrome (HIV/AIDS), and terminal illness; (5) prevention services and primary care services for women, children, and the elderly; and (6) a federally mandated bill to provide quality care and safe staffing ratios.
- Roles and opportunities for nurses in the field of policy development and politics are changing, and nursing can benefit from this "window of opportunity."
- Becoming politically active is as easy as signing your name in support of an issue, registering to vote, organizing a project, or speaking out on an issue.
- Political involvement is empowering; one person *can* make a difference.
- The involvement of nurses in the political process benefits nurses, the nursing profession, and the recipients of health care.

CRITICAL THINKING QUESTIONS

1. Conduct a class poll. Of those in the class who are eligible to vote, how many are registered? How many voted in the last local, state, or national election? Challenge those not registered to become registered before the end of the current school term.
2. List three types of power. How can nurses use these types of power on behalf of their profession and the health care system?
3. Because nurses have differing personal and political values, it has been a challenge to get them all united behind a single issue or candidate. If you were the president of the American Nurses Association, what techniques would you use to convince the 2.7 million American nurses to use the power of their numbers, their knowledge, and their commitment on behalf of their profession?
4. Identify policy issues in which nurses should take particular interest. What evidence do you see that nurses are actively involved in these issues in your community?
5. Find out whether the members of your state board of nursing are elected or appointed. What is the makeup of the board (how many registered nurses, licensed practical nurses, consumers, and so forth)? Do nurses hold most of the

seats on the state board? Are there any other health professionals, such as physicians, on the board of nursing? If so, are there any nurses on the state board of medicine?

REFERENCES

ABC News: Presidential race: real-time vote results, ABC 2000: the vote, Online November, 12, 2003 *(www.abcnews.go.com/sections/politics/2000vote/general/president.html)*.

American Association of Nurse Anesthetists: Fact sheet concerning the November 2001 CMS rule, Capitol Corner, 2001, Online November 7, 2003 *(www.aana.com/capcorner/fact-sheet_111301.asp)*.

Congressional Quarterly: *The 49th annual CQ almanac,* Washington, D.C., 1993, Congressional Quarterly.

Eagleton Institute of Politics, Rutgers University: 2000 Presidential election, Online October, 8, 2003 *(www.rci.rutgers.edu/~eagleton/e-gov/e-politicalarchive-2000.htm)*.

Kaiser Family Foundation: Issue spotlight on the uninsured, Online November 12, 2003 *(www.kaisernetwork.org/static/spotlight_uninsured_index.cfm)*.

Mason D, Leavitt J, Chaffee M, editors: *Policy and politics in nursing and health care,* ed 4, St. Louis, 2002, WB Saunders.

Mooney MM: Hog-housed! *Reflect Nurs Leadersh* 29(4):8-9, 2003.

Posner R: *Breaking the deadlock: the 2000 election, the Constitution and the courts,* Princeton, NJ, 2001, Princeton University Press, p 48.

Sigma Theta Tau International: *Woodhull study on nursing and the media,* Indianapolis, 1997, Center Nursing Press.

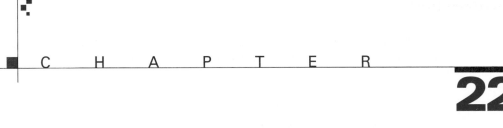

CHAPTER 22

Nursing's Future Challenges

Kay Kittrell Chitty

Key Terms

Alternative Treatment
Assisted Suicide
Bioterrorism
Birthrate
Centenarian
Cultural Diversity
Demography
Designer Medicines
Differentiated Practice
Disaster
Disenfranchised

Distance Learning
Epidemiologist
Euthanasia
Futurist
Heterogeneous
Homogeneous
Hospitalist
Human Genome
   Project
Managed Care
Medically Indigent

Morbidity Rate
Mortality Rate
Multidrug Resistant
   Strains
Multiskilled Worker
Nursing Informatics
Shared Governance
Telehealth
Urbanization
Vulnerable Population
Working Poor

Learning Outcomes

After reading this chapter, students will be able to:

- Review societal influences on the nursing profession anticipated during the next decade.
- Recognize the impact that changes in the health care system will have on the practice of nursing.
- Explain trends in nursing education needed to meet society's future nursing needs.
- Describe major challenges that the nursing profession must resolve to ensure it remains in control of its destiny.
- Explain trends in nursing education needed to meet society's future nursing needs.
- Describe the major components of *Nursing's Agenda for the Future.*

As you have seen throughout this textbook, the nursing profession is profoundly affected by a rapidly changing world. The challenges nurses face today relate to a variety of factors: changes in demographics, unhealthy lifestyles of many Americans, the continued deterioration of the environment, rapid change in the health care system brought about by cost containment initiatives, advances in technology, notably in genomics and informatics, bioterrorism, natural and man-made disasters, cultural diversity within both nursing and the population, blurring of professional boundaries and increasing interdisciplinary collaboration, and issues within nursing itself.

It is painfully clear that even in the United States, the wealthiest of the industrialized nations, we fall far short of the goal of having a healthy nation. Millions of Americans still have no health insurance, and many more have less than enough. Infant mortality rates remain unacceptably high. The fitness level of citizens, including young people, continues to decline as obesity climbs at an alarming rate. Smoking in youth continues to increase. And the threat of bioterrorism is a new challenge we must face as a profession and as a nation.

All these negative trends continue even though the United States spends more of its gross domestic product on health than any nation in the world. Complete overhaul of the health care system, believed by many Americans to be essential if these problems are to be addressed, has been stalled in Congress since 1994.

Nursing enjoys high levels of respect and public confidence. It is a profession in heavy demand, and its practitioners enjoy more autonomy than ever. As the health care profession with the highest number of practitioners, nursing has enormous but largely untapped political power that would allow nurses to influence societal changes—rather than simply be influenced by them—if they were unified in their efforts. Yet turf issues, lack of focus, and inaction continue to divide nurses, diminishing their influence at every level.

You might wonder what purpose is served by thinking about the future. The purpose of "futures work" is "to study potential developments, using tools and certain attitudinal alignments, to effect change in a desired direction. A deliberated future may be personal, professional or organizational, but the process is the same: creating an image of a desired result to serve as a blueprint for action. … It allows us to avert, encourage, or *direct* the course of events" (Dickenson-Hazard, 2003), rather than simply *reacting* to them.

This chapter explores some of nursing's challenges and opportunities in the future.

SOCIETAL CHALLENGES

At least six societal influences are expected to have major impact on the future of the nursing profession: demographic changes, environmental deterioration, the recently recognized need to prepare for large-scale public health disasters, unhealthy lifestyles and resulting illnesses, continuing need for cost containment, and regulation of health care. Each of these influences is examined briefly.

Demographics

Demography is the science that studies vital statistics and social trends. Demographers examine vital statistics such as **birthrates** (births per thousand people), **morbidity rates** (illness), **mortality rates** (deaths), marriages, the ages of various populations, and migration patterns. From this wealth of information, **futurists,** people who try to project what will occur, draw conclusions about what these trends mean for the future.

Four demographic trends are particularly important to the future of nursing: the aging population, poverty, the cultural diversity of the population, and urbanization, including increasing levels of violence. Each has implications for nursing.

Aging population

Estimates vary, but demographers have predicted that the number of people over the age of 75 in the United States by the year 2020 will exceed 21.8 million. The number of aging "baby boomers" will create an additional strain on the U.S. health care system. These "boomers" will be different from patients in the past because they will "expect more and tolerate less"(Wolf, 2003, p. 32). They will be the most knowledgeable health care consumers ever and will keep their caregivers on their toes.

Centenarians, people over 100 years of age, represent one of the fastest-growing groups in the United States. The World Future Society predicts that by the end of the twenty-first century, the average life span will approach 100 years (Hendrick, 1995). Many elderly people are healthy, but the likelihood of illness becomes greater as people age. For example, indications are that by the age of 90, one of two people will develop Alzheimer's disease (Herbert, Scherr, Beckett, et al., 1995). In general, the elderly are greater users of health care than any other population segment (Valentino, 2002). Clearly, nurses of the future must be prepared to work effectively with the rising numbers of elderly patients.

Ethical issues such as **euthanasia** and **assisted suicide** will become increasingly important as technology enables people to sustain life far beyond the point of useful, meaningful existence. Society's views of assisted suicide and euthanasia are changing, as evidenced by the fact that juries acquitted Dr. Jack Kevorkian of charges of murder in the assisted deaths of several terminally ill people before he was ultimately convicted and sentenced to prison. Additionally, the citizens of Oregon passed an assisted suicide referendum. Two countries, The Netherlands and Belgium, have legalized assisted suicide and a number of other nations are considering it. The future will gradually bring further changes in laws and attitudes toward giving individuals control over the timing and manner of their own deaths.

Poverty

Even though the United States is considered the world's wealthiest nation, the number of Americans living below the poverty line is increasing. This is particularly true of women, children, and the elderly. Another large group of Americans are employed yet cannot make enough money to provide adequately for their families' needs. They are known as the **working poor.** This group has grown since "welfare reform" legislation passed in 1996. The gap between the "haves" and the "have-nots" in the United States continues to widen, creating discontent and disillusionment.

When basic needs for food, clothing, and shelter are unmet or uncertain, health care becomes a luxury. Children's immunizations, prenatal care for pregnant women, nutritious meals, and a variety of other health-maintaining factors are neglected. **Medically indigent** people, those who do not qualify for Medicaid but nevertheless cannot pay for health care, tend to put off seeking care until illness is advanced and thus harder to treat. Conditions that can be prevented often are not because of lack of education, poor sanitation, crowded living conditions, improper shelter, homelessness, and a host of other poverty-related factors.

It is a sad reality that poverty will continue to rise in the future, creating increasing numbers of **disenfranchised** people, that is, people who have no power in the political system, with limited access to health care. As their numbers grow, both federal and state governments will be forced by limited resources to implement more strategies that limit health care expenditures for these **vulnerable populations.**

Nursing, as a profession, values providing care to all people, regardless of social and economic factors. The increasing numbers of medically disenfranchised people and pressure to limit health care expenditures will collide to create an intense values conflict for nurses of the future.

Cultural diversity

Cultural diversity refers to the array of people from different racial, ethnic, religious, social, and geographic backgrounds who make up a particular entity. Some countries, such as Japan, are **homogeneous** in culture. This means the citizens have similar cultural beliefs and practices. Others, such as the United States, have a **heterogeneous** cultural mix. The cultural beliefs and practices of our citizens are quite different and becoming more so with every passing year.

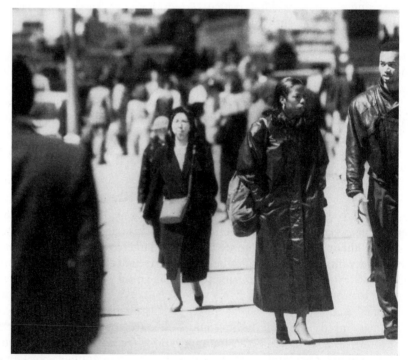

Figure 22-1
Immigration to the United States from Southeast Asia, the Middle East, Central America, Mexico, and islands of the Caribbean is expected to continue in the next decade, contributing to sweeping demographic changes. (Courtesy *Tennessee Nurse,* photo by Thomas Sconyers.)

Immigration to the United States from Southeast Asia, Central America, the Middle East, Mexico, and the islands of the Caribbean has increased in recent years as a result of civil unrest, wars, and poor economic conditions (Figure 22-1). People from these countries are the latest wave of newcomers to the United States and join the European-Americans, African-Americans, and others whose ancestors came to this country in the twentieth century and earlier. Each group has its own nutritional practices, health beliefs, folk remedies, childcare practices, and conventional wisdom about health and illness.

Nurses need to take cultural beliefs, values, and practices into consideration when planning and implementing nursing care for individuals of diverse cultural backgrounds. Culturally competent care will be more important in the future than ever before. Speaking a second language, particularly Spanish, will be an important skill that will increase nurses' ability to communicate with patients and their value to health care organizations.

The nursing profession itself will become increasingly diverse as its membership reflects a heterogeneous society. This will create the need for nurses to understand, respect, and value the contributions of co-workers of all cultural backgrounds.

Urbanization

Urbanization, that is, people moving from rural, farming areas to cities, has increased since the time of the Industrial Revolution. That trend continues today and is expected to go on well into the new century.

As cities grow, suburbs flourish, and many people who can afford to do so move away from the business centers of cities. Decaying inner cities with large populations of poor people create major social problems such as homelessness, drugs, gangs, single-parent households, mental illness, violence, and crime. Despite the increase in public-private partnerships designed to revitalize inner cities and programs formulated to deal effectively with urban issues, social problems continue to grow and spill over into the suburbs and rural areas, creating further social changes. Nurses of the future will be increasingly confronted with health problems resulting from these social phenomena.

Violence is of particular concern to members of the nursing profession. Violence is present in our homes, workplaces, schools, and communities, causing untold chaos and loss. Violence is becoming a major public health problem in the United States and elsewhere, and we see the results in offices, clinics, and trauma units. Because the nursing profession cannot turn a blind eye to this problem, we will see nurses as individuals and as a professional group increasingly take action against the rising tide of violence to protect basic societal principles.

Environment

Every newspaper, news magazine, and television news program brings disturbing reports of the deterioration of our environment. There are major environmental tragedies, such as a nuclear power plant incident in Japan and floodwaters spreading effluent from hundreds of pig farms in eastern North Carolina. These overshadow the less dramatic but insidious gradual decline in the quality of the world's air, water, and plant and animal life.

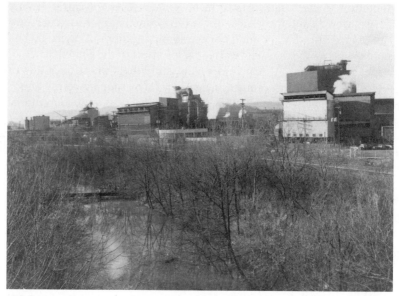

Figure **22-2**
This manufacturing plant, while providing jobs to scores of workers, has polluted the air and the ground around it, as well as a nearby stream. Although the plant is slated for closure, it will take years to clean up the ground and water contaminated during its decades of operation. (Photo by Kelly Whalin.)

Acute and chronic respiratory diseases are increasing, as are debilitating allergic reactions to chemicals in the environment and cancers of all types (Figure 22-2). Reports of worsening of the hole in the ozone layer, accidental lead and mercury poisonings, toxic shellfish beds, truckloads of pesticides spilling into streams and rivers, and accidental release of radioactive steam from nuclear power plants all occur with distressing regularity. Meanwhile, clear-cutting of forests, destruction of wetlands by development, and relaxing of standards for polluting industries have become "business as usual."

Epidemiologists, who study the origins of diseases, believe that there is a relationship between environmental decline and increases in certain diseases, including epidemic diseases such as Hantavirus and Ebola virus. Emerging diseases and **multidrug resistant strains** of organisms currently under control, such as tuberculosis, will increasingly challenge health care resources.

Humans are responsible for destroying the environment, and the more human beings there are, the faster the environment will decline. Overpopulation contributes to the deterioration of the world's environment, yet too few countries are dealing effectively with issues of overpopulation, including the United States.

In December 2003 the world population reached the record number of 6.3 billion people. The U.S. Census Bureau has projected that the world's population will increase to 8.8 billion by the end of 2025 (U.S. Census Bureau, 2003). Feeding, immunizing, providing potable water, and caring for this many human beings threatens to destroy the environmental, economic, social, and medical systems of the world. In the United States alone there is one birth every 8 seconds, one international migrant every 22 seconds, and one death every 13 seconds—for a net gain of 1 person every 10 seconds (U.S. Census Bureau, 2003).

At the most recent Earth Summit Conference held in Johannesburg, South Africa, in 2002, the analogy of the overloaded lifeboat was frequently used. World overpopulation, overdevelopment, and overconsumption by wealthy nations threaten to deplete the resources and destroy the environment of the entire world, not just overpopulated countries. The related problems of environmental deterioration and overpopulation are health care issues that future nurses will face, and there are no easy answers.

Disasters and Bioterrorism

Since September 11, 2001, and its aftermath, many professions have reevaluated their disaster preparedness. Nurses are often at the forefront in emergency and disaster situations, but few U.S. schools of nursing include disaster training in their curricula. As we have all so sadly witnessed, this needs to change in the future.

A **disaster** is defined as "an event or situation that is of greater magnitude than an emergency; disrupts essential services such as housing, transportation, communications, sanitation, water, and health care; and requires the response of people outside the community affected" (Gebbie and Qureshi, 2002). Disasters can be natural or man-made and range from earthquakes, hurricanes, and major fires to wars and major environmental contamination.

Regardless of the cause of a disaster situation, no two of which are alike, the basic competencies nurses need in disaster preparedness are essentially the same. The Centers for Disease Control and Prevention collaborated with a nurse, Dr. Kristin M. Gebbie, to develop a set of core emergency preparedness competencies for public health workers. This served as a basis upon which Dr. Gebbie and another nurse, Kristin Qureshi, developed core competencies for nurses (Gebbie and Qureshi, 2002). The core disaster preparedness competencies for nurses are found Box 22-1.

Until recently, nurses weren't expected to know much about the specific type of disaster caused by bioterrorism. **Bioterrorism** refers to the use of a biological or chemical agent as a weapon. Now nurses must be able to recognize the signs and symptoms of biological agents such as anthrax and smallpox or chemical agents such as Ricin. They must know how to notify the proper authorities; "assist with diagnosis, postexposure prophylaxis, and treatment; and participate in infection control" (Coleman, 2001).

Nurses are encouraged to keep up with emerging information to improve their readiness for possible bioterrorism by referring to the CDC's bioterrorism website *(www.bt.cdc.gov)*. You can register for the CDC's free email updates and training opportunities via the CDC's Clinician Registry *(www.bt.cdc.gov/clinregistry/index.asp)*.

Nursing organizations are taking an active role in improving the preparedness of professional nurses. The American Nurses Association (ANA) worked with the Office of Emergency Response, U.S. Department of Health & Human Services, in the establishment of the *National Nurses Response Team (NNRT)*. According to the

Box 22-1 Core Nursing Competencies for Disaster Preparedness

To consider themselves prepared for a major emergency or a disaster, nurses should be able to perform the following:

- Describe the agency's (your place of employment's) role in responding to a range of emergencies that might arise.
- Describe the chain of command in emergency response (to whom you would report).
- Identify and locate the agency's emergency response plan (or the pertinent portion of it).
- Describe emergency response functions or roles and demonstrate them in regularly performed drills.
- Demonstrate the use of equipment (including personal protective equipment) and the skills required in emergency response during regular drills.
- Demonstrate the correct operation of all equipment used for emergency communication.
- Describe communication roles in emergency response within your agency, with news media, with the general public (including patients and families), and with personal contacts (one's own family, friends, and neighbors).
- Identify the limits of your own knowledge, skills, and authority, and identify key system resources for referring matters that exceed these limits.
- Apply creative problem-solving skills and flexible thinking to the situation, within the confines of your role, and evaluate the effectiveness of all actions taken.
- Recognize deviations from the norm that might indicate an emergency and describe appropriate action. Participate in continuing education to maintain up-to-date knowledge in relevant areas.
- Participate in evaluating every drill or response and identify necessary changes to the plan.

In addition, nurses with managerial or leadership responsibilities should be able to perform the following:

- Ensure that there is a written plan for major categories of emergencies.
- Ensure that all parts of the emergency plan are practiced regularly.
- Ensure that identified gaps in knowledge or skills are filled.

From Gebbie KM, Qureshi K: Emergency and disaster preparedness: core competencies for nurses, *Am J Nurs* 102(1):46-51, 2002.

ANA, "The NNRT creates an excellent opportunity for registered nurses who on September 11 were asking themselves, 'What can I do to help my country?'" (ANA, 2003a). The NNRT will be composed of 10 regionally based teams of 200 registered nurses who could be called upon to assist in chemoprophylaxis or vaccination of hundreds of thousands or even millions of Americans, or in other scenarios requiring large numbers of nurses. Team members will be enrolled in the National Disaster Medical System. You can learn more on the ANA website (*www.nursingworld.org/news/disaster/biocare.htm*).

Unhealthy Lifestyles

Despite the focus on wellness in contemporary American society, unhealthy lifestyles still predominate; this trend shows no signs of changing.

Obesity

Every year public health officials report that there are more obese Americans than ever, even though obesity has long been known to predispose people to a number of illnesses, including diabetes, heart disease, high blood pressure, and arthritis. The accompanying News Note tells of a distressingly rapid increase in the number of Americans who are more than 100 pounds overweight.

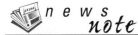 *n e w s note*

Extreme Obesity Ballooning: 1 in 50 Adults in U.S. at Least 100 Pounds Too Heavy

Americans are not just getting fatter; they are ballooning to extremely obese proportions at an alarming rate. The number of extremely obese American adults, those who are at least 100 pounds overweight, has quadrupled since the 1980s to about 4 million. That works out to about 1 in every 50 adults.

Extreme obesity once was thought to be a rare, distinct condition whose prevalence remained relatively steady over time. The new study contradicts that thinking and suggests that it is at least partly due to the same kinds of behaviors, overeating and underactivity, that have contributed to the epidemic number of Americans with less severe weight problems.

In fact, the findings by a RAND Corporation researcher show that the number of extremely obese adults has surged twice as fast as the number of less severely obese adults.

On the scale of obesity, "as the whole population shifts to the right, the extreme categories grow the fastest," said RAND economist Roland Sturm. He added, "These people have the highest health costs."

Sturm said health problems associated with obesity—including diabetes, heart disease, high blood pressure and arthritis—probably affect the extremely obese disproportionately and at young ages. "There is no evidence that it (the obesity rate) is flattening out," Sturm said. "It's full speed ahead." He has done projections showing that if nothing is done, the number of obese Americans will jump from about 20 percent of adults today to 80 percent by 2040, and the proportion of normal-weight people will drop from 42 percent today to 5 percent in 2040.

Sturm's study, which appeared in the *Archives of Internal Medicine,* is based on nationwide telephone surveys conducted by the U.S. Centers for Disease Control and Prevention, in which people were asked their height and weight. His report covers surveys from 1986 through 2000.

Continued

news note—cont'd

In 1986, 1 in 200 adults reported height and weight measurements reflecting extreme obesity, or a body-mass index of at least 40. By 2000 that had jumped to 1 in 50, Sturm found. Body-mass index is a ratio of height to weight.

The prevalence of the most extreme obesity, people with a BMI of at least 50, grew fivefold—from 1 in 2,000 to 1 in 400—Sturm said. By contrast, ordinary obesity, a BMI of 30 to 35, doubled—from about 1 in 10 to 1 in 5—based on the same surveys.

Americans tend to understate their weights, and a recent study based on actual measurements found an obesity rate of nearly 1 in 3, or almost 59 million people. Sturm said his findings probably understate the problem for the same reason.

The average man with a BMI of 40 in the study was 5 feet 10 inches and 300 pounds, while the average woman was 5 feet 4 inches and 250 pounds. Sturm said the trend largely is the result of the increasing affordability of calorie-dense food. "We've reached Nirvana," he said. "Food is cheap and plentiful. You can stuff yourself on less than a half-hour of minimum wage."

The trend is also fueled by a substantial reduction in the amount of physical activity that Americans engage in, said Linda Baumann, a nursing professor at the University of Wisconsin-Madison. School physical education budgets have been cut, suburban neighborhoods have been built without sidewalks, and "children are driven instead of walking to school," said Baumann, who is also is president of the Society of Behavioral Medicine.

Obesity researchers say the trend has to be reversed, or the health consequences will be devastating. "How can we put up with having this many people that large?" said James Hill, an obesity expert at the University of Colorado. "We have to do something quick."

From Extreme Obesity Ballooning, *The Post and Courier* [Charleston, SC] 103(287): 1A, 8A, 2003.

Futurists predict that Americans will eat more meals in restaurants in the future, but ordering a nutritious, well-balanced meal in a restaurant is a major challenge, even to people with a working knowledge of nutritional science. In a distressing sign that indicates acquiescence to the fast-food mentality of many families, nutritional consultants are now being hired by public school districts to teach cafeteria workers how to make nutritious school lunches look and taste more like fast foods. Apparently, many modern children refuse to eat anything else.

As a result of pressure from health-conscious consumers, many of whom are now aging "baby boomers," some restaurant chains have introduced grilled foods and other "low-fat" items. On examination, however, the fat content of some of these foods is unacceptably high. Restaurant owners report that even when they include low-fat meals on the menu, few people order them. The majority of regular menu items are still loaded with animal fats (long known to cause cardiovascular disease) and sodium (known to aggravate a variety of health conditions). A taco salad, for example, can contain as many as 30 grams of fat.

Tobacco use

Yet another lifestyle issue is tobacco use. Smoking continues to increase among the young, especially females and minorities, both of whom are targeted for higher levels of marketing by tobacco companies. For decades, smoking has been known to cause lung cancer, emphysema and other chronic lung diseases, low-birth-weight babies, and a host of other health problems.

Lung cancer is a leading cancer killer in both men and women. There were an estimated 164,100 new cases of lung cancer and an estimated 156,900 deaths from lung cancer in the United States in 2000. The rate of lung cancer cases appears to be dropping among white and African-American men in the United States, while it continues to rise among both white and African-American women (American Lung Association, 2003).

The use of smokeless tobacco is rising, creating unhealthy oral mucous membranes and predisposing users to oral cancer. All these trends ensure that tobacco-related illnesses and deaths will rise in the future.

Lack of exercise

Lack of exercise is a troubling lifestyle issue for Americans of the future, particularly the young. The ready availability of entertainment on television is at least partly to blame. Studies show that the more television people of all ages watch, the more likely they are to be overweight. Snacking and television watching usually go hand in hand. Entire generations of Americans, raised watching several hours of television each day, are unlikely to give up the habit in the future, especially because more options are added yearly. Others spend hours in front of computer screens, playing video games, or in other sedentary pursuits. These habits are expected to continue in the future.

Lack of exercise is not limited to the young, however. For every middle-aged jogger seen pounding the roadways, legions of sedentary adults remain unseen at home, gradually becoming less fit and more susceptible to disease. Browsing through mail-order catalogs aimed at the affluent middle-aged population reveals a plethora of labor-saving devices being developed and marketed to make Americans even less active in the future.

Eating disorders

Advertising affects yet another lifestyle risk factor. With the emphasis on thinness in fashion advertising, many girls and young women resort to unhealthy habits such as starving or binging and purging. Rather than eating sensibly and engaging in exercise to maintain normal weights, they assume bizarre eating habits in the pursuit of the fashionable, if unnatural, degree of gauntness. Barring a dramatic change in the fashion industry, eating disorders and their resulting health hazards will continue to increase.

Stress

Another lifestyle issue is stress. The rapid pace of modern life creates stress, yet Americans continue to step up the pace with cellular telephones, fax machines, satellite communications, personal computers, paging devices, call-waiting options, and all the other fruits of modern technology. Although many Americans mourn the loss of leisure time, indications are that when given more leisure time, many people spend it working. This evidence indicates that stress-related diseases are on the increase.

HIV/AIDS and drug abuse

The twin epidemics of acquired immunodeficiency syndrome (AIDS) and drug abuse are two issues that will profoundly affect the future of nursing. When the AIDS epidemic began in the United States early in the 1980s, many of those affected were homosexual men. A few years later, infection rates among intravenous drug users began to rise. By the mid-1980s, AIDS moved into the general population of heterosexual adults, a trend already seen in other countries and now well established in the United States. The spread of AIDS to adolescents and rural Americans now causes considerable concern.

Even optimists in the medical community no longer predict a vaccine against human immunodeficiency virus (HIV), believing that it will be many years before a vaccine is discovered, if ever. Meanwhile, millions of Americans are already infected, and no cure is on the horizon.

Substance-abusing people suffer more accidents and illness than their nonabusing counterparts, thus requiring more medical and nursing care. They are also more likely to have unprotected sex, putting them at risk for acquiring HIV and other sexually transmitted diseases. Other health risks include hepatitis, noninfectious liver disorders, and kidney failure, among others. Nurses of the future will be called on to provide intensive nursing care to increasing numbers of substance abusers and people with AIDS.

Nurses' own lifestyle choices will come under increasing scrutiny as the issue of HIV and hepatitis infections in physicians, dentists, nurses, and other health care workers becomes a focus of public concern. Nurses will be involved in the development of sound public policies concerning these issues.

Given the predominance of unhealthy lifestyle choices, it is clear that nurses will play an increasingly important role in educating people about wellness and self-care in the years ahead. Nurses will also be instrumental in educating the public about how to be informed consumers of health care services. Nurses will continue to provide nursing care in acute care settings, such as hospitals, to those who choose not to listen.

Cost Containment

During the last 30 years, governmental budget deficits reached all-time highs. At federal, state, and local levels, governments spent more money than was generated through taxes, and the pressure for health care for the elderly and poor created a significant part of those budgetary problems.

Our nation leads the world in health care costs but ranks 21st in life expectancy and 27th in infant mortality (Wolf, 2003). Our drug costs are the highest in the world. Society's poor, homeless, elderly, substance abusers, AIDS patients, and mentally ill are increasing in number and will continue to increase. The question yet to be answered is "How can we pay for health care for these vulnerable populations now and in the future when their numbers are even greater?"

Federal and state governments are seeking to answer that question. In many states, Medicaid is the largest and fastest-growing single state expense. Although welfare reform efforts have effectively removed thousands from welfare rolls, the aging of America will continue to create huge numbers of social security–eligible and Medicare-eligible citizens. The decrease in the ratio of these individuals to the number of those working and paying social security and income taxes will place an additional burden on the federal government's budget.

The future may bring hospital closings, continued pressures from the business community to force changes in health care financing, and significant health care reform, piece by piece if not by sweeping legislative mandate. The nursing profession stands to benefit because nursing has been shown to be a cost-conscious yet high-quality alternative to traditional medical care. In addition, nurses are well equipped to provide managed care. As a profession, nursing is expected to benefit from health care woes in the United States by expanding roles in prevention and community-based nursing.

One cost-effective method of providing basic health care to children is through school nurses. As the burden of providing care continues to shift from federal agencies to state and local agencies, local school boards will recognize the economies to be realized through school nursing. Health care reform will likely provoke a dramatic rise in state-mandated health "safety net" services for children. Many of these services will be delivered by nurses.

Regulation of Health Care

Even if the cost of health care can be contained, health care expenses in the United States will continue to rise. This rise is anticipated owing to the large number of aging Americans and the growing number of impoverished ones. As more citizens are covered by government-sponsored medical programs such as Medicare and Medicaid, even greater governmental regulation of health care will be required.

Nurses will become increasingly active in developing health policies that improve access, quality, and value in the delivery of health services. Legislation mandating the direct reimbursement of nurses for their services will be a feature of most government-funded programs, despite the opposition of organized medicine and hospitals. Private **managed care** programs will increasingly use advanced practice registered nurses to provide primary health care.

Nursing, through its professional associations, will continue to be a player in health care politics in the United States. Nurses will form coalitions with consumer groups to influence consumer-friendly legislation at state and national levels. Individual nurses will become more politically active as voters, campaign workers, community health activists, and political candidates. As nursing's public profile becomes higher, public scrutiny of the profession will increase. Consumers of nursing services will exercise their political power to ensure that nurses and other primary care providers consistently offer first-class health care.

CHALLENGES IN NURSING PRACTICE

The societal changes just reviewed will necessarily create changes in nursing practice. Nurses in the next decade will face an ever-widening array of practice opportunities in hospital and community-based health care settings, each of which will bring its own set of challenges.

Differentiating Practice Levels

There has been considerable resistance to differentiating levels of nursing practice, even though visionary nursing leaders have pointed out the need to do so for years. **Differentiated practice** means that nurses prepared in associate degree, baccalaureate degree, and higher degree programs should have different, well-defined roles and possibly even different levels of licensure. The competencies of nurses at each level could be clearly demonstrated, and nurses at each level could be held accountable for practice standards at that level. If differentiated practice became a reality, educational programs could be streamlined, employers and consumers could understand the differences, and patient care delivery systems could be reorganized to capitalize on the strengths of each level.

In the past, nurses prepared in diploma and associate degree programs opposed efforts to differentiate educational and practice levels in nursing, believing that they would be disenfranchised. Nursing leaders have been unwilling to take the risk of tacking such a potentially divisive issue. The result is that nursing is the only health care profession for which entry into practice is less than a baccalaureate degree. Many professions currently require a master's degree as the credential for entry into a profession, and educational standards are rising in all fields but nursing. This has hampered nursing in its quest for professionalism and equal status among the health care professions.

In addition to improving educational standards, differentiated practice could help nurses be more cost-effective by determining who is best suited to perform certain nursing actions. Differentiated practice can be realized in the future only if practicing nurses are willing to give up the notion that "a nurse is a nurse is a nurse" and acknowledge that different educational programs do and should prepare different types of nursing practitioners. Nurses must be willing to see the larger picture and recognize that advances in the profession benefit all nurses. They are being encouraged in these efforts by the American Association of Colleges of Nursing (AACN), which refers to differentiated practice as one of the "hallmarks of the professional nursing practice environment" in its white paper by the same title. You can read the entire document at AACN's website *(www.aacn.nche.edu/Publications/ positions/hallmarks.htm)*.

Cost Containment's Impact

During the 1990s, cost-containment initiatives in hospitals eliminated layers of middle-management nurses. This represented a crisis for individual nurse managers but created an opportunity for a stronger voice for nurses involved in direct patient care. Future cost-containment measures such as managed care and capitation will require nurses to demonstrate the cost-effectiveness of the care they provide. The "bottom line" will be an increasing focus of concern in all health care settings, and nurses will need resource management skills more than ever before. Nurses will find that they need business expertise as much as they need clinical expertise.

Increasingly, nurses will work with unlicensed assistive personnel and delegate tasks to deliver patient care. They will need communication, interpersonal, and management skills to make the new partnerships work. **Multiskilled workers** will take their place alongside nurses in all settings. Nurses will be challenged to expand their skills into areas formerly the domain of specialized workers, such as respiratory therapists and physical therapists. This will be essential if nurses are to cope with the periodic variations in supply and demand for traditional nursing positions. In addition, a variety of new health care job opportunities in quality care, case management, advanced practice, and primary care will present themselves as a result of economic pressures of managed care and health reforms (Perla, 2002).

Autonomy and Accountability

Shared governance, that is, participation by nurses on strong policymaking hospital committees, is a trend already seen and mandated by accreditation bodies such as the Joint Commission on the Accreditation of Healthcare Organizations (JCAHO). Along with the empowerment of nurses, however, will come increased demand for accountability. Effective nursing care will be measured by patient outcomes. Continuous quality improvement of nursing care will be emphasized more than ever. Nurses must be able to show evidence that the care they provide makes a demonstrable difference in patient outcomes.

As more and more nursing care is provided in community settings, autonomy and accountability will become increasingly important. Nurses who function independently in homes and other community-based practice settings need additional education and experience. When the supervisory guidance of better-prepared colleagues is not readily available, novice or inexperienced nurses must assume responsibility for knowing the limits of their expertise and for seeking consultation to ensure patient safety. Professional nurses of the future will increasingly pursue baccalaureate and advanced degrees to prepare them for autonomous practice.

Technology and Nursing Informatics

All types of technology will continue to advance at a dizzying pace, as they have in the first years of the twenty-first century. Areas expected to impact nursing are nursing informatics, telecommunications, genetic engineering, alternative treatments, and the Internet.

Nursing informatics

Nursing informatics, the organization and use of nursing data, continues to change nursing practice dramatically. Computerized health information networks (CHINs) will allow immediate access to all patient data needed in refining the plan of care. The increased access to patient data will reinforce the need for patient confidentiality.

Voice-activated bedside computers already allow nurses to record patient information literally "at the bedside," rather than making written notes and transferring them to the patient's chart at a later time. This practice will become widespread.

Telecommunications

Advances in telecommunications will improve access to medical services for rural and elderly Americans. Nurses and physicians will examine and treat patients who are hundreds of miles away using two-way television systems. They will evaluate and prescribe treatments via telephone. Telemedicine will become routine for those who live in remote areas or are homebound. Nurses will be increasingly involved in **telehealth.**

Genetic engineering

Genetic engineering has become more common as the scientists participating in the **Human Genome Project** work to complete the mapping and sequencing of a composite set of human genes. This will make it possible to treat and prevent many more genetically transmitted and genetically predisposed diseases. It will also create ethical dilemmas of gigantic proportions as the ability to clone individuals and predetermine characteristics of human infants becomes a reality. Genetic research will also make possible individualized medications, or designer medicines. **Designer medicines** are drugs tailor-made to treat patients based on their individual genetic makeup. A new role for nurses, the Genomics Nurse Case Coordinator, has already been proposed (Lea and Monsen, 2003). Programs preparing nurses for basic practice have been encouraged to include knowledge and skills to prepare graduates for "family history assessments, screening, and case coordination for clients receiving genetic testing and gene-based therapies" (Lea and Monsen, 2003, p. 75).

Alternative treatments

More Americans will turn away from mainstream medical care in the future and seek **alternative treatments** as they take responsibility for their own health (Figure 22-3). Nontraditional care, such as chiropractic, homeopathy, acupuncture, massage, therapeutic touch, and herbal remedies, will increasingly become a focus of interest, study, research, practice, and publication (McKenna, 1995).

The Internet

The Internet will create major changes in the way Americans view health care and their role as partners in their own care. The proliferation of websites designed to provide reliable medical and health information to the lay public will continue. Nurses will be called on to educate patients about how to evaluate and appropriately use the information they obtain from these sites.

As a result of these and other unforeseen technological advances, nurses of the future will continue to fight the dehumanizing tendency of technological advances such as patient monitoring devices while valuing and providing a holistic, "high-touch" environment for patients. Nurses will realize that advanced technology and traditional nursing values are not mutually exclusive. Patients can have both if nurses stay focused on the patient rather than on the machine or monitor. Advances in technology will bring new ethical dilemmas. Nurses will be more active

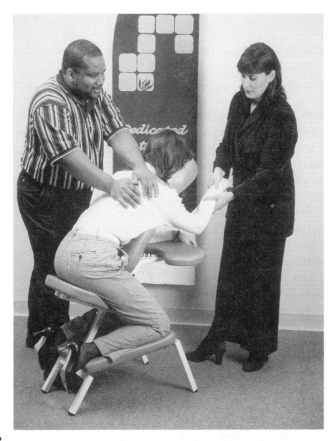

Figure **22-3**
Alternative treatments, such as massage therapy, are appealing to more Americans as they take responsibility for their own health. This trend to natural healing is expected to increase in the future. (Courtesy Memorial Hospital, Chattanooga, Tennessee.)

in exploring ethical aspects of patient care, and their unique ethical perspective will be valued by other professionals. As a result, nurses will sit on ethics committees and serve as ethics consultants in greater numbers.

Practice in Community Settings

Community-based primary health care will continue to expand as cost-effectiveness remains a high priority. Nurse-managed clinics will increasingly serve underserved populations in inner city and rural areas. School nurses will be needed in large numbers, as will hospice nurses and those specializing in gerontology and chronic illnesses. For nurses who are willing to work outside traditional settings and their own "comfort zones," there will be no end to the available opportunities.

Flexible scheduling and job sharing will increase in all professions and will become commonplace in nursing. Nurse entrepreneurship will flourish in the future as a result of changes in restrictive legislation, the resourcefulness and self-confidence of better-educated nurses, and the trust the public places in the nursing profession. Increasing numbers of nurses will own clinics and other health-related businesses, such as independent practice associations, free-standing wellness programs, adult day care centers, dialysis care services, and worksite health programs.

Cultural Competence

Providing culturally competent nursing care will become even more important in the future as the nation's demographics change even more dramatically than they have in the past. Nurses of the future must recognize that cultural sensitivity begins with one's fellow health care providers. If relationships within the team are strained by insensitivity and prejudice, patient care cannot be culturally sensitive. Meaningful dialogue must become a vehicle for building relationships within the work group. A united team will be capable of providing respectful, understanding, and dignified care to patients.

Effective nursing leaders of the future will provide cultural support groups and mentoring to ensure that "faculty, providers, students, patients, and others can become less inhibited about individuals who are culturally different. They can foster the courage to engage in conversations, to get to know each other, to share our worldviews, to speak out, and to trust that interactions about our specific and particular culture, on a personal level, will make a difference" (Gary, Sigby, and Campbell, 1998, p. 277). Nurses who are unable or unwilling to become culturally aware, culturally sensitive, and culturally competent will unnecessarily limit their career potential.

Maintaining a Healthy Work Environment

No profession is free from hazards, and no work place can ever ensure absolute security. Nursing is no exception to this sad fact of contemporary life. Occupational health hazards in nursing include needlestick injuries and possible infection with hepatitis and HIV; exposure to chemicals such as disinfectants and chemotherapeutic agents; and violence in the workplace, among others.

Additional hazards include latex allergy, a continuing concern for nurses, with a prevalence rate of approximately 8 to 12 percent in frequent glove users (American Nurses Association, 2003b). Injuries from accidents and back strain also occur too frequently, with pain, disability, lost income, absenteeism, and decreased productivity only a few of the results.

Shift work itself is a hazard to nurses, causing a variety of physical and psychological problems, including exhaustion, depression, interpersonal problems, and accidents. Stress from work overload, inadequate staffing, and the intense feelings generated by caring for acutely ill and dying patients adds to the mix of workplace hazards faced by nurses.

In addition, nurses increasingly find themselves at risk for violence in the workplace. This is not a new phenomenon, but it is being discussed more openly than in the past, as evidenced by the fall 1999 issue of Sigma Theta Tau International's membership publication, *Reflections* (now named *Reflections on Nursing Leadership*), being devoted entirely to the issue of workplace violence.

Among the articles in that issue of *Reflections* was a report of a 1997 survey by the Colorado Nurses Association's Task Force on Violence, which conducted a seven-state survey examining nurse safety. There were 586 respondents, one third of whom disclosed "that they were victims of workplace violence in 1996. Most nurses indicated patients were the assailants. … Yet half of the nurses acknowledged that violence went unreported at work" (Carroll and Goldsmith, 1999, p. 26).

Assuring nurses of a healthy work environment is a major challenge for the next decade. It is not, however, a problem that nurses can expect will be solved by others. Clearly, nurses of the future must themselves take positive, effective, united action to ensure the basic dignity and safety of practicing nurses everywhere. They must demand and use safer needlestick devices and disposal containers; high-efficiency ventilation systems; alternatives to latex gloves and products; adequate housekeeping support; adequate lifting assistance with devices or additional personnel; reduction or elimination of shift rotation; and appropriate occupational safety and health training. Nurses themselves must use impeccable handwashing techniques and personal protective equipment such as gloves, gowns, and masks when needed. And they must demand that adequate security be provided to protect them against violent patients and family members.

CHALLENGES IN NURSING EDUCATION

As the profession of nursing matures, more nurses will recognize the value of bachelor's degrees for beginning professional practice and master's degrees for advanced practice. More nurses will pursue doctoral degrees to prepare for leadership roles in research, theory development, and teaching. In response, colleges of nursing will expand flexible educational programs to improve access. They will also develop differentiated levels of nursing education that correspond to differentiated levels of practice.

Outcome-Based Education

The quality of educational programs will continue to be judged by student competencies—that is, what students can actually do as a result of education. Nursing educational programs will monitor their graduates' activities and achievements as professional nurses. They will be required to report on graduates' accomplishments as part of the accreditation process. The emphasis on accountability of nursing education programs will increase as measures of competence in graduates are refined.

Just as nursing practice is being challenged to measure patient outcomes and adopt evidence-based practice, nursing education will be challenged to develop student outcomes and adopt evidence-based education. Faculty will modify age-old teaching/learning strategies and adopt new pedagogies (teaching methods) proven effective through research (i.e., evidence-based teaching). Passive learning, such as lectures, will be deemphasized. Critical thinking, independent decision making, and creative problem solving will assume even greater importance, fostered by role playing, simulations, and group problem solving (Huston and Fox, 1998). Faculty will be required to document evidence-based teaching as part of accreditation processes.

Accreditation of nursing education programs will become more difficult to achieve as national accrediting bodies come under increasing pressure to raise standards and to apply standards consistently. Substandard programs will be closed. This will strengthen nursing but will not help the nursing shortage.

Diversity

Students in nursing education programs will reflect the demographics of the United States and become more diverse than ever before. More men, older students, and students with baccalaureate degrees in other fields will come into nursing because of the emotional rewards, economic stability, and professional image it offers. Student bodies will become more culturally diverse, reflecting the diversity of the nation's population.

Access to education for nontraditional and traditional students will be an even greater issue. Schools will expand nontraditional curricula that enable adults to work and go to school simultaneously. Nursing courses delivered by **distance learning** technologies, such as telecommunications and satellite linkages, will increase access for students living in remote areas. Cost-minded legislators will require that state-supported schools offer fully articulated programs in order to qualify for state funding. Schools that fall behind in distance learning offerings will have difficulty filling their classes as more and more students seek nonresidential education.

Changes in demographics will affect the content of curricula, as well as the methods by which content is delivered. As the population ages, the need for nurses prepared in gerontology, chronic disease management, and hospice care will give emphasis to educational programs at both undergraduate and graduate levels. Curricula will emphasize community-based care instead of traditional hospital-based care. Educational programs will develop and expand multicultural courses. Foreign languages will again become a graduation requirement in baccalaureate programs. International educational opportunities will increase as the global village concept becomes a reality. Every nursing program will have the provision of culturally competent care as an outcome criterion for its graduates.

Technology and Nursing Informatics' Impact

Technological advances and the growth of nursing knowledge will create the need for informatics expertise in nursing education as well as in nursing practice. Computer competence will not suffice for nurses of the future. Students will need to master sophisticated information systems to use the wealth of available knowledge to improve and document patient care.

Faculty will be challenged to keep pace with students' acquisition of knowledge from the World Wide Web. Students of the future will become increasingly active in obtaining information from a vast array of sources available to them at the touch of a computer key. This will enable students to be more engaged in their own learning process and foster active learning.

Nursing faculty will be required to practice the profession actively to keep up with rapidly changing technologies. Maintaining faculty currency will become a greater focus in higher education. Active practice in addition to teaching will become an expected part of the faculty role. Students will be incorporated into faculty practices to obtain clinical experience. In this regard, nursing education will resemble medical education.

It will be impossible for nursing education programs to include in their curricula everything nurses of the future need to know. If, for example, genomics and disaster nursing are to be added to curricula, what will be removed? Nursing students already are overwhelmed with the amount of material they must master.

The solution to this problem is that all nurses must be educated to become lifelong learners. They must be taught to expect change and be prepared to adapt or retool their skills quickly to respond to health care marketplace demands (Huston and Fox, 1998). They must become active on their own behalf, pursuing knowledge and refreshing their knowledge base through vigorous, self-motivated continuing education efforts.

Licensing examinations will change to reflect the expansion of nursing knowledge and the increase in community-based practice and resulting autonomy. Licensure at multiple levels will become a reality. Employers of new graduates will expect to provide internships designed to enable novices to make the transition from student to practicing nurse effectively.

Collaboration

As nurses acquire more education, the resulting knowledge and self-confidence will enable them to develop collaborative relationships on an equal footing with physicians and other highly educated health care professionals. This will enable nurses to be more assertive in patient advocacy and will improve patient care and strengthen the profession.

Nursing faculty, nurse managers, and practicing nurses will join forces to strengthen educational experiences and mentorships for tomorrow's nurses. They will collaborate on clinical research that demonstrates the effectiveness of nursing care in terms of patient outcomes. They will collaborate with other nurses and consumer groups to remove regulatory restrictions that impede advanced clinical practice.

Nurse educators will recognize the need to treat students as professionals in training and will transform nursing education attitudes from controlling students to collaborating with them. This will create a new generation of empowered nursing professionals.

Disciplinary boundaries are becoming blurred as knowledge from all disciplines is brought to bear on problems of mutual concern, such as breast cancer, domestic violence, and AIDS. Nursing must become more interdisciplinary in its focus. Only nurses with a strong sense of personal and professional identity will be able to enter fully into multidisciplinary collaboration. Those nurses who understand the value of collaboration will become the managers of care using a case-management model, and they will thrive.

Reforms in Health Care and Higher Education

As a result of health care reform and cost-containment initiatives, nurses of the future will need to be well versed in the costs, budgeting, and financing of health care. Business education will be increasingly emphasized, particularly at the graduate level, as nurses pursue entrepreneurial and intrapreneurial roles. Nursing faculty will either return to school to prepare themselves to teach business courses or will create interdisciplinary alliances with business schools to provide nursing students with the necessary business courses.

Higher education will undergo public scrutiny and reform. It already suffers from serious underfunding. As governmental grants are reduced or eliminated to help balance the national budget and state tax revenues decline, educational programs will experience budgetary constraints. Several nursing education programs, including some well-regarded ones, had closed as a result of funding shortfalls. In many universities, autonomous schools and colleges of nursing were combined with health and human service programs into one administrative unit to save money. This often weakened the nursing program's voice on the campus. Budgets for operating expenses, equipment, and faculty salaries are under par in many locations, even though the demand for nursing education remains high.

For a time, it appeared that hospitals could be a source of support for nursing education programs, but with their own significant budgetary constraints, it is unlikely that this will be a long-term solution. Hospitals, however, will support nursing education for as long as possible with financial aid to students, subsidies of faculty salaries, joint appointments of faculty, and other forms of assistance.

Graduate education programs will change to produce practitioners who can meet consumer demands. Changes in hospital-based nursing practice will force a reexamination of the clinical nurse specialist and nurse practitioner roles. The need for efficiency and cost-effectiveness will lead to a revision of advanced practice models, and educational programs will combine the two roles and emphasize community-based practice.

Curricula at all levels will be standardized and streamlined to reduce cost and confusion and improve student mobility. The trend toward use of multiskilled workers will force nursing faculty to identify unique aspects of nursing and to educate students for broader roles in the delivery of patient care.

Faculty Shortage/Student Shortage

In the next decade, many long-time nursing faculty members, educated at the master's level during the nurse-traineeship funding heyday of the 1960s, will retire. There will be no one to replace many of them because relatively few younger nurses are entering teaching because nursing education salaries lag behind those in practice settings. By the year 2010, there will be a serious shortage of nursing faculty. This will force a major restructuring of nursing education programs and negatively affect the already problematic shortage of nurses.

Colleges of nursing already report turning away qualified applicants, often because of a lack of faculty to teach them. These two problems, too few faculty members and fewer students in the pipeline, combine to create a negative synergy and downward spiral in the number of practicing nurses. The nursing profession, working in collaboration with public and private funding sources policy makers, and employers of nurses must find a solution to these twin problems in the near future if nursing is to thrive as a profession. Creating a more desirable work environment for practicing nurses, thereby retaining nurses who might otherwise leave the profession, will attain a greater and much-needed focus (Valentino, 2002).

As the faculty shortage in nursing is translated into a student shortage—and therefore to a worsening of the nursing shortage—medical schools are increasing their output of physicians. Of particular concern is the trend toward physician role expansion in the area of inpatient care by **hospitalists.** These are physicians who are hospital-based and care for patients only while they are hospitalized. They "are predicted to care for many nonsurgical patients by 2005, thus decreasing demand for advanced practice nurses" (Wolf, 2003, p. 32). Since advanced practice nursing is the goal of many of today's undergraduate nursing students, this is a troubling trend that bears monitoring.

A CHALLENGE TO THE ENTIRE NURSING PROFESSION: FOCUS, UNITE, ACT!

Most of the important issues the nursing profession will face in the next decade cannot be resolved by any one group of nurses. These concerns will require the attention of the entire profession, working in a focused, united, active manner through nursing's professional associations. Although collective power is the only way nursing will effectively resolve these issues, fewer than 10 percent of all nurses belong to their professional association, a sad commentary on the priorities most nurses place on this vital aspect of professionalism.

As the largest health care profession in the United States, with over 2.7 million registered nurse members, nursing *can* and *should* have a powerful voice and presence at every table where substantive health care issues are discussed. However, nurses have historically been unwilling to throw their support behind their professional organizations. They have allowed issues of educational background, political philosophies, abortion, and other concerns to divide them.

If you think for a moment about other groups to which you belong—for example, a political party, church, or parent-teacher association—you do not expect to agree with every position taken by the organization or its leaders. Nurses seem to have such an expectation of their professional association, however, and use that as a reason for lack of unity. This is naïve and unrealistic. With nursing and society becoming increasingly diverse, nurses of the future must become more tolerant of differences and work hard to find common ground with their colleagues in the profession. If we fail to do so, nursing will not prosper, nor will its practitioners.

Nursing's Agenda for the Future

An encouraging development was the coming together in 2001 of 19 major nursing organizations at the Nursing Profession Summit. A $100,000 grant from the American Nurses Foundation, a branch of the American Nurses Association, enabled the ANA to convene this group, which formed a steering committee. The steering committee took leadership in identifying 10 domains (areas) that describe the work needed to accomplish the vision they set forth in a document titled *Nursing's Agenda for the Future*. This document identifies what the steering committee envisioned: how nursing should look and where it should be by the year 2010.

In other words, this committee developed a desired future vision for nursing and set forth areas that must be addressed to achieve the desired vision.

The steering committee called on all nurses to review *Nursing's Agenda for the Future* "and to find those objectives that match with the mission, priorities and resources of their own entities. The intent is to involve as many nurses as possible in charting their own future. It is this critical ... step that will bring the strategic plan to life, move it forward and make progress toward the desired future state" (Nursing's Agenda Steering Committee, 2002, pp. 6-7). You can download the report in PDF form from the ANA website, Nursing World *(www.nursingworld.org/ naf)*. I challenge you to do so and to decide how *you* will participate in achieving the vision.

You, the readers of this book, are the future of the nursing profession. You represent our best hope for building nursing into an even more powerful force for good. Look around at the other members of your class. Whether you have 25 fellow students or 125, you can accomplish far more working together than you can working in isolation. So it is with nursing's future: we can accomplish far more by working collectively. All nurses, individually and as a profession, will benefit from the results.

Summary of Key Points

- Future societal changes will occur in the following areas: demographics, the environment, potential for disasters such as bioterrorism, lifestyles, economics, and governmental regulation of health care.
- Both nursing practice and nursing education will be affected by these changes.
- Today's nurses should be prepared to serve effectively as members of an emergency and disaster response team.
- Nursing roles will be differentiated.
- Nursing practice will become more community-based with new roles continually emerging.
- Nurses will be able to demonstrate that the care they provide makes a positive difference in patient outcomes.
- Nurses will continue to provide a warm, humanizing influence on patient care in potentially dehumanizing high-tech environments.
- Effective nurses will become culturally competent.
- The major challenges for nursing education will be to respond to societal changes rapidly with appropriate curricular modifications; to produce a steady supply of well-prepared graduates in the face of an aging faculty; to adapt to rapidly changing technology; to acquire competency needed to respond to increasing cultural diversity of students and patients; and to address the lack of human and budgetary resources in higher education.
- Active membership in professional associations is the best way for nurses to focus, unite, and act to solve the challenges facing the profession.

CRITICAL THINKING QUESTIONS

1. As the number of elderly Americans rises, the rate of chronic illness also rises. What challenges does this present for nurses of the future?

2. Take a position on the statement "Nurses of the future will have an impact on the environment that exceeds that of the ordinary citizen." Be prepared to defend your position.

3. Describe economic issues that will affect nurses of the future. How can you begin now to prepare yourself to deal with these issues?

4. Initiate a classroom debate on the issue "HIV-positive nurses should not be limited in how they practice nursing."

5. As a class, brainstorm ways a school health nurse could improve pupils' health status. Then design an educational program to prepare school nurses. Compare your curriculum with that of an existing school health nurse program.

6. Interview faculty members to identify components of your educational program that will prepare you for the culturally competent nursing needed in the twenty-first century. Report your findings to the class.

7. Using the core competencies listed in Box 18-1, evaluate your own disaster preparedness and devise a plan to become better prepared.

8. Using the GeneTests website as a resource *(www.genetests.org)*, learn all you can about testing, counseling, and treatment for a genetic condition. These might include albinism, sickle cell disease, hereditary breast or ovarian cancer, hemophilia, hemochromatosis, Marfan's syndrome, cystic fibrosis, or others of interest to you or your family. Report your findings to the class.

REFERENCES

American Lung Association: Facts about lung cancer, Online, 2003 *(www.lungusa.org/diseases/lungcanc.html)*.

American Nurses Association: Bioterrorism website, 2003a *(www.nursingworld.org/news/disaster/biocare.htm)*.

American Nurses Association: Workplace issues: occupational safety and health, Online, 2003b *(www.nursingworld.org/osh/latex.htm)*.

Carroll V, Goldsmith J: One-third of nurses are abused in the workplace, *Reflections* 25(3):24-27, 1999.

Coleman EA: Anthrax: know the guidelines for management, *Am J Nurs* 101(12):48-52, 2001.

Dickenson-Hazard N: Future study or the Magic 8 Ball? *Reflect Nurs Leadersh* 29(4):4, 2003.

Gary FA, Sigsby LM, Campbell D: Preparing for the 21st century: diversity in nursing education, research, and practice, *J Prof Nurs* 14(5), 272-279, 1998.

Gebbie KM, Qureshi K: Emergency and disaster preparedness: core competencies for nurses, *Am J Nurs* 102(1):46-51, 2002.

Hendrick B: The coming millennium, *The Atlanta Journal/The Atlanta Constitution,* July 16, A12, 1995.

Herbert LE, Scherr PA, Beckett LA, et al: Alzheimer's disease, *JAMA* 273(17):1354-1359, 1995.

Huston CJ, Fox S: The changing health care market: implications for nursing education in the coming decade, *Nurs Outlook* 46(3):109-114, 1998.

Lea DH, Monsen RB: Preparing nurses for a 21st century role in genomics-based health care, *Nurs Ed Perspect* 24(2):75-80, 2003.

McKenna MAJ: Going mainstream, *The Atlanta Journal/The Atlanta Constitution*, May 17, C8, 1995.

Nursing's Agenda for the Future Steering Committee: *Nursing's agenda for the future: the future vision for nursing,* Washington, DC, 2002, American Nurses Publishing.

Perla L: The future role of nurses, *J Nurses Staff Dev* 18(4):194-197, 2002.

U.S. Census Bureau: Population clock, U.S. and International, 2003 *(www.census.gov/main/www/popclock.html).*

Valentino LM: Future employment trends in nursing, *AJN 2002 career guide,* New York, 2002, Lippincott Williams and Wilkins.

Wolf G: Coming of age in health care: changes, challenges, choices, *Reflect Nurs Leadersh* 29(4):32-34, 2003.

Epilogue

You, our readers, are inheriting a rich legacy of achievement and progress in the nursing profession. While appreciating the accomplishments of those who paved the way for us, let us not lose sight of the fact that much remains to be done. As health care professionals, you will be challenged to lead your communities in addressing the complex issues of health care costs, access to health care for the disenfranchised, and other not-yet-imagined concerns. You will be part of the solution.

It is the hope of all the nurses who have participated in preparing this textbook that through this book you have been stimulated to develop values, beliefs, knowledge, professionalism, and desire to become a nursing leader of the future and a positive force for change in the nursing profession.

You can begin exerting your influence to improve the profession by evaluating this book. If you are willing to help in this way, please email me and I will send you a brief questionnaire. I also encourage you to share any opinions you have about the helpful and unhelpful aspects of the current edition. With your help we can continue to improve the textbook to better meet the needs of future students.

KayKChitty1@comcast.net

Glossary

AACN American Association of Colleges of Nursing.

Acceptance See Nonjudgmental acceptance.

Accountability Responsibility for one's behavior.

Accreditation A voluntary review process of educational programs or service agencies by professional organizations.

Action language A developmental phase in language development of older infants. Examples include reaching for or crawling toward a desired object or of closing the lips and turning the head when an undesired food is offered.

Active collaborator One who is engaged as a participant with another person.

Active listening A method of communicating interest and attention using such signals as good eye contact, nodding, and encouraging the speaker.

Acuity Degree of illness.

Acute illness Sudden, steadily progressing symptoms that subside quickly with or without treatment, such as influenza.

Adaptation A change or coping response to stress of any kind.

Adaptation model A conceptual model that focuses on the patient as an adaptive system; that is, one that strives to cope with both internal demands and external demands of the environment.

Adjudicate To decide or sit in judgment, as in a legal case.

Administrative law Law created by a governmental agency to meet the intent of statutory law.

Advance directives Written instructions recognized by state law that describe individuals' preferences in regard to medical intervention should they become incapacitated.

Advanced degrees Degrees beyond the bachelor's degree; master's and doctoral degrees.

Advanced practice Nursing roles that require either a master's degree or specialized education in a specific area.

Aesthetics Branch within philosophy that studies the nature of beauty.

Affective goal Effort directed toward a change in a patient's feelings, values, or belief system.

Alternative educational programs Programs other than basic nursing programs, such as baccalaureate programs for registered nurses and the Excelsior Program, formerly known as the New York Regents' External Degree Program.

Alternative treatment Treatment other than traditional Western medical treatment.

Altruism Unselfish concern for the welfare of others.

Ambulatory care Health services provided to those who visit a clinic or hospital as outpatients and depart after treatment on the same day.

American Assembly for Men in Nursing (AAMN) Professional organization that seeks to encourage, support, and advocate for men in nursing.

American Association of Colleges of Nursing A national organization devoted to advancing nursing education at the baccalaureate and graduate levels.

American Nurses Association A professional organization that addresses ethics, clinical standards, public policy, and the economic and general welfare of nurses. Membership is limited to nurses.

American Organization of Nurse Executives (AONE) An organization for high-level nursing managers, such as chief nurses. Leaders in nursing education can be associate members.

ANA Position Paper A 1965 paper published by the American Nurses Association concluding that baccalaureate education should become the basic foundation for professional practice.

Analysis The second step in the nursing process during which various pieces of patient data are analyzed. The outcome is one or more nursing diagnoses.

Ancillary workers Nonprofessional auxiliary health care workers, such as nursing assistants.

Androcentric Male-centered cultural bias.

Anxiety A diffuse, vague feeling of apprehension and uncertainty.

Applied science Use of scientific theory and laws in a practical way that has immediate application.

Appropriateness A criterion for successful communication in which the reply fits the circumstances and matches the message, and the amount is neither too great nor too little.

Articulation An educational mobility system providing for direct movement from a program at one level of nursing education to another without significant loss of credit.

Assault A threat or an attempt to make bodily contact with another person without the person's consent.

Assessment The first step in the nursing process involving the collection of information about the patient.

Assisted suicide Suicide by a person with help from another person, such as a health care provider.

Associate degree program   The newest form of basic nursing education program, leading to the associate degree (AD), consisting of 3 or fewer years, and usually offered in technical or community colleges.

Association   An organization of members with common interests.

Authority   Possessing both the responsibility for making decisions and the accountability for the outcome of those decisions.

Autonomy   Self-governing; freedom from the influence of others.

Baccalaureate degree in nursing (BSN)   Degree offered by programs that combine nursing courses with general education courses in a 4- or 5-year curriculum in a senior college or university.

Balance of power   A distribution of forces among the branches of government so that no one branch is strong enough to dominate the others.

Ball, Mary Ann   A Civil War woman who cared for the wounded and was known as "Mother Bickerdyke." She lived from 1817 to 1901.

Barton, Clara   A famous Civil War nurse and founder of the American Red Cross who lived from 1821 to 1912.

Basic program   Any nursing education program preparing beginning practitioners.

Battery   The impermissible, unprivileged touching of one person by another.

Belief   The intellectual acceptance of something as true or correct.

Belief system   Organization of an individual's beliefs into a rational whole.

Beneficence   The ethical principle of doing good.

Benner, Patricia   Nursing theorist who proposed seven domains of nursing practice based on her research into the nature of nurses' knowledge.

Mother Bickerdyke   Affectionate nickname given by soldiers to Mary Ann Ball, a Civil War lay nurse.

Biculturalism   A term used to describe a nurse's ability to balance the ideal nursing culture learned about in school and the real one experienced in practice, using the best of both.

Bioethics   An area of ethical inquiry focusing on the dilemmas inherent in modern health care.

Biomedical technology   Complex machines or implantable devices used in patient care settings.

Bioterrorism   The use of a biological or chemical agent as a weapon.

Birthrate   The number of births in a particular place during a specific time period, usually expressed as a quantity per 1,000 people in a year.

Breckinridge, Mary   Founder of the Frontier Nursing Service in 1925.

BRN   Baccalaureate registered nurse, a term sometimes used to describe a registered nurse who has returned to school to earn a bachelor's degree.

Brown Report   A 1948 report recommending that basic schools of nursing be placed in universities and colleges and that efforts be made to recruit large numbers of men and minorities into nursing education programs.

Burnout   A state of emotional exhaustion due to cumulative stress.

Cadet Corps   A government-created entity designed during World War II to rapidly increase the number of registered nurses being educated to assist in the war effort.

Capitation   A cost management system in which a certain amount of money is paid to a provider annually to take care of all of an individual's or group's health care needs.

"Captain of the ship" doctrine   A legal principle that implies that the physician is in charge of all patient care and, thus, should be financially responsible if damages are sought.

Caring   Watching over, attending to, and providing for the needs of others.

Case management   Systematic collaboration with patients, their significant others, and their health care providers to coordinate high-quality health care services in a cost-effective manner with positive patient outcomes.

Case management nursing   A growing field within nursing in which nurses are responsible for coordinating services provided to patients in a cost-effective manner.

Case manager   An individual responsible for coordinating services provided to a group of patients.

CCNE   Commission on Collegiate Nursing Education, the accrediting arm of the American Association of Colleges of Nursing.

Centenarian   A person who has reached the age of 100 or more years.

Centers for Medicare and Medicaid Services (CMS)   Federal cost-containment program that establishes standards and monitors care in the Medicare and Medicaid programs. Formerly known as Health Care Financing Administration (HCFA).

Certificate of need (CON)   A cost-containment measure requiring health care agencies to apply to a state agency for permission to construct or substantially add to an existing facility.

Certified nurse-midwife   A nationally certified nurse with advanced specialized education who assists women and couples during uncomplicated pregnancies, deliveries, and postdelivery periods.

Certified Registered Nurse Anesthetist (CRNA)   A nationally certified nurse with advanced education who specializes in the administration of anesthesia.

Certification   Validation of specific qualifications demonstrated by a registered nurse in a defined area of practice.

Change agent   An individual who recognizes the need for organizational change and facilitates that process.

Chief executive officer (CEO)   The senior administrator of an organization.

Chief nurse executive   The senior nursing administrator of an organization.

Chief of staff   A physician in a health care facility, generally elected by the medical staff for a specified term, who is responsible for overseeing the activities of the medical staff organization.

Chronic illness   Ongoing health problems of a generally incurable nature, such as diabetes.

Civil law   Law involving disputes between individuals.

Clarification   A therapeutic communication technique in which the nurse seeks to understand a patient's message more clearly.

Clinical coordinator   See Clinical director.

Clinical director   Middle management nurse who has responsibility for multiple units in a health care agency.

Clinical judgment   The ability to make consistently effective clinical decisions based on theoretical knowledge, informed opinions, and prior experience.

Clinical ladder   Programs allowing nurses to progress in the organizational hierarchy while staying in direct patient care roles.

Clinical nurse specialist   A nurse with an advanced degree who serves as a resource person to other nurses and often provides direct care to patients or families with particularly difficult or complex problems.

Closed system   A system that does not interact with other systems or with the surrounding environment.

Coalition   A temporary alliance of distinct factions.

Code of Academic and Clinical Conduct   Code of ethics of the National Student Nurses Association.

Code of Ethics for Nurses   A formal statement of the nursing profession's code of ethics.

Code of ethics   A statement of professional standards used to guide behavior and as a framework for decision making.

Cognitive   Pertaining to intellectual activities requiring knowledge.

Cognitive goal   Effort directed toward a desired change in a patient's knowledge level.

Cognitive rebellion   A stage in the educational process wherein students begin to free themselves from external controls and to rely on their own judgment.

Collaboration   Working closely with another person in the spirit of cooperation.

Collective action   Activities undertaken by or on behalf of a group of people who have common interests.

Collective bargaining   Negotiating as a group for improved salary and work conditions.

Collective identity   The connection and feeling of similarity individuals in a particular group feel with one another; group identification.

Collegiality   The promotion of collaboration, cooperation, and recognition of interdependence among members of a profession.

Common law   Law that comes about as a result of decisions made by judges in legal cases.

Communication   The exchange of thoughts, ideas, or information; a dynamic process that is a primary instrument through which change occurs in nursing situations.

Community-based nursing   Nursing care provided for individuals, families, and groups in a variety of settings, including homes, workplaces, schools, and other places.

Community health nursing   Formerly known as public health nursing; a nursing specialty that systematically uses a process of delivering nursing care to improve the health of an entire community.

Competency   Refers to the capability of a particular patient to understand the information given and to make an informed choice about treatment options.

Concept   An abstract classification of data; for example, "temperature" is a concept.

Conceptual model or framework   A group of concepts that are broadly defined and systematically organized to provide a focus, a rationale, and a tool for the integration and interpretation of information.

Confidentiality   Ensuring the privacy of individuals participating in research studies or being treated in health care settings.

Congruent   A characteristic of communication that occurs when the verbal and nonverbal elements of a message match.

Constituent Member Association (CMA)   Organizational members of the American Nurses Association, such as state nurses associations or specialty nursing organizations.

Consultation   The process of conferring with patients, families, or other health professionals.

Consumerism   A movement to protect consumers from unsafe or inferior products and services.

Contact hour   A measurement used to recognize participation in continuing education offerings, usually equivalent to 50 minutes.

Context   An essential element of communication consisting of the setting in which an interaction occurs, the mood, the relationship between sender and receiver, and other factors.

Continuing education (CE)   Informal ways, such as workshops, conferences, and short courses, in which nurses maintain competence during their professional careers.

Continuous quality improvement (CQI)   A management concept focusing on excellence and employee involvement at all levels of an organization.

Contracts   Documents agreed to by workers and management that include provisions about staffing levels, salary, work conditions, and other issues of concern to either party.

Copayment   The portion of a provider's charges that an insured patient is responsible for paying.

Coping   The methods a person uses to assess and manage demands.

Coping mechanisms   Psychological devices used by individuals when a threat is perceived.

Cost containment   An attempt to keep health care costs stable or increasing only slowly.

Criminal law   Law involving public concerns against unlawful behavior that threatens society.

Critical paths   Multidisciplinary care plans.

Cross-functional team   People from all parts of an organization who contribute to a particular activity and outcome.

Cross-training   Preparing a single worker for multiple tasks that formerly were performed by multiple specialized workers.

Cultural assessment   The process of determining a patient's cultural practices and preferences in order to render culturally competent care.

Cultural care, theory of   A nursing theory focusing on the importance of incorporating a patient's culturally determined health beliefs and practices into care.

Cultural competence   The integration of knowledge, attitudes, and skills that enhance cross-cultural communication and appropriate interactions with others.

Cultural diversity Social, ethnic, racial, and religious differences in a group.

Culturally competent care Nursing care that incorporates knowledge, attitudes, and skills that enhance cross-cultural communication and appropriate interactions with others.

Culture The attitudes, beliefs, and behaviors of social and ethnic groups that have been perpetuated through generations.

Culture of nursing The rites, rituals, and valued behaviors of the nursing profession.

Curtis, Namahyoke The first trained African-American nurse employed as a military hospital nurse during the Spanish-American War of 1898.

Data Information or facts collected for analysis.

Davis, Mary E. One of the founders of the *American Journal of Nursing*.

Deaconess Institute A large hospital and planned training program for deaconesses established in 1836 by Pastor Theodor Fliedner at Kaiserswerth, Germany.

Decentralization An organizational structure in which decision-making authority is shared with employees most affected by the decisions rather than being retained by top executives.

Deductible The out-of-pocket amount individuals must pay before their health insurance begins to pay for health care.

Deductive reasoning A process through which conclusions are drawn by logical inference from given premises; proceeds from the general case to the specific.

Defining characteristics Signs and symptoms of disease.

Delegate To refer a task to another.

Delegation The practice of assigning tasks or responsibilities to other persons.

Demographics The study of vital statistics and social trends.

Demography The science that studies vital statistics and social trends.

Deontology The ethical theory that the rightness or wrongness of an action depends on the inherent moral significance of the action.

Dependency The degree to which individuals adopt passive attitudes and rely on others to take care of them.

Dependent intervention Nursing actions on behalf of patients that require knowledge and skill on the part of the nurse but may not be done without explicit directions from another health professional, usually a physician, dentist, or nurse practitioner.

Designer medicines Pharmacological agents developed for an individual, based on his or her genetic makeup.

Developmental theory A theory in which growth is defined as an increase in physical size and shape toward a point of optimal maturity.

Diagnosis Identification of a disease or condition.

Diagnosis-related groups (DRGs) A method of classifying and grouping illnesses according to similarities of diagnosis for reimbursement purposes.

Dietitian Bachelor's-educated nutrition expert who specializes in therapeutic diet preparation and nutrition education.

Differentiated practice Nursing practice at two levels, professional and technical, with differences in both educational preparation and clinical responsibilities.

Diploma program The earliest form of formal nursing education in the United States; usually based in hospitals, require 3 years of study, and lead to a diploma in nursing.

Disaster An event or situation that is of greater magnitude than an emergency; disrupts essential services such as housing, transportation, communications, sanitation, water, and health care; and requires the response of people outside the community affected.

Disease A pathological alteration at the tissue or organ level.

Disease management A process of helping patients understand and manage their chronic conditions more effectively through phone calls, coaching and education, symptom prevention and management and collaboration with the patient's health care provider.

Disenfranchised The state of having no power or no voice in a political system.

Disseminate Publish or widely distribute scientific information, such as the findings of a research study.

Dissonance Lack of harmony.

Distance learning The process of taking classes and earning academic credit through technological means such as televised or online classes. The teacher and student may be many miles apart.

Dix, Dorothea L. A Boston schoolteacher, devoted to the care of the mentally ill, who served as the first superintendent of the Women Nurses of the Army during the Civil War.

Dock, Lavinia A well-known early twentieth-century nurse who was actively involved in women's rights issues and the suffragette movement.

Documentation Written communication about patient care, usually found in the patient record.

Dominant culture Mainstream culture that contains one or more subcultures.

Double effect Ethical concept encompassing the belief that there are some situations in which it is necessary to inflict potential harm in an effort to achieve a greater good.

Duty of care The responsibility of a nurse or other health professional for the care of a patient.

Duty to report The requirement, according to state law, for health professionals to report certain illnesses, injuries, and actions of patients.

Economic and general welfare Employment issues relating to salaries, benefits, and working conditions.

Educative instrument A tool for increasing the knowledge and power of another person.

Efficiency A criterion for successful communication that consists of using simple, clear words timed at a pace suitable to participants.

Electoral process The procedures that must be followed to select someone to fill an elected position.

Elliott, Francis Reed The first African-American nurse accepted by the American Red Cross Nursing Service in 1918.

Emotional intelligence Awareness of and sensitivity to the feelings of others.

Empathy Awareness of, sensitivity to, and identification with the feelings of another person.

Entrepreneur A person who sees a need for, organizes, manages, and assumes responsibility for a new enterprise or business.

Environment All the many factors, such as physical or psychological, that influence life and survival.

Epidemiologist A scientist who studies the origins and transmission of diseases.

Epistemology The branch of philosophy dealing with the theory of knowledge.

Ethical decision making The process of choosing between actions based on a system of beliefs and values.

Ethics The branch of philosophy that studies the propriety of certain courses of action.

Ethnocentric The belief that one's own culture is the most desirable.

Ethnographic research A type of qualitative research.

Euthanasia The act of painlessly putting to death a person suffering from an incurable disease; also called mercy killing.

Evaluation Measuring the success or failure of the outputs and consequently the effectiveness of a system. It is the final step in the nursing process wherein the nurse examines the patient's progress to determine whether a problem is solved, is in the process of being solved, or is unsolved. In communication theory, the analysis of information received.

Evidence-based practice Using research findings as a basis for practice rather than trial and error, intuition, or traditional methods.

Exacerbation Reemergence or worsening of the symptoms of a chronic illness.

Executive branch The branch of government responsible for administering the laws of the land.

Experimental design Research design that provides evidence of a cause-and-effect relationship between actions.

Expert power Strength that derives from knowledge that can influence an outcome.

Expert witness An individual called on to testify in court because of special skill or knowledge in a certain field, such as nursing.

Extended care Medical, nursing, or custodial care provided to an individual over a prolonged period of time.

Extended family A term used to describe nonnuclear family members such as grandparents, aunts, and uncles.

External degree program An alternative program in which learning is independent and is assessed through highly standardized and validated examinations.

External factors Values, beliefs, and behaviors of significant others that have an impact on an individual.

False reassurance A nontherapeutic form of communication.

Family system The group of individuals who comprise the basic unit of family living and their interactions with one another and the larger society.

Famous trio Three famous schools of nursing founded in 1873: the Bellevue Training School, the Connecticut Training School, and the Boston Training School.

Feedback The information given back into a system to determine whether or not the purpose of the system has been achieved. A major element in the communication process.

Feminism Belief in the value and equality of women.

Fidelity An ethical principle that values faithfulness to one's responsibilities.

Flexibility A criterion for successful communication that occurs when messages are based on the immediate situation rather than preconceived expectations.

Flexible staffing A mechanism whereby nurses may work at times other than the traditional hospital shifts.

Flexner Report A 1910 study of medical education that provided the impetus for much needed reform.

Ford, Loretta With Dr. E. K. Silver, founded the nurse practitioner movement in the United States in the mid-1960s.

Formal socialization The process by which individuals learn a new role through what others purposely teach them.

For-profit agency A health care agency established to make a profit for the owners or stockholders.

Franklin, Martha Founder, in 1908, of the National Association of Colored Graduate Nurses (NACGN).

Frontier Nursing Service Founded in Kentucky in 1925 and provided the first organized midwifery service in the United States.

Functional nursing A system of nursing care delivery in which each worker has a task, or function, to perform for all patients.

Futurist An individual who studies trends and makes predictions about the future.

Galileo An Italian physicist and astronomer who lived from 1564 to 1642.

Gatekeeper An individual, generally a primary care physician, who controls patients' access to diagnostic procedures, medical specialists, and hospitalization.

Gender-role stereotyping The practice of automatically and routinely linking positive or negative characteristics to either males or females; also called sex-role stereotyping.

General election An election in which all registered voters may vote and may choose a candidate from any party on the ballot.

General systems theory A theory promulgated by Ludwig von Bertalanffy in the late 1930s to explain the relationship of a whole to its parts.

Generalizable Research findings that are transferable to other situations.

Generic master's degree An accelerated master's degree in nursing for people with nonnursing bachelor's degrees.

Generic nursing doctorate A doctoral degree program designed for individuals who are not already registered nurses and who possess baccalaureate degrees in other fields.

Genetic counseling Health and reproductive advice given to individuals based on their genetic makeup.

Goldmark Report A major study of nursing education published in 1923 and named *The Study of Nursing and Nursing Education in the United States*.

Goodrich, Annie Served as assistant professor of nursing at Teachers College, head of the Army School of Nursing (formed in 1918), president of the American Nurses Association, and first dean of the school of nursing at Yale University.

Governmental (public) agency An agency primarily supported by taxes, administered by elected or appointed officials, and tailored to the needs of the communities served.

Grassroots activism The involvement of a large number of people, generally widely dispersed, who are concerned about a particular issue.

Growth An increase in physical size and shape toward a point of optimal maturity.

Hardiness A personality characteristic that enables people to manage the changes associated with illness and to have fewer physical illnesses resulting from stress.

Health An individual's physical, mental, spiritual, and social well-being; a continuum, not a constant state.

Health behaviors Choices and habitual actions that promote or diminish health.

Health beliefs Culturally determined beliefs about the nature of health and illness.

Health care network A corporation with a consolidated set of facilities and services for comprehensive health care.

Health Insurance Portability and Accountability Act (HIPAA) Federal law, passed in 1996, designed to protect health insurance coverage for workers and their families when they change or lose their jobs.

Health maintenance Preventing illness and maintaining maximal function.

Health maintenance organization (HMO) A network or group of providers who agree to provide certain basic health care services for a single predetermined yearly fee.

Health promotion Encouraging a condition of maximum physical, mental, and social well-being.

Health promotion model A theoretical nursing model that uses illness prevention and health promotion as a basic framework.

Helping professions Professions such as social work, teaching, and nursing that emphasize meeting the needs of clients.

Henderson, Virginia An influential twentieth-century nursing author and theorist who was widely known for her nursing textbooks, insightful definition of nursing, and identification of 14 basic patient needs.

Henry Street Settlement A clinic for the poor founded by Lillian Wald and her colleague Mary Brewster on New York's Lower East Side.

Heterogeneous Composed of parts of differing kinds.

High-level wellness Functioning at maximum potential in an integrated way within the environment.

High-tech nursing Nursing care that involves the use of technologies such as monitors, pumps, and ventilators.

High-touch nursing Nursing care that involves the use of interpersonal skills such as communication, listening, and empathy.

Hill-Burton Act A 1946 federal law that called for and funded surveys of states' needs for hospitals, paid for planning hospitals and public health centers, and provided partial funding for constructing and equipping them.

Hippocrates (400 B.C.) A Greek physician who believed that disease had natural, not magical, causes; known as the father of medicine.

Holism A school of health care thought that espouses treating the whole patient: body, mind, and spirit.

Holistic communication Sharing both emotional and factual information and appreciating another individual's point of view.

Holistic nursing care Nursing care that nourishes the whole person—that is, the body, mind, and spirit.

Holistic nursing research Nursing research that considers the whole person—that is, the body, mind, and spirit.

Holistic values The approach to nursing practice that takes the physical, emotional, social, economic, and spiritual needs of the person into consideration.

Home health agency An organization that delivers various health services to patients in their homes.

Home health nursing Rapidly growing field of nursing in which nursing care is provided to patients in their own homes.

Homeostasis A relative constancy in the internal environment of the body.

Homogeneous Composed of parts of the same or similar kinds.

Hospice An agency that provides services to terminally ill patients and their families.

Hospice care nursing A specialized nurse who provides end-of-life care to patients and their families in homes and residential facilities.

Hospitalist Hospital-based physicians who care for patients only while they are hospitalized.

Human caring, theory of Nursing theory emphasizing the nurturing aspects of professional nursing through which curative strategies are implemented.

Human Genome Project A scientific project designed to map the genetic structure of composite human DNA.

Human motivation Abraham Maslow's conceptualization of human needs and their relationship to the stimulation of purposeful behavior.

Human needs theory Theory proposed by Abraham Maslow that human motivation is determined by the drive to meet intrinsic human needs.

Human responses The problems an individual experiences as a result of a disease process.

Humanistic nursing care Care that includes viewing professional relationships as human-to-human rather than nurse-to-patient.

Humanistic nursing values The approach to professional relationships as human-to-human experiences rather than nurse-to-patient experiences.

Hypothesis A statement predicting the relationship among various concepts or events.

Illness An abnormal process in which an individual's physical, emotional, social, or intellectual functioning is impaired.

Illness prevention All activities aimed at diminishing the likelihood that an individual's physical, emotional, social, and intellectual functions become impaired.

Implementation A stage of the nursing process during which the plan of care is carried out.

Incongruent Describes a confusing form of communication that occurs when the verbal and nonverbal elements of a message do not match.

Independent intervention Actions on behalf of patients for which the nurse requires no supervision or direction.

Inductive reasoning The process of reasoning from the specific to the general. Repeated observations of an experiment or event enable the observer to draw general conclusions.

Inertia Disinclination to change.

Informal socialization The process through which individuals learn a new role by observing how others behave.

Informatics nurse A nurse who combines nursing science with information management science and computer science to manage and make accessible information nurses need.

Information technology (IT) Hardware and software used to manage and process information.

Informed consent The process of asking individuals who are scheduled to undergo diagnostic procedures or surgery or who are potential research subjects to sign a consent form once the procedures and risks have been explained and their privacy has been ensured.

Infrastructure Basic support mechanisms needed to ensure that an activity can be conducted.

Input The information, energy, or matter that enters a system.

Institutional review board A committee that ensures that research is well designed and ethical and does not violate the policies and procedures of the institution in which it is conducted.

Institutional structure The way in which the workers within an agency are organized to carry out the functions of the agency.

Interdependent intervention Actions on behalf of patients in which the nurse must collaborate or consult with another health professional before or while carrying out the action.

Interdisciplinary team Group composed of individuals representing various disciplines who work together toward a common end.

Internal factors Personal feelings and beliefs that influence an individual.

Internalize The process of taking in knowledge, skills, attitudes, beliefs, norms, values, and ethical standards and making them a part of one's own self-image and behavior.

International Council of Nurses (ICN) The federation of national nurses associations, currently representing nurses in more than 100 countries.

Internship An apprenticeship under supervision.

Irrational belief A fixed idea that is not affected by information to the contrary.

Issues management Assisting a group to resolve a particular question about which there are significant differences of opinion.

Job hopping Moving rapidly from job to job.

Johnson, Dorothy Nursing theorist who proposed a system of nursing based on observation of patient behavior.

Judicial branch The branch of government that decides cases or controversies on particular matters.

Justice An ethical principle stating that equals should be treated the same and that unequals should be treated differently.

King, Imogene Nursing theorist who proposed a theory of goal attainment.

Knowledge-based power Authority or control based on the way information is used to effect an outcome.

Knowledge technology The use of computer systems to transform information into knowledge and to generate new knowledge; expert systems.

Latent power Untapped ability.

Law All the rules of conduct established by a government and applicable to the people, whether in the form of legislation or custom.

Learned resourcefulness An acquired ability to use available resources in one's behalf.

Legal authority A group of people in whom power is vested by law, such as the powers vested in state boards of nursing by nursing practice acts.

Legislative branch The branch of government consisting of elected officials who are responsible for enacting the laws of the land.

Leininger, Madeleine Nurse theorist best known for her theory of cultural care.

Length of stay (LOS) The number of days a patient stays in an inpatient setting, such as a hospital.

Levine, Myra Nursing theorist who proposed a model based on principles of wholeness, adaptation, and conservation.

Licensure The process by which an agency of government grants permission to qualified persons to engage in a given profession or occupation.

Licensure by endorsement A system whereby registered nurses or licensed practical/vocational nurses can, by submitting proof of licensure in another state and paying a licensure fee, receive licensure from the new state without sitting for a licensing examination.

Lobby An attempt to influence the vote of legislators.

Locus of control The place an individual believes the power in his life resides, either within himself or outside of himself.

Logic The field of philosophy that studies correct and incorrect reasoning.

Long-term care Care provided to individuals, such as people with Alzheimer's disease, who require lengthy assistance in the maintenance of activities of daily living.

Long-term goals Major changes that may take months or even years to accomplish.

Lysaught Report A 1970 report entitled *An Abstract for Action* that made recommendations concerning the supply and demand for nurses, nursing roles and functions, and nursing education.

Mahoney, Mary Eliza America's first African-American "trained nurse," who lived from 1845 to 1926.

Malpractice An unintentional tort that occurs when a professional fails to act as a reasonably prudent professional would under specific circumstances.

Managed care A process in which an individual, often a nurse, is assigned to review patients' cases and coordinate services so that quality care can be achieved at the lowest cost.

Managed care organization (MCO) Any of a number of organizations that attempt to coordinate subscriber services to ensure quality care at the lowest cost.

Mandatory continuing education The requirement that nurses complete a certain number of hours of continuing education as a prerequisite for relicensure.

Maslow, Abraham An American humanistic psychologist who formulated a theory of human motivation in the 1940s.

Maximum health potential The highest level of well-being that an individual is capable of attaining.

Medicaid A jointly funded federal and state public health insurance that covers citizens below the poverty level and those with certain disabling conditions; established in 1965.

Medical paternalism The attitude that health care providers know best and that "good" patients simply follow directions without asking questions.

Medically indigent Individuals and families who do not qualify for Medicaid or Medicare but cannot afford health insurance or medical care.

Medicare A federally funded form of public health insurance for citizens 65 years of age and above; established in 1965.

Members In professional associations, members may be individuals, agencies such as schools of nursing, or other associations. For example, in the ANA, the members are the state associations, whereas in the NLN, members may be either individuals or organizations.

Mentor An experienced nurse who shares knowledge with less experienced nurses to help advance their careers.

Message An essential element of communication consisting of the spoken word, plus accompanying nonverbal communication.

Metaparadigm The most abstract aspect of the structure of knowledge; the global concepts that identify the phenomena of interest for a discipline.

Metaphysics The branch of philosophy that considers the ultimate nature of existence, reality, and experience.

Milieu Surroundings or environment.

Mission The special task(s) to which an organization devotes itself.

Model A symbolic representation of a concept or reality.

Modeling An informal type of socialization that occurs when an individual chooses an admired person to emulate.

Montag, Dr. Mildred Originator, in 1952, of the concept of associate degree nursing education.

Moonlighting The practice of working a second job in addition to the regular one.

Moral development The ways in which a person learns to deal with moral dilemmas from childhood through adulthood.

Morals Established rules or standards that guide behavior in situations in which a decision about right and wrong must be made.

Morbidity rate The incidence or occurrence of a certain illness in a particular population during a specific period of time; usually expressed as a quantity per 1,000 people in a specific year.

Mortality rate The number of deaths in a particular population during a specific period of time; usually expressed as a quantity per 1,000 people in a specific year.

Multidrug resistant strains Microorganisms, such as tuberculosis, that have become immune to the effects of drugs that formerly were effective against them.

Multiskilled worker Individual who has been cross-trained to perform a number of tasks formerly performed by multiple specialized workers.

Mutuality Sharing jointly with others.

Mutual recognition model A system whereby a registered nurse may be licensed in the state of residency yet practice in other states, after being recognized by them, without additional licenses.

NANDA International (formerly North American Nursing Diagnosis Association) Group working since 1970 to establish a comprehensive list of nursing diagnoses.

National League for Nursing National organization that seeks to advance the profession of nursing through advocacy and improving educational standards for nurses. Nonnurses may be members.

National Practitioner Data Bank A national clearinghouse containing reports of adverse incidents involving physicians, nurses, and other health care providers that may be useful to potential employers or patients.

National Student Nurses Association National organization devoted to developing leadership skills in nursing students.

NCLEX-PN National Council Licensing Examination for Practical Nurses; the examination that graduates of practical nursing programs must take to become licensed to practice as licensed practical nurses (LPNs) or licensed vocational nurses (LVNs).

NCLEX-RN National Council Licensing Examination for Registered Nurses; the examination that graduates of basic nursing programs must take to become licensed to practice as registered nurses (RNs).

Negligence The failure to act as a reasonably prudent person would have acted in specific circumstances.

Network A system of interconnected individuals; useful to develop contacts or exchange information to further a career.

Neuman, Betty Nursing theorist who developed a systems model of nursing.

Newman, Margaret Nursing theorist who developed a theory of health as expanding consciousness.

Newton, Isaac English philosopher and mathematician who lived from 1642 to 1727.

Nightingale, Florence Nineteenth-century English woman known as the founder of modern nursing and nursing education.

NLN National League for Nursing.

NLNAC The National League for Nursing Accreditation Commission.

Nonexperimental design Research design in which the research subjects are not influenced in any way.

Nonjudgmental Describes an attitude that conveys neither approval nor disapproval of patients' beliefs and respects each person's right to his or her beliefs.

Nonjudgmental acceptance An accepting attitude that conveys neither approval nor disapproval of patients or their personal beliefs, habits, expressions of feelings, or chosen lifestyles.

Nonmaleficence The duty to inflict no harm or evil.

Nonverbal communication Communication without words; consists of gestures, posture, facial expressions, tone and loudness of voice, actions, grooming, and clothing, among other things.

Not-for-profit agency An organization that does not attempt to make a profit for distribution to owners or stockholders. Any profit made by such organizations is used to operate and improve the organization itself or to extend its services.

Nuclear family Term used to describe a mother and father and their children.

Nurse activist A nurse who works actively on behalf of a political candidate or certain legislation.

Nurse anesthetist A nurse with specialized advanced education who administers anesthetic agents to patients undergoing operative procedures.

Nurse citizen A nurse who exercises all the political rights accorded citizens, such as registering to vote and voting in all elections.

Nurse executive The top nurse in the administrative structure of a health care organization.

Nurse Licensure Compact An agreement among states, authorized by legislation, that they will honor licenses issued to registered nurses by one another.

Nurse manager A nurse who is in charge of all activities in a unit, including patient care, continuous quality improvement, personnel selection and evaluation, and resource (supplies and money) management. Formerly known as a head nurse.

Nurse-based practice A clinic, office, or home practice in which nurses carry their own caseloads of patients with physical or emotional needs.

Nurse-midwife A nurse with advanced specialized education who assists women and couples during uncomplicated pregnancies, deliveries, and postdelivery periods.

Nurse-patient relationship The mode of connection between a nurse and patient.

Nurse politician A nurse who runs for political office.

Nurse practice act Law defining the scope of nursing practice in a given state.

Nurse practitioner A nurse with advanced education who specializes in primary health care of a particular group, such as children, pregnant women, or the elderly.

Nursing The provision of health care services, focusing on the maintenance, promotion, and restoration of health.

Nursing diagnosis A process of describing a patient's response to health problems that either already exist or may occur in the future.

Nursing informatics The branch of nursing that manages knowledge and data through technology with the goal of improving patient care.

Nursing information system A software system that automates the nursing process.

Nursing interventions classification (NIC) A classification system describing more than 400 treatments that nurses perform in all specialties and all settings.

Nursing orders Actions designed to assist the patient in achieving a stated patient goal.

Nursing outcomes classification (NOC) A classification system describing patient outcomes sensitive to nursing interventions.

Nursing process A cognitive activity that requires both critical and creative thinking and serves as the basis for providing nursing care. A method used by nurses in dealing with patient problems in professional practice.

Nursing research The systematic investigation of events or circumstances related to improving nursing care.

Nutting, Adelaide M. An early twentieth-century nurse activist, first professor of nursing in the world, and a cofounder of the *American Journal of Nursing.*

Objective data Factual information obtained through observation and examination of the patient or through consultation with other health care providers.

Occupation A person's principal work or business.

Occupational health nurse A nurse specializing in the care of a specific group of workers in a given occupational setting.

Open-ended question An inquiry that causes the patient to answer fully, giving more than a "yes" or "no" answer.

Open posture Bodily position, squarely facing another person, with arms in a relaxed position.

Open system A system that promotes the exchange of matter, energy, and information with other systems and the environment.

Orem, Dorothea Nursing theorist known for her model focusing on patients' self-care needs and nursing actions designed to meet patients' needs.

Orientation phase The beginning phase of a nurse-patient relationship in which the parties are getting acquainted with one another.

Orlando, Ida Nursing theorist who proposed a theory of nursing process.

Outcome criteria Patient goals.

Out-of-pocket payment Direct payment for health services from individuals' personal funds.

Output The end result or product of a system.

Palliative care nursing A rapidly developing specialty in nursing dedicated to improving the experience of seriously ill and dying patients and their families.

Palmer, Sophia First editor of the *American Journal of Nursing.*

Paramedical Having to do with the field of medicine; generally used to describe ancillary workers such as emergency medical technicians.

Parental modeling A type of socialization that occurs when parents' behavior and responses to various stimuli influence a child's future behaviors and responses.

Parish nurse A specialized nurse that focuses on the promotion of health within the context of the values, beliefs, and practices of a faith community.

Parse, Rosemarie Nursing theorist who proposed a theory of human becoming.

Patient acuity The degree of illness of a particular patient or group of patients; used to determine staffing needs.

Patient advocate One who promotes the interest of patients. A nursing role.

Patient classification system (PCS) Identification of patients' needs for nursing care in quantitative terms.

Patient-focused care A system that emphasizes coordinating patient care to maximize patient comfort, convenience, and security.

Patient interview A face-to-face interaction with the patient in which an interviewer elicits pertinent information.

Patient Self-Determination Act Effective December 1, 1991, this law encourages patients to consider which life-prolonging treatment options they desire and to document their preferences in case they should later become incapable of participating in the decision-making process.

Patients' rights Responsibilities that a hospital and its staff have toward patients and their families during hospitalization.

Pay equity Equal pay for work of comparable value.

Peer review process The process of submitting one's work for examination and comment by colleagues in the same profession.

Pember, Phoebe A Southern nurse during the Civil War who was made Matron of the huge Chimborazo Hospital in Richmond, Virginia.

Pender, Nola A nurse theorist best known for her health promotion model of professional nursing.

Perception The selection, organization, and interpretation of incoming signals into meaningful messages.

Performance improvement (PI) Organizational efforts to improve corporate performance, incorporating aspects of quality management.

Person An individual—man, woman, or child.

Personal payment Direct payment for health services from individuals' personal funds.

Personal space The amount of space surrounding individuals in which they feel comfortable interacting with others; usually culturally determined.

Personal value system The social principles, ideals, or standards held by an individual that form the basis for meaning, direction, and decision making in life.

Petry, Lucille The first woman appointed (in 1949) to the position of Assistant Surgeon General of the United States Public Health Service.

Pew Health Professions Commission One of three major national groups that in 1993 issued reports or studies of nursing education in the United States.

Phenomenon An occurrence or circumstance that is observable.

Phenomenological inquiry/research A qualitative research approach focusing on what people experience in regard to a particular phenomenon, such as grief, and how they interpret those experiences.

Philosophy The study of the truths and principles of being, knowledge, or conduct.

Physician hospital organization (PHO) A separate corporation formed by a hospital and a group of its medical staff for the purpose of joint contracting with managed care organizations and businesses.

Planning The third step in the nursing process, which begins with the identification of patient goals.

Point-of-care technology Information system used for entering patient data directly from the bedside.

Point-of-service organization (POS) A hybrid preferred provider organization in which the consumer selects service providers within the defined network or may go outside the network and pay a higher deductible or copayment.

Policy The principles and values that govern actions directed toward given ends. Policy sets forth a plan, direction, or goal for action.

Policy development The generation of principles and procedures that guide governmental or organizational action.

Policy outcome The result of decisions made by governmental or organizational leaders who choose a certain course of action.

Political action committees (PACs) Groups that raise and distribute money to candidates who support their organization's stand on certain issues.

Politics The area of philosophy that deals with the regulation and control of people living in society; in government, it includes the allocation of scarce health care resources.

Population The entire group of people possessing a given characteristic; for example, all brown-eyed people over the age of 65.

Position power Authority and control accorded to an individual who holds an important role in an organization, profession, or government.

Posttraumatic stress disorder (PTSD) An anxiety disorder characterized by an acute emotional response to a traumatic event or situation.

Power grabbing Hoarding control, taking it from others, or wielding it over others.

Power sharing A process of equalizing resources, knowledge, or control.

Powers of appointment The authority to select the people who serve in positions such as judges, ambassadors, and cabinet officials.

Practical nurse (LPN/LVN) program A 1-year educational program preparing individuals for direct patient care roles under the supervision of a physician or registered nurse.

Preceptor A teacher; in nursing, usually an experienced nurse who assumes responsibility for teaching a novice.

Preferred provider organization (PPO) A form of HMO that contracts with independent providers such as physicians and hospitals for a negotiated discount for services provided to its members.

Premium The amount paid for an insurance policy, usually in installments.

Primary care Basic health care, including promotion of health, early diagnosis of disease, and prevention of disease.

Primary election An election in which voters who are declared members of a political party choose among several candidates of that same party for a particular office.

Primary nursing A system of nursing care delivery in which one nurse has responsibility for the planning, implementation, and evaluation of the care of one or more clients 24 hours a day for the duration of the hospital stay.

Primary source The patient is considered the primary source of data about himself or herself.

Private insurance Insurance obtained from a privately owned company, as opposed to public or governmental insurance.

Private practice Nursing practice engaged in by some nurses with advanced education; usually provided on a fee-for-service basis, as in most medical practices.

Privileged communications The principle that information given to certain professionals is so confidential in nature that it is not to be disclosed even in court.

Problem solving A method of finding solutions to difficulties specific to a given situation and designed for immediate action.

Profession Work requiring advanced training and usually involving mental rather than manual effort.

Professional A person who engages in one of the professions, such as law or medicine.

Professional accountabilities In the shared governance model, a basic set of responsibilities of all professional nurses regardless of practice setting.

Professional association An organization consisting of people belonging to the same profession and thereby having many common interests.

Professional boundary The dividing line between the activities of two professions. The area in which a professional person functions to avoid both underinvolvement and overinvolvement, maintaining the patient's needs as the focus of the relationship.

Professional governance The concept that health care professionals have a right and a responsibility to govern their own work and time within a financially secure, patient-centered system.

Professional outcomes The impact on a profession from political action by its practitioners.

Professional practice advocacy Includes activities such as education, lobbying, and advocating individually and collectively to advance a profession's agenda.

Professionalism Professional behavior, appearance, and conduct.

Professionalization A process through which an occupation evolves to professional status.

Professional review organization (PRO) Organizations that review Medicare hospital admissions and Medicare patients' lengths of stay.

Professional socialization The process of developing an occupational identity.

Proposition A statement about how two or more concepts are related.

Prospective payment system (PPS) A cost-containment mechanism wherein providers, such as physicians and hospitals, receive payment on a per-case basis, regardless of the cost of delivering the services.

Protocol A written plan specifying the procedure to be followed.

Provider A deliverer of health care services—hospital, clinic, nurse, or physician.

Proximate cause Action occurring immediately before an injury, thereby assumed to be the reason for the injury.

Psychomotor goal Effort directed toward a change in motor skills or actions by a patient.

Pure science Information that summarizes and explains the universe without regard for whether the information is immediately useful; also known as "basic science."

Qualitative research Research that seeks to answer questions that cannot be answered by quantitative designs and that must be addressed by more subjective methods.

Quality management See Total quality management.

Quantitative research Research that is objective and uses data-gathering techniques that can be repeated by others and verified. Data collected are quantifiable—that is, they can be counted, measured with standardized instruments, or observed with a high degree of agreement among observers.

Receiver An essential element of communication; the person receiving the message.

Reengineering Radical redesign of business processes and thinking to improve performance.

Referendum An election resulting from registered voters being asked by a legislative body to express a preference on a policy issue.

Reflection A communication technique that consists of directing questions back to patients, thereby encouraging patients to think through problems for themselves.

Reflective thinking The process of evaluating one's thinking processes during a situation that has already occurred, as opposed to evaluating one's thinking during the situation as it occurs.

Registered nurse (RN) An individual who has completed a basic program for registered nurses and successfully completed the licensing examination.

Rehabilitation services Those activities designed to restore an individual or a body part to normal or near-normal function following a disease or an accident.

Reliable Yielding the same values dependably each time an instrument is used to measure the same thing.

Reality shock The feelings of powerlessness and ineffectiveness often experienced by new nursing graduates; usually occurs as a result of the transition from the educational setting to the "real world" of nursing in an actual health care setting.

Remission A period of chronic illness during which symptoms subside.

Replication The process of repeating a research study as closely as possible to the original.

Research process Prescribed steps that must be taken to plan and conduct meaningful research properly.

Research question A statement, question, or hypothesis that a research study is designed to answer.

Resilience A pattern of successful adaptation despite challenging or threatening circumstances.

Resocialization A transitional process of giving up part or all of one set of professional values and learning new ones.

Resolution A written position on an issue presented to the voting members of an association for their consideration, discussion, and vote.

Respondeat superior Legal theory that attributes the acts of employees to their employer (Latin term).

Retrospective reimbursement Insurance payment made after services are delivered.

Richards, Linda In 1873, she became the first "trained nurse" in the United States.

Risk management A program that seeks to identify and eliminate potential safety hazards, thereby reducing patient injuries.

RN-to-baccalaureate in nursing Programs enabling registered nurses who hold associate degrees or diplomas in nursing to acquire baccalaureate degrees in nursing.

Robb, Isabel Hampton An outstanding turn-of-the-century American nurse who was instrumental in forming the forerunners of the National League for Nursing and the American Nurses Association, as well as cofounding the *American Journal of Nursing*.

Role A goal-directed pattern of behavior learned within a cultural setting.

Role model An individual who serves as an example of desirable behavior for another person.

Role strain Stress created by difficulty experienced in adjusting to a life or occupational role.

Rogers, Martha Nursing theorist who developed a model known as the "science of unitary human beings."

Roy, Sister Callista Nursing theorist who developed an adaptation model based on general systems theory.

Salary compression A phenomenon in which pay increases are limited during an individual's career, so that the salary of a veteran nurse may be little higher than that of a recently hired novice nurse.

Sample A subset of an entire population that reflects the characteristics of the population.

Sanger, Margaret Founder in 1916 of the first birth control clinic in the United States and an ardent proponent of women's rights to use contraception.

Scales, Jessie Sleet In 1900 she became the first African-American public health nurse.

School nurse Nurse specializing in the care of school-age children or adolescents and practicing in school settings.

Scientific discipline A branch of instruction or field of learning based on the study of a body of facts about the physical or material world.

Scientific method A systematic, orderly approach to the gathering of data and the solving of problems.

Scope of practice The boundaries of a practice profession's activities as defined by law.

Secondary care An intermediate level of health care performed in a hospital having specialized equipment and laboratory facilities.

Secondary source Sources of data such as the nurse's own observations or perceptions of family and friends of the patient.

Self-actualization A process of realizing one's maximum potential and using one's capabilities to the fullest extent possible.

Self-awareness Understanding of one's own needs, biases, and impact on others.

Self-insurance Coverage in which an individual or business pays for care directly rather than purchasing insurance.

Self-care model Nursing theoretical model based on the concept of ability to care for self.

Self-directed work team A method of decentralizing decision making using cross-functional groups united around common goals.

Self-efficacy A belief in self as possessing the ability to perform an activity, such as administering daily insulin.

Sender An essential element of communication; the person sending a message.

Separation of powers Under the U.S. Constitution, each branch of the federal government has separate and distinct functions and powers.

Set A group of circumstances or situations joined and treated as a whole.

Sex-role stereotyping The practice of automatically and routinely linking positive or negative characteristics to either males or females; also called gender-role stereotyping.

Sexual assault nurse examiner (SANE) Nurse trained to collect forensic evidence and provide initial counseling following rape or other sexual assault.

Shared governance Incorporation of unit-based decision making in nursing practice models. Generic term used to describe any organization in which decision making is shared throughout.

Short-term goals Specific, small steps leading to the achievement of broader, long-term goals.

Sick role A culture's criteria that must be met before people can qualify as being "sick."

Sigma Theta Tau International (STTI) The international honor society for nursing.

Sign Outward evidence of illness visible to others; for example, a rash.

Skill mix The ratio of registered nurses to licensed practical nurses and nursing assistants in a hospital unit.

Socialization The process whereby values and expectations are transmitted from generation to generation.

Social services Services designed to assist individuals and families in obtaining basic needs, such as housing, food, and medical care.

Somatic language Language used by infants to signal their needs to caretakers—for example, crying; reddening of the skin; fast, shallow breathing; facial expressions; and jerking of the limbs.

Spellman Seminary Site of the first nursing program for African-Americans; founded in Atlanta, Georgia, in 1886.

Spirituality Belief in and sense of connectedness with a higher power.

Staff nurse The bedside nurse who cares for a group of patients but has no management responsibilities for the nursing unit.

Stage theory A theory that views human development as a series of identifiable stages through which individuals and families pass.

Standard of care A guideline stating what the reasonably prudent nurse, under similar circumstances, would have done.

Standards of practice Formal statements by a profession of the accountability of its practitioners.

State Board of Nursing The regulatory body in each state that regulates and enforces the scope of practice and discipline of the members of the nursing profession.

Statutory law Law established through formal legislative processes.

Stereotypes Prejudiced attitudes developed through interactions with family, friends, and others in an individual's social and cultural system.

Stereotyping Erroneous belief that all people of a certain group are alike.

Stress Any emotional, physical, social, economic, or other type of factor that requires a response or change.

Stressors Stimuli that tend to disturb equilibrium.

Subacute care A level of care between hospital-based acute care and long-term residential care.

Subjective data Information obtained from patients as they describe their needs, feelings, and strengths, as well as their perceptions of the problem.

Subjects The individuals who are studied in a research project.

Subsystems The parts that make up a system.

Supervision The initial direction and periodic inspection of the actual accomplishment of a task.

Suprasystem The larger environment outside a system.

Symptom An indication of illness felt by the individual but not observable to others, such as pain.

Synergy Combined action that is greater than that of the individual parts.

System A set of interrelated parts that come together to form a whole.

Systems theory See General systems theory.

Taxonomy A framework for classifying and organizing information.

Taylor, Susie An African-American Civil War nurse who knew and was influenced by Clara Barton; lived from 1848 to 1912.

Team nursing A system of nursing care delivery in which a group of nurses and ancillary workers are responsible for the care of a group of patients during a specified time period, usually 8 to 12 hours.

Telehealth The practice of providing health care by means of telecommunication devices, such as telephone lines or televisions.

Telehealth nursing The delivery of nursing care services and related health care activities through telecommunication technology, such as telephones, video conferencing, and others.

Termination phase The final phase of the nurse-patient relationship wherein a mutual evaluation of progress is conducted.

Tertiary care Specialized, highly technical level of health care provided in sophisticated research and teaching hospitals.

Tertiary source Sources of data including the medical records and health care providers, such as physical therapists, physicians, or dietitians.

Theory A general explanation scholars use to explain, predict, control, and understand commonly occurring events.

Therapist Any of several health care workers with differing educational backgrounds who work with patients with specific deficits; examples include physical therapists and occupational therapists.

Third-party payment Payment for health services by an entity other than the patient or the provider of services, such as the government or insurance companies.

Throughput The processes a system uses to convert raw materials into a form that can be used, either by the system itself or by the environment.

Tort A civil wrong against a person; may be intentional or unintentional.

Total quality management (TQM) Management philosophy and activities directed toward achieving excellence and employee participation in all aspects of that goal.

Transcultural nursing Nursing care that is based on the patient's culturally determined health values, beliefs, and practices.

Transmission The expression of information verbally or nonverbally.

Truth, Sojourner A famous African-American nurse and former slave who was an abolitionist and underground railroad agent during the Civil War; lived from 1797 to 1881.

Tubman, Harriet Ross An African-American Civil War nurse who helped more than 300 slaves reach freedom through the underground railroad; lived from 1820 to 1913.

Unitary human beings, science of A nursing theory developed by Martha Rogers.

Universal care Provision of health care to all people.

Unlicensed assistive personnel Health care personnel, such as nursing assistants and home care aides, who do not function under their own licenses but are supervised by licensed individuals, such as nurses or physicians.

Urbanization The process of population migration to cities.

Utilitarianism An ethical theory asserting that it is right to maximize the greatest good for the happiness or well-being of the greatest number of people.

Valid Measuring what it is intended to measure, as in a valid test question or research instrument.

Values The social principles, ideals, or standards held by an individual, class, or group that give meaning and direction to life.

Ventilation The verbal "letting off steam" that occurs when people talk about concerns or frustrations.

Veracity Truthfulness.

Verbal communication All language, whether written or spoken; represents only a small part of communication.

Value ethics Ethical beliefs and behaviors that arise from the character of the decision maker.

Voluntariness The degree to which an action is brought about by an individual's own free choice.

Voluntary (private) agency An agency supported entirely through voluntary contributions of time and/or money.

Wald, Lillian Founder of the Henry Street Settlement and public health nursing in the United States. She later formed the National Organization of Public Health Nurses (1912), marking the beginning of specialization in nursing.

Watson, Jean Nursing theorist who emphasizes human caring as a focus of nursing.

Whistle-blower A person who speaks out against unfair, dishonest, or dangerous practices by a company or agency.

Whole system shared governance System in which people at all levels within the organization are included in decision making.

Woodhull Study on Nurses and the Media A comprehensive 1997 study of nursing in the print media.

Workers' compensation A federally mandated insurance system covering workers injured on the job.

Work ethic A belief in the importance of work; an appreciation for the characteristics employers desire in employees and a commitment to providing it.

Working phase The middle phase of the nurse-patient relationship, wherein goals are achieved.

Workplace advocacy Action ensuring that workers have a voice in the issues that concern them, either through collective action or other effective means.

Yale School of Nursing The first school of nursing in the world to be established as a separate university department with an independent budget and its own dean, Annie W. Goodrich.

Index

Page numbers followed by f indicate figures; t, tables; b, boxes

A

AARP. *See* American Association of Retired Persons (AARP).
Abuse. *See specific types.*
Acceptance, 459, 496, 498
Accountability
  as criteria for professionalism, 169, 171-172
  increased demand for, 615
  in nursing delegation, 562-563
  of nursing education programs, 619-620
  in primary nursing, 194, 365
  in shared governance, 379b, 380-381
Accreditation
  of educational programs, 44-45, 557, 620
  for hospitals, 192
  Joint Commission on Accreditation of Healthcare Organizations (JCAHO), 337-338, 355, 471, 615
  National League for Nursing Accreditation Commission (NLNAC), 41, 44, 124
Acquired immunodeficiency syndrome (AIDS), 109-110, 612, 618
Action language, 502
Active collaborator, 186
Active listening, 504-506, 507f
Activism
  environmental, 254
  legislative lobbying as, 129
Acuity, 96
Acute respiratory distress syndrome (ARDS), 146
Adaptation, 247, 281, 284-285
Adaptation Model of Nursing, 179b, 284-285
Adler, Mortimer, 506
Administrative law, 553
Advance directives, 538-539, 571
Advanced degrees, 154-159.
  See also specific degrees.
Advanced Practice Nurses (APNs)
  certification for, 50-51
  cost containment and, 614-615
  malpractice statistics on, 575
  opposition to, 158-159
  reimbursement for, 130, 157, 570-571, 582
  role in managed care, 613-614
  types of, 139, 154-159
Advocacy
  in case management nursing, 368b
  Center for Nursing Advocacy, 81-82
  failure to advocate, 561b

Advocacy *(Continued)*
  for nursing legislation, 582
  as nursing role, 377-378
  in work situations, 129
Aesthetics, 229
African-Americans
  attitudes toward cancer of, 294
  in clinic nursing, 13-14
  cultural differences and, 27
  culturally competent communication with, 514b
  discrimination against, 22
  famous women, 5
  Jessie Sleet Scales, 15f
  in military nursing, 19-20
  National Black Nurses Association, 22
  population demographics of, 88-89, 137
  rate of lung cancer in, 611
Age of Reason, 301
Age/aging
  chronic illness and, 85-86, 321, 333, 457
  effects on health care finance, 424, 603, 613
  effects on nursing, 85-86, 159, 603, 620
  elder abuse, 94
  of nurses, 137
  nursing shortage and, 97-98, 603
  See also Geriatrics/gerontology.
Agency/traveling nurses, 97, 557-558
Agenda for Health Care Reform (1992), 26-27
AIDS. *See* Acquired immunodeficiency syndrome (AIDS).
Aiken, Linda, 569
AJN. *See American Journal of Nursing* (AJN).
Alcohol, 258-259
Alexander, JoAnn, 444
Alfaro-LeFevre, Rosalinda, 409, 410b-411b
Allergies, 606, 618
Alternative treatments, 616, 617f
Altruism, 166, 171, 173
Alzheimer's disease, 603
AMA. *See* American Medical Association (AMA).
Ambulatory care, 139
American Assembly for Men in Nursing (AAMN), 70
American Association of Colleges of Nursing (AACN)
  on differentiated practice, 614
  Journal of Professional Nursing, 107
  legislative initiatives of, 131
  mission of, 125
  Nursing Education's Agenda for the 21st Century (report), 53
  Peaceful Death (document), 149
  position statement of, 38
  report on faculty shortage (2003 white paper), 57

American Association of Retired Persons (AARP), 87
American Board for Occupational Health Nurses (ABOHN), 147
American Cancer Society, 370
American Heart Association (AHA), 335f
American Hospital Association (AHA), 86-87, 446
American Journal of Nursing (AJN), 13-14, 107, 585
American Medical Association (AMA)
  Journal of the American Medical Association (JAMA), 443
  labor union of, 348
  opposition to health care reform, 446
American Nurses Association (ANA)
  American Journal of Nursing (AJN), 13-14, 107, 585
  The American Nurse (newspaper), 107, 123
  on assisted suicide, 111b
  Capitol Update (online newsletter), 591
  Center for American Nurses of, 129
  Code of Ethics for Nurses of. *See as main heading.*
  Competencies for Telehealth Technologies in Nursing, 151
  Constituent Member Associations (CMAs) of, 109, 116, 582-583
  definition of nursing, 190b-191b
  definition of parish nursing, 151
  on disaster preparedness, 607-608
  discrimination in, 22
  on Equal Rights Amendment, 67-68
  "Every Patient Deserves a Nurse" campaign, 440-441
  federal appointment project of, 593
  formation of, 10
  importance of membership in, 174
  legislative initiatives of, 119, 129-131
  mission of, 116, 122-124
  Model Practice Act of, 555
  Nurses Strategic Action Teams (N-STAT), 130, 591
  on nursing education, 23
  Nursing's Agenda for the Future vision statement, 58, 623-624
  Nursing's Social Policy Statement, 176, 187, 195, 227, 392
  political action committee of (ANA-PAC), 591-593
  position papers of, 37-38, 110-111b, 149
  Scope and Standards of Hospice and Palliative Care Nursing Practice, 149
  Scope and Standards of Practice, 392, 574
  Standards of Clinical Nursing Practice, 195
  on unlicensed assistive personnel, 568
American Nurses Association, Political Action Committee (ANA-PAC), 591-593
American Nurses Credentialing Center (ANCC), 50-52, 150, 485-486

American Organization of Nurse Executives (AONE)
  mission of, 126
  Nurse Leader (newsletter), 107
  on recruitment and retention of nurses, 113
American Red Cross, 7, 15-17, 16f
Americans for Nursing Shortage Relief (ANSR), 119
Americans, uninsured, 432-434, 433f, 590, 602
ANA. *See* American Nurses Association (ANA).
Andrews, M.M., 513, 514b
Androcentrism, 65
Anesthetists. *See* Certified Registered Nurse Anesthetist
  (CRNA).
Anger, 459, 473, 483
Anglo-Americans, 88-89
Anthrax, 607
Antibiotics, 17
Antisepsis, 4
Anxiety
  control of, 482-483
  learning and, 479
  of nursing students, 199
  symptoms of, 473-476
Arant, Matthew, 121-122
Army Nurse Corps, 13, 19-20, 71
Army School of Nursing, 15
Aroskar, Mila A., 524-525
Articulated program, 41-42
Asian-Americans, 88-89
Assaults, 95, 562-563
Assessment skills, 393-396, 395f
Assisted suicide, 111b, 603
Associate Degree in Nursing (ADN), 22
  development of, 40-41, 97
  differentiated practice with, 372, 614
  level of nursing theory in, 290b
  popularity of, 39-40, 138
Associations. *See* Professional associations.
Asthma, 259-260
Attitudes
  of acceptance, 459, 496, 498
  nonjudgemental, 223-224, 258, 461, 498
  toward cancer diagnosis, 294
Autonomy
  advance directives and, 538-539
  for Advanced Practice Nurses, 158
  as criteria of professionalism, 165-166, 169, 171-173
  ethics and, 529-531
  increased demand for, 615
  legal aspects of, 560
  of nurse entrepreneurs, 144
  opposition to, 158-159
  Patient Self-Determination Act, 538-543, 571
  of patients, 498-499, 527, 529-531
  in primary nursing, 365, 602

B

"Baby boom," 21, 85, 333, 603
Baccalaureate degree in nursing (BSN)
  criticism of, 38
  curricula development for, 39, 290
  differentiated practice with, 372, 614, 615
  foreign language requirement in, 620
  level of nursing theory in, 290b
  for nonnursing postbaccalaureate students, 43
  opposition to, 581b
  popularity of, 36, 39, 138
  Registered Nurses (RNs) in, 42-43, 198, 205, 208
  as research preparation, 322-323

Bachelor of Science in Nursing (BSN). *See* Baccalaureate
  degree in nursing (BSN).
Balance of power, 587, 588f
Balanced Budget Act (of 1997), 337, 348, 429-430, 570
Bandura, Albert, 201, 204, 263
Bandura's Concept of Modeling, 204
Barton, Clara, 7
Battery, 95, 562-564
Baumann, Linda, 610
Becker, Patricia, 305
Behaviors
  changing of, 321
  coping ability and, 462
  dependency, 461-462
  ethics and, 528
  illness behavior, 459-470
  incontinence, 319
  infant sucking, 304
  of patients, 261-266, 279-280, 459-470
  of peers and professionals, 537-538
  resilience, 463
Behaviors System Model of Nursing, 279-280
Beliefs
  about health, 261-266
  about nurses/nursing, 443
  belief systems, 223, 250, 522b
  categories of, 224
  cultural, 250, 466
  definition of, 223
  development of, 200-201
  Health Beliefs Model (HBM), 262-264
  irrational/illogical, 497-498
  spiritual, 151-152, 464-465
Bellevue Hospital Training School for Nurses, 5, 9, 33
Beneficence/nonmaleficence, 527, 530-531
Benner, Patricia, 201, 204, 278, 387
Benner's Stages of Nursing Proficiency, 204-205, 206b
Benson, Herbert, 464
Beth Israel Deaconess Medical Center Philosophy of Nursing,
  231-232
Beth Israel Medical Center, 255
Betts, Virginia Trotter, 593
Bickerdyke, Mary Ann "Mother," 6-7
Bickford, Carol, 375
Biculturalism, 213-215
Bioethics, 230, 522, 524-525
Biomedical technology, 90-91
Bioterrorism, 27, 131, 373, 602, 607
Birth control movement, 14
Birthrates, 602
Bishop, Peggy and Barbara, 20f
Bixler, Genevieve and Roy, 170
Blakeney, Barbara A., 122-124, 123f
Block grants, 426, 447b
Boards of Trustees, 338, 339b
Body language, 449, 469b, 500f, 502
Body mass index (BMI), 610
Bok, Sissela, 524
Bolton Act, 19
Bolton, Frances Payne, 19
Boston Training School for Nurses, 9
Boundaries, professional, 496-497
Boynton, Mary, 291f
Brain, 301
Breast cancer, 294
Breckinridge, Mary, 17-18
Brody, Charlotte, 255
Brown, Esther Lucille, 37
Brown Report, 20, 37
Bureau of Labor Statistics, 159

Burnout, 212-216
Bush, George W., 439, 586, 593

C

CABG. *See* Coronary artery bypass graft (CABG).
Cadet Nurse Corps, 19, 20f
Callahan, Daniel, 524
Cancer
  American Cancer Society, 370
  children with, 305
  death rates, 259-260
  environmental causes of, 606
  ethnic attitudes toward, 294
  See also Oncology; *specific cancer types.*
Capitation, 348, 615
Capps, Lois, 123f, 595-596
"Captain of the ship" doctrine, 560
Cardiology
  American Heart Association, 335f
  cardiac arrhythmias, 23
  cardiac surgery, 21
  coronary artery bypass graft, 93
  coronary care nursing, 23-24
  drugs for, 21
  heart disease, 259-260
  HeartCare, 93
Career choice
  financial security and, 66, 72
  gender roles and, 65-67, 76b, 169
  longterm commitment to, 74, 167-168
  reasons for, 72, 96
  trends in, 68-70
Caregiving
  caregiver role strain, 485
  impact on nurses, 484-488
  See also Nursing.
Caring technology, 92
Carondelet St. Mary's Hospital and Health Center, 369
Carr, Sandra H., 522b
Case management nursing
  advantages and disadvantages of, 370b
  cost containment and, 614-615
  definition of, 150, 366
  functions of, 150, 366-369, 368b
  models of, 366-370, 369f
Case Management Society of America (CMSA), 366, 368b
Case Western Reserve, 323
Cates, Tressa, 19
CCU. *See* Coronary Care Unit (CCU).
Center for American Nurses, 129
Center for Nursing Advocacy, 81-82
Centers for Disease Control and Prevention (CDC), 607,
  609-610
Centers for Medicare and Medicaid Services (CMS), 347,
  425, 582
Centre for Evidence-Based Medicine (EBM), 324
Certificate of Need (CON), 422
Certification programs
  characteristics of, 49-50
  through professional associations, 118-119
  types of, 50-52
Certified Nurse Midwife (CNM)
  function of, 157
  legal issues of, 567
  liability insurance for, 574
  malpractice statistics on, 575
  percentage of, 155f
  reimbursement for, 570-571

Certified Nursing Assistant (CNA)
  collaboration with, 516-518
  licensing of, 568-570
  response to nursing shortage, 22
  role of, 361-365
Certified Registered Nurse Anesthetist (CRNA)
  function of, 158
  malpractice statistics on, 575
  percentage of, 155f
  reimbursement for, 570-571, 582
Change agent, 377, 378b
Chater, Shirley, 593
Chemicals, 618
Chief Executive Officer (CEO), 339
Chief of staff, 339
Children
  with cancer, 305
  child psychiatry, 320b
  communication with, 316
  eating habits of, 610-611
  health insurance for, 430
  language development in, 502
  parental modeling and, 460, 465, 536b
  in poverty, 603
  of registered nurses, 138
  self-esteem in, 316-317
  See also Infants; School nursing.
Children's Health Insurance Program (CHIP), 430
Cholera, 9
Christianity, 237
Civil Works Administration (CWA), 18
Cleanliness, 275, 276
Clinical judgment, 406, 408-409, 410b-411b
Clinical ladder, 140
Clinical Nurse Specialist (CNS), 46-47, 140, 155f, 157, 622
Clinical Pastoral Educator (CPE), 153
Clinical pathways, 367
Clinton, Bill
  1996 election results, 586
  health care reform efforts of, 585
  support of ANA for, 591, 593
CMAs. See Constituent Member Associations (CMAs).
CNS. See Clinical Nurse Specialist (CNS).
Code of Academic and Clinical Conduct, 111, 112b
Code of Ethics for Nurses
  on confidentiality, 564-565
  on delegation, 562
  on end-of-life care, 110
  history of, 523-526
  on non-biased nursing, 199
  posession of, 195
  preface to, 187-188
  professionalism and, 176-177
  on stereotypes, 498
  values of, 222-223
Codes of ethics
  "do no harm" in, 527, 531, 559
  history of, 523-526
  professionalism and, 173-177
  purpose of, 106
  See also specific code name.
Cognitive rebellion, 202
Cognitive skills, 390t
Cohen, H.A., 202, 203b
Cohen's Model of Basic Student Socialization, 202, 203b
Collaboration
  active collaborator, 186
  among nursing students, 108-109
  elements of, 513, 515
  function of, 377

Collaboration (Continued)
  gender differences in, 515-516
  of nursing professionals, 621, 623
  in nursing research, 319, 321
Collective action, 106-113
Collective bargaining, 21-22, 119, 129
Collective identity, 167
Collegiality, 177
Colorado Nurses Association Task Force on Violence, 619
Commission on Collegiate Nursing Education (CCNE), 45
Common law, 553
Commonwealth research foundation, 434-435
Communication
  breakdown of, 509-510
  in case management nursing, 150
  with children, 316
  congruent and incongruent, 449
  criteria for, 502-508
  cultural influence on, 466
  culturally competent, 508-509, 514b
  development of, 502
  in disaster response, 608b
  documentation as, 573, 576b
  elements of, 499-502, 501f
  foreign language fluency, 480, 605, 620
  holism in, 512, 576
  listening skills in, 504-506, 507f
  negligent failure of, 561b
  nonverbal, 449, 469b, 500f, 502
  in office nursing, 146-147
  open-ended questioning in, 507-508
  privileged, 565
  in professional associations, 107
  responding techniques in, 506-512
  self-assessment of, 493b
  silence/reflection in, 508
  in team nursing, 362
  theory of, 499-504
  veracity in, 531-532
  in work relationships, 363f, 512-518, 573, 575
Communication theory, 499-504
Community-based nursing, 139, 141-144, 440, 613, 615, 620
Competence/competencies
  in core disaster preparedness, 607, 608b
  cultural competence, 90, 250, 563, 605, 618
  five stages of, 278
  in informed consent, 564
  for leadership, 118b
  of nursing education programs, 41, 372, 619-620
  of nursing students, 205, 206t
Competencies for Telehealth Technologies in Nursing, 151
Compliance/noncompliance, 461
Computed tomography (CT) scans, 332, 343
Computerized health information networks (CHINs), 615
Concepts of Nursing (Orem), 283
Conceptual models, 200-208, 279-286
Confidentiality/privacy, patient
  advanced technology and, 565-566, 615
  as ethical and legal issue, 91
  HIPAA and, 429
  in informed consent, 311
  of patient data, 395-396
Conflicts
  institutional and societal, 540-543
  of patient's rights, 538-539
  of peers and professionals, 537-538
  resolution of, 213
Conservation Model of Nursing, 281-282
Constituent Member Associations (CMAs), 109, 116, 582-583, 590-591

Consultation skills, 394-395
Consumerism, 86-88
Consumers
  demands on food industry, 610-611
  education of, 349, 442
  expectations of, 349-350, 417b
  -oriented health care, 460
  power of, 349
Contact hour, 53
Continuing Education (CE), 52-53, 54b, 574
Continuing Education Unit (CEU), 53
Continuous quality improvement (CQI), 355-356f
Cooper, Barbara Medoff, 304
Copayments (insurance), 422
Coping ability, 462, 477-479
Corcoran, Ruth, 124
Coronary artery bypass graft (CABG), 93
Coronary Care Unit (CCU), 23-24
Cost containment
  budget and, 612
  capitation for, 348, 615
  effects on educational programs, 622
  effects on nursing, 357, 524, 614-615
  ethical dilemmas of, 540
  factors affecting, 423-424, 613-614
  in health care finance, 99, 422-427
  in hospitals, 99, 439-445
  incentives for, 438
  LPNs/LVNs and, 44
  managed care for, 26, 614-615
  obesity effects on, 609-610
  of prescription drugs, 438-439
  quality management and, 440-445, 568
  strategies for, 424-427
  unlicensed personnel for, 568-570
Council of National Defense, Committee on Nursing, 15
Credentials committees, 339
Crime in America, 94, 94-96
Criminal law, 553
Critical path, 150, 402
Critical thinking skills
  exercise in, 391
  in nursing process, 387-391
  in nursing theory, 272, 279-280
  in student socialization, 202-204
Croke, E.M., 560, 561b
Cross-functional teams, 351
Crossing the Quality Chasm: A New Health System for the 21st Century (report), 572
Cultural assessment, 460, 467-470, 469b
Cultural competence, 90, 250, 563, 605, 618
Cultural diversity, 27, 88-90, 256-257, 604-605, 618, 620
Culture
  biculturalism, 213-215
  cultural assessment, 460, 467-470, 469b
  cultural diversity, 27, 88-90, 256-257, 604-605, 618, 620
  culturally competent care, 460, 471-473
  culturally competent communication, 508-509, 514b
  effect on illness behavior of, 465-470
  gender culture, 516
  homogeneous/heterogeneous, 604-605
  influence on learning, 480
  multicultural workplaces, 513-518
  of nursing, 198
  Theory of Culture Care Diversity and Universality, 286-287, 288f
  transcultural nursing, 89, 250, 287, 466-467, 472
Curie, Marie and Pierre, 302b

Curricula
  development of, 36, 39, 53, 128, 185, 622
  effects of demographics on, 620

D

Dartmouth-Hitchcock Medical Center, 255
Data, patient
  analysis of, 396-399
  confidentiality of, 395-396
  organization of, 395
  sources and collection of, 394-395
  types of, 394
Data, research
  analysis of, 313
  collection instruments for, 309-310, 312
  triangulation of, 535
Daughters of the American Revolution (DAR), 12
Davidhizar, R., 208-209
Davis, Mary E., 13
Day, Hughes, 23
Decentralization, 351
Deductible (insurance), 422
Deductive reasoning, 301-303
Defibrillators, 21, 24f
Delano, Jane A., 15, 16f
Delegates, nursing, 108f
Delegation
  accountability in, 562-563, 576b
  Five Rights of Delegation, 562
  function of, 362, 560-561
  increased use of, 615
Deming, W. Edwards, 355
Demographics/statistics
  Bureau of Labor Statistics, 159
  on cultural diversity in America, 88-89, 137
  definition of, 602
  future trends in, 603-605
  on malpractice, 575
  on Medicare/Medicaid funding, 421f, 424
  on men in nursing, 20-22, 70, 136
  on needlestick injuries, 110
  on obesity, 609-610
  on population growth and aging, 85-86, 424
  on registered nurses, 136-138
  on single-parent families, 249
  on uninsured Americans, 432-434, 433f, 590, 602
  on violence in America, 94-95
  on world population, 606-607
Deontology, 526-527
Dependency, 461-462
Depression, 317, 459
Designer medicines, 616
Dewar, Anne, 457
Diabetes, 259-260
Diagnosis, medical
  medical versus nursing, 398-399
  by nurses. *See* Nursing diagnoses.
Diagnosis-related groups (DRGs), 422, 426
Dietitians, 341-342
Diet/nutrition
  dietitians, 341-342
  eating disorders, 611
  fast foods, 610-611
  fat in American diet, 610-611
  healthy, 487b
  in patient needs philisophy, 275, 276
  See also Obesity.
Differentiated practice, 371-373, 614, 615

Diploma programs, 33, 35-36, 138, 614
Disasters/emergencies, 607-608
Discharge planning, 249-250
Disciplinary action, 496
Discrimination
  against African-Americans, 20-22
  in communication skills, 514b
  disparities in health care, 321
  against men in nursing, 70-71, 73-74
Disease. *See* Illness/disease.
Disease management companies, 333, 337
Distance learning (DL), 54-55, 200-201
Dix, Dorothea L., 5, 7
Dock, Lavinia Lloyd, 11-13, 12f, 27
Doctor of Nursing Science (DNS), 48-49, 138
Doctor of Philosophy (PhD) in nursing
  level of nursing theory in, 290b
  as research preparation, 322-323
Documentation, nursing
  advanced directives in, 571
  as communication, 573, 576b
  failure to document, 561b
  importance of, 357
  informatics nursing, 153-154, 375, 376b
  mechanics of, 444
  role in research, 535
  by voice-activated computers, 215, 616
  See also Medical records.
Domestic abuse, 94-95
Dominant culture, 68
Double effect principle, 531
Downsizing, 352
Drugs
  abuse of. *See* Substance abuse/addictions.
  antibiotics, 17
  costs of, 438-439
  designer medicines, 616
  development of, 21
  effects on health care costs, 423
  ethical dilemmas about, 544-547
  imported, 439
  lifestyle drugs, 423
  multi-drug resistant strains, 606
  narcotics, 581
  nurse prescriptive rights, 156-158, 567-568, 592
  penicillin, 17
  pharmacists roles, 342, 343f
  psychotropic, 320b
Dunbar, Sandra, 323
Duty of care, 559
Duty to report, 565

E

Earth Summit Conference, 607
Eating disorders, 611
Ebola virus, 606
Economic issues
  basic economic theory, 415-418
  for hospitals, 34, 46
  inflation of health care, 423
  for nurses, 69
  of nursing care, 439-443
  See also Health care finance.
Education, nursing
  challenges in, 55-59
  curricula development for, 127-128, 185
  faculty shortages in, 57-58
  funding for, 72

Education, nursing *(Continued)*
  learning theories of, 200-208
  reform of, 164
  research on, 127-128
  shortage of graduates, 55-56, 57t
  theory-based, 290-291
Educational programs
  accountability in, 619-620
  accreditation of, 44-45, 557, 620
  advanced degrees, 45-49, 154-159, 614
  alternative programs, 42-43
  articulated programs, 41-42
  associate degree program, 22, 41, 56, 97, 138
  baccalaureate program, 36-39, 42-43, 56, 138
  basic programs, 35
  business education for nurses, 621-622
  certification program, 49-52
  competence in, 41, 372, 619-620
  continuing education, 52-53, 54b
  curricula development for, 36, 39, 53, 185
  demographics of, 35t
  development of, 17, 20, 33-34, 39
  diploma program, 33, 35-36, 56, 138
  distance learning, 54-55
  doctoral program, 48-49, 138
  in early nursing, 4-5, 8
  evidence-based, 619-620
  external degree program, 41
  future directions in, 53-55
  master's program, 43, 46-48, 138
  men's nursing schools, 71
  for nonnursing postbaccalaureate students, 43
  nursing theory in, 290-291
  practical nursing program, 43-44, 97
  recruitment goals for, 76
  reform of, 622
  returning to (resocialization), 205-209
  scholarships for, 585
  studies on quality of, 34-35
  teachers colleges, 34, 46, 48
  training schools, 2, 4-5, 8-9
  types of, 32, 138
Educative instrument, 186
Elder abuse, 94
Electoral College, 586
Electoral process
  electoral college, 586
  function of, 587
  third party candidates in, 588-589
  types of elections, 589, 603
Emory University, 323
Emotional intelligence, 92
Emotions
  anger, 459, 473, 483
  anxiety, 199, 471, 473-476, 482-483
  burnout, 212-216
  chronic illness and, 458-459, 473-475
  nurse as counselor, 375-376
  reality shock, 212-216
Empathy, 507
Emphysema, 611
Employers
  employer-provided insurance, 433-436, 447b
  expectations of, 44, 214-216
Employment opportunities
  for advanced degrees, 154-159
  in case management, 150
  in community health nursing, 139, 141-144
  future of, 159
  in hospice and palliative care, 149

Employment opportunities (*Continued*)
  hospital-based, 139-141
  in informatics nursing, 153-154
  as nurse entrepreneur, 144-145
  in occupational health, 147
  office-based, 145-147
  in parish nursing, 151-153
  in schools, 147-149
  in telehealth, 150-151
  variety of, 138-139
  See also Work.
End-of-life issues, 110b-111b, 149, 322, 540-542, 571
Entrepreneur, 144-145, 194, 377
Environment/suprasystem
  activism for, 254
  effects on health, 605-607
  epidemiological reports on, 606
  patient behavior and, 280, 284-285
  systems and subsystems of, 245, 248-251, 253
Epidemiology, 606
Epistomology, 229
Equal Rights Amendment (ERA), 67-68
Equipment, medical
  costs of, 423
  life support systems, 540-542, 571
  proper use of, 561b, 573
  for technical personnel, 343-344
ERA. *See* Equal Rights Amendment (ERA).
Ethical decision making
  models of, 543-546
  personal accounts of, 524-525, 546b-547b
  research on, 535
  steps in, 544-546
Ethical dilemmas
  about drugs, 545-547
  about pain, 545-547
  of cost containment, 540
  in families, 540-542
  in nursing practice, 534-538
  Patient Self-Determination Act and, 538-543, 571
  from technology, 523, 565-566, 616-617
Ethics
  bioethics, 230, 522, 524-525
  codes written for, 523-526
  committees on, 543
  decision-making in. See Ethical decision making
  definition of, 523
  dilemmas of. See Ethical dilemmas
  patient privacy and, 91, 564-565
  Patient Self-Determination Act and, 538-543, 571
  as philosophy, 230
  principles of, 528-532
  in research, 312b, 528
  theories of, 526-528, 529t
  virtue ethics, 528
  work ethic, 215
Ethnicity/race, 137, 321
  See also Culture; Stereotypes.
Ethnocentrism, 467
Etiology, 397-398
Euthanasia/assisted suicide, 603
Evaluation, 242, 501, 616
"Every Patient Deserves a Nurse" campaign, 440-441
Evidence-based practice, 127, 172, 305-306, 323-324, 325b, 456
Excelsior College, 41
Executive branch, 552, 587, 588f
Exercise
  breathing exercises, 477b
  in critical thinking, 391

Exercise (*Continued*)
  lack of, 610, 611
  plan for, 262f, 487b
  relaxation exercises, 478b
Expert power, 584
Expert witness, 559
Extended care, 139
External degree program, 41

F

Faculty Loan Program, 111, 131
Faculty, nursing
  in active nursing practice, 620-621
  demographics of, 154
  Faculty Loan Program, 111, 131
  professional development of, 125
  quality of, 39
  shortage of, 57, 111, 622-623
  teaching methods of, 619
Family
  ethical dilemmas of, 540-542
  impact of illness on, 470, 480-484
  nuclear and extended, 248-249
  role in rehabilitation, 333
  single-parent, 249-250
Farrand Training School for Nurses, 173
Fatigue, physical, 211
Fats, dietary, 610-611
FDA. *See* Federal Drug Administration (FDA).
Fear, 459, 474
Federal Drug Administration (FDA), 581
Federal Trade Commission (FTC), 350
Feedback, 242, 500, 502-503
Feminism, 67-70, 68
Fenwick, Bedford, 10
Ferguson, Vernice L., 59b
Fidelity, 532
Fish, 255-256
Fitness, 487b, 602
Five Rights of Delegation (document), 562
Flexible staffing, 141
Flexner Report, 164
Florence Nightingale Pledge, The, 173-174
Flores, Robert, 96
Florida Supreme Court, 586
Flu epidemic (1917-1919), 15, 17
Food. *See* Diet/nutrition.
Ford, Lorretta, 24
Ford-Roegner, Pat, 593
Free-market economy, 416-418, 417b
Frontier Nursing Service, 17-18

G

G. I. Bill, 72
Galbraith, John Kenneth, 504-505
Galileo, 301
Gallup Polls, 78-79
Gardner, Marilyn, 504-506
Gastrointestinal stromal tumor (GIST), 484
Gatekeeper, 348
Gebbie, Kristin M., 593, 607, 608b
Gender roles
  effects on nursing, 65-76
  feminine traits, 65
  gender culture work styles, 516, 517b
  language of, 526

Gender roles (*Continued*)
  professionalism and, 169
  of registered nurses, 136
  role strain, 72
  stereotypes of women, 66b
General elections, 589
Genetic engineering, 302b, 616
Genetic traits, 245
Genetics, 302b, 321-322, 524
Genomics Nurse Case Coordinator, 616
Georgetown University, 406
Geriatrics/gerontology
  AARP and, 87
  centenarians, 603
  elder abuse, 94
  end-of-life issues in, 11b-111b, 149, 322
  euthanasia/assisted suicide in, 111b, 603
  growth of, 86, 424, 617, 620
  hospice and palliative care in, 149, 617, 620
  prevalence of falls in, 305
  retirement, 435
  tai chi research in, 318
Germ theory, 4
Gilligan, Carol, 533-534
Gleevec, 484
Goals, patient, 399-401, 400f
Goldmark Report, 17, 34
Goldwater, Marilyn, 437
Goodrich, Annie W., 15, 34
Gore, Albert, 586, 591, 593
Government
  federal, 552-553, 587, 591-593
  levels of, 587
  local, 587
  shared governance, 117
  state. See State government.
  structure within nursing, 378-381
  three branches of, 586
  voter participation in, 586
"Graying of America," 85-86
Great Depression, 18
Gretter, Lystra Eggert, 173
Guilt, 473

H

Hale, Sarah J., 8-9
Hall, Richard H., 165
Halle, Judith Noble, 319
Hamilton Medical Center, 192-193, 485
Hantavirus, 606
Harrison, Emily Haines, 7
Harvey, William, 302b
Hazardous materials, 254
Health
  of Americans, 602
  beliefs about, 250, 261-266
  as a continuum, 254, 256-257
  definitions of, 256-257, 287-289
  effects of lifestyle and behavior on, 321
  Health Beliefs Model (HBM), 262-264
  maximum health potential, 187
  protection and promotion of, 257-261, 331, 332b
  ten leading indicators of, 261b
Health Beliefs Model (HBM), 262-264
Health care
  aging population and, 85-86, 603
  alternative treatments in, 616-617
  as big business, 336

Health care *(Continued)*
community-based, 87, 91
consumer movement in, 86-88, 460
distribution of resources in, 529
high-level wellness, 257, 265-266
holism in, 187, 188f
home health agencies, 337
increased demand for, 424
legislation for, 590-593
news coverage of, 80
patient-focused, 351
prayer in, 303, 304
price sensitivity in, 416-417
primary, 336
promotion and maintenance of health, 185-186
public health, 17, 18, 248
rationing of, 448b
regulation of, 590-593
responses to change in, 350-354
as right versus privilege, 416
secondary, 336-337
self-care, 283
services provided by, 331-333, 336-338
subacute, 337-338
technological advances in, 90-93, 184
Health care agencies
accreditation of, 355
classifications of, 333-338
government (public), 333-334
home health services, 337
local, 334-335
maintaining quality in, 354-356
not-for-profit and for-profit, 335-336
state, 334
structure of, 338-341
voluntary (private), 335
Health care delivery system
agencies within, 333-341, 354-356
forces of change in, 346-350
future of, 330
objectives and goals of, 330
personnel within, 340-346
services provided by, 336-338
Health care finance
block grants for, 426, 447b
case study on, 431
Centers for Medicare and Medicaid Services (CMS), 425
Children's Health Insurance Program (CHIP), 430
cost containment in, 99, 422-427
crisis in, 414-415
diagnosis-related groups (DRGs) and, 426
employer-provided insurance, 433-436, 447b
fraud and abuse in, 424
funding sources in dollars, 421f
government appropriation for, 587
Hill Burton Act, 21, 421
history of, 21, 420-423
malpractice costs and, 439
managed care plans. *See specific plans by name.*
Medicaid Program, 418-419, 420t, 421f, 425, 447b
Medicare Program, 418, 419b, 420t, 421f, 425, 447b
national health insurance, 443-449
payment methods in, 418-420
personal (out-of-pocket) payments, 418, 421f
premium increases, 434-435
private insurance, 419, 420, 421f
professional review organizations (PROs), 425-426
reimbursement for clinical nurse specialists, 157
reimbursement for nurse practitioners, 156
reimbursement for nurses, 27, 570-571

Health care finance *(Continued)*
research funding in, 306, 321-323
during retirement, 435
retrospective reimbursement in, 422
two-tiered system of, 449b
uninsured Americans, 432-434, 433f, 590
universal health insurance, 446, 447b
Workers' Compensation Program, 418, 420, 424
Health care insurance. *See* Health care finance.
Health care networks, 428b, 447b
Health care reform
1990's attempts at, 590
American Nurses Association support of, 122
legislation for, 427, 429-430
of Medicare Program, 130
need for, 443, 445
Nursing's Agenda for Health Care Reform, 591
opposition to, 446, 585, 602
proposals for, 446-449
in school nursing, 613
Health care teams
components of highly effective, 383b
cross-functional, 351
interdisciplinary, 340, 381-382
key members of, 340-346
nurse's role on, 373-378
Health Care Without Harm, 255-256
Health insurance. *See* Health care finance.
Health Insurance Portability and Accountability Act (HIPAA)
online information for, 566
privacy provisions of, 565-566
purpose of, 427, 429
Health maintenance organizations (HMOs)
definition of, 348, 428b
reimbursement for nurses from, 570-571
Healthfinder (report), 265
Healthy People 2000/2010 (report)
future of, 259-261, 260b-261b
goals of, 257-259, 260b, 330-331
health promotion priorities of, 258
initiatives of, 258
ten leading health indicators from, 261b
Heart disease, 259-260
HeartCare, 93
Henderson, Virginia, 186, 187, 190b, 275-277, 276b
Henry Ford Health System, 427
Hepatitis, 109-110, 618
High-level wellness, 257, 265-266
Hill Burton Act, 21, 421
Hill, James, 610
Hinshaw, Ada Sue, 202
Hinshaw-Davis Model of Basic Student Socialization, 202-204
Hippocrates, 301, 302b
Hippocratic Oath, 174, 530
Hispanic-Americans, 88-89, 137, 514b
History, nursing
in American Civil War, 4-8
in Crimean War, 3
in early England, 2-4
early nursing textbooks, 186
of educational programs in, 33-34
Florence Nightingale Pledge, The, 174b
during flu epidemic, 15-17
during Great Depression, 18
influences on professionalism from, 169-170
in Korean War, 23
lessons of, 27
men in, 70-72
in Spanish-American War, 12-13

History, nursing *(Continued)*
state licensure in, 13
in Vietnam War, 26, 81, 95
in World War I, 15-17
in World War II, 18-21, 43, 72
"Hi-tech" versus "hi-touch," 616
HIV. *See* Human immunodeficiency virus (HIV).
Holism/holistic care
in case management, 150
in communication skills, 512, 576
definition of, 187, 245, 256-257
in nursing practice, 188f, 304, 402, 455-456
in primary nursing model, 364-365
for yourself, 487b-488b
Hollinger, Paula, 592
Home health agencies, 337
Home health care. *See* Visiting Nursing.
Homeostasis, 244, 247-248
Homophobia, 72
Hospice and palliative care, 149, 617, 620
Hospital-based nursing, 139-141
Hospitalists, 623
Hospitals
accreditation of, 192
advance directives in, 538-539, 571
advanced practice nursing in, 613-615, 622
American Hospital Association (AHA), 86-87, 446
board of directors responsibilities in, 339b
cost containment in, 99, 439-443
definition of nursing by, 192-193
economics of, 34, 46
expansion of, 21-22
history of, 2, 7-8, 17
hospitalist physicians, 623
managers roles in, 354
negligence in, 560, 561b
organizational models of, 352-354
as producers of waste, 254
reengineering of, 350-352
specialty units of, 140-141
support for nursing education, 622
technological advances in, 91-92
HP 2000/2010, See Healthy People 2000/2010 (report).
Human Genome Project, 524, 616
Human immunodeficiency virus (HIV), 109-110, 612, 618
Human needs theory
definition of, 245-248, 271-272
Maslow's hierarchy of needs, 246f, 398
Hume, David, 527
Hypothesis, 308-309

I

ICN. *See* International Council of Nurses (ICN).
ICU. *See* Intensive care units (ICUs).
Illness/disease
acute, 456
aging and, 85-86
behavior during. *See* Behavior: illness behavior.
beliefs about, 250
chronic, 321, 470
description of, 456-458
emotions and, 473-475
personal account of, 458b
definition of, 277, 456
diagnosis and treatment of, 331-332
disease management, 333, 337
early detection of, 332b
emotions and, 375-376, 458-459, 473-475

Illness/disease *(Continued)*
impact on families, 470, 480-485
impact on patients, 470, 473-480
patient acuity (degree of illness), 96
patient's environment and, 275
phases of coping with, 457
prevention of, 282, 331, 332b
remission/exacerbation of, 458, 459
social change and, 249-250
stages of, 458-460
stress-related, 249-250, 477, 479b
Imagery, 305
Immigration, 10-11, 604f, 605
Immunizations, 148, 446
Incontinence, 319
Indigent, medically, 603
Inductive reasoning, 301-303
Industrial Revolution, 71, 249-250, 605
Inertia, 218
Infants
low birth weight in, 305
mortality rate of, 259-260, 446, 602
oxygen deprivation in, 319
sucking reflex of, 304
Inflation, 423
Informatics nursing, 153-154, 375, 376b
Information technology (IT), 91, 153-154, 349-350, 395, 615
Informed consent
battery and, 563-564
competence in, 564
research in, 311
witness of signature on, 565f
Infusion Nurses Society, 108
Institute of Medicine (IOM), 572-573
Institutional review board, 311-312
Institutional structure, 338
Instructive Visiting Nursing Association, 17
Insurance. *See* Health care finance; Malpractice.
Intensive care units (ICUs), 18, 23-24
Interacting Systems Framework and Theory of Goal Attainment Model of Nursing, 280-281
Internal Revenue Service (IRS), 420
International Council of Nurses (ICN), 10, 116-117
Code of Ethics for Nurses, 106, 110, 173-177, 187-188, 526
definition of nursing, 187-189, 191b
Internet
fraudulent claims on, 350
health care information on, 349-350, 375, 484
for nurses/nursing students, 375, 620
referring patients to, 375, 376b, 616
support groups on, 253, 482-483
See also Online information.
Internship, 218
Interpersonal Relations in Nursing (Peplau), 492
Intrapreneur, 377, 378b
Intravenous therapy, 107-108
IT. *See* Information technology (IT).

J

Jenner, Edward, 302b
Johns Hopkins School of Nursing, 9, 81
Johnson & Johnson, 99, 585
Johnson, Dorothy, 279-280
Johnson, Eddie Bernice, 595
Joint Commission on Accreditation of Healthcare Organizations (JCAHO)
on cultural competence, 471
function of, 355

Joint Commission on Accreditation of Healthcare Organizations (JCAHO) *(Continued)*
on shared governance, 615
on subacute care, 337-338
Journal of Nursing Research, 22
Journal of Nursing Scholarship, 107, 127
Journal of Professional Nursing, 107
Journal of the American Medical Association (JAMA), 443
Journal of Transcultural Nursing, 466
Judicial branch, 552, 587, 588f

K

Kaiser Permanente, 255, 429, 432-433
Kant, Immanuel, 229, 526
Kasper, Christine, 319, 321
Kassebaum, Nancy, 437
Kellogg Foundation, 372
Kentucky Committee for Mothers and Babies, 17-18
Kevorkian, Jack, 603
Killeen, Maureen, 315f, 316-317
King, Imogene, 279b
Interacting Systems Framework and Theory of Goal Attainment Model of Nursing, 280-281
Kipnis, Laura, 542
Koch, Heinrich, 9
Koch, Robert, 302b
Kohlberg, Laurence, 532-533, 534
Koop, C. Everett, 264, 350
Korean War, 23
Krupnick, Catherine, 505-506

L

Labor unions
within American Medical Association, 348
collective bargaining by, 21-22, 119, 129
contracts of, 109
United American Nurses, 129
Laborotory technologists/technicians, 343, 344f
Lang, Norma, 184
Language
development in children, 502
fluency in foreign, 480, 605, 620
gender-related, 526
types of, 449, 469b, 500f, 502
"ventilation" (verbal), 504
vocabulary of nursing, 198, 292, 404, 406
Laparoscopy, 332
Latent power, 584
Law, branches of American, 552f, 553
Lawrence, David, 256
Lead, 606
Leadership
American Organization of Nurse Executives support of, 126
competence in, 117-118
training in, 381
Learning
active versus passive, 619-621
basic teaching techniques, 481b
coping with stress of, 462, 478
critical thinking in, 202-204, 272, 279-280, 387-391, 389b
cultural influence on, 480
distance learning, 54-55, 200-201
effects of anxiety on, 479
learned resourcefulness, 463
life-long, 488b, 621

Learning *(Continued)*
principles of, 480b
theories of, 200-208
See also Educational programs.
Lee, Elizabeth, 457
Legal aspects in nursing
future of, 566-571
licensure of nurses, 555-558
malpractice, 558-560
negligence, 558-560, 561b
nurse practice acts, 553-555
patient privacy as, 91, 564-565
preventing problems in, 576b
standard of care, 561b
standard of care as, 558-560
state boards of nursing, 553-554
torts, 558-560
Legal system, American, 552-553
Legislation
affecting hospital reimbursement, 348
Balanced Budget Act (of 1997), 337, 348, 429-430, 570
consumer influence on, 87-88
to fund hospital construction, 421
for health care reform, 427, 429-430, 448b
history in health care, 590-593
for hospital staffing, 109
lobbying for, 119, 129-131
maternity stay laws, 436-437
nurse practice acts, 185, 193, 195, 553-555, 581
for nursing education, 130
pathway through congress, 588f
on patient's rights, 538-539
to promote nursing, 99, 109, 111, 193-194, 597
for travel nursing and telehealth, 557-558
for welfare reform, 603
Legislative branch, 552, 586, 588f
Leininger, Madeleine
Culture Care Theory and the Health Belief Model of, 294
interview with, 471-473
photo of, 291f
Theory of Culture Care Diversity and Universality of, 286-287, 288f
transcultural nursing and, 89, 250, 468
Length of stay (LOS), 150, 159
Leone, Lucile Petry, 19
Levine, Myra, 279b
Conservation Model of Nursing, 281-282
Licensed practical/vocational nurse (LPN/LVN)
cost containment and, 44
licensure of, 43-44, 557
response to nursing shortage, 22
role of, 361-365
serving in congress, 595
supervision of, 568-570
Licensure, state
definition of, 49, 532
by endorsement, 557
examinations for, 557, 621
history of, 13
multiple levels of, 621
Nurse Licensure Compact, 557-558
requirements for, 35, 43, 556-557
suspension or revocation of, 556
trends in, 557-558
Life expectancy, 259
Life support, 540-542, 571
Lifestyles
attitudes toward, 223-224, 258, 461
balanced plan for, 486-488
changing of, 321

Lifestyles *(Continued)*
  lifestyle drugs, 423
  of nurses, 612
  -related diseases, 331
  sedentary/unhealthy, 258, 457, 609-612
  stressful, 612
Listening, 504-506, 507f
Lister, Joseph, 4
Literature review, 308
Livermore, Mary, 5
Lobbying, 119, 129-131, 582-583, 590-592
Locus of control, 263
Long, Kathleen Ann, 125
Long-term care, 333
LPN. *See* Licensed practical/vocational nurse (LPN/LVN).
Lung cancer, 611
Lupus Erythematosis, 458b
LVN. *See* Licensed practical/vocational nurse (LPN/LVN).
Lynch, Thomas, 542
Lysaught Report, 38

M

Magnet Recognition Program, 485-486
Magnetic resonance imaging (MRI), 343, 345f
Malone, Beverly, 593
Malpractice
  costs of, 439
  documentation and, 573
  examples of, 560, 561b
  professional liability insurance, 574, 575b, 576b
  statistics on registered nurses, 575
Managed care
  advanced practice nursing in, 613-614
  for cost containment, 615
  definition of, 347
  expansion of, 427
  in health networks, 428b, 447b
  impact on health services, 435-439
  legislation on, 448b
  for Medicare/Medicaid recipients, 570
  nursing roles in, 26-27, 349
  for vulnerable populations, 437-438, 448b
Managed care organizations (MCOs)
  definition and function of, 347-349
  future of, 448b
  peer review in, 425-426
  quality of care in, 358
  types of, 428b
Marital status, 138
MASH units. *See* Mobile Army Surgical Hospital
  (MASH) units.
Maslow, Abraham, 245-247, 398
Massachusetts General Hospital, 33
Master of Science in Nursing (MSN)
  characteristics of program, 46
  differentiated practice with, 614
  generic degree in, 43
  level of nursing theory in, 290b
  as research preparation, 322-323
  role preparation breakdown in, 47f, 48, 138
Master's of Business Administration (MBA), 340
Maternity stay laws, 436-437
Maximum health potential, 187
Mayo Clinic, 23
McCarthy, Carolyn, 595
McGee, Anita N., 12
McLean Asylum Training School, 71
McNeely, Elizabeth, 305, 318

Media
  Internet, 585
  power of, 584-585
  print/publications, 75, 79, 81-82, 585, 605-607
  reports on environment, 605-607
  talk radio, 585
  television, 67, 69, 79-82, 585, 605-607
Medicaid Program
  Centers for Medicare and Medicaid Services (CMS),
    347, 425, 582
  costs of, 423b
  description of, 418-419, 420t
  effects of aging on, 613
  fraud and abuse in, 424
  future of, 447b
  initiation of, 23, 421
  managed care for, 437-438, 570
  nursing support for, 590
  percentage of health care from, 421f
  reimbursement for nurses from, 130, 570
Medical paternalism, 87
Medical records
  advance directives in, 571
  as legal evidence, 573
  patient's right to, 566
  personnel for, 346
Medicare Program
  Centers for Medicare and Medicaid Services (CMS),
    347, 425, 582
  costs of, 423b
  description of, 418, 420t
  drug coverage by, 130, 419b, 439
  effects of aging on, 613
  fraud and abuse in, 424
  future of, 447b
  initiation of, 23, 421
  legislation to expand, 580
  managed care for, 437-438, 570
  nursing reform of, 130
  nursing support for, 590
  percentage of health care from, 421f
  reform of, 130
  reimbursement for nurses from, 570, 582
Meiman, Colleen, 437
Meltzer, Lawrence, 23
Memorial Health Care System Philosophy of Nursing, 233-234
Men
  American Assembly for Men in Nursing, 70
  discrimination of, 71, 73-74
  gender culture of, 516, 517b
  as nurse anesthetists, 158
  in nursing, 20-21, 22, 70, 75-76, 136
  nursing schools for, 71
  rate of lung cancer in, 611
Mendel, Gregor, 302b
Mentors/role models
  characteristics of, 218-219
  for ethical decision making, 535
  for male nurses, 75-76
  for nursing research, 316-317
  for political action, 598-599
  role models, 204
Mercury, 255-256, 606
Metaparadigm, 274
Metaphysics, 230
Midwives. *See* Certified Nurse Midwife (CNM).
Military nursing
  in American Civil War, 4-8, 5, 8
  in Crimean War, 3
  in Korean War, 23

Military nursing *(Continued)*
  men in, 20-21, 71-72
  nurse corps, 13, 19
  in Spanish-American War, 12-13
  in Vietnam War, 26, 81, 95
  in World War I, 15-17, 16f
  in World War II, 18-21, 43, 186
Mill, John Stuart, 527
Miller's Wheel of Professionalism in Nursing, 174-176, 175f
Mills School of Nursing for Men, 71
Mind/Body Medical Institute, 464
Minor, Nannie, 17
Minorities. *See specific cultural group.*
Mobile Army Surgical Hospital (MASH) units, 23
Model Practice Act, 555
Models
  of behavior systems, 279-280
  of case management, 366-370, 369f
  conceptual models, 200-208, 279-286
  for distributing health care, 529
  for ethical decision making, 543-546
  for interstate nursing, 373
  Model Practice Act, 555
  of mutual recognition, 557-558
  for nursing practice, 555
  organizational models, 352-354
  parental modeling, 460, 465, 536b
  of political power, 584, 598-599
  of professional socialization, 200-208
  role models, 204, 218-219
  of shared governance, 379b, 380-381
  systems models, 244
  See also specific model name.
Montag, Mildred, 39
Montoya, Pat, 593
Moore, Kathryn, 436
Morals/morality
  definition of, 522-523
  in deontology, 527
  theories of, 532-534
  women and, 533
Morbidity/mortality rates, 259-260, 446, 569, 602
Morphine sulfate, 545-547
Morris, Mitchell, 349
Motivation and Personality (Maslow), 245
MSN. *See* Master of Science in Nursing (MSN).
Multi-drug resistant strains, 606
Multiskilled workers, 351, 615, 622
Mutual recognition model, 557-558
Mutuality, 202

N

Nader, Ralph, 588
Names, patient, 77-78, 514b
NANDA International, 392, 397-399
Narcotics, 581
National Black Nurses Association, 22
National Board for Certification of School Nurses
  (NBCSN), 148
National Center for Complimentary and Alternative
  Medicine, 334
National Committee for Quality Assurance (NCQA), 358
National Council Licensing Examination for Practical
  Nurses (NCLEX-PN), 43, 557
National Council Licensing Examination for Registered
  Nurses (NCLEX-RN), 35, 557
National Council of State Boards of Nursing (NCSBN),
  373, 496, 557, 562

National Institute for Occupational Safety and Health (NIOSH), 96, 147
National Institute of Nursing Research (NINR), 131, 301, 303-304, 321
National Institutes of Health (NIH)
  on end-of-life care, 322
  Nurses Health Study, 313
  on women in research, 312b
National League for Nursing Accreditation Commission (NLNAC), 41, 44
National League for Nursing (NLN)
  as accrediting organization, 41, 44
  mission of, 124
  Nursing and Health Care Perspectives (report), 107
  position papers of, 38, 41
  Transforming the Landscape for Nursing Education, 58
  Vision for Nursing Education (report), 53
National Nurses Response Team (NNRT), 607-608
National Nurses Week, 592f
National Organization of Public Health Nursing, 14
National Practitioner Data Bank, 574-575
National Student Nurses Association (NSNA)
  Code of Academic and Clinical Conduct of, 111-112b
  collective action of, 107-108
  leadership development in, 117, 118b
  mission of, 121-122
  Student Bill of Rights and Responsibilities of, 111
Native Americans, 88-89
Navy Nurse Corps, 13, 19-20, 71
NCLEX-PN. *See* National Council Licensing Examination for Practical Nurses (NCLEX-PN).
NCLEX-RN. *See* National Council Licensing Examination for Registered Nurses (NCLEX-RN).
Needlestick injuries, 109-110, 618
Needlestick Safety and Prevention Act, 110
Needs. *See* Human needs theory.
Negligence
  categories of, 560, 561b
  definition of, 558
Networking, 107
Neuman, Betty, 279b
  Systems Model of Nursing, 282-283
New England Hospital for Women and Children, 33
New England Medical Center, 366-368
Newman, Margaret, 287-288
  theory of Health as Expanding Consciousness, 287-289
Newton, Sir Isaac, 301
Nightingale, Florence
  background of, 2-3
  in the Crimean War, 3
  definition of nursing by, 185-186
  Florence Nightingale Pledge, The, 173-174
  on men in nursing, 71
  nursing philosophy of, 4, 274-275
  as political activist, 3, 598
  principles of nursing education, 33
  at St. Thomas' Hospital, 4, 9, 33
Nightingale School, The, 4
Nineteenth Amendment, 17
NIOSH. *See* National Institute for Occupational Safety and Health (NIOSH).
NLN. *See* National League for Nursing (NLN).
NNN Alliance, 406
Noise, 275, 276
Nonexperimental designs, 309
North American Nursing Diagnosis Association (NANDA), 397-398, 404, 406
North Dakota State University (NDSU), 581b
NP. *See* Nurse Practitioner (NP).
Nuclear power plants, 606

Nurse activist
  in Civil War, 5
  Lavinia Dock as, 11-12
  for legislation, 582-583
  Margaret Sanger as, 14
  monitoring of media by, 83-84
  opportunities for, 95, 594-596
Nurse citizen, 594
Nurse Education Act, 130
Nurse educator
  in activism, 594-596
  in advanced practice, 157
  of coping skills, 463, 478-481
  on health care team, 373-375
  of lifestyle changes, 612
  in nursing education, 154, 621
  in parish nursing, 147, 151-152
  teaching tips for, 481b
Nurse entrepreneur, 144-145, 194, 377, 617-618
"Nurse extender" positions, 97, 568
Nurse Licensure Compact, 557-558
Nurse managers, 140
Nurse midwives. *See* Certified Nurse Midwife (CNM).
Nurse politician, 595-598
Nurse practice acts
  changes in, 581
  function of, 553-555
  of Missouri, 567
  need for, 195
  of North Dakota, 555
  of Ohio, 193
  of Tennessee, 554f
  of Utah, 558
Nurse Practitioner (NP)
  advice from, 522b
  function of, 24-25
  in hospitals, 622
  malpractice statisitcs on, 575
  from MSN programs, 46
  Nurse Practitioner (journal), 155, 158
  prescriptive authority of, 156-158, 567-568, 592
  reimbursement for, 570-571, 582
  scope of practice for, 155-156, 449b, 622
Nurse Reinvestment Act, 99, 111, 131, 585, 591-592
Nurse researcher
  education for, 48
  function of, 304-307
  interviews with, 315-318
  process of, 311
  roles of, 322-323, 376-377
Nurse, role of
  as activist. *See* Nurse activist.
  as administrator, 47
  in advanced practice, 50-51, 66, 139, 154-159
  as anesthetist, 23, 155f, 157
  as attorney, 47-48
  as businessperson, 144-145, 194, 340, 377, 617-618
  as caregiver, 484-488
  as case manager, 349
  as certified informatics nurse, 375, 376b
  as change agent, 377, 378b
  as chief nurse executive, 340
  as citizen, 594
  as collaborator, 377
  as counselor, 148-149, 151-152, 375-376
  cultural beliefs about, 467
  as educator. *See* Nurse educator.
  as entrepreneur, 144-145, 194, 377, 617-618
  as executive, 376
  in industry, 147

Nurse, role of *(Continued)*
  in informed consent, 564
  as intrapreneur, 377, 378b
  as leader, 598
  as manager, 140, 150, 376
  as midwife, 155f, 157
  as new graduate, 209-212
  partial listing of, 380b
  as patient advocate, 377-378
  in political action, 579, 591-599
  as politician, 595-597
  as practitioner, 24-25
  as research subject, 313
  as researcher. *See* Nurse researcher.
  in sexual assault, 94-95
  stereotypes of, 9
  as student nurse. *See* Student nurses.
  as supervisor of personnel, 568-570
  as utilization manager, 357
  See also specific nursing title.
Nurse-based practices, 144
Nurse-patient relationships
  emotional needs of nurse in, 496-497
  orientation phase of, 492-494
  social versus professional, 495b
  termination phase of, 494-495
  Theory of Human Relatedness, 498-499
  working phase of, 494
Nurses Health Study, 313
Nurses' March on Washington, 583f
Nurses of America (NOA), 79-81
Nurses Strategic Action Teams (N-STAT), 130, 591
Nursing
  activism. *See* Nurse activist.
  with advanced degrees, 154-159
  in advanced practice, 50-51, 66, 139, 154-159, 613-614
  African-Americans in, 5, 12-14, 15f, 19-20, 22, 27
  in American Red Cross, 7, 15-17, 16f
  attitudes toward, 74
  in case management, 150, 365-370
  certification programs in, 49-52, 50b
  challenges in, 614-619
  clinical judgment in, 406, 408-411b
  codes of ethics for, 106, 110, 173-177
  communication in. *See* Communication.
  community-based, 139, 141-144, 440, 613, 615, 617, 620
  competence in, 90
  conceptual models of, 244, 279-286
  in the Confederacy, 7
  conflicts/rivalry in, 170, 173
  continuing education in, 52-53, 54b
  in coronary care, 23-24
  cost containment in, 357, 439-443, 614-615
  critical thinking skills in, 387-391, 389b
  cultural diversity in, 604-605
  culturally competent care in, 460, 468, 471-473, 509, 604-605, 618, 620
  culture of, 198
  definition of
    development of, 191-193
    evolution of, 185-191, 189b-191b
    need for, 184-185
  differentiated practice in, 614
  documentation in, 215, 357
  economics of care in, 439-443
  education. *See* Educational programs; Nurse educator.
  employment prospects in, 138-154, 159
  entrepreneurial, 144-145, 194
  ethics in. *See* Ethics.
  evidence-based, 127, 172, 305-306, 323-324, 325b, 456

Nursing *(Continued)*
  feminism and women's movements in, 67-70
  functional, 361-362
  future of, 148, 352
  gender roles in, 64-67, 66b, 169
  health beliefs models and, 263-264
  health promotion in, 265-267
  "high-tech" versus "high-touch," 91-93
  history of. *See* History, nursing.
  holism in, 187, 188f, 266-267, 304, 455-456
  hospice and palliative care in, 149, 617, 620
  hospital-based, 139-141
  image of, 76-85, 78b
  individualized care in, 247
  influences on development of, 2
  informatics nursing, 91, 153-154, 615-616, 620
  in intensive care, 23-24
  language of, 198, 292, 404, 406
  leadership in, 117-118, 126, 598
  legal aspects of. *See* Legal aspects in nursing.
  licensure requirements for. *See* Licensure, state.
  limitations of scientific method in, 303
  managed care and, 26-27
  men in
    advantages for, 74
    attitudes toward, 20-22, 72-74
    history of, 70-72
    promotion of, 74-76, 75f
  in the military. *See* Military nursing.
  nonhospital positions in, 98
  nurse-patient ratio, 99
  nurse-patient relationships. *See* Nurse-patient relationships.
  in occupational health, 147
  office-based, 145-147
  outcomes and interventions in, 400-402
  parish nursing, 151-153, 374, 465
  philosophies of, 230-238, 274-278
  political action in, 582-583
  primary care in, 24, 364-365, 366b, 602, 614-615
  process of. *See* Nursing process.
  as a profession, 164
  professional boundaries in, 496-497
  in public health, 17
  quality management in, 440-445, 568
  research on, 21, 67, 78-82, 185, 201, 208-209
  salaries. *See* Salary, nursing.
  in schools, 95, 147-149, 274, 375, 594, 613, 617
  as science and art, 284
  scope of practice for, 194-195, 614-615
  shortages in, 21-22, 36, 96-100, 98t, 113, 622-623
  societal influences on, 85-96, 601-614
  specialization in, 23, 46-47, 99, 194
  spiritual aspects of, 151-152, 276-278, 464-465
  staff retention in, 113
  state regulation of, 35, 185, 193-194, 373, 553-558
  stress in, 26, 484-488, 618
  structure of knowledge in, 272-274
  systems models, 244
  team nursing, 351, 362-364, 363f, 516-518, 618
  in telehealth, 150-151, 557-558
  theory of. *See* Theory, nursing.
  three major concepts of, 241, 268f
  training schools for, 2, 4-5, 8-9
  transcultural, 89, 250, 287, 466-467, 472
  travel nursing, 97, 557-558
  in the Union, 5-7
  values in, 226-229, 226b, 466-467, 522b, 534-537
  visiting nursing, 10-11, 18, 142-143, 159, 337
  vocabulary of, 198, 292, 404, 406
  women's movement and, 11, 17, 67-70

Nursing *(Continued)*
  working conditions in, 21
  writing skills in, 398b, 399, 401, 402
Nursing and Health Care Perspectives (report), 107
Nursing delivery systems
  case management nursing, 365-370
  certified nursing assistant role in, 361, 363
  functional nursing, 361-362
  licensed practical/vocational nurse role in, 361, 363
  primary nursing, 364-365, 366b
  registered nurse role in, 361-370
  team nursing, 362-364, 363f
Nursing diagnoses
  classification of, 392
  definition and process of, 397-399
Nursing Doctorate (ND), 48
Nursing Education's Agenda for the 21st Century (report), 53
Nursing homes
  advance directives in, 571
  demand for, 430
Nursing informatics, 91, 153-154, 615-616, 620
Nursing interventions, 401-402
Nursing Interventions Classification (NIC), 402, 404, 406
Nursing orders, 401
Nursing Outcomes Classification (NOC), 400-401,
    404, 406
Nursing practice
  advanced practice, 50-51, 66, 139, 154-159
  challenges in, 614-619
  differentiated, 371-373, 614, 615
  evidence-based, 127, 172, 305-306, 323-324, 325b, 456
  five stages of, 204-205
  legal authority for, 566-567
  legal problems in, 576b
  levels of, 371-373, 372b
  nurse practice acts, 553-555, 581
  philosophy of, 237-238
  public policy impact on, 580-581
  research-induced changes in, 317
  standards of, 195, 559
  stress in, 26, 484-488, 618
  theory-based, 272-274, 291-292
Nursing process
  case study in, 405b
  definition of, 172
  dynamic nature of, 404
  goals and outcomes in, 399-401
  history of, 390, 392
  nursing diagnosis in, 397-399
  phases of
    analysis, 396-399
    assessment, 393-396
    evaluation, 403
    implementation, 402-403
    planning, 399-402
  reality shock and, 215
  taxonomy of, 406-408
  traditional steps of, 281
  use of patient data in, 394-396
Nursing students. *See* Student nurses.
Nursing's Agenda for the Future vision statement, 58, 90,
    623-624
Nursing's Social Policy Statement, 176, 187, 195, 227, 392
Nutting, Mary Adelaide, 13, 15, 34

O

Obesity, 258-261, 602, 609-610
Occupational health, 147, 618-619

Occupational therapists, 345, 618-619
Office-based nursing, 145-147
Oncology, 140-141
Online information
  for American Nurses Credentialing Center, 119
  for Centers for Disease Control and Prevention, 607
  about critical thinking skills, 388
  for Department of Health and Human Services
    Healthfinder, 265
  detecting validity of, 265b
  on diversity in nursing, 90
  for Evolve for WebLinks, 99
  on faculty shortage, 111
  on future research themes, 322
  for Health Insurance Portability and Accountability Act
    (HIPAA), 566
  about new nursing graduates, 212
  for Nurse Licensure Compact, 558
  on nurse mentoring, 219
  on nursing advocacy, 82
  about nursing outcomes and interventions, 401-402
  for nursing publications, 149
  on nursing scholarships, 585
  on nursing systems, 244
  for *Nursing's Agenda for the Future*, 90
  for online support groups, 253, 482-483
  for Patient's Bill of Rights, 86
  on popularity of internet, 264
  on professional associations, 114-116b
  on professional boundaries, 497
  about stress management, 478
  on telemedicine, 151
  for unlicensed assistive personnel, 568
Operation Restore Trust, 424
Orem, Dorothea
  Concepts of Nursing by, 283
  definition of nursing, 186, 190b
  Self-Care Model of Nursing by, 279b, 283
Organizational structures, 352-354
Orientation periods, 212-218
Orlando, Ida, 286
OSHA. *See* National Institute for Occupational Safety and
    Health (NIOSH).
Outcome criteria, 399
Overpopulation, 424, 606-607
Oxford University, 324
Ozone layer, 606

P

Pacifiers, 305
PACs. *See* Political action committees (PACs).
Pain
  cultural expression of, 467
  ethical dilemmas about, 544-547
Palmer, Sophia, 13
Paramedical staff, 343-346
Parental modeling, 460, 465, 536b
Parish nursing, 151-153, 374, 465
Parse, Rosemarie, 289
Parsons, Talcott, 257, 460
Pasteur, Louis, 302b
Patient acuity (degree of illness), 96, 142, 439
Patient classification system (PCS), 439
Patient Self-Determination Act, 538-543, 571
Patient-focused care, 351
Patients
  as active collaborators, 186
  advocates for, 368b, 377-378, 561b

Patients (Continued)
autonomy of, 498-499, 527, 529-531
basic needs of, 276b
behaviors of, 261-266, 279-280
beliefs about nurses of, 443
called "clients," 526
confidentiality/privacy of, 91, 311, 395-396, 429, 564-566, 615
coping ability of, 462
data on, 394-396, 399
definition of excellent nursing care, 371
dependence and independence of, 461-462
environment of, 4, 275, 280, 284-285
expectations of, 349-350
goals of, 399-401, 400f
hardiness/resilience of, 463
impact of illness on, 470, 473-480
interviewing of, 394
names of, 514b
patient outcomes, 615
Patient Self-Determination Act, 538-543, 571
patient-focused care, 351
Patient's Bill of Rights, 86-87, 446, 448b, 538
positioning of, 146
rights of, 86-87, 538-539, 566
socialization with, 496-497
violence toward nurses by, 619
See also Consumers.
Patient's Bill of Rights, 86-87, 446, 448b, 538
Peaceful Death (document), 149
Pearl Harbor, 19
Pediatrics, 21f, 22f
Peer review, 314, 425-426
Pellom, Hiroko, 367
Pember, Phoebe, 7-8
Pender, Nola, 257
Penicillan, 17
Peplau, Hildegard, 186, 190b, 474, 492
Performance improvement (PI), 355-356
Persistent vegetative state, 110-111b
Personal space, 466
Personhood/self-awareness
beliefs/value systems, 223-230, 534, 536-537
development of, 495-497
human responses, 398, 459
personality characteristics, 461-465
respect for persons, 528
as a system, 244-248
theories of, 279-285, 287-289
PES format, 397-398
Pesut, Daniel J., 126-127
Pew organizations, 53, 79, 349, 373
Pharmacists, 342, 343f
Phenomena
definition of, 306
found in nursing, 271-272
phenomenological research, 311
social, 10-11, 85-86
Philosophy
branches of, 229-230
definition of, 229, 274
ethics principles in, 528-531
Philosophy and Science of Caring, (Watson), 277-278
Philosophy, nursing
beliefs and values in, 223-229
carative versus curative, 277-278
ethics principles in, 528-531
examples of, 230-237, 274-278
personal development of, 237-238

Philosophy of the Department of Nursing, Central Missouri State University, 236
Philosophy of the School of Nursing, Palm Beach Atlantic University, 237
Philosophy of the School of Nursing, University of North Florida, 234-235
Physical examination, 395, 396f
Physical therapists, 345
Physician hospital organizations (PHOs), 348-349
Physicians
bonus plans for, 438, 448b
"captain of the ship" doctrine, 560
credentials committees for, 339
function of, 341
"gag rules" for, 438, 448b
as hospital medical staff, 339-340
as hospitalists, 623
-nurse relationships, 66, 76-79, 170, 515-516, 567
-patient relationships, 87
as primary care gatekeepers, 348
role in case management, 367
Pinneo, Rose, 24f
Planning skills, 399-402
Point of care technology, 91
Point-of-service (POS) organizations, 348, 428b
Policy, health
function of, 580-581
nurses influence on, 590-591, 594-598
nursing research for, 584
policymakers in, 595b
Political action
of the American Nurses Association, 590-592
types of involvement in, 594-597
Political action committees (PACs), 590-591
Politics, 230, 580, 623
Pollution, environmental, 605-607, 606f, 618
Populations
aging of America, 603
definition of, 310
disenfranchised, 604
medically indigent, 603
population growth, 424, 606-607
"vulnerable populations," 437-438, 447b, 448b, 604
Positioning, patient, 146
Positron emission tomography (PET), 343
Post-traumatic stress disorder (PTSD), 26, 95
Poverty
correlation to crime, 94, 605
effects on families, 249, 603, 605
effects on health, 438, 605
Power
balance of power, 587, 588f
definition of, 583
of the media, 584-585
position power, 584
powers of appointment, 587
separation of powers, 586
types of, 584, 623
Power grabbing/power sharing, 584
Powers of appointment, 587
Practical nurses (LPNs/LVNs)
educational programs for, 43-44, 97
licensure of, 43
scope of practice for, 44
Prado, Marta, 593
Prayer, 303, 304
Preceptors, 214, 218-219, 535
Preferred provider organizations (PPOs), 348, 428b, 570-571
Pregnancy, teenage, 375
Premiums, insurance, 419, 435

Prescriptive authority, 156-158, 567-568, 592
Press-Ganey Patient Satisfaction Survey, 353
Prevention, illness, 282, 331, 332b
Price sensitivity, 416-417
Priestly, Joseph, 300, 302b
Primary care nursing, 24, 365, 602, 614-615
Primary elections, 589
Privileged communication, 565
Professional associations
activities of, 107-113
certification through, 118-119
choosing of, 113-116, 120
collective action in, 106-113
communication in, 107
constituents of, 106-107
in electoral process, 590-591
function of, 106-107
issues addressed by, 127-131
labor unions and, 119, 129, 348
list of, 114-116b
lobbying of, 119, 129-131, 582-583, 590-592
membership benefits of, 117-120, 120, 174, 623
missions of, 120-127
networking opportunities in, 107
support of, 567
types of, 113-117
See also specific association by name.
Professional liability insurance, 574, 575b, 576b
Professional review organizations (PROs), 425-426
Professional socialization
consumer's guide to, 210b-211b
definition of, 198
education and, 198-200
models of, 200-208
personal participation in, 209-210
postgraduate resocialization, 208-212
Professionalism, nursing
barriers to, 168-170
biases and, 200
boundaries and, 496-497
characteristics of, 165-166
commitment to, 69, 167-168, 173
criteria for, 170-176, 178
differentiated practice and, 614
in educational programs, 34, 36-39, 290
media images of, 82-85
Miller's Wheel of Professionalism in Nursing, 174-176, 175f
policy outcomes for, 582
promotion of, 9-10
socialization within, 197-219
state licensure and, 13
through research, 300, 319
titles and uniforms in, 76-78
unprofessional behavior, 574-575
See also Professional associations.
Professions
commitment to, 167-168
criteria for, 164-165
versus family time, 200
versus jobs, 166-167, 178
Prospective payment system (PPS), 422
Protecting by Degrees (report), 255
Protocol, 310, 401
Proximate cause, 559
Psychiatry, 320b
PTSD. See Post-traumatic stress disorder (PTSD).
Public Health Service
American Nurses Association support of, 123
environment and, 248
flu epidemic and, 17

Public Health Service *(Continued)*
  Great Depression and, 18
  HP2000/2010 initiatives for, 258
  levels of, 333-335
Publications
  of professional associations, 107
  promoting nursing, 75, 79
  studies on nursing in media, 79, 81-82
Pure science, 300-301

Q

Quackwatch (report), 265
Quad-Council Organizations, 79-80
Qualitative research, 307, 311, 313
Quality management
  cost containment and, 440-445, 614-615
  Institute of Medicine on, 572-573
  nursing involvement in, 403, 445
  for safety, 572
  staffing issues and, 109, 113
Quantitative research, 307-308
Quereshi, Kristin, 607, 608b
Quiggle, James, 434

R

Radio, 585
Radiology technologists/technicians, 343-344
Radwin, Laura, 371
Ramsey, Paul, 524
Reach to Recovery program, 370
Reality shock, 212-216
Recovery rooms, 18
Recruitment
  for educational programs, 76
  of foreign nurses, 97
  of registered nurses, 74-75
Reengineering, 350-353
Referendum, 589, 603
Reflections on Nursing Leadership (news magazine), 127
Reflective thinking, 387
Registered Nurse Population, The: March 2000 (document),
    136-138
Registered Nurses (RNs)
  African-American, 137
  age distribution of, 137
  in baccalaureate programs, 198, 205, 208
  bedside care and, 22
  BSN programs for, 42-43
  characteristics of, 136-138
  children of, 138
  commitment to profession, 69, 167-168
  employment opportunities for, 138-154, 159
  future challenges of, 613-614
  gender of, 136, 169
  Hispanic-American, 137
  identification of, 77-78
  impact of caregiving on, 484-488
  licensure of, 13, 35, 43, 49, 555-558, 556
  malpractice statisitcs on, 575
  marital status of, 138
  payment mechanisms for, 570-571
  -physician relationships, 66, 76-79, 170, 515-516, 567
  race/ethnicity of, 89f, 137
  recruitment of, 74-75
  shortages of, 96-100, 98t
  See also Nurse, role of.

*Registered Nurse Utilization of Unlicensed Assistive
    Personnel* (position statement), 568
Rehabilitation services, 332-333, 556
Reimbursement, insurance
  for Advanced Practice Nurses, 130, 157, 570-571, 582
  for hospitals, 348
  for Nurse Anesthetists, 570-571, 582
  for Nurse Midwives, 570-571
  for Nurse Practitioners, 570-571, 582
  for nurses, 27, 130, 570-571, 582, 613-614
  retrospective, 422
Relationships, interpersonal
  communication in professional, 573, 575-576
  mentoring/preceptorship. *See* Mentors/role models.
  in multicultural workplaces, 513-518
  nurse-coworker, 512-518
  nurse-patient, 277-278, 492-499
  nurse-physician, 66, 76-79, 170, 515-516
  nurse-to-patient ratios, 441, 582
  physician-patient, 87
  Theory of Human Relatedness, 498-499
Relaxation response, 464, 478b
Reliability/validity, 302, 309-310, 456, 483b, 616
Religion
  Christianity, 237
  Jehovah's Witnesses, 223-224
  parish nursing, 151-153
  versus spirituality, 464
Research
  conceptual framework for, 308
  conclusions from, 314
  on coping with illness, 249-250, 457
  dissemination of findings in, 314-315
  ethics in, 312b, 528
  ethnographic, 304
  on gender role stereotypes, 67
  genetic, 616
  "gold standard" in, 324
  hypothesis formation in, 308-309
  on illness and families, 482
  on organizational restructuring, 353
  on patient mortality, 569
  phenomenological, 311
  protocol for, 310
  quantitative versus qualitative, 307-308
  reliability in, 309-310
  review of literature/documentation in, 308, 535
  on sham health insurance, 434
  subjects, populations, and sample groups in, 310
  validity in, 302, 310
Research, nursing
  agencies for, 306, 322-323
  based on scientific method, 303-306
  changes in practice from, 317
  collaboration in, 319, 321
  criteria for, 306
  definition of, 185
  ethnographic, 304
  funding for, 21, 321-322
  journals of, 314
  National Institute of Nursing Research, 131, 301,
    303-304, 321
  nurse researchers. *See* Nurse researcher.
  on nurse-patient ratio, 441
  on nursing education, 128
  on nursing image, 78-82
  on nursing quality, 371
  organizations for, 321-322
  on outcomes classification, 400-401
  process of, 307-308

Research, nursing *(Continued)*
  on professional socialization, 201, 208-209
  for public policy, 584
  on socialization, 205-208
  theory-based, 292-294
  three sources of, 315, 317
  See also Research.
Resilience, 463
Resocialization, 205-208, 205-212
Respiratory technologists, 344
Respondeat superior, 560
Retirement, 435
Retrospective reimbursement, insurance, 422
Rheumatoid arthritis, 304
Richards, Melinda Anne (Linda), 33
Richey, Ann, 375
Ricin, 607
Risk management, 572
RN. *See* Registered Nurses (RNs)
Robb, Isabel Hampton, 9-10, 12-13, 34, 106
Robert Wood Johnson Foundation (RWJF), 99, 149, 585
Robertson, Charlene, 444
Robson, Judy, 592
Roentgen, Wilhelm K., 302b
Rogers, Martha, 187, 190b
  Science of Unitary Human Beings, 279b, 283-284,
    285b
Role models. *See* Mentors/role models.
Role strain, 72, 194, 208
Ross, Perot, 587-588
Roy, Callista, 284-285
  Adaptation Model of Nursing, 179b, 284-285
Royal College of Nursing (RCN), 188, 191b
Ruesch, Jurgen, 499-502
Ryan, Judith, 593

S

Sachs, Sadie, 14
Safford, Mary, 7
Salary, nursing
  for Advanced Practice Nurses, 160
  for female vs. male, 74
  overtime pay, 131
  pay equity in, 582
  reimbursement for. *See* Reimbursement, insurance
  statistics and demographics on, 159-161, 160f
Salk, Jonas, 302b
Sanger, Margaret, 14
SARS. *See* Severe Acute Respiratory Syndrome (SARS).
Scahill, Larry, 319-320
Scherzer, Norman and Anita, 484
Schiavo, Terri, 540-542
School nursing, 95, 147-149, 375, 594, 613, 617
Science
  health related events in, 302b
  pure versus applied, 13, 300
Science of Unitary Human Beings, 279b, 283-284, 285b
Scientific method
  definition of, 300
  history of, 301
  inductive and deductive reasoning in, 301-303
  limitations of, 303
*Scope and Standards of Hospice and Palliative Care Nursing
    Practice*, 149
Scope and Standards of Parish Nursing Practice, 153
Scope and Standards of Practice, 392, 574
Scope of practice, 194, 392, 574
Self-actualization, 246

Self-Care Model of Nursing, 279b, 283
Self-efficacy, 263
Self-esteem, 316-317
Semiprofessions, 164
Separation of powers, 586
Severe Acute Respiratory Syndrome (SARS), 27
Sexual assault, 94-95
Sexual Assault Nurse Examiner (SANE), 94-95
Shafer, Patricia, 593
Shalala, Donna, 259
Sham health insurance, 434
Shannon, Virginia G., 20
Shared governance, 379b, 380-381, 615
Sharps. *See* Needlestick injuries.
Shephard-Towner Act, 17
Sigma Theta Tau International (SSTI)
    Journal of Nursing Scholarship, 107, 127
    mission of, 126-127
    position statement of, 325
    Reflections on Nursing Leadership (news magazine), 127,
        484-488
    support of nursing research, 324, 325b
Single-parent families, 249
Sisters of Charity, 3
Sisters of Mercy, 5
Sisters of the Holy Cross, 5, 12-13
Sleep, 487b
Sleet-Scales, Jesse, 14, 15f
Smallpox, 131, 607
Smith, Janna Malamud, 541
Smoking/tobacco use
    effects on health, 262-263, 611
    increase in, 602
    laws limiting, 580
Smuts, Jan Christian, 256-257
Social workers, 344-345
Socialization
    effects on nursing, 67-76
    formal, 198, 199f
    gender roles in, 64-67
    influences on, 200-201, 460, 465, 516
    informal, 198
    between nurses and patients, 496-497
    parental modeling and, 460, 465, 536b
    professional, 197-219
    resocialization, 205-209
    studies on, 201, 208-209
Society of Rogerian Scholars, 284
Society/social systems, 250-251, 602-607
Soldier's Aid Societies, 5
Somatic language, 502
Spanish-American War, 12-13
Specialization, 23, 46-47, 99, 194
Speizer, Frank, 313
Spirituality
    beliefs and, 151-152
    illness and, 464-465
    in nursing philosophy, 276-278
    versus religion, 464
    role of prayer in, 304
    for yourself, 487b
St. Thomas' Hospital, 4, 9, 33
Staffing
    for cost containment, 449b
    development of, 18
    flexible scheduling and job sharing, 141
    of hospitals, 109, 340-346
    retention of staff, 113
    shortages in, 194
    with students, 36

Standard of care
    documents defining, 194-195
    failure to follow, 561b
    legal aspects in, 558-560
Standards of Clinical Nursing Practice (document), 195, 559
Standards of practice, 106, 195, 559, 573-574
State boards of nursing
    appointments to, 593
    definition of, 553-554
    function of, 555-556
State government
    boards of nursing, 553-556
    function of, 587
    licensure for nurses by, 13, 35, 43, 49, 555-558
    nurse practice acts of, 553-555, 581
    nursing regulations by, 185, 193-194, 553-558
    political action in, 591-593
Statutory law, 553
Stelmack, Pamela G., 357-358
Stenson, Julia C., 19
Stereotypes
    avoidance of, 497-498, 514b
    of cultures, 466
    of gender roles, 9, 64-67, 66b
Stewart, Isabel M., 11
Stewart, Maitland, 27
Stillman House, 14
Stress/stressors
    coping techniques for, 477-479
    effects on families, 249-253
    illness-caused, 475-480
    of military nursing, 26
    personal inventory of, 479b, 487b-488b
    questionnaire for, 251b-253b
    responses to, 476-477
Stroke, 259-260
Student nurses
    Code of Academic and Clinical Conduct for, 111, 112b
    competence of, 205, 206t, 620
    expectations versus reality of, 203, 205, 210-211
    Imprint (newsletter), 107
    National Student Nurses Association (NSNA), 107-108,
        117, 119, 121-122
    shortage of, 622-623
    socialization of, 198-209
Sturm, Roland, 609
Substance abuse/addictions
    AIDS epidemic and, 612
    alcohol and drugs, 258-261
    of nurses, 537-538, 556
Suffrage movement, 11, 17, 67, 584
Suffrage Party, 11
Suicide, assisted, 111b, 603
Sullivan, Louis, 249
Sulmasy, Daniel, 540-541
Supply and demand, 415-416
Support, moral, 253, 457, 482-483
Synergy, 243
Systems
    of American government, 586-590
    American health care system, 330-355
    of beliefs, 223, 250, 522b
    components of, 242, 243f
    court systems, 587
    culture as, 250
    dynamic nature of, 244, 245b
    environment/suprasystem, 245, 248-254
    family as, 248-250, 480
    King's theory of, 280-281
    in Neuman's model of practice, 282-283

Systems *(Continued)*
    of nursing language, 404, 406, 439
    payment systems, 422, 424
    people as, 244-248
    pricing systems, 417b
    subsystems, 280
    types of, 242-243
    of values, 534, 536-537
Systems Model of Nursing, 282-283

T

Tai chi, 305, 318
Talk radio, 575
Taxonomy, 406-408
Teachers colleges, 34, 46, 48
Team-building, 326-364, 351, 363f, 516-518, 618
Technology
    appeal for men, 72
    biomedical, 90-91, 149
    of caring, 92
    dehumanizing aspects of, 332, 616
    development of, 22, 321-322
    for distance learning, 620
    for documentation, 215, 357, 444
    effects on health care, 184, 423
    ethical dilemmas from, 523, 565-566
    future trends in, 615-617, 620
    impact on nursing, 90-93
    information technology, 153-154, 349-350, 395
    knowledge technology, 91
    point-of-care technology, 91
    recent advances in medical, 90-92, 331-332
    stress caused by, 612
    for telecommunication/telehealth, 150-151
    virtual reality, 55
    voice-activated computers, 215, 616
Telecommunication, 150-151, 616
Telehealth, 150-151, 557-558, 616
Television
    influence on gender roles, 67
    nursing's image on, 69, 79-82
    sedentary nature of viewing, 611
Tenet Healthcare, 424
Terminology. *See* Language.
Textbook of Nursing (Shaw), 186
Textbook of the Principles and Practices of Nursing
    (Harmer), 186
The American Nurse (newspaper), 107
The Registered Nurse Population: March 2000
    (report), 136
Theories
    of basic economics, 415-418
    behavior theory, 319
    of belief systems, 224, 287-289
    classification of, 286
    of communication, 499-504
    of ethics, 526-528, 529t
    germ theory, 4
    of human relatedness, 498-499
    of learning, 200-208
    middle-range theory, 286
    of moral development, 532-534
    nursing theories. *See* Theory, nursing.
    of systems. *See* Systems.
Theory, nursing
    conceptual models in, 279-286
    examples of, 286-293
    need for, 272-273

Theory, nursing *(Continued)*
  philosophies of, 274-278
  textbooks on, 273-274
Theory of Culture Care Diversity and Universality,
  286-287, 288f
Theory of Health as Expanding Consciousness, 287-289
Theory of Human Becoming, 289
Theory of Human Relatedness, 498-499
Third-party payments, 416-417
Thompkins, Sallie, 7
Throwe and Fought's Model for Socialization, 205-208
Time management, 216-218
To Err Is Human: Building a Safer Health System (report), 572
Torts, 558-560
Tourette syndrome, 320b
Training schools, 2, 4-5, 8-9
Transcultural nursing, 89, 250, 287, 466-467, 472
Transcultural Nursing Society, 466
Transforming the Landscape for Nursing Education
  (project), 58
Trautman, E. Neil, 436-437
Triage, 527-528
Trigger event, 263
Trust, patient, 403, 492-493, 597, 618
Truth, Sojourner, 5
Tuberculosis, 9, 13-14, 606
Tubman, Harriet, 5
Turley, Rita, 126

U

Ultrasonography, 332
Underground Railroad, 5
Uniforms, 76-77, 78b
Uninsured Americans, 432-434, 433f, 590, 602
Union, The, 5-7
United American Nurses (UAN), 129
United States Census Bureau, 606-607
United States of America, 2-8
United States Sanitary Commission, 6f, 8
Universal health care, 446, 447b
Unlicensed assistive personnel, 22, 109, 119, 568-570, 615
Urbanization, 605
Urination, 319
U.S. Congress
  function of, 586, 588f
  nurses serving in, 595-596
  terms of service in, 589
U.S. Constitution, 530, 537, 586-587
U.S. Department of Health and Human Services
  Federal Drug Administration (FDA) of, 581
  on life expectancy, 321
  nurses serving in, 593
  on nursing salaries, 160
  Office of Emergency Response of, 607-608
  Practitioner Data Bank of, 575
  Registered Nurse Population, The: March 2000
    (report), 136-138
U.S. House of Representatives, 586, 588f, 595-596
U.S. Senate, 586, 588f

U.S. Supreme Court, 587
Utilitarianism, 527-528
Utilization, 349, 357
Utterback, Karen, 593
Uustal, Diann, 225, 485-486

V

Vaginal birth after cesarean (VBAC), 157
Values
  clarification of, 227, 228b-229b, 522b
  cultural differences in, 466-467
  definition of, 225-226
  family versus professional, 200
  holistic, 304, 364-365, 402, 487b-488b, 512, 576
  nonjudgemental, 223-224
  Nursing's Social Policy Statement, 227
  parental modeling of, 460, 465, 536b
  systems of, 522b, 534, 536-537
Vassar Training Camp for Nurses, 15
Ventouse, 250
Veracity, 531-532
Vesalius, Andreas, 302b
Viagra, 423
Vietnam War, 26, 81, 95
Violence in America
  assault and battery, 95, 562-563
  causes and types of, 93-95, 605
  HP 2000/2010 on, 258-261
  against nurses, 95-96, 618-619
Virginia Henderson International Nursing Library, 127
Virtual reality, 55
Virtue ethics, 528
Viruses, 606
Vision for Nursing Education (report), 53
Visions: The Journal of Rogerian Science, 284
Visiting nursing
  associations for, 17
  future of, 159
  history of, 10-11, 18
  as home health care, 142-143, 337
Vollman, Kathleen, 146
Voluntariness, 564
Von Bertalanffy, Ludwig, 242

W

Wakefield, Mary, 593
Wald, Lillian, 11, 27
War. *See specific conflict.*
Watson, Jean
  definition of caring, 485
  definition of nursing, 190b
  The Philosophy and Science of Caring (Watson), 277-278
  philosophy of nursing, 277-278
Weakland, Rembert, 505-506
Weapons
  biological/chemical, 607-608
  firearms, 94-95, 595

Web sites. *See* Online information.
Wellness. *See* Health.
Whistle-blower protection, 109
Whitfield, Ed, 123f
WHO. *See* World Health Organization (WHO).
Willett, Walter, 313
Women
  eating disorders in, 611
  gender culture of, 516, 517b
  lung cancer rates in, 611
  as research subjects, 312b
  workplace violence and, 619
Women Nurses of the Army, 5
Women's Central Relief Committee, 5
Women's Movement
  effects on nursing, 67-70
  suffrage, 11, 17, 584
Woodhull, Nancy, 81
Woodhull Study on Nursing and the Media, 81-82,
  584-585
Work
  conditions and environment of, 129-131
  downsizing in, 352
  employer-provided insurance, 433-436
  employment opportunities in nursing, 138-154, 159
  environment at, 618-619
  flexible scheduling and job sharing, 617
  full-time versus part-time, 136
  multicultural relationships at, 513-518
  multiskilled workers, 351, 615, 622
  orientation phase of, 212-218
  postgraduate resocialization to, 209-212
  profession versus occupation, 166-167, 178
  violence at, 618-619
  work ethic, 215
  workplace advocacy, 129
Workers' Compensation Program, 418, 420, 424
Working poor, the, 603
Workplace advocacy, 129
World Future Society, 603
World Health Organization (WHO), 256
World War I, 15-17, 16f
World War II
  effects on families, 249
  male nurses in, 72
  nursing in, 18-21, 43, 186
  rebuilding after, 355
World Wide Web. *See* Online information.
Writing skills, 398b, 399, 401, 402
Wykle, May, 323

Y

Yale School of Nursing, 34

Z

Zoloft, 423